Hematopoietic Stem Cell Transplantation

Cancer Treatment and Research

Steven T. Rosen, M.D., ***Series Editor***

Bishop, M.R. (ed): *Hematopoietic Stem Cell Transplantation.* 2009. ISBN 978-0-387-78579-0.

Blake, M., Kalra, M. (eds): *Imaging in Oncology.* 2008. ISBN 978-0-387-75586-1.

Gradishar, W.J., Wood, W.C. (eds): *Advances in Breast Care Management, Second Edition.* 2008. 978-0-387-73160-5.

Ansell, S. (ed): *Rare Hematological Malignancies.* 2008. ISBN 978-0-387-73743-0.

Angelos, P. (ed): *Ethical Issues in Cancer Patient Care, Second Edition.* 2008. ISBN 978-0-387-73638-9.

Woodruff, T., Snyder, K.A. (eds): *Oncofertility.* 2007. ISBN 978-0-387-72292-4.

Raizer, J., Abrey, L.E. (eds): *Brain Metastases.* 2007. ISBN 978-0-387-69221-0.

Leong, S.P.L. (ed): *Cancer Metastasis and the Lymphovascular System: Basis for rational therapy.* 2007. ISBN 978-0-387-69218-0.

Ceelen, W.P. (ed): *Peritoneal Carcinomatosis: A Multidisciplinary Approach.* 2007. ISBN 978-0-387-48991-9.

Meyers, C. (ed): *Aids-Associated Viral Oncogenesis.* 2007. ISBN 978-0-387-46804-4.

Leong, S.P.L. (ed): *Cancer Clinical Trials: Proactive Strategies.* 2006. ISBN 0-387-33224-3.

Leonard, J.P., Coleman, M. (eds): *Hodgkin's and Non-Hodgkin's Lymphoma.* 2006. ISBN 0-387-29345.

Haefner, B., Dalgleish, A. (eds): *The Link Between Inflammation and Cancer.* 2006. ISBN 0-387-26282-2.

Small, Jr. W., Woloschak, G. (eds): *Radiation Toxicity: A Practical Guide.* 2005. ISBN 1-4020-8053-0.

Leong, S.P.L., Kitagawa, Y., Kitajima, M. (eds): *Selective Sentinel Lymphadenectomy for Human Solid Cancer.* 2005. ISBN 0-387-23603-1.

Platanias, L.C. (ed.): *Cytokines and Cancer.* 2005. ISBN 0-387-24360-7.

Abrey, L.E., Chamberlain, M.C., Engelhard, H.H. (eds): *Leptomeningeal Metastases.* 2005. ISBN 0-387-24198-1

Balducci, L., Extermann, M. (eds): *Biological Basis of Geriatric Oncology.* 2004. ISBN

Khleif, S. (ed.): *Tumor Immunology and Cancer Vaccines.* 2004. ISBN 1-4020-8119-7.

Farid, N. (ed.): *Molecular Basis of Thyroid Cancer.* 2004. ISBN 1-4020-8106-5.

Finn, W.G., Peterson, L.C. (eds.): *Hematopathology in Oncology.* 2004. ISBN 1-4020-7919-2.

Verweij, J., Pinedo, H.M. (eds): *Targeting Treatment of Soft Tissue Sarcomas.* 2004. ISBN 1-4020-7808-0.

Kumar, R. (ed.): *Molecular Targeting and Signal Transduction.* 2004. ISBN 1-4020-7822-6.

Keller, E.T., Chung, L.W.K. (eds): *The Biology of Skeletal Metastases.* 2004. ISBN 1-4020-7749-1.

For further volumes:
http://www.springer.com/5808

Michael R. Bishop
Editor

Hematopoietic Stem Cell Transplantation

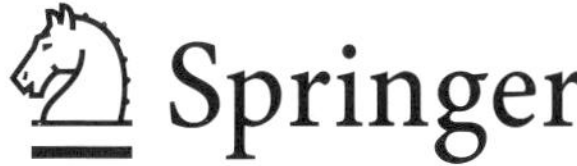

Editor
Michael R. Bishop
National Cancer Institute
Bethesda, MD, USA
mbishop@mail.nih.gov

ISSN: 0927-3042
ISBN: 978-0-387-78579-0 e-ISBN: 978-0-387-78580-6
DOI 10.1007/978-0-387-78580-6

Library of Congress Control Number: 2008921984

Printed on acid-free paper

springer.com

Contents

Introduction

> The dogmas of the quiet past are inadequate to the stormy present. The occasion is piled high with difficulty, and we must rise with the occasion. As our case is new, so we must think anew and act anew.
>
> Abraham Lincoln, 1862

When I came across this quote, it made me recall my first participation at an international meeting on bone marrow transplantation, at a time when this was the only term that was used to describe the field. During a particular session there was a presentation on the use of peripheral blood as the sole source of stem cells for transplantation, and a member of the audience rose to state that it was medically unethical to consider such treatment, as it certainly could not contain stem cells. Now nearly twenty years later, peripheral blood is the predominant source of stem cells used for hematopoietic stem cell transplantation. In the same period of time there have been several other dogmatic opinions, which permeate all of medicine, that have come and gone in the field of hematopoietic stem cell transplantation, and will continue to do so with advancements from basic and clinical research.

It is within this context that the format of this book was devised. Traditionally reviews on specific topics related to hematopoietic stem cell transplantation reflect the views of a single author or a research group. Although that view may be correct, it is rare within this field that the view is universally accepted, and with continued advances in research, opinions and views are quickly challenged or disproved. As such, each chapter within this text is authored by at least two individuals, both respected authorities on their respective topic, who do not necessarily share the same opinion or have direct research ties. The goal was to bring two perspectives to the same topic resulting in a more comprehensive and balanced review on relevant topics related to the field of hematopoietic stem cell transplantation. The danger in using such an approach was either a predominant review of one author or a particularly sanitized presentation on only areas where the authors had total agreement would emerge. However, the results of this "little experiment" were quite pleasing, as the reader will find in the following chapters contained within this text. They offer broad and often contrasting opinions on specific topics, highlighting the expertise of all the authors. More often than not, the collaboration between the various authors, who had not worked together previously, resulted in truly unique reviews.

The topics covered within this text cover general principles of hematopoietic stem cell transplantation, application of hematopoietic stem cell transplantation to specific diseases, and the biology and treatment of transplant-related complications. In addition specific chapters cover topics in which further understanding of the underlying biology and advancements within the laboratory or emerging topics which are currently or likely having major clinical implications on the field filed of hematopoietic stem cell transplantation.

This collection is meant to complement more encyclopedic texts on the subject of hematopoietic stem cell transplantation. Each chapter is more detailed than a standard review, yet adequately concise and focused to provide comprehensive information relative to biology, clinical results, and treatment recommendations to meet the needs of students, scientists, and clinicians interested in the field of hematopoietic stem cell transplantation. It is hoped that those needs will be met and result in the improved care and outcomes of patients undergoing hematopoietic stem cell transplantation.

Michael R. Bishop, M.D.

Contributors

Joseph H. Antin
The Dana-Farber Cancer Institute, Harvard University, Boston, MA, USA, jantin@partners.org

Lee Ann Baxter-Lowe
Department of Surgery, University of California, San Francisco, CA, USA, LeeAnn.BaxterLowe@ucsfmedctr.org

Philip J. Bierman
Department of Internal Medicine, Section of Oncology-Hematology, University of Nebraska Medical Center, 987680 Nebraska Medical Center, Omaha, NE, USA, pjbierma@unmc.edu

Michael R. Bishop
Experimental Transplantation and Immunology Branch, National Cancer Institute, Bethesda, MD, USA, mbishop@mail.nih.gov

Mark Bridges
University of Alabama Bone Marrow Transplantation Program, University of Alabama Comprehensive Cancer Center Birmingham, Alabama, USA

Claudio Brunstein
University of Minnesota, Minneapolis, Minnesota, USA

Benedetto Bruno
Assistant Professor of Hematology, Bone Marrow Transplantation Unit Program Head University of Torino, Italy School of Medicine, bruno@unito.it

Mitchell S. Cairo
Morgan Stanley Children's Hospital of New York-Presbyterian, Columbia University, Columbus, OH, USA, mc1310@columbia.edu

Sarah Cooley
Division of Hematology, Oncology and Transplantation, University of Minnesota Cancer Center, Minneapolis, MN 55445

Anne M. Dickinson
Newcastle University, a.m.dickinson@ncl.ac.uk

John F. DiPersio
Division of Oncology, Siteman Cancer Center, Washington University School of Medicine, St Louis, MO, USA, jdipersi@im.wustl.edu

Matthias Edinger
Department of Hematology and Oncology, University Hospital Regensburg, Regensburg, Germany, matthias.edinger@klinik.uni-regensburg.de

Sherif S. Farag
Division of Hematology and Oncology, Indiana University School of Medicine, Indianapolis, IN, USA, ssfarag@iupui.edu

Stephen Forman
The City of Hope National Medical Center, Duarte, CA, USA, sforman@coh.org

Francine Foss
Medical Oncology and Bone Marrow Transplantation, Yale University School of Medicine, New Haven, CT, USA, Francine.Foss@yale.edu

Daniel Fowler
Experimental Transplantation and Immunology Branch, Center for Cancer Research, National Cancer Institute, Bethesda, MD, USA, fowlerda@mail.nih.gov

Juan C. Gea-Banacloche
Experimental Transplantation and Immunology Branch, National Cancer Institute, National Institutes of Health, Bethesda, MD, USA, banacloj@mail.nih.gov

Sergio Giralt
M.D. Anderson Cancer Center, Houston, TX, USA, sgiralt@mdanderson.org

Ajay K. Gopal
Division of Medical Oncology, Department of Medicine, University of Washington and Clinical Research Division, Fred Hutchinson Cancer Research Center, Seattle, WA, USA, agopal@u.washington.edu

Thomas G. Gross
Nationwide Children's Hospital, Ohio State University, Columbus, OH, USA,

Elizabeth O Hexner
Division of Hematology-Oncology and Abramson Cancer Center, University of Pennsylvania Medical Center, Philadelphia, PA 19106

Petra Hoffmann
Department of Hematology and Oncology, University Hospital Regensburg, Regensburg, Germany

Carolyn Katovich Hurley
Department of Oncology, Georgetown University Medical Center, Washington, DC, USA, hurleyc@georgetown.edu

Armand Keating
Department of Hematology and Medical Oncology, Princess Margaret Hospital, Toronto, Ontario, Canada, armand.keating@uhn.on.ca

Robert Korngold
The Cancer Center, Hackensack University Medical Center, Hackensack, NJ, USA, RKorngold@humed.com

Aviva C. Krauss
Pediatric Oncology Branch, National Cancer Institute, NIH Bethesda, Maryland, USA

Mary Laughlin
Case Western Reserve University, Cleveland, OH, USA, mjl13@case.edu

Crystal L. Mackall
Pediatric Oncology Branch, National Cancer Institute, NIH, Bethesda, MD, USA, mackallc@mail.nih.gov

Paul J. Martin
Fred Hutchinson Cancer Research Center, Seattle, WA, USA, pmartin@fhcrc.org

Vikram Mathews
Department of Haematology, Christian Medical College, Vellore, India 632004

Jeffrey S. Miller
Division of Hematology, Oncology and Transplantation, University of Minnesota Cancer Center, Minneapolis, MN, USA, mille011@tc.umn.edu

Jeffrey Molldrem
Transplant Immunology, M.D. Anderson Cancer Center, Houston, TX, USA, jmolldre@mdanderson.org

Craig Moskowitz
Memorial Sloan-Kettering Cancer Center, New York, NY, USA, moskowic@mskcc.org

Steven Z. Pavletic
Experimental Transplantation and Immunology Branch, National Cancer Institute, Bethesda, MD, USA, pavletis@mail.nih.gov

Karl S. Peggs
Royal Free and University College London Medical Schools, London, UK, k.peggs@ucl.ac.uk

Gordon L. Phillips II
Wilmot Cancer Center, Department of Medicine, University of Rochester Medical Center, Rochester, NY, USA, Gordon_Phillips@URMC.Rochester.edu

David L. Porter
Division of Hematology-Oncology and Abramson Cancer Center, University of Pennsylvania Medical Center, Philadelphia, PA, USA, david.porter@uphs.upenn.edu

Stanley Riddell
Clinical Research Division, Fred Hutchinson Cancer Research Center, Professor of Medicine, University of Washington, Seattle, WA, USA, sriddell@fhcrc.org

Loredana Ruggeri
University of Perugia, Perugia, Italy, loredana.ruggeri@unipg.it

Tara Seshadri
Department of Hematology and Medical Oncology Princess Margaret Hospital, Toronto, Ontario, Canada

Roberto Sorasio
Chief Resident University of Torino, Italy School of Medicine

John Sweetenham
Taussig Cancer Institute, The Cleveland Clinic, Cleveland, OH, USA, sweetej@ccf.org

Martin S. Tallman
Division of Hematology-Oncology, Northwestern University Feinberg School of Medicine, Chicago, IL, USA, mtallman@northwestern.edu

Guido Tricot
University of Utah School of Medicine, tricotguidoj@uams.edu

William Tse
Case Western Reserve University, Cleveland, Ohio, USA.

Koen van Besien
Section of Hematology/Oncology, University of Chicago, Chicago, IL, USA, kvbesien@medicine.bsd.uchicago.edu

William Vaughn
University of Alabama Bone Marrow Transplantation Program, University of Alabama Comprehensive Cancer Center, Birmingham, AL, USA, WVaughan@uabmc.edu

James C. Wade
Medical College of Wisconsin, Milwankee, WI, USA, jwade@mcw.edu

John E. Wagner
University of Minnesota, Minneapolis, MN, USA,
wagne002@maroon.tc.umn.edu

Daniel Weisdorf
University of Minnesota Blood and Marrow Transplant Program,
Minneapolis, MN, USA, weisd001@umn.edu

Eva M. Weissinger
Hannover Medical School, mischak-weissinger.eva@mh-hannover.de

Jane N. Winter
Division of Hematology/Oncology, Department of Medicine, and Robert H. Lurie Comprehensive Cancer Center, Feinberg School of Medicine, Northwestern University, Chicago, IL, USA, jwinter@northwestern.edu

Maurizio Zangari
Professor of Medicine, University of Utah School of Medicine

Shuhong Zhang
Division of Hematology and Oncology, Indiana University School of Medicine Indianapolis, Indiana, U.S.A.

Chapter 1
Principles and Overview of Allogeneic Hematopoietic Stem Cell Transplantation

Sergio Giralt and Michael R. Bishop

1.1 Introduction and Historical Perspectives

Hematopoietic stem cell transplantation (HSCT) is the process and intravenous infusion of hematopoietic stem and progenitor cells to restore normal hematopoiesis and/or treat malignancy [1, 2]. The term "hematopoietic stem cell transplantation" has replaced the term "bone marrow transplantation" (BMT) because hematopoietic stem cells can be derived from a variety of sources other than the bone marrow, including the peripheral blood and umbilical cord blood [2, 3]. Stem cells used for HSCT are distinguished as being of hematopoietic origin, as there is growing interest in using more primitive stem cells for regenerative therapy due to their plasticity and unique biologic characteristics [4]. Hematopoietic stem cells are further characterized according to their source, that is, from whom they are obtained. Hematopoietic stem cells obtained from the patient him- or herself are referred to as autologous [1, 3]. Hematopoietic stem cells obtained from an identical twin are referred to as syngeneic obtained, and hematopoietic stem cells from someone other than the patient or an identical twin are referred to as allogeneic, which is the focus of this chapter.

The clinical application of HSCT originated in the clinical observations of the severe myelosuppressive effects of radiation among nuclear bomb survivors at Hiroshima and Nagasaki [5]. Intensive research efforts were made in the 1950s and early 1960s to develop methods to reverse the myelosuppressive effects of radiation, including the infusion of bone marrow [6–11]. The subsequent determination and understanding of the major histocompatibility complex (MHC) and human leukocyte antigens (HLA) as the major determinants of graft rejection significantly advanced laboratory studies and clinical application of allogeneic HSCT [12–14]. The first successful reports of clinical bone marrow transplantation, utilized for patients with severe combined immunodeficiency disorders, severe aplastic anemia, and advanced acute leukemias, occurred in the late 1960s and

S. Giralt (✉)
M.D. Anderson Cancer Center, Houston, TX, USA
e-mail: sgiralt@mdanderson.org

M.R. Bishop (ed.), *Hematopoietic Stem Cell Transplantation*,
Cancer Treatment and Research 144, DOI 10.1007/978-0-387-78580-6_1,

Table 1.1 Clinical indications for allogeneic hematopoietic stem cell transplantation

Malignant disorders
Acute myeloid leukemia
Acute lymphoblastic leukemia
Chronic myeloid leukemia
Myelodysplastic syndromes
Myeloproliferative disorders
Non-Hodgkin's lymphoma
Hodgkin's disease
Chronic lymphocytic leukemia
Multiple myeloma
Juvenile chronic myeloid leukemia
Non-malignant disorders
Aplastic anemia
Paroxysmal nocturnal hemoglobinuria
Fanconi's anemia
Blackfan–Diamond anemia
Thalassemia major
Sickle cell anemia
Severe combined immunodeficiency
Wiskott–Aldrich syndrome
Inborn errors of metabolism

Modified from Copelan EA. N Engl J Med. 2006;354:1813–26

early 1970s [15–20]. Allogeneic HSCT has become a standard treatment option for a variety of hematologic malignancies (Table 1.1) [21]. In addition, allogeneic HSCT is a standard treatment for many immunodeficiency states, metabolic disorders (e.g., Hurler's syndrome), and defective hematopoietic states (e.g., severe aplastic anemia, thalassemia). This chapter focuses primarily on the rationale for the application of allogeneic HSCT in the treatment of malignancy.

The distinctive characteristics of allogeneic HSCT are that the stem cell graft is free of contamination by malignant cells and contains immunologically competent lymphocytes that are capable of mediating a reaction against foreign antigens. This latter characteristic can be a major advantage if the immunologic response is directed against malignant cells, referred to as the graft-versus-leukemia or graft-versus-tumor (GvT) effect, thus potentially eradicating disease and reducing the chance of disease relapse [22–24]. However, if the immunologic response is directed against antigens present on normal tissues, it can lead to the destruction of normal organs, described clinically as graft-versus-host disease (GvHD). The risk of both graft rejection (host-versus-graft reaction) and GvHD rises with HLA disparity.

The GvT effect was first recognized in animal models and subsequently was noted among patients undergoing allogeneic HSCT for acute and chronic leukemias [22–25]. The clinical importance of the interactions between immunocompetent donor T cells and tumor cells in mediating a GvT effect is supported by an increased rate of relapse in allogeneic stem cell grafts from which T cells have been removed (T-cell depletion), an inverse correlation between relapse and severity of GvHD, and a comparatively increased rate of relapse after syngeneic or autologous HSCT using the same myeloablative conditioning regimen [25]. Finally, the most compelling evidence for a T cell-mediated GvT effect originates from the observation that infusion of allogeneic lymphocytes, a donor lymphocyte infusion (DLI), at a time remote from the transplant conditioning regimen, can treat leukemia relapse successfully after allogeneic HSCT [26–29]. The DLI, without any additional cytotoxic therapy, resulted in sustained cytogenetic and molecular remissions. Over time it became increasingly apparent that a significant part of the curative potential of allogeneic HSCT could be directly attributed to the GvT effect.

1.2 Technical Aspects of Allogeneic Hematopoietic Stem Cell Transplantation

1.2.1 Donor Selection

In allogeneic HSCT, stem cells are obtained from a donor other than the recipient. Donor and recipient usually are identical or "matched" for HLA, which is derived from the MHC located on chromosome 6 [30]. A single set of MHC alleles, described as a haplotype, is inherited from each parent, resulting in HLA pairs. The most important HLAs include HLA-A, HLA-B, HLA-C, HLA-DR, and HLA-DQ loci. Among siblings, the genes which encode for HLA-B and HLA-C are located so close to each other in the MHC that one is rarely inherited without the other. As a result, an HLA match among siblings is referred to a "6 of 6," as they are matched for HLA-A, -B, and -DR; however, in actuality they are matched for all of the HLA antigens [3]. The other antigens, such as HLA-C, become more important in alternative sources of hematopoietic stem cells, such as unrelated donors and cord blood, which are described in more detail later in this chapter [31, 32].

The choice of donor for an allogeneic HSCT takes into account several factors, including the patient's disease, disease state, and urgency in obtaining a donor. When allogeneic HSCT is being considered for a patient, a fully HLA-matched sibling is the preferred donor source, because the risk of graft rejection and GvHD is lowest with this source of allogeneic stem cells. As described earlier, a haplotype is inherited from each parent, and by simple Mendelian genetics it would be expected that the probability that two siblings would share the same haplotypes would be 1:4. The probability of having an HLA-matched sibling increases with the number of siblings within a specific family. The probability can be estimated using the following formula: The chance of having an HLA-matched sibling = $1-(0.75)^n$, where n is the number of potential sibling donors [3]. There is an approximately 1% chance of crossing over (i.e., genetic material switched between chromosomes during meiosis), primarily between the HLA-A and the HLA-B loci. The clinical outcomes for allogeneic HSCT using a sibling with a single HLA mismatch are similar to those with a fully HLA-matched sibling [33].

For patients who lack a fully HLA-matched sibling donor, the preferred alternative sources for allogeneic stem cells include an unrelated fully HLA-matched donor, a partially HLA-matched cord blood unit, or a partially HLA-matched family member [34–36]. A closely HLA-matched volunteer hematopoietic stem cell donor may be identified through a bone marrow donor registry, such as the National Marrow Donor Program (NMDP) in the United States, which includes about six million potential donors. Many HLA phenotypes are possible, which sometimes makes the identification of a matched unrelated donor difficult and time consuming. Depending on the ethnic descent of both patient and donor, the probability of identifying an HLA-matched unrelated donor is between 50% and 80%. Due to advances in HLA-typing (reviewed in Chap. 4 by Baxter-Lowe and Hurley) through the use of molecular typing techniques and improved supportive care over the last decade, current results of matched unrelated donor transplants for malignancy are not significantly different when compared to HSCT from matched sibling donor transplant [32, 37].

One major disadvantage of using an unrelated donor is that the average time required to identify and procure an HLA-matched unrelated donor is approximately 2–3 months, which may be too long for patients with rapidly progressive malignancies [38]. The alternative stem cell source to an unrelated bone marrow donor for allogeneic HSCT is umbilical cord blood [35–39]. The major advantages of umbilical cord stem cells (reviewed in Chap. 10 by Wagner, Brunstein, Tse, and Laughlin) is that they can be obtained in less than 4 weeks and that even cord blood units mismatched in up to 2 of 6 HLA may be used for allogeneic HSCT. This degree of HLA mismatching is acceptable because the overwhelming percentage of T cells within the cord blood unit are naïve, and the incidence of acute GvHD is comparable to or less than that associated with an HLA-matched unrelated bone marrow donor. The major disadvantage of umbilical cord blood units is they are associated with a relatively high degree of graft rejection, especially in adults [35, 39]. Engraftment and treatment-related mortality appear to be directly related to umbilical cord cell dose; the small volume usually available (50–150 mL) of cord blood results in low stem cell doses in adult patients. It may be that the limitation of cell dose can be overcome by the use of more than one cord blood unit or the transient support from $CD34^+$ cells from haploidentical family members [40, 41]. The other significant disadvantage is that once the cord blood unit is used, there is no way to go back and get additional cells for a donor lymphocyte infusion or in the event of graft failure.

The other alternative source of allogeneic hematopoietic stem cells is to identify partially HLA-matched family among the patient's first-degree relatives who share at least one haplotype (haploidentical) with the potential recipient [36, 42]. The major advantage with the use of a haploidentical family member is that the donor is readily available for almost all patients. The major disadvantages are an increased risk of graft rejection, GvHD, and severe immune dysregulation, which rises with higher degrees of HLA-mismatching. Haplo-identical allogeneic HSCT has been limited primarily to use in children, although the use of less intense conditioning regimens (discussed below) has increased its applicability in adults [36, 43].

1.2.2 Stem Cell Acquisition

Hematopoietic stem cells for allogeneic HSCT may be obtained from the bone marrow, the peripheral blood, and umbilical cord blood. Bone marrow hematopoietic stem cells usually are harvested by repeated aspirations from the posterior iliac crest until an adequate number of cells have been removed [44]. If sufficient cells cannot be obtained from the posterior iliac crest, marrow also can be harvested from the anterior iliac crest and sternum. The minimal number of nucleated marrow cells required for long-term repopulation in humans is not precisely known. In practice, the number of nucleated marrow cells harvested is usually $1–3\times10^8$/kg of recipient weight, depending on the diagnosis (i.e., higher for aplastic anemia), the type and intensity of pre-transplant conditioning, and whether the marrow graft will be modified in vitro. Marrow sometimes is treated in vitro to remove unwanted cells before it is returned to the patient. In allogeneic HSCT with major ABO incompatibility between donor and recipient, it is necessary to remove the mature erythrocytes from the graft to avoid a hemolytic transfusion reaction [45]. Peripheral blood hematopoietic stem cells are used in approximately 60–70% of allogeneic HSCT [46]. In steady-state, the concentration of hematopoietic stem cells and myeloid progenitor cells is quite low, and prior to collection of peripheral blood hematopoietic stem cells by apheresis, attempts are made to increase or "mobilize" the number of circulating hematopoietic stem cells by administering hematopoietic growth factors, primarily granulocyte colony-stimulating factor (G-CSF; filgrastim) to the donor. The procedure is associated with a very low incidence of complications and can generally be done as an outpatient. In both the autologous and the allogeneic settings, the use of peripheral blood stem cells has been associated with accelerated recovery of hematopoiesis when compared to traditional BMT. In the allogeneic setting, the presence of higher numbers of T cells in the peripheral blood stem cell graft initially raised the concern for greater frequency and severity of GvHD. Several large studies have now demonstrated that the use of peripheral blood in the allogeneic HSCT setting is associated with a decreased relapse rate in hematologic malignancies and improvement in overall and disease-free survival in patients with late-stage disease [47]. However, the use of peripheral blood has been associated with a significant risk of extensive chronic GvHD. After collection and processing, hematopoietic stem cells from bone marrow, peripheral blood, or cord blood may be directly infused or they may be processed with dimethylsulfoxide

(DMSO) with or without hydroxyethylstarch and then stored in liquid nitrogen until needed for transplantation [48].

1.2.3 Conditioning

Once an allogeneic stem cell source has been identified, patients are put on regimens with the intent of "conditioning" or "preparing" them for the infusion of hematopoietic stem cells. Most conditioning or preparative regimens use a combination of radiation and chemotherapy [1, 3]. They also may contain radio-immunoconjugates and/or monoclonal antibodies that target T cells (e.g., alemtuzumab) [49]. The choice of a specific conditioning regimen depends on the disease that is being treated. The earliest conditioning regimens were designed to permit the administration of maximum doses of chemotherapy and/or radiation (i.e., "high-dose" regimens) for the eradication of disease and to be adequately immunosuppressive to prevent graft rejection. The most commonly used chemotherapy agents in these regimens are alkylating agents (e.g., cyclophosphamide and/or etoposide) with or without total lymphoid or total body irradiation (TBI) at doses varying between 800 and 1440 cGy. The doses of chemotherapy and radiation used in these regimens are referred to as "myeloablative" because they result in a degree of myelosuppression and immunosuppression that is nearly universally fatal without the infusion of hematopoietic stem cells as a rescue product [50].

Though efficacious, TBI is associated with a number of short and long-term complications including secondary malignancies, cataracts, and endocrine dysfunction. More recently a low-dose non-fractionated mode of administration of TBI with 200 cGy has been incorporated in the setting of nonmyeloablative transplants [51]. The toxicities of TBI-containing conditioning regimens led to the development of radiation-free regimens. Of these, the most commonly used chemotherapy is the combination of busulfan and cyclophosphamide, developed initially by Santos and coworkers and subsequently modified by Tutschka et al. [52, 53]. Busulfan is traditionally administered orally as 4mg/kg divided into four daily doses and given on each of four successive days (total dose $= 16 \times$mg/kg) but this oral administration is limited by the erratic absorption of the drug. High plasma levels are associated with increased incidence of hepatic veno-occlusive disease (VOD) and other toxicities [53]. More recently, an intravenous formulation of busulfan has become available which allows more predictable drug delivery [54].

Allogeneic HSCT with myeloablative conditioning regimens has been performed successfully in patients older than 60 years of age; however, survival after these transplants declines with increasing age, limiting the application of allogeneic transplantation to a minority of patients who potentially could benefit from this procedure. The substantial toxicities associated with traditional, myeloablative conditioning regimens have limited the application of allogeneic transplantation to relatively young patients with good performance status. However, the demonstration that an immune-mediated GvT effect plays a central role in the therapeutic efficacy of allogeneic HSCT led to the hypothesis that myeloablative conditioning regimens were not essential for tumor eradication. This idea subsequently led investigators to develop less intense, "nonmyeloablative" conditioning regimens, which were adequately immunosuppressive to permit the engraftment of donor hematopoietic stem cells, while sparing the patient many of the toxicities related to traditional high-dose therapy. A variety of nonmyeloablative and "reduced-intensity" conditioning regimens have been reported [51, 55, 56]. These regimens have been associated with decreased early post-transplant morbidity and mortality and have permitted allografting in older and medically debilitated patients. However, the important clinical question is whether this reduction in toxicity comes at the cost of a loss of anti-tumor activity within the conditioning regimen.

1.2.4 Treatment-Related Toxicities

There are a variety of acute and late toxicities, which can result in significant morbidity and mortality, that are associated with and specific to allogeneic transplantation [57]. The basic principle underlying the supportive care of the transplanted patient is prevention. Most transplant complications have a temporal relation to the conditioning regimen and the transplant. A simple index, based on pre-transplant comorbidities, has been developed that reliably predicts non-relapse mortality and survival [58]. This comorbidity index is useful for patient counseling prior to allogeneic HSCT.

1.2.4.1 Rejection and Graft Failure

The failure to recover hematologic function or the loss of marrow function after initial reconstitution constitutes graft failure. Graft rejection occurs when immunologically competent cells of host origin destroy the transplanted cells of donor origin [59]. Graft failure can occur in 5–11% of HLA-identical recipients and may be mediated by immunologic graft rejection by the host immune system, infections, drugs, or an inadequate stem cell dose. Graft failure generally takes place within 60 days of transplantation, though late graft failure has been known to occur. A number of factors are known to increase the graft failure rate after allografting, among them, low nucleated cell count infused, T-cell depletion, HLA mismatching, and the use of nonmyeloablative conditioning. This complication occurs more commonly in patients who receive transplants from alternative or HLA-mismatched donors, in T-cell–depleted transplants, and in patients with aplastic anemia who receive a non-TBI-containing regimen. Graft rejection is less likely to occur in non-transfused patients with aplastic anemia.

1.2.4.2 Infections

Due to the utilization of post-transplantation immunosuppressive agents, patients undergoing allogeneic HSCT are at increased risk, particularly to fungal and viral infections, as compared to patients undergoing autologous stem cell transplantation (reviewed in Chap. 21 by Wade and Gea-Banacloche). Infection prophylaxis is routinely employed to guard against bacterial, fungal, and viral pathogens. Fluconazole has been shown to reduce the incidence of systemic and superficial fungal infections, but does not affect the incidence of resistant Candida species; intraconazole has been demonstrated to decrease mold infections [60, 61]. Aspergillosis is the most common cause of death due to infection after allogeneic HSCT, and the risk of invasive fungal infections is increased in patients receiving prolonged, systemic corticosteroid for the treatment of GvHD. However, newer anti-fungal agents (e.g., voriconazole, caspofungin) have been demonstrated to successfully treat invasive aspergillosis in the transplant setting. Clinical infections with cytomegalovirus (CMV) have been significantly reduced utilizing a strategy of monitoring for CMV reactivation by detection of CMV DNA in leukocytes, plasma, or serum and upon detection, the pre-emptive administration of ganciclovir before overt CMV disease [62].

1.2.4.3 Genito-Urinary Toxicities

The development of hemorrhagic cystitis is associated with high-dose cyclophosphamide within the conditioning regimen. This complication has been largely abrogated by the use of mesna (sodium 2-sulfanylethanesulfonate) and aggressive hydration. Acute renal failure requiring dialysis during the transplant occurs infrequently [63]. Thrombotic microangiopathy, either idiopathic or associated with the administration of calcineurin-inhibitors (e.g., cyclosporine) can be a serious complication after allogeneic HSCT, posing a high mortality risk or resulting in end-stage renal disease [64]. Nephrotic syndrome and membranous nephropathy have been described in long-term survivors; these complications seem to be associated more commonly with chronic GvHD and nonmyeloablative conditioning [65].

1.2.4.4 Hepatic Toxicities

The most common liver complication associated with transplantation is veno-occlusive disease (VOD)/sinusoidal obstruction syndrome of the liver [66, 67]. VOD is caused by endothelial damage in the hepatic sinusoids, and is characterized any unexplained weight gain, painful hepatomegaly, and ascites; severe VOD is associated with a high mortality rate. Beneficial treatments for VOD are relatively limited; however, there have been encouraging reports on the treatment of VOD with defibrotide [68]. The prophylactic use of ursodiol has decreased hepatic complications following allogeneic HSCT, especially among patients receiving conditioning regimen containing busulfan [69].

1.2.4.5 Acute Graft-Versus-Host Disease

Graft-versus-host disease represents the most important barrier to allogeneic HSCT. Graft-versus-host disease is described as either acute, generally presenting within the first 100 days post-transplant (reviewed in Chap. 11 by Antin and Korngold), or chronic, generally presenting after the first 100 days post-transplant (reviewed in Chap. 12 by Martin and Pavletic). Risk factors for the development of acute GvHD include a female donor (particularly a multiparous donor), more advanced age in the patient and the donor, and cytomegalovirus sero-positivity of the donor or patient and use of an unrelated donor. Acute GvHD is manifested by symptoms in several organ systems, including the skin, gastrointestinal tract, and liver (Table 1.2) [70]. The skin manifestations range from a maculopapular rash up to generalized erythroderma or desquamation. The severity of liver GvHD is scored on the basis of the bilirubin and the gastrointestinal severity on the quantity of diarrhea per day. Organs may be involved in isolation or simultaneously. However, delayed de novo presentations of acute GvHD are reported. A clinical grading system (Table 1.2) correlates with clinical outcome. Severity is described as Grade I (mild) to Grade IV (severe). The incidence of clinically significant GvHD (Grades II–IV) in recipients of HLA-genotypically identical grafts (T cell replete) and using cyclosporine and methotrexate for GvHD prophylaxis is approximately 40%. Increasing HLA disparity increases both the incidence and severity of resultant GvHD, with recipients of

Table 1.2 Classification of patients with acute graft-versus-host disease

Clinical staging

Stage	Skin	Liver	Gut
+	Rash < 25%	BSA Total bilirubin 2–3 mg/dL	Diarrhea 500–1000 mL/day
+ +	Rash 25–50% BSA	Total bilirubin 3–6 mg/dL	Diarrhea 1000–1500 mL/day
+ + +	Generalized erythroderma	Total bilirubin 6–15 mg/dL	Diarrhea > 1500 mL/day
+ + + +	Desquamation and bullae	Total bilirubin > 15 mg/dL	Pain, with or without ileus

Clinical grading

		Stage		
Grade	Skin	Liver	Gut	PS
0 (none)	0	0	0	0
I	+ to + +	0	0	0
II	+ to + + +	+	+	+
III	+ + to + + +	+ + to + + +	+ + to + + +	+ +
IV	+ + to + + + +	+ + to + + + +	+ + to + + + +	+ + +

BSA = body surface area, PS = performance status

phenotypically matched unrelated donor grafts experiencing a 50–80% incidence of grade II–IV GvHD. Other risk factors for acute GvHD include older age, a parous or alloimmunized donor, less intense immunosuppression, or the use of a T cell replete versus T cell depleted graft.

Acute GvHD can often be diagnosed on the basis of clinical findings. Histologic confirmation can be valuable in excluding other possibilities such as infection. Mild GvHD of the skin may demonstrate vacuolar degeneration and infiltration of the basal layer by lymphocytes. With more advanced disease, histologic findings of necrotic dyskeratotic cells with acantholysis may progress to frank epidermolysis. In the liver, early GvHD may be difficult to distinguish from hepatitis of other causes.

The best therapy for GvHD is prophylaxis. The prophylactic use of cyclosporine and methotrexate are effective in reducing the incidence of acute GvHD as well as the survival of transplant patients and is the most commonly used form of GvHD prophylaxis. Cyclosporine is a cyclic polypeptide that prevents T cell activation by inhibiting interleukin-2 (IL-2) production and IL-2 receptor expression. While effective as GvHD prophylaxis, cyclosporine imparts significant toxicities including hypertension, nephrotoxicity, hypomagnesemia, a risk for seizures, hypertrichosis, gingival hyperplasia, tremors, and anorexia. Tacrolimus is a macolide lactone which closely resembles cyclosporine in mechanism of action, spectrum of toxicities, and pharmacologic interactions. The combination of tacrolimus and methotrexate was demonstrated to be superior to cyclosporine and methotrexate in reducing Grade II–IV acute GvHD when used as prophylaxis.

Moderate to severe GvHD (Grades II–IV) requires appropriate treatment. The mainstay of therapy has long been corticosteroid therapy. Treatment for acute GvHD includes high-dose corticosteroids, anti-thymocyte globulin (ATG), or various monoclonal antibodies [71–73]. Methylprednisolone, at a dose of 2 mg/kg/d, can be expected to achieve responses in 40–60% of patients. Higher doses of steroids have not been shown to be of greater benefit. Steroid refractory GvHD responds poorly to second line therapies and is associated with increased mortality. ATG is commonly used as a second line treatment with limited success. Novel treatments showing efficacy in preliminary studies include extracorporeal photo-therapy and the combination of mycophenolate mofetil and tacrolimus. In general, acute GvHD of the skin is most responsive to treatment while GvHD of the liver is least responsive. The fatality rate for acute GvHD may be as high as 50%.

1.2.4.6 Chronic Graft-Versus-Host Disease

Chronic GvHD occurs in 20–50% of long term survivors. Chronic GvHD occurs most commonly between 100 days and 2 years from the transplant and has polymorphic features similar to a number of autoimmune diseases [74]. It is most likely to develop in older patients who also had acute GvHD or received peripheral blood rather than bone marrow grafts; in 20% of cases there is no history of prior acute GvHD [75]. Adverse prognostic factors include thrombocytopenia, a progressive clinical presentation, extensive skin involvement, and an elevated bilirubin [76]. Common manifestations include the sicca syndrome, lichen planus-like skin rash, scleroderma-like skin changes, esophageal and intestinal fibrosis, obstructive lung disease with or without pneumonitis, and elevated alkaline phosphatase with or without hyperbilirubinemia. Underlying immunologic deficiencies including hypogammaglobulinemia are common, placing patients at increased risk for infectious events.

Chronic GvHD may be limited or extensive [76]. Limited disease implies localized skin involvement with minimal or no liver involvement while extensive disease suggests generalized skin involvement with or without other organ involvement. Patients with limited disease have a good prognosis with 60–70% long-term survival while those with extensive disease experience 20–30% long-term survival. Treatment for chronic GvHD is guided by the extent of disease. Initiation of therapy prior to functional impairment is of critical importance. Treatments for chronic GvHD include corticosteroids, cyclosporine, thalidomide, ultraviolet light treatments, or other immunosuppressive agents [77, 78]. Alternatives include azathioprine, UV light, psoralen-UV-A, extracorporeal photopheresis, and thalidomide. The most common cause of death in patients with chronic GvHD remains infection so all should receive prophylactic antibiotics with or without intravenous immunoglobulin [78].

1.2.4.7 Late Complications

These include endocrine toxicities such as hypothyroidism, hypogonadism, or growth hormone deficiency in younger patients; pulmonary effects may include obstructive lung disease or pulmonary fibrosis; and other late effects including cataracts and leukoencephalopathy [57].

1.3 Current Indications for Allogeneic Hematopoietic Stem Cell Transplantation for Patients with Malignancy

There is clinical evidence that allogeneic HSCT can provide benefit, defined as freedom of progression or overall survival, for most hematologic malignancies. However, the beneficial effects of allogeneic HSCT vary greatly with each type of malignancy. Data indicate that due to their relative responsiveness to cytotoxic therapy, myeloablative conditioning regimens with allogeneic HSCT result in higher response rates than cytotoxic or conventional agents for almost all hematologic malignancies. However, the durability of these responses and their effect on survival varies from disease to disease. Similarly, there is evidence of a clinical GvT effect in almost every hematologic disease; however, its potency and clinical relevance are highly variable. Interpretation of the results of trials of HSCT always is complicated by issues of patient selection. This can lead to either underestimating the efficacy of allogeneic HSCT if it is used after exhausting all other available therapies or overestimating its efficacy if only the patients with favorable prognostic characteristics are selected. The specific indications for allogeneic HSCT are covered in the chapters for each respective disease. This section briefly addresses the outcomes for malignancies with allogeneic HSCT.

1.3.1 Acute Myeloid Leukemia

With the exception of acute promyelocytic leukemia there is no doubt that allogeneic HSCT offers the highest anti-leukemic activity after a conventional induction and intensification therapy for acute myeloid leukemia (AML; a.k.a. acute myelogenous leukemia) patients in first remission. Randomized controlled trials comparing autologous and allogeneic HSCT to conventional chemotherapy in patients with AML in first complete remission have demonstrated improved leukemia-free survival with both forms of HSCT; however, there has been no significant improvement in overall survival due to increased treatment related mortality with allogeneic HSCT [79, 80]. The one exception has been in pediatric AML, where allogeneic HSCT has been demonstrated to improve both leukemia-free and overall survival for patients transplanted in first complete remission [81]. For AML patients with poor prognostic features (adverse cytogenetics, secondary leukemias, presence of minimal residual disease) there are strong indications for allogeneic HSCT in first complete remission (CR1) [82]. The outcome of HSCT for patients beyond CR1 is worse when compared to the use of transplant while in CR1, but for these patients allografting still remains the most effective strategy to obtain long-term disease control. Reduced-intensity and nonmyeloablative conditioning regimens may increase the applicability of allogeneic HSCT for older AML patients [83].

1.3.2 Acute Lymphoblastic Leukemia

For adult patients with poor-risk acute lymphoblastic leukemia (ALL), most investigators recommend an allogeneic transplant [84–86]. The results for patients in later remissions, early relapse, or primary refractory disease are clearly inferior to those of patients in CR1, but in nearly all of these circumstances if an HLA donor is available, an allogeneic HSCT is associated with improved outcomes when compared to prior therapy [87].

1.3.3 Chronic Myeloid Leukemia

Before the development of imatinib mesytale chronic myeloid leukemia (CML; a.k.a. chronic myelogenous leukemia) was one of the major indications for allogeneic HSCT, and a well established curative strategy for CML with 5-year disease-free survival rates of 85% [88]. After the advent of imatinib and the new tyrosine kinase inhibitors (TKI), allogeneic transplantation is no longer the first option for CML patients [89]. Use of allogeneic HSCT is limited to those patients in chronic phase who failed one, or in some instances, two lines of TKI [90]. The GvT effect is critical in the potential cure of CML with allogeneic transplantation, thus nonmyeloablative and reduced-intensity conditioning regimens in this group of patients would seem an attractive strategy. However it is not yet possible to conclude that for younger patients, those younger than 40–50 years, either nonmyeloablative or reduced-intensity allogeneic HSCT offers a major advantage to patients who would otherwise be candidates for an allografting with conventional, myeloablative conditioning [90]. Patients with accelerated, blastic or second chronic phase CML can not be cured with imatinib or the new TKI dasatinib, and responses are usually of short duration. Although clinical results of allogeneic HSCT are poor for these advanced phases of CML, it continues to be the only potential curative approach [91].

1.3.4 Myelodysplastic Syndromes

Allogeneic HSCT is the only curative treatment for myelodysplastic syndromes (MDS). Because of the older age of patients with MDS, transplantation has generally been reserved for patients with higher risk MDS or MDS transforming to AML. The best results have been obtained in relatively younger patients, who are earlier in their disease course and have not received any prior therapy. To identify factors influencing transplantation outcome for MDS, the International Bone Marrow Transplantation Registry (IBMTR) studied 452 recipients of HLA-identical sibling transplants for MDS [92]. Three-year transplantation-related mortality, relapse, disease-free survival, and overall survival rates were 37%, 23%, 40%, and 42%, respectively. Multivariate analyses showed that young age and platelet counts higher than 100,000 at transplantation were associated with lower transplant-related mortality and higher disease-free and overall survival rates. Because the optimal timing for transplantation for MDS is unknown, the IBMTR constructed a Markov model to examine three transplantation strategies for newly diagnosed MDS: transplantation at diagnosis, transplantation at leukemic progression, and transplantation at an interval from diagnosis but prior to leukemic progression [93]. Analyses using individual patient risk-assessment data from transplantation and non-transplantation registries were performed using the International Prognostic Scoring System (IPSS) for MDS with adjustments for quality of life. For low and intermediate-1 IPSS groups, delayed transplantation maximized overall survival. Transplantation prior to leukemic transformation was associated with a greater number of life years than transplantation at the time of leukemic progression. In a cohort of patients under the age of 40 years, an even more marked survival advantage for delayed transplantation was noted. For intermediate-2 and high IPSS groups, transplantation at diagnosis maximized overall survival. There is evidence that reduced-intensity allogeneic HSCT may benefit older patients with MDS [94, 95].

1.3.5 Non-Hodgkin Lymphoma and Hodgkin Lymphoma

Although allogeneic HSCT has been reported to yield long-term disease-free survival for patients with intermediate and high-grade non-Hodgkin's lymphomas (NHL), the demonstration of a potent GvT effect against NHL is less clear, and the efficacy of donor lymphocyte infusion in lymphoma is anecdotal at best [96–99]. Consequently, the specific role of allogeneic HSCT has not been defined. There are data that nonmyeloablative and reduced-intensity allogeneic HSCT may provide benefits for patients with recurrent follicular NHL; however, the data indicate that this approach requires that the disease remains chemotherapy-sensitive [98].

Allogeneic HSCT has had a limited role in the treatment of Hodgkin lymphoma (HL; a.k.a. Hodgkin's disease) due to the efficacy of autologous HSCT, the treatment-related toxicities associated with myeloablative allogeneic HSCT, and a relative lack of evidence of a GvT effect against HL. However, recent data indicate that reduced-intensity allogeneic HSCT may benefit patients with recurrent HL, and a GvT effect against HD may exist [100].

1.3.6 Multiple Myeloma

A graft-versus-myeloma effect has been demonstrated, but the use of allogeneic HSCT for multiple myeloma had been limited since transplant-related mortality in this group of patients with conventional myeloablative regimens was very high, 30–50% [101]. Data with nonmyeloablative regimens are encouraging, and based on the high transplant-related mortality, multiple myeloma was a good model for investigating the feasibility of nonmyeloablative transplants in this type of patients. Although several studies have demonstrated that transplant-related mortality was decreased with nonmyeloablative conditioning regimens, the relapse rate is greater when compared to standard allografting [90]. Results of a prospective biologically assigned study suggest, however, that the use of nonmyeloablative allogeneic HSCT may be superior to autologous HSCT in newly diagnosed myeloma patients [102].

1.3.7 Solid Tumors

There has been considerable interest in investigating the presence of a GvT effect in a variety of solid tumors, including renal cell carcinoma and breast cancer [103–105]. Childs and colleagues reported on a series of 19 patients with metastatic renal cell carcinoma who underwent nonmyeloablative allogeneic stem cell transplantation [103]. Nine patients had responsive disease (47%), of which three were complete responses.

1.4 Conclusion

There has been tremendous success since the 1980s in the increased safety of allogeneic HSCT and in the expanding application of this treatment to more patient populations. Areas currently under development that may further improve the use and efficacy of transplantation include continuous improvements in supportive care for transplant patients, broadened use of alternative donors, more refined graft manipulations, and further improvements in the nonmyeloablative transplantation techniques and GvHD prevention. Future progress depends on our ability to identify safer and better-targeted anti-tumor therapies that can be incorporated in the transplantation regimens without attenuating the GvT responses. This remains a challenge for future clinical research.

References

1. Thomas E, Storb R, Clift RA, et al. Bone-marrow transplantation (two parts). N Engl J Med. 1975;292:832–43, 895–902.
2. Weissman IL. Translating stem and progenitor cell biology to the clinic: barriers and opportunities. Science 2000;287:1442–6.
3. Armitage JO. Bone marrow transplantation. N Engl J Med. 1994;330:827–38.
4. Rafii S, Lyden D. Therapeutic stem and progenitor cell transplantation for organ vascularization and regeneration. Nat Med. 2003;9:702–12.
5. Clark ML, Lynch FX. Clinical symptoms of radiation sickness, time to onset and duration of symptoms among Hiroshima survivors in the lethal and median lethal ranges of radiation. Mil Surg. 1952;111:360.
6. Jacobson LO, Marks EK, Robson MJ, et al. Effect of spleen protection on mortality following X-irradiation. J Lab Clin Med. 1949;34:1538–43.
7. Rekers PE, Coulter MP, Warren S. Effects of transplantation of bone marrow into irradiated animals. Arch Surg. 1950;60:635.
8. Lorenz E, Uphoff DE, Reid TR, Shelton E. Modification of irradiation injury in mice and guinea pigs by bone marrow injections. J Natl Cancer Inst. 1951;12:197–201.
9. Barnes DW, Corp MJ, et al. Treatment of murine leukaemia with X rays and homologous bone marrow; preliminary communication. Br Med J. 1956;2:626–7.
10. Dameshek W. Bone marrow transplantation; a present-day challenge. Blood 1957;12:321–3.
11. Groth CG, Brent LB, Calne RY, et al. Historic landmarks in clinical transplantation: conclusions from the consensus conference at the University of California, Los Angeles. World J Surg. 2000;24:834–43.

12. Van Rood JJ, Eernisse JG, et al. Leucocyte antibodies in sera from pregnant women. Nature 1958;181:1735–6.
13. Wilson RE, Henry L, Merrill JP. A model system for determining histocompatibility in man. J Clin Invest. 1963;42:1497–503.
14. Dausset J, Rapaport FT, et al. A leucocyte group and its relationship to tissue histocompatibility in man. Transplantation 1965;3:701–5.
15. Mathé G, Amiel JL, Schwartzenberg L, et al. Successful allogeneic bone marrow transplantation in man: chimerism, induced specific tolerance and possible antileukemic effects. Blood 1965:25:179–96.
16. Bach FH, Albertini RJ, et al. Bone-marrow transplantation in a patient with the Wiskott–Aldrich syndrome. Lancet 1968;2:1364–6.
17. Gatti RA, Meuwissen HJ, et al. Immunological reconstitution of sex-linked lymphopenic immunological deficiency. Lancet 1968;2:1366–9.
18. De Koning J, Van Bekkum DW et al. Transplantation of bone-marrow cells and fetal thymus in an infant with lymphopenic immunological deficiency. Lancet 1969;1:1223–7.
19. Thomas ED, Buckner CD, et al. Aplastic anemia treated by marrow transplantation. Lancet 1972;i:284–9.
20. Thomas ED, Buckner CD, et al. One hundred patients with acute leukemia treated by chemotherapy, total body irradiation, and allogeneic marrow transplantation. Blood 1977;49:511–33.
21. Copelan EA. Hematopoietic stem-cell transplantation. N Engl J Med. 2006;354:1813–26.
22. Weiden PL, Flournoy N, Thomas ED, et al. Antileukemic effect of graft-versus-host disease in human recipients of allogeneic-marrow grafts. N Engl J Med. 1979;300: 1068–73.
23. Weiden PL, Sullivan KM, Flournoy N, et al. Anti-leukemic effect of chronic graft-versus-host disease: contribution to improved survival after allogeneic marrow transplantation. N Engl J Med. 1981;304:1529–33.
24. Butturini A, Bortin MM, et al. Graft-versus-leukemia following bone marrow transplantation. Bone Marrow Transplant. 1987;2:233–42.
25. Horowitz MM, Gale RP, Sondel PM, et al. Graft-versus-leukemia reactions after bone marrow transplantation. Blood 1990;75:555–62.
26. Kolb HJ, Mittermüller J, Clemm C, et al. Donor leukocyte transfusions for treatment of recurrent chronic myelogenous leukemia in marrow transplant patients. Blood 1990;76: 2462–5.
27. Porter DL, Roth MS, McGarigle C, et al. Induction of graft-versus-host disease as immunotherapy for relapsed chronic myeloid leukemia. N Engl J Med. 1994;330:100–6.
28. Kolb HJ, Schattenberg A, Goldman JM, et al. Graft-versus-leukemia effect of donor lymphocyte transfusions in marrow grafted patients. European Group for Blood and Marrow Transplantation Working Party Chronic Leukemia. Blood 1995;86:2041–50.
29. Collins RH Jr, Shpilberg O, Drobyski WR, et al. Donor leukocyte infusions in 140 patients with relapsed malignancy after allogeneic bone marrow transplantation. J Clin Oncol. 1997;15:433–44.
30. McCluskey J, Peh CA. The human leucocyte antigens and clinical medicine: an overview. Rev Immunogenet. 1999;1:3–20.
31. Hurley CK, Wade JA, Oudshoorn M, et al. A special report: histocompatibility testing guidelines for hematopoietic stem cell transplantation using volunteer donors. Tissue Antigens. 1999;53:394–406.
32. Flomenberg N, Baxter-Lowe LA, Confer D, et al. Impact of HLA class I and class II high-resolution matching on outcomes of unrelated donor bone marrow transplantation: HLA-C mismatching is associated with a strong adverse effect on transplantation outcome. Blood 2004;104:1923–30.
33. Beatty PG, Clift RA, Mickelson EM, et al. Marrow transplantation from related donors other than HLA-identical siblings. N Engl J Med. 1985;313:765–71.

34. Kernan NA, Bartsch G, Ash RC, et al. Analysis of 462 transplantations from unrelated donors facilitated by the National Marrow Donor Program. N Engl J Med. 1993;328:593–602.
35. Rubinstein P, Carrier C, Scaradavou A, et al. Outcomes among 562 recipients of placental-blood transplants from unrelated donors. N Engl J Med. 1998;339:1565–77.
36. Aversa F, Tabilio A, Velardi A, et al. Treatment of high-risk acute leukemia with T-cell-depleted stem cells from related donors with one fully mismatched HLA haplotype. N Engl J Med. 1998;339:1186–93.
37. Yakoub-Agha I, Mesnil F, Kuentz M, et al. Allogeneic marrow stem-cell transplantation from human leukocyte antigen-identical siblings versus human leukocyte antigen-allelic-matched unrelated donors (10/10) in patients with standard-risk hematologic malignancy: a prospective study from the French Society of Bone Marrow Transplantation and Cell Therapy. J Clin Oncol. 2006;24:5695–702.
38. Grewal SS, Barker JN, Davies SM, Wagner JE. Unrelated donor hematopoietic cell transplantation: marrow or umbilical cord blood? Blood 2003;101:4233–44.
39. Laughlin MJ, Eapen M, Rubinstein P, et al. Outcomes after transplantation of cord blood or bone marrow from unrelated donors in adults with leukemia. N Engl J Med. 2004;351:2265–75.
40. Barker JN, Weisdorf DJ, Wagner JE. Creation of a double chimera after the transplantation of umbilical-cord blood from two partially matched unrelated donors. N Engl J Med. 2001;344:1870–1.
41. Fernandez MN, Regidor C, et al. Unrelated umbilical cord blood transplants in adults: early recovery of neutrophils by supportive co-transplantation of a low number of highly purified peripheral blood CD34+ cells from an HLA-haploidentical donor. Exp Hematol. 2003;31:535–44.
42. Henslee-Downey PJ, Abhyankar SH, Parrish RS, et al. Use of partially mismatched related donors extends access to allogeneic marrow transplant. Blood 1997;89:3864–72.
43. O'Donnell PV, Luznik L, Jones RJ, Vogelsang GB, Leffell MS, Phelps M, Rhubart P, Cowan K, Piantados S, Fuchs EJ. Nonmyeloablative bone marrow transplantation from partially HLA-mismatched related donors using posttransplantation cyclophosphamide. Biol Blood Marrow Transplant. 2002;8:377–86.
44. Buckner CD, Clift RA, Sanders JE, et al. Marrow harvesting from normal donors. Blood 1984;64:630–4.
45. Seebach JD, Stussi G, Passweg JR, Loberiza FR Jr, Gajewski JL, Keating A, Goerner M, Rowlings PA, Tiberghien P, Elfenbein GJ, Gale RP, van Rood JJ, Reddy V, Gluckman E, Bolwell BJ, Klumpp TR, Horowitz MM, Ringdén O, Barrett AJ; GVHD Working Committee of Center for International Blood and Marrow Transplant Research. ABO blood group barrier in allogeneic bone marrow transplantation revisited. Biol Blood Marrow Transplant. 2005;11:1006–13.
46. Gratwohl A, Baldomero H, Frauendorfer K, Urbano-Ispizua A; Joint Accreditation Committee, International Society for Cellular Therapy; European Group for Blood and Marrow Transplantation. EBMT activity survey 2004 and changes in disease indication over the past 15 years. Bone Marrow Transplant. 2006;37:1069–85.
47. Stem Cell Trialists' Collaborative Group. Allogeneic peripheral blood stem-cell compared with bone marrow transplantation in the management of hematologic malignancies: an individual patient data meta-analysis of nine randomized trials. J Clin Oncol. 2005;23: 5074–87.
48. Rowley SD, Feng Z, Chen L, et al. A randomized phase III clinical trial of autologous blood stem cell transplantation comparing cryopreservation using dimethylsulfoxide vs dimethylsulfoxide with hydroxyethylstarch. Bone Marrow Transplant. 2003;31:1043–51.
49. Simpson D. T-cell depleting antibodies: new hope for induction of allograft tolerance in bone marrow transplantation? BioDrugs 2003;17:147–54.
50. Baranov A, Gale RP, Guskova A, et al. Bone marrow transplantation after the Chernobyl nuclear accident. N Engl J Med. 1989;321:205–12.

51. Niederwieser D, Maris M, et al. Low-dose total body irradiation (TBI) and fludarabine followed by hematopoietic cell transplantation (HCT) from HLA-matched or mismatched unrelated donors and postgrafting immunosuppression with cyclosporine and mycophenolate mofetil (MMF) can induce durable complete chimerism and sustained remissions in patients with hematological diseases. Blood 2003;101:1620–9.
52. Santos GW, Sensenbrenner LL, et al. HL-A-identical marrow transplants in aplastic anemia, acute leukemia, and lymphosarcoma employing cyclophosphamide. Transplant Proc. 1976;8:607–10.
53. Tutschka PJ, Copelan EA, et al. Bone marrow transplantation for leukemia following a new busulfan and cyclophosphamide regimen. Blood 1987;70:1382–8.
54. Andersson BS, Kashyap A, et al. Conditioning therapy with intravenous busulfan and cyclophosphamide (IV BuCy2) for hematologic malignancies prior to allogeneic stem cell transplantation: A phase II study. Biol Blood Marrow Transplant. 2002;8:145–54.
55. Giralt S, Estey E, Albitar M, et al. Engraftment of allogeneic hematopoietic progenitor cells with purine analog-containing chemotherapy: harnessing graft-versus-leukemia without myeloablative therapy. Blood 1997;89:4531–6.
56. Slavin S, Nagler A, Naparstek E, et al. Nonmyeloablative stem cell transplantation and cell therapy as an alternative to conventional bone marrow transplantation with lethal cytoreduction for the treatment of malignant and nonmalignant hematologic diseases. Blood 1998;91:756–63.
57. Antin JH. Clinical practice. Long-term care after hematopoietic-cell transplantation in adults. N Engl J Med. 2002;347:36–42.
58. Sorror ML, Maris MB, Storb R, et al. Hematopoietic cell transplantation (HCT)-specific comorbidity index: a new tool for risk assessment before allogeneic HCT. Blood 2005;106:2912–9.
59. Champlin RE, Horowitz MM, van Bekkum DW, et al. Graft failure following bone marrow transplantation for severe aplastic anemia: risk factors and treatment results. Blood 1989;73:606–13.
60. Goodman JL, Winston DJ, Greenfield RA, Chandrasekar PH, Fox B, Kaizer H, Shadduck RK, Shea TC, Stiff P, Friedman DJ, et al. A controlled trial of fluconazole to prevent fungal infections in patients undergoing bone marrow transplantation. N Engl J Med. 1992;326: 845–51.
61. Winston DJ, Maziarz RT, Chandrasekar PH, Lazarus HM, Goldman M, Blumer JL, Leitz GJ, Territo MC. Intravenous and oral itraconazole versus intravenous and oral fluconazole for long-term antifungal prophylaxis in allogeneic hematopoietic stem-cell transplant recipients. A multicenter, randomized trial. Ann Intern Med. 2003;138: 705–13.
62. Sullivan KM, Dykewicz CA, Longworth DL, Boeckh M, Baden LR, Rubin RH, Sepkowitz KA; Centers for Disease Control and Prevention; Infectious Diseases Society of America; American Society for Blood and Marrow Transplantation Practice Guidelines and beyond. Preventing opportunistic infections after hematopoietic stem cell transplantation: the Centers for Disease Control and Prevention, Infectious Diseases Society of America, and American Society for Blood and Marrow Transplantation Practice Guidelines and beyond. Hematology Am Soc Hematol Educ Program. 2001: 392–421.
63. Gruss E, Bernis C, Tomas JF, et al. Acute renal failure in patients following bone marrow transplantation: prevalence, risk factors and outcome. Am J Nephrol. 1995;15:473–9.
64. Ruutu T, Barosi G, Benjamin RJ, Clark RE, George JN, Gratwohl A, Holler E, Iacobelli M, Kentouche K, Lämmle B, Moake JL, Richardson P, Socié G, Zeigler Z, Niederwieser D, Barbui T; European Group for Blood and Marrow Transplantation; European LeukemiaNet. Diagnostic criteria for hematopoietic stem cell transplant-associated microangiopathy: results of a consensus process by an International Working Group. Haematologica. 2007;92:95–100.

65. Srinivasan R, Balow JE, Sabnis S, et al. Nephrotic syndrome: an under-recognised immune-mediated complication of non-myeloablative allogeneic haematopoietic cell transplantation. Br J Haematol. 2005;131:74–9.
66. Bearman SI, Anderson GL, Mori M, et al. Venoocclusive disease of the liver: development of a model for predicting fatal outcome after marrow transplantation. J Clin Oncol. 1993;11:1729–36.
67. DeLeve LD, Shulman HM, McDonald GB. Toxic injury to hepatic sinusoids: sinusoidal obstruction syndrome (veno-occlusive disease). Semin Liver Dis. 2002;22:27–42.
68. Richardson PG, Murakami C, Jin Z, Warren D, Momtaz P, Hoppensteadt D, Elias AD, Antin JH, Soiffer R, Spitzer T, Avigan D, Bearman SI, Martin PL, Kurtzberg J, Vredenburgh J, Chen AR, Arai S, Vogelsang G, McDonald GB, Guinan EC. Multi-institutional use of defibrotide in 88 patients after stem cell transplantation with severe veno-occlusive disease and multisystem organ failure: response without significant toxicity in a high-risk population and factors predictive of outcome. Blood 2002;100:4337–43.
69. Essell JH, Schroeder MT, Harman GS, Halvorson R, Lew V, Callander N, Snyder M, Lewis SK, Allerton JP, Thompson JM. Ursodiol prophylaxis against hepatic complications of allogeneic bone marrow transplantation. A randomized, double-blind, placebo-controlled trial. Ann Intern Med. 1998;128(12 Pt 1):975–81.
70. Przepiorka D, Weisdorf D, Martin P, et al. 1994 Consensus Conference on Acute GVHD Grading. Bone Marrow Transplant. 1995;15:825–8.
71. Martin PJ, Schoch G, Fisher L, et al. A retrospective analysis of therapy for acute graft-versus-host disease: initial treatment. Blood 1990;76:1464–72.
72. Kennedy MS, Deeg HJ, Storb R, et al. Treatment of acute graft-versus-host disease after allogeneic marrow transplantation: randomized study comparing corticosteroids and cyclosporine. Am J Med. 1985;78:978–83.
73. Jacobsohn DA, Vogelsang GB. Novel pharmacotherapeutic approaches to prevention and treatment of GVHD. Drugs 2002;62:879–89.
74. Shulman HM, Kleiner D, Lee SJ, Morton T, Pavletic SZ, Farmer E, Moresi JM, Greenson J, Janin A, Martin PJ, McDonald G, Flowers ME, Turner M, Atkinson J, Lefkowitch J, Washington MK, Prieto VG, Kim SK, Argenyi Z, Diwan AH, Rashid A, Hiatt K, Couriel D, Schultz K, Hymes S, Vogelsang GB. Histopathologic diagnosis of chronic graft-versus-host disease: National Institutes of Health Consensus Development Project on Criteria for Clinical Trials in Chronic Graft-versus-Host Disease: II. Pathology Working Group Report. Biol Blood Marrow Transplant. 2006;12:31–47.
75. Lee SJ, Vogelsang G, Flowers ME. Chronic graft-versus-host disease. Biol Blood Marrow Transplant. 2003;9:215–33.
76. Filipovich AH, Weisdorf D, Pavletic S, Socie G, Wingard JR, Lee SJ, Martin P, Chien J, Przepiorka D, Couriel D, Cowen EW, Dinndorf P, Farrell A, Hartzman R, Henslee-Downey J, Jacobsohn D, McDonald G, Mittleman B, Rizzo JD, Robinson M, Schubert M, Schultz K, Shulman H, Turner M, Vogelsang G, Flowers ME. National Institutes of Health consensus development project on criteria for clinical trials in chronic graft-versus-host disease: I. Diagnosis and staging working group report. Biol Blood Marrow Transplant. 2005;11:945–56.
77. Vogelsang GB. How I treat chronic graft-versus-host disease. Blood 2001;97:1196–201.
78. Couriel D, Carpenter PA, Cutler C, Bolaños-Meade J, Treister NS, Gea-Banacloche J, Shaughnessy P, Hymes S, Kim S, Wayne AS, Chien JW, Neumann J, Mitchell S, Syrjala K, Moravec CK, Abramovitz L, Liebermann J, Berger A, Gerber L, Schubert M, Filipovich AH, Weisdorf D, Schubert MM, Shulman H, Schultz K, Mittelman B, Pavletic S, Vogelsang GB, Martin PJ, Lee SJ, Flowers ME. Ancillary therapy and supportive care of chronic graft-versus-host disease: National Institutes of Health consensus development project on criteria for clinical trials in chronic Graft-versus-host disease: V. Ancillary Therapy and Supportive Care Working Group Report. Biol Blood Marrow Transplant. 2006;12:375–96.

79. Zittoun RA, Mandelli F, et al. Autologous or allogeneic bone marrow transplantation compared with intensive chemotherapy in acute myelogenous leukemia. European Organization for Research and Treatment of Cancer (EORTC) and the Gruppo Italiano Malattie Ematologiche Maligne dell'Adulto (GIMEMA) Leukemia Cooperative Groups. N Engl J Med. 1995;332:217–23.
80. Cassileth PA, Harrington DP, et al. Chemotherapy compared with autologous or allogeneic bone marrow transplantation in the management of acute myeloid leukemia in first remission. N Engl J Med. 1998;339:1649–56.
81. Woods WG, Neudorf S, Gold S, et al. Children's Cancer Group: a comparison of allogeneic bone marrow transplantation, autologous bone marrow transplantation, and aggressive chemotherapy in children with acute myeloid leukemia in remission. Blood 2001;97:56–62.
82. Gale RP, Park RE, Dubois RW, Herzig GP, Hocking WG, Horowitz MM, Keating A, Kempin S, Linker CA, Schiffer CA, Wiernik PH, Weisdorf DJ, Rai KR. Delphi-panel analysis of appropriateness of high-dose therapy and bone marrow transplants in adults with acute myelogenous leukemia in 1st remission. Leuk Res. 1999;23:709–18.
83. Aoudjhane M, Labopin M, Gorin NC, et al. Comparative outcome of reduced intensity and myeloablative conditioning regimen in HLA identical sibling allogeneic haematopoietic stem cell transplantation for patients older than 50 years of age with acute myeloblastic leukaemia: a retrospective survey from the Acute Leukemia Working Party (ALWP) of the European group for Blood and Marrow Transplantation (EBMT). Leukemia 2005;19:2304–12.
84. Gale RP, Park RE, Dubois RW, Herzig GP, Hocking WG, Horowitz MM, Keating A, Kempin S, Linker CA, Schiffer CA, Wiernik PH, Weisdorf DJ, Rai KR. Delphi-panel analysis of appropriateness of high-dose therapy and bone marrow transplants in adults with acute lymphoblastic leukemia in first remission. Leuk Res. 1998;22:973–81.
85. Thomas X, Boiron JM, Huguet F, Dombret H, Bradstock K, Vey N, Kovacsovics T, Delannoy A, Fegueux N, Fenaux P, Stamatoullas A, Vernant JP, Tournilhac O, Buzyn A, Reman O, Charrin C, Boucheix C, Gabert J, Lhéritier V, Fiere D. Outcome of treatment in adults with acute lymphoblastic leukemia: analysis of the LALA-94 trial. J Clin Oncol. 2004;22:4075–86.
86. Hunault M, Harousseau JL, Delain M, Truchan-Graczyk M, Cahn JY, Witz F, Lamy T, Pignon B, Jouet JP, Garidi R, Caillot D, Berthou C, Guyotat D, Sadoun A, Sotto JJ, Lioure B, Casassus P, Solal-Celigny P, Stalnikiewicz L, Audhuy B, Blanchet O, Baranger L, Béné MC, Ifrah N; GOELAMS (Groupe Ouest-Est des Leucémies Airguës et Maladies du Sang) Group. Better outcome of adult acute lymphoblastic leukemia after early genoidentical allogeneic bone marrow transplantation (BMT) than after late high-dose therapy and autologous BMT: a GOELAMS trial. Blood 2004;104:3028–37.
87. Fielding AK, Richards SM, et al. Outcome of 609 adults after relapse of acute lymphoblastic leukemia (ALL); an MRC UKALL12/ECOG 2993 study. Blood 2007;109:944–50.
88. Radich JP, Gooley T, et al. HLA-matched related hematopoietic cell transplantation for chronic-phase CML using a targeted busulfan and cyclophosphamide preparative regimen. Blood 2003;102:31–5.
89. Giralt SA, Arora M, et al. Impact of imatinib therapy on the use of allogeneic haematopoietic progenitor cell transplantation for the treatment of chronic myeloid leukaemia. Br J Haematol. 2007;137:461–7.
90. Crawley C, Iacobelli S, et al. Reduced-intensity conditioning for myeloma: lower nonrelapse mortality but higher relapse rates compared with myeloablative conditioning. Blood 2007;109:3588–94.
91. Weisser M, Schleuning M, et al. Allogeneic stem-cell transplantation provides excellent results in advanced stage chronic myeloid leukemia with major cytogenetic response to pre-transplant imatinib therapy. Leuk Lymphoma. 2007;48:295–301.
92. Sierra J, Perez WS, Rozman C, et al. Bone marrow transplantation from HLA-identical siblings as treatment for myelodysplasia. Blood 2002;100:1997–2004.

93. Cutler CS, Lee SJ, Greenberg P, et al. A decision analysis of allogeneic bone marrow transplantation for the myelodysplastic syndromes: delayed transplantation for low risk myelodysplasia is associated with improved outcome. Blood 2004;104:579–85.
94. Tauro S, Craddock C, Peggs K, et al. Allogeneic stem-cell transplantation using a reduced-intensity conditioning regimen has the capacity to produce durable remissions and long-term disease-free survival in patients with high-risk acute myeloid leukemia and myelodysplasia. J Clin Oncol. 2005;23:9387–93.
95. Martino R, Iacobelli S, et al. Retrospective comparison of reduced-intensity conditioning and conventional high-dose conditioning for allogeneic hematopoietic stem cell transplantation using HLA-identical sibling donors in myelodysplastic syndromes. Blood 2006;108:836–46.
96. Ratanatharathorn V, Uberti J, Karanes C, et al. Prospective comparative trial of autologous versus allogeneic bone marrow transplantation in patients with non-Hodgkin's lymphoma. Blood 1994;84:1050–5.
97. Bierman PJ, Sweetenham JW, Loberiza FR Jr, et al. Syngeneic hematopoietic stem-cell transplantation for non-Hodgkin's lymphoma: a comparison with allogeneic and autologous transplantation–The Lymphoma Working Committee of the International Bone Marrow Transplant Registry and the European Group for Blood and Marrow Transplantation. J Clin Oncol. 2003;21:3744–53.
98. Robinson SP, Goldstone AH, Mackinnon S, et al. Chemoresistant or aggressive lymphoma predicts for a poor outcome following reduced-intensity allogeneic progenitor cell transplantation: an analysis from the Lymphoma Working Party of the European Group for Blood and Bone Marrow Transplantation. Blood 2002;100:4310–6.
99. Grigg A, Ritchie D. Graft-versus-lymphoma effects: clinical review, policy proposals, and immunobiology. Biol Blood Marrow Transplant. 2004;10:579–90.
100. Peggs KS, Hunter A, Chopra R, et al. Clinical evidence of a graft-versus-Hodgkin's-lymphoma effect after reduced-intensity allogeneic transplantation. Lancet 2005;365:1934–41.
101. Barlogie B, Kyle RA, et al. Standard chemotherapy compared with high-dose chemoradiotherapy for multiple myeloma: final results of phase III US Intergroup Trial S9321. J Clin Oncol. 2006;24:929–36.
102. Bruno B, Rotta M, Patriarca F, et al. A comparison of allografting with autografting for newly diagnosed myeloma. N Engl J Med. 2007;356:1110–20.
103. Childs R, Chernoff A, Contentin N, et al. Regression of metastatic renal-cell carcinoma after nonmyeloablative allogeneic peripheral-blood stem-cell transplantation. N Engl J Med. 2000;343:750–8.
104. Bishop MR, Fowler DH, Marchigiani D, et al. Allogeneic lymphocytes induce tumor regression of advanced metastatic breast cancer. J Clin Oncol. 2004;22:3886–92.
105. Carella AM, Beltrami G, Corsetti MT, et al. Reduced intensity conditioning for allograft after cytoreductive autograft in metastatic breast cancer. Lancet 2005;366:318–320.

Chapter 2
The Principles and Overview of Autologous Hematopoietic Stem Cell Transplantation

William Vaughan, Tara Seshadri, Mark Bridges, and Armand Keating

2.1 Introduction

Autologous hematopoietic stem cell transplantation (HSCT) refers to the use of self-renewing progenitor cells derived either from the patient's own marrow or peripheral blood, as opposed to cells from an allogeneic or syngeneic donor, to repopulate the hematopoietic system after administration of chemotherapy. This treatment modality enables very high ("myeloablative") doses of chemotherapy to be administered in the hope of eradicating tumors while avoiding the serious side effect of prolonged myelosuppression or even marrow ablation. Autologous HSCT is best viewed as one step in the treatment strategy for malignant (usually hematological) diseases and not a therapeutic entity in itself.

Almost half a century has passed since the first report of the infusion of autologous bone marrow into a human to facilitate hematopoietic reconstitution following high-dose chemotherapy [1], although interest in the therapeutic use of marrow dates back much further. Brown-Sequard and d'Arsonaval made the earliest known attempts, when they administered marrow by mouth to patients with anemia related to leukemia [2]. Other methods of delivering marrow followed, including the use of intramuscular [3] and intramedullary [4] injection in the 1930s and the first report of intravenous infusion of viable bone marrow in 1939, in an unsuccessful attempt to treat a patient with aplastic anemia [5]. The first uses of marrow therapeutically were exclusively with marrow derived from an allogeneic source, a concept that might seem counterintuitive given the relative frequencies of autologous and allogeneic transplants today.

These early attempts were carried out largely in isolation, and it was not until the world entered the "atomic age" in 1945 that a concerted research effort developed rapidly in the area of toxicity related to massive doses of radiation and how these toxicities might be treated. Bone marrow suppression was one of

W. Vaughan (✉)
University of Alabama Bone Marrow Transplantation Program, University of Alabama Comprehensive Cancer Center, Birmingham, AL, USA
e-mail: WVaughan@uabmc.edu

M.R. Bishop (ed.), *Hematopoietic Stem Cell Transplantation*,
Cancer Treatment and Research 144, DOI 10.1007/978-0-387-78580-6_2,

the principal effects, occurring at exposure levels lower than for other significant toxicities. Early murine studies by Jacobson et al. published in 1949 showed that by shielding the spleen (which is hematopoietic in the mouse), the hematological effects of large doses of radiation could be ameliorated [6]. Subsequent studies demonstrated that the implantation of a non-irradiated autologous spleen into a lethally irradiated mouse could accomplish the same objective [7]. Much of the subsequent work again focused on using marrow derived from an allogeneic or syngeneic source, and clinical reports of the use of allogeneic marrow to treat leukemia followed in the mid-1950s [8, 9]. These were largely unsuccessful, presumably due to an immune response against the infused marrow, as histocompatibility antigens were not yet known.

It was not until the mid to late 1950s that interest developed in the use of one's own hematopoietic system to repopulate an ablated marrow. It was known at the time that a steep dose–response curve existed for some malignancies, but use of very high doses of chemotherapy or radiation was precluded by profound toxicity to organs and tissues, particularly myelosuppression. To circumvent this toxicity, while at the same time avoiding an immune response against foreign marrow cells, attempts were made to harvest bone marrow from patients with a terminal malignancy and then re-infuse the marrow after treatment with massive doses of radiation or chemotherapy.

The first report of this method was published by Kurnick et al. [1] in 1958. Other reports soon followed in 1959 by McFarland et al. [10], McGovern et al. [11], and Newton et al. [12]. These early attempts were in patients with very advanced solid and hematologic malignancies and showed that the autologous marrow infusion appeared to be capable of regenerating a lethally damaged bone marrow. They did not, however, demonstrate any significant benefit to high-dose therapy over conventional dose therapy and the use of autologous transplantation fell out of favor for more than a decade. In the 1960s and 1970s, led principally by Dr. E. Donnall Thomas and colleagues, allogeneic transplantation again dominated the landscape, owing to the identification of histocompatibility antigens and the development of improved anti-infective agents and supportive measures. Initial successes were in patients with immunodeficiency syndromes, soon followed by patients with hematological malignancies.

Allogeneic transplantation, however, presented significant and unique problems, principally graft-versus-host disease (GvHD) and the lack of a suitable donor in many cases. In part because of these challenges, there was a renewed interest in autologous transplantation in the late 1970s, with the first successful cure of lymphoma using this method reported by Appelbaum and colleagues in 1978 [13]. At that time methods for storage of transplant products were not well developed, limiting autologous transplant regimens to those with a very short marrow toxicity half life such as total body irradiation (TBI) [14], cyclophosphamide [15], melphalan [16], BCNU (1,3-bis(2-chloroethyl)-1-nitroso-urea) [17], and nitrogen mustard [18]. The development of cryoprotectants such as dimethyl sulfoxide (DMSO) [19] in conjunction with controlled-rate freezing techniques permitted the cryopreservation and storage of autologous bone marrow for extended periods of time [19, 20]. The availability of cryopreserved bone marrow enabled clinicians to utilize both drugs with longer half-lives and multi-agent, multi-day, intensive therapy regimens, resulted in the explosion of interest in autologous bone marrow transplantation in the 1980s.

The next major advance in transplantation technology was based on the recognition that hematopoietic precursor cells circulated in the peripheral blood in man [20]. Goldman et al. in 1979 demonstrated that peripheral blood cells collected from patients in chronic phase of chronic myelogenous leukemia (CML) appeared to be capable of restoring chronic phase CML in patients treated with marrow ablative therapy for acute phase CML [21]. Later, Juttner and colleagues [22] reported high numbers of progenitor cells in the blood of patients with acute leukemia recovering from induction chemotherapy and that these cells were capable of producing prompt but incomplete hematopoietic reconstitution after high dose melphalan chemotherapy. In 1984, Kessinger et al. [23] performed the first successful autologous transplant with recovery of hematopoiesis after marrow ablative therapy using cells collected from steady-state peripheral blood in a patient with breast cancer. That same year, Korbling and colleagues reported successful engraftment with normal hematopoiesis in a patient given peripheral blood cells following high dose chemotherapy for Burkitt's lymphoma [24]. In a later report, Kessinger et al. [25] described a series of 10 consecutive lymphoma and breast cancer patients who received autologous peripheral blood stem cell grafts, resulting in partial engraftment in all patients and full and sustained engraftment in the eight patients who did not die early from transplant-related toxicity or progressive disease. Adequacy of the product was determined by peripheral mononuclear cell counts and colony-forming unit (CFU) assays. Two subsequent critical advances, the use of hematopoietic growth factors [e.g., granulocyte colony-stimulating factor (G-CSF), granulocyte-macrophage colony-stimulating factor (GM-CSF)] for progenitor and stem cell mobilization [26] and stem and progenitor cell enumeration with the anti-CD34 monoclonal antibody developed by Civin et al. [27], eventually resulted in peripheral blood stem cell collection becoming the standard source for autologous HSCT by the early 1990s. Today, the number of autologous transplants far outpaces the number for its allogeneic counterpart, and autologous HSCT has now become standard therapy for many hematological malignancies.

2.2 Current Concepts and Evolving Rationale for Autologous HSCT

2.2.1 Patient Selection

The experience with autologous HSCT in metastatic breast cancer serves as a strong reminder of the importance of patient selection and the need for randomized trials to accurately evaluate the role of such therapy. Early encouraging results of prolonged disease-free survival (DFS) in 30% of patients with metastatic breast cancer treated with autologous HSCT fueled emotional debates world-wide about the appropriateness of the therapy in this patient population. There was considerable pressure both to treating doctors and insurance companies to offer autologous HSCT; consequently many patients were treated off-trial. Hence, it was some time before well-designed randomized controlled trials (RCT) accrued sufficient numbers of patients to appropriately evaluate autologous HSCT in metastatic breast cancer. Several RCTs demonstrated improved progression-free survival (PFS) with autologous HSCT for metastatic breast cancer; however, none showed an advantage in overall survival (OS). Moreover, up to 10% of patients succumbed to treatment-related mortality [28]. This experience highlights the disadvantages of deferring an evidence-based approach in favor of treating individual patients with a potentially promising but unproven therapy. The prevailing climate after the release of the negative RCT results has discouraged other clinical trials of autologous HSCT to be designed and performed in selected patients with breast cancer, who might conceivably have benefited.

Despite the experience with autologous HSCT for breast cancer, we have learned some important principles of the use of autologous HSCT. The efficacy of autologous HSCT is dependent on chemotherapy sensitivity, timing, and tumor biology, and these concepts are critical in ascertaining who and when to transplant. As such, the indications and timing for autologous HSCT have slowly evolved, and recommendations for when and on whom to perform the procedure for specific diseases are changing. A summary of the current indications for autologous HSCT is provided in Table 2.1.

2.2.2 Chemotherapy Sensitivity

Response to salvage chemotherapy is a very important predictor of outcome after autologous HSCT; patients with non-Hodgkin's lymphoma (NHL) who were sensitive to salvage chemotherapy had a significantly improved 5-year PFS (49% vs. 13%) following autologous HSCT compared to patients whose are resistant [43, 44]. Studies with aggressive NHL show that patients frankly refractory to salvage chemotherapy derive little benefit from autologous HSCT [45], thus establishing chemotherapy sensitivity as a general requirement before proceeding. It is noteworthy that many autologous HSCT trials in follicular NHL [36], aggressive NHL [29] and Hodgkin lymphoma (HL, a.k.a. Hodgkin's disease) [30, 46] only include patients responding to chemotherapy. Response to salvage therapy is also a predictor of outcome. Patients with either NHL or HL achieving a complete remission after salvage chemotherapy were observed to have a 75% failure-free survival at 2 years after autologous HSCT compared with 40% for patients who achieved a partial remission [47]. As autologous HSCT works on the principle of using large doses of chemotherapy

Table 2.1 Indications for autologous hematopoietic stem cell transplantation

Disease	Autologous HSCT indicated?	When to perform Autologous HSCT	Reference
Aggressive NHL	Yes	Relapsed/refractory	[29]
Hodgkin's Lymphoma	Yes	Relapsed/refractory	[30, 31]
Multiple Myeloma	Yes	After induction therapy	[32–34]
Mantle Cell Lymphoma	Yes	In first remission	[35]
Follicular Lymphoma	Possibly	In second/subsequent remission	[36]
Chronic Lymphocytic Leukemia	possibly	In second/subsequent remission	[37]
Acute Myeloid Leukemia	Yes	In second remission if allogeneic donor is unavailable	[38, 39]
Acute Lymphoblastic leukemia	Investigational		[140]
Breast Cancer	Controversial	Consider in metastatic disease in context of trial	[141–143]
Germ Cell Tumors	Yes	Relapsed/refractory	[144]
Autoimmune disease	Investigational		[40]

to eradicate disease, it follows logically that patients refractory to induction or salvage chemotherapy are less likely to have a favorable outcome compared with those sensitive to chemotherapy.

2.2.3 Timing of Autologous HSCT

The timing of autologous HSCT is also critically important in determining an optimum outcome. For example, although autologous HSCT is unlikely to be of benefit in aggressive NHL as part of primary therapy [48], its use in treating relapsed and refractory disease that is chemotherapy sensitive became widespread after the publication of the PARMA trial in 1995 [43]. Of note, most trials demonstrating the benefits of autologous HSCT in aggressive B-cell NHL, either upfront or in relapsed patients, were performed in the pre-rituximab era. The inclusion of rituximab as part of salvage chemotherapy improves response rates in rituximab-naïve patients [49], thereby increasing the eligibility of patients for autologous HSCT.

In contrast to aggressive NHL, autologous HSCT for mantle cell lymphoma (MCL) appears to be of most benefit when performed as part of primary therapy in patients sensitive to anthracycline-based chemotherapy. Several case series show that autologous HSCT in first remission is associated with an improved OS and progression-free survival (PFS) when compared with historical controls [35, 50, 51].

Unlike MCL, autologous HSCT is generally not performed as part of initial therapy for follicular or other low-grade NHL. These diseases are generally associated with a long OS, and although autologous HSCT may improve PFS [52] when performed early in the disease course, OS is not altered. There is a suggestion that improvements in both PFS and OS can be made when autologous HSCT is performed in second relapse [53]. Despite the consistent results of autologous HSCT in second relapse, its place in the treatment of follicular NHL remains to be defined, especially in view of the impressive results of rituximab maintenance after second-line chemotherapy [54]. The role of rituximab as maintenance therapy after autologous HSCT also warrants further investigation in NHL.

Several phase III trials have demonstrated that the use of autologous HSCT early in the disease course for multiple myeloma results in improved complete remission, event-free survival (EFS), and OS rates as compared to conventional chemotherapy alone [32–34]. However, patients with adverse cytogenetic features such as p53 deletion, t(4:14), and del 13q continue to have a poor outcome after autologous HSCT [55, 56]. Responses to autologous HSCT have also been shown to be an important predictor of outcome in multiple myeloma. Patients achieving complete remission (CR) post-autologous HSCT having a higher likelihood of surviving 5 years compared to those achieving partial remission (PR). This has led to the investigation of tandem autologous HSCT in multiple myeloma in an attempt to improve complete remission rates [57].

2.2.3.1 Tumor Biology

One of the best examples in using tumor biology to decide therapy has been the experience with acute myeloid leukemia (AML). Currently, therapy for AML is heavily stratified according to cytogenetics. Patients with favorable-risk AML, defined by the presence of t(15:17)(q22;q12) or a translocation involving the core binding factors, have a good outcome with chemotherapy alone. Thus, autologous HSCT or allogeneic transplantation is not recommended in first complete remission (CR1) for this subgroup. Patients relapsing can be effectively salvaged with an allotransplant or autologous HSCT should a donor not be available. Patients with poor-risk AML, defined by adverse cytogenetics or those who require more than one induction to obtain a complete remission, have a 5-year probability of relapse of 75–90%. These patients are generally offered an allogeneic transplant in first remission if an appropriate donor is available, as this approach appears to confer a survival advantage [58, 59]. The best treatment approach for patients with intermediate-risk AML, the most common subgroup of AML, is undefined. Trials with subgroup analyses of patients with intermediate-risk AML did not demonstrate an advantage of autologous HSCT in CR1 [60, 61]. Therefore, the role of autologous HSCT in AML is best reserved for patients in second remission who lack an allogeneic donor.

2.2.4 Hematopoietic Progenitor Cells

Hematopoietic progenitor cells (HPC) have a variable ability to self renew and are able to terminally differentiate into mature cells of the erythroid, myeloid, megakaryocytic and lymphoid lineages. They form the corner stone in autologous HSCT as they re-establish normal hematopoiesis following myeloablative chemotherapy. They are immunophenotypically characterized by the expression of CD34, and this antigen is used to identify them in flow cytometric assays. They can be subdivided into mature and immature subsets. Mature forms express HLA-DR, CD33, and CD38 and lack CD90, while the immature subset expresses CD90 and lacks CD33, CD38, and HLA-DR [62].

Hematopoietic progenitor cells are located primarily in the bone marrow with only very small numbers circulating in the peripheral blood. Bone marrow microenvironmental cells express numerous cell adhesion molecules and elaborate cytokines, which interact with progenitors and stem cells and participate in hematopoietic regulation and cell-microenvironment interactions. The capacity of intravenously infused stem cells to migrate to the bone marrow was established in 1970s. The mechanisms involved in bone marrow homing are complex. Transplanted HPC interact with bone marrow stromal cells and the extra-cellular matrix. Adhesion molecules such as integrins, CD44, CD62, and c-kit expressed on progenitor cells and selectins expressed on endothelial cells mediate this process. Subsequent rolling and firm adhesion of stem/progenitor cells to the endothelial cell occurs [39]. A key factor in signaling is the chemokine, SDF-1 (CXCL12). This is produced by osteoblasts and marrow stromal cells and interacts with the receptor CXCR4 present on stem/progenitor cells. Disruption of this pathway appears, in part, to be involved in the mechanism behind HPC mobilization with G-CSF.

2.2.4.1 Hematopoietic Progenitor Cell Mobilization

The vast majority of autologous HSCT is performed using peripheral blood progenitor cells and obviates the need for a bone marrow harvest, hence saving the patient a general anesthetic. Furthermore, the use of mobilized peripheral blood progenitors results in rapid engraftment of platelets and granulocytes [63]. Initial concerns that peripheral blood stem cells confer an inferior survival over bone marrow-derived stem cells [42] have been put to rest following a cohort analysis [64] and two prospective RCTs, which showed no survival advantage with marrow HPC [65, 66]. Thus, it is unlikely that graft source alters survival outcome to any significant degree.

Hematopoietic progenitor cells can be mobilized from the bone marrow into the peripheral blood via cytokines or chemotherapy. Chemotherapy was first found to increase progenitors in the peripheral blood in 1976 [67]. Following administration of chemotherapy, leukopheresis can be initiated during the hematological recovery phase. This mobilization chemotherapy is usually myelosuppressive and results in a brief episode of severe neutropenia. Cyclophosphamide, either as a single agent or in combination, is frequently used as a mobilizing agent [68]. Alternatively, leukopheresis can be performed after combination chemotherapy for the primary disease process when hematological recovery commences. A disadvantage of chemotherapy alone relates to logistics. More leukophereses are required after chemotherapy alone and hematological recovery may be delayed because of the mobilization of insufficient numbers of $CD34^+$ cells. As a consequence, chemotherapy alone is rarely used for mobilization.

Cytokines such as G-CSF and to a much lesser extent, GM-CSF, are used for progenitor cell mobilization. G-CSF is more effective [68] and is well tolerated. The most common side effects are bone pain and headaches. G-CSF is generally administered subcutaneously at a dose of 10 μg/kg/day and the HPC collection commences after 5 days of administration. The main advantage of this method is that the day of collection is more reliably predicted and there is avoidance of side effects induced by chemotherapy.

Combination chemotherapy with cytokines results in excellent progenitor cell collections [69]. In patients who have had considerable prior chemotherapy exposure this approach may be successful especially if insufficient HPC were obtained after cytokines alone. AMD 3100 (plerixafor), a bicyclam derivative, has been shown to be an effective progenitor cell-mobilizing agent [70]. This drug reversibly blocks SDF-1 from binding CXCR4 and hence interrupts the hematopoietic stem cell–bone marrow stromal cell interaction. Like G-CSF, AMD 3100 is administered subcutaneously. In phase II trials in patients with NHL, multiple myeloma and HL the combination of AMD 3100 and G-CSF resulted in superior collections compared to G-CSF alone, with 84% of patients having a 50% increase in their daily $CD34^+$ cell collections; blocking CXCR4 does not appear to affect engraftment since delayed engraftment. AMD 3100 may also be useful in conjunction with chemotherapy to reduce bone marrow tumor load; the SDF-1–CXCR4 pathway plays a role in tumor cell homing to the bone marrow in diseases such as multiple myeloma.

2.2.4.2 Factors Affecting Hematopoietic Progenitor Cell Mobilization

Despite the overall success of chemotherapy and cytokines in mobilizing progenitor cells, in a small proportion of patients collecting adequate numbers of $CD34^+$ cells remains problematic. The most important factor determining a successful HPC mobilization is the amount of myelosuppressive chemotherapy a patient has received prior to collection [71]. In addition, prior exposure to certain agents such as melphalan, busulphan, procarbazine, platinum compounds and fludarabine are associated with impaired progenitor cell mobilization. Univariate analysis has also identified prior pelvic radiotherapy, age greater than 60 years, bone marrow involvement with disease, and underlying disease histology to be associated with inadequate $CD34^+$ cell collections.

Methods to improve poor mobilization of HPC are lacking. Re-mobilizing patients using a different strategy such as chemotherapy combined with G-CSF instead of G-CSF alone are effective in some [69]. Stem cell factor has synergistic effects on mobilization when combined with G-CSF, resulting in higher $CD34^{+}$ cell yields [72, 73]. However, in a non-randomized study of patients who previously failed progenitor cell collection with traditional methods, the addition of stem cell factor did not result in a successful collection [74]. The utility of AMD 3100, either as a single agent or in combination with G-CSF, in this patient population remains to be established.

Collection of HPC from bone marrow to supplement an inadequate HPC collection from the peripheral blood has been investigated. Collection of HPC from bone marrow is performed under a general anesthetic and, overall, is a safe procedure with an incidence of life threatening complications of 0.5%. Pain at the collection site is frequent and affects up to 80% of patients [75]. Several studies demonstrate the feasibility of this approach resulting in sustainable engraftment [76, 77].

2.2.4.3 Hematopoietic Progenitor Cell Collection from Peripheral Blood

Collection of HPC from the peripheral blood is performed using apheresis machines, which work on the principle of centrifugation which separates anticoagulated blood into various component layers based on specific gravity and the stem/progenitors are located between the platelets and granulocytes [78]. A continuous blood flow of 60–100 ml/min is required and can be achieved with the use of 16–18 gauge needles for the draw and return of blood. Alternatively, placement of a double lumen large bore catheter into the femoral, subclavian or jugular vein can be performed if peripheral vascular access is poor.

In some centers, HPC collection following mobilization is initiated when the white blood cell (WBC) count is greater than $1 \times 10^{9}/l$, although the WBC does not correlate well with the $CD34^{+}$ cell yield. Direct quantification of $CD34^{+}$ cell levels in the peripheral blood is preferable and correlates well with the number of progenitors actually collected [79]. When the peripheral blood $CD34^{+}$ cell count is more than $20 \times 10^{3}/ml$ there is a 94% chance of obtaining an adequate HPC from a single apheresis [80, 81]. $CD34^{+}$ cell enumeration is generally performed by flow cytometry, and there can be considerable variation in $CD34^{+}$ cell enumeration when different protocols and analyzers are used [82]. Generally, a $CD34^{+}$ cell dose of greater than $2 \times 10^{6}/kg$ will provide with adequate hematopoietic recovery following high-dose therapy [83]; $CD34^{+}$ cell doses of $1–2 \times 10^{6}/kg$ results in significantly delayed platelet engraftment while generally preserving neutrophil recovery. More rapid hematopoietic recovery is associated with the total number of $CD34^{+}$ cells infused [62], while long term platelet engraftment is more dependent on the immature CD34 ($CD90^{+}$, $CD33^{-}$, $CD38^{-}$, HLA-DR^{-}) infused [84, 85].

2.2.4.4 Hematopoietic Progenitor Cell Storage

The vast majority of hematopoietic progenitor cell collections are cryopreserved after collection. Following collection, a cryoprotectant, usually dimethylsulfoxide (DMSO) at 10% concentration, is added. A 5% concentration of DMSO may be used when combined with hydroxyethylstarch [86]. These agents protect against the freezing damage to living cells and has been proven to be non-toxic to stem cells. After the addition of the cryoprotectant, the cells are frozen in a controlled manner to −156°C. Subsequent thawing is usually carried out at the bedside using a 37°C water bath [81]. The infusion of DMSO is frequently associated with nausea and vomiting, however other cardiovascular and respiratory toxicities have also been reported. Microbial contamination of autografts is rare (1–4.5%) and is more likely with a bone marrow harvest compared with an apheresis product [87–89]. After infusion of a contaminated graft the risk of serious sequelae is extremely low; there has been one death reported following infusion of an autograft contaminated with Pseudomonas cepacia [87]. Standard operating procedures need to be in place to ensure microbial contamination remains low, and recommended guidelines have been published [90]. If the opportunity to re-collect the graft is not available (i.e., the intensive therapy regimen has been administered) re-infusing a graft contaminated with skin organisms would appear to be safer than subjecting the patient to a prolonged period of pancytopenia. The role of prophylactic antibiotics in this circumstance is unclear.

Non-cryopreserved autografts have been used successfully [91]. An advantage is that toxicity from DMSO is avoided and infrastructure and resource issues relating to cryopreservation are unnecessary, allowing more institutions to perform autologous HSCT. Studies with non-cryopreserved autografts demonstrate a near 100% hematopoietic recovery rate. Non-cryopreserved stem/progenitor cells remain viable for only 3–5 days, which limits the intensive therapy regimen that can be employed.

2.2.4.5 Purging of Hematopoietic Progenitor Cell Grafts

With autologous HSCT there is always a concern that the re-infused hematopoietic progenitor cells will be contaminated with tumor cells and thus contribute to relapse of disease. In a gene marking study on 20 patients with AML or neuroblastoma, harvested progenitor cells were marked with neomycin resistant gene. This gene was detected by polymerase chain reaction (PCR) assay in the recurrent malignant cells of all five patients who relapsed after transplant [92]. Hence, various methods to remove or “purge” residual tumor cells from the hematopoietic progenitor cell grafts have been tried. In NHL, B-cell specific antibodies with subsequent complement-mediated lysis or immunomagnetic beads to negatively or positively select for tumor cells or stem cells respectively have been employed in vitro [93]. In vivo purging can result in grafts, which are negative for tumor contamination by polymerase chain reaction (PCR) testing, and impressive EFS and OS rates have been seen in both MCL and follicular lymphoma when PCR-negative grafts are used. Alternatively, in vivo purging strategies using rituximab combined with chemotherapy have been developed for NHL [94, 95]. Despite the theoretical risk of contaminated grafts, the main factor contributing to relapse following autologous HSCT is incomplete tumor eradication following intensive therapy. Thus purging will not significantly alter outcome until intensive therapies are improved to the point where all minimal residual disease is eliminated.

2.2.5 *Intensive Therapy Regimens*

The most important aspect of autologous HSCT is that it allows for dose-escalation of chemotherapeutics beyond usual the maximal tolerated dose (MTD) by mitigating an important dose-limiting toxicity (delayed or even absent recovery of hematopoiesis). This dose intensification, particularly involving agents with steep-dose response curves, enables a greater killing of malignant cells than can be achieved with lower doses of the same agent [96]. Conventional chemotherapy regimens have been designed in accordance with the Norton–Simon model; that is, multiple cycles of chemotherapy are more likely to eradicate residual cancer cells than a single treatment [97]. There are a variety of intensive or "high-dose" therapy regimens that are used for autologous HSCT, and these are outlined in Table 2.2. Randomized controlled trials on the efficacy of varying intensive therapy regimens are lacking. From the available literature it appears that they do not appear to lead to differences in PFS and OS, but have widely divergent toxicity profiles.

For autologous HSCT in HL and NHL, regimens generally include agents such as BCNU, cyclophosphamide, etoposide, and melphalan [107]. In MCL, TBI has often been used as part of the intensive therapy regimen [108]; however, an analysis of autologous HSCT for MCL from the European Blood and Bone Marrow Transplant Registry showed that TBI was not associated with improved outcome [51]. High-dose, single-agent melphalan is the most common intensive therapy regimen used in autologous HSCT for multiple myeloma, and the addition of TBI has not shown to result in superior efficacy and thus is not used on a routine basis [100].

Intensive therapy regimens for AML are generally based on data from myeloablative allogeneic transplants. The two traditional regimens are TBI or busulfan, both combined with cyclophosphamide. TBI has the advantage of being non-cross resistant with chemotherapy; however, issues relating to patient scheduling and equipment availability make the widespread use of TBI difficult. The combination of busulfan and cyclophosphamide is also effective in AML [109].

Monoclonal antibodies have been investigated as part of intensive therapy regimens. The humanized anti-CD52 monoclonal antibody alemtuzumab has been utilized in high-dose regimens for chronic lymphocytic leukemia. However, the use of alemtuzumab in this setting can result in a syndrome of severe

Table 2.2 Intensive therapy regimens used in autologous HSCT

Regimen	Dose	Disease	Reference
Carmustine	300 mg/m^2 D1	NHL	[98]
Etoposide	200 mg/m^2 BD D2-5	HL	[99]
Cytarabine	200 mg/m^2 BD D2-5		
Melphalan	140 mg/m^2 D5		
Carmustine	300 mg/m^2 D1	NHL	[29]
Etoposide	100 mg/m^2 BD D2-5		
Cytarabine	100 mg/m^2 BDD2-5		
Cyclophosphamide	35 mg/kg D2-5		
Melphalan	200 mg/m^2	MM	[100]
Etoposide	60 mg/kg D-4	NHL	
Melphalan	140 mg/m^2 D-3	HL	[101]
±TBI		MCL	
		AML	[102]
Busulfan		AML	[103]
Cyclophosphamide			
Cyclophosphamide		AML	[104, 105]
TBI			
Cyclophosphamide	100 mg/kg D-2	NHL	[106]
Etoposide	60 mg/kg D-4		
BCNU	15 mg/kg		

autologous GvHD, attributed to auto-effector T cells, which clinically presents similarly to allogeneic GvHD [110]. Rituximab has been used successfully as part of the intensive therapy regimens for patients with MCL and other NHL. Unlike with alemtuzumab, there was no increase in toxicity or engraftment, and an improved EFS was observed in MCL [112].

Radio-immunoconjugates such as yttrium-90 (^{90}Y) ibritumomab tiuxetan (Zevalin®) and iodine-131 (^{131}I) tositumomab (Bexxar®) are anti-CD20 monoclonal antibodies conjugated to radioisotpes to deliver cytotoxic radiation to tumor cells (reviewed in Chap. 13 by Gopal and Winter). ^{90}Y ibritumomab tiuxetan has been given in addition to high-dose chemotherapy in relapsed/refractory B-cell NHL. This approach did not result in increased toxicity, and 2-year relapse-free survival and OS for patients with aggressive B-cell NHL was 74% and 93%, respectively [113]. Similarly, ^{131}I tositumomab tiuxetan has been combined with high-dose chemotherapy in chemotherapy-resistant B-cell NHL patients; the resulting EFS and OS rates were 39% and 55%, respectively, at 3 years [114].

Within the past decade or so, advances in the collection of hematopoietic progenitor have made it possible to administer high-dose therapy in sequential cycles each supported by hematopoietic progenitor cell infusion. This approach has most notably been applied in the pediatric tumors (e.g., medulloblastoma and neuroblastoma [115, 116]), but it also has been utilized in adult patients with germ cell tumors [117] and hematological malignancies [118, 119], particularly multiple myeloma [57]. A randomized trial performed by the Intergroupe Francophone du Myelome (IFM) demonstrated an overall survival advantage for the group treated with tandem transplants [24]. Another approach in multiple myeloma has been the use of high-dose therapy and autologous HSCT as a method of cytoreduction, followed by a nonmyeloablative allogeneic hematopoietic stem cell transplant [127, 128].

The intensive therapy regimen is designed to eradicate tumors, but in reality it generally just induces a state of minimal residual disease. Even when molecular negativity has been established, relapse after autologous HSCT continues to occur, implying that our methods for minimal residual disease detection need to be further refined. Furthermore, targeting patients at most risk of relapse after autologous HSCT, using, for example, post-transplant therapy, is required.

2.2.6 Complications Following Autologous HSCT

2.2.6.1 Early Complications

Complications associated with autologous HSCT can be subdivided into early and late. High-dose chemotherapy or TBI results in mucositis and pancytopenia. The incidence of mucositis after autologous HSCT ranges from 75% to 100%, and the severity can range from slight erythema to rarely, severe ulcerations involving the entire gastrointestinal tract requiring the need for total parenteral nutrition. The pathogenesis of mucositis involves direct epithelial damage and may also include more complex mechanisms such as induction of oxygen free radicals, up-regulation of pro-inflammatory cytokines and micro-vascular damage [111]. Generally, mucositis is managed with supportive measures such as analgesia, mouthwashes and fluid replacement. Palifermin, a recombinant human keratinocyte growth factor has been shown in a randomized controlled trial to decrease the duration and severity of mucositis in patients receiving TBI-based intensive therapy [129].

Infections in the peri-transplant period are due to the immunosuppression induced by the high-dose chemotherapy, as well as other risk factors such as the presence of central lines, catheters and the breakdown of mucosal integrity. Fungal infections can occur after autologous HSCT but the incidence is low. In an analysis of almost 1200 patients in Finland receiving autologous HSCT, the incidence of an invasive fungal infection was 1.5%, with the majority comprising invasive aspergillosis infections [130].

Engraftment syndrome is characterized by fever, rash, fluid retention, and pulmonary infiltrates and is seen shortly after engraftment occurs [131]. Pathogenesis is multi-factorial with interactions among T cells, monocytes, cytokines, and complement activation combined with epithelial injury from the high-dose regimen playing contributing roles. On neutrophil recovery, the release of cytokines and other mediators of oxidative damage triggers the clinical manifestations. While management is largely supportive, corticosteroids are particularly helpful in patients with pulmonary symptoms [131].

Organ toxicity is another cause of early treatment related mortality, responsible for up to 2% of all early deaths. Cardiac (from failure, arrhythmias, or infarction) and pulmonary complications (secondary to adult respiratory distress syndrome or pneumonia) predominate; however, liver failure from veno-occlusive disease still occurs occasionally. Patients undergoing autologous HSCT for amyloid, particularly patients with cardiac involvement, are particularly prone to early treatment-related mortality with an incidence of death approaching 25% [132].

2.2.6.2 Late Complications

The immune system after autologous HSCT is severely depressed with reduced numbers of T cells, particularly CD4$^+$ cells, reduced B cell production, and disordered immunoglobulin production. These factors predispose transplanted patients to develop infections, particularly with encapsulated organisms. Current recommendations are that all autologous HSCT should have repeat vaccinations against pneumococcus, diphtheria, tetanus, pertussis, and polio (inactivated vaccine) 12 months after autologous HSCT. Vaccinations against hepatitis A, B and H and Influenzae B can occur at 6 months while the combined measles, mumps and rubella vaccines should be administered 24 months post-autologous HSCT [133].

The rate of hypogonadism after autologous HSCT is high with one study reporting that 97% of females and 19% of males showing hypogonadism [134]. Infertility in women after autologous HSCT is very common; return of ovarian function does occur in approximately 30% of females undergoing autologous HSCT, with younger women (age $<$ 25 years) and those not receiving TBI more likely to have menses return [135]. In addition, normal healthy pregnancies have been reported after autologous HSCT [136]. After autologous HSCT, reduced libido is present in up to 25% of men and appears to correlate with reduced testosterone levels [137]. Long-term spermatozoa damage is common in men after high dose therapy regimens, especially those that include TBI, consequently pretreatment sperm banking is recommended for those with viable sperm.

Pulmonary complications relating to TBI; chemotherapy agents such as busulfan, etoposide or melphalan; and infections can occur after autologous HSCT and present as interstitial pneumonitis. After autologous HSCT, regular clinical reviews and emphasis on cessation of smoking are suggested [120]. Other late complications after autologous HSCT include hypothyroidism, often related to TBI, renal and bladder dysfunction due to TBI and/or cyclophosphamide, osteopenia and osteoporosis [121], and psychosocial complaints [122]. Quality of life in the first few months after autologous HSCT is impaired and may be due to ongoing fatigue, nausea, and anorexia; however, with time QOL usually improves.

An increased incidence of acute myeloid leukemia or myelodysplastic syndrome (MDS) is associated in patients undergoing autologous HSCT for lymphoma.

A multicenter case controlled study examined over 2700 patients with NHL or HL undergoing autologous HSCT. The cumulative incidence of therapy-related MDS or AML of the entire cohort was 3.7% at 7 years after autologous HSCT [123]. Risk factors for the development of therapy-related MDS or AML include age greater than 35 years, TBI, and the amount of pretransplant chemotherapy, especially alkylating agents [124].

Nonrelapse mortality represents 10% of all deaths after 100 days from transplant and occurs in approximately 5% of all autologous HSCT recipients [125]. The most common causes of late non-relapse mortality are second cancers or, less commonly, late infections with an incidence that is similar regardless of whether TBI was used or not. Long-term follow up of patients undergoing autologous HSCT, therefore, is important.

2.2.7 Post-Autologous HSCT Therapy

Relapse of disease after autologous HSCT is likely due to the resurgence of incompletely eradicated tumor cells. Thus, therapy after autologous HSCT to eradicate minimal residual disease has been proposed to improve overall survival. Rituximab administered in the post-transplant period for follicular NHL and MCL is associated with conversion to a molecular remission [126] and may result in improved EFS. The role of post transplant rituximab in aggressive NHL is currently being investigated in two international multicenter trials.

Several types of maintenance therapy have been studied in multiple myeloma [138]. In a randomized three-arm trial (arm A was observation, arm B was pamidronate, and arm C was thalidomide and pamidronate) of maintenance therapy in multiple myeloma, thalidomide administration resulted in an improved event-free survival at 3 years post transplant (52% vs. 36%) but given its toxicities, its routine use cannot be justified and may be more appropriate in patients who have a suboptimal response to transplant. [139] Bortezomib and lenalidomide are currently under investigation as maintenance therapy after autologous HSCT [138]. The notion that therapy should cease following autologous HSCT is simplistic. Autologous HSCT is but one method of achieving minimal residual disease. Innovative post-autologous HSCT therapies are needed to eradicate minimal residual disease and hence, ultimately, achieve cure.

2.3 Conclusion

Autologous HSCT is a safe, frequently used treatment modality that has made significant improvements in both OS and PFS for many conditions. Provided autologous HSCT is undertaken in institutions with sound policies and protocols, the mortality and morbidity of autologous HSCT should be low. The advent of new therapies targeting components of tumor proliferation, differentiation, and survival is exciting and is waiting to be explored in conjunction with autologous HSCT.

References

1. Kurnick NB, Montano A, Gerdes JC, et al. Preliminary observations on the treatment of postirradiation hematopoietic depression in man by the infusion of autogenous bone marrow. Ann Intern Med. 1958;49:973–8.
2. Quine WE. The remedial application of bone marrow. JAMA 1896;26:1012–3.
3. Schretzenmayr A. Anamiebehandlung mit knochemarksinjektionen. Klin Wochenschr. 1937;16:1010–2.
4. Migdalska KZ. Special section—transplantation of bone marrow. Blood 1958;13:300–1.
5. Osgood EE, Riddle MC, Mathews TJ. Aplastic anemia treated with daily transfusions and intravenous marrow. Ann Intern Med. 1939;13:357–67.
6. Jacobson LO, Marks EK, Gaston EO, et al. Effect of spleen protection on mortality following x-irradiation. J Lab Clin Med. 1949;34:1538–43.
7. Jacobson LO, Simmons EL, Marks EK, et al. Recovery from radiation injury. Science 1951;113:510–1.
8. Thomas ED, Lochte HL, Lu WC, et al. Intravenous infusion of bone marrow in patients receiving radiation and chemotherapy. N Engl J Med. 1957;257:491–6.
9. Thomas ED, Lochte HL, Cannon JH, et al. Supralethal whole body irradiation and isologous marrow transplantation in man. J Clin Invest. 1959;38:1709–16.
10. McFarland W, Granville NB, Dameshek W. Autologous bone marrow infusion as an adjunct in therapy of malignant disease. Blood 1959;14:503–21.
11. McGovern JJ, Russell PS, Atkins L, et al. Treatment of terminal leukemic relapse by total-body irradiation and intravenous infusion of stored autologous bone marrow obtained during remission. N Engl J Med. 1959;260:675–83.
12. Newton KA, Humble JG, Wilson CW, et al. Total thoracic supervoltage irradiation followed by the intravenous infusion of stored autogenous marrow. Br Med J. 1959;1: 531–5.
13. Appelbaum FR, Herzig GP, Ziegler JL. Successful engraftment of cryopreserved autologous bone marrow in patients with malignant lymphoma. Blood 1978;52:85–95.
14. Kurnick NB. Autologous and isologous bone marrow storage and infusion in the treatment of myelo-suppresson. Transfusion 1962;2:178–87.
15. Buckner CD, Rudolph RH, Fefer A. High dose cyclophosphamide therapy for malignant disease—Toxicity, tumor response, and effects of stored autologous marrow. Cancer 1972;29:357–65.
16. McElwain TJ, Hedley DW, Burton G, et al. Marrow autotransplantation accelerates haematological recovery in patients with malignant melanoma treated with high-dose melphalan. Br J Cancer. 1979;40:72–80.
17. Aronin PA, Mahaley MS Jr, Rudnick SA, et al. Prediction of BCNU pulmonary toxicity in patients with malignant gliomas: an assessment of risk factors. N Engl J Med. 1980;303:183–8.
18. Herzig GP. Autologous marrow transplantation in cancer therapy. In: Brown EB, editor. Progress in hematology. New York: Grune and Stratton; 1981. p. 1–23.
19. Dicke KA, Zander A, Spitzer G, et al. Autologous bone-marrow transplantation in relapsed adult acute leukaemia. Lancet 1979;1:514–7.
20. McCredie KB, Hersh EM, Freireich EJ. Cells capable of colony formation in the peripheral blood of man. Science 1971;171:293–4.
21. Goldman JM, Catovsky D, Hows J, et al. Cryopreserved peripheral blood cells functioning as autografts in patients with chronic granulocytic leukaemia in transformation. Br Med J. 1979;1:1310–3.

22. Juttner CA, To LB, Haylock DN, et al. Circulating autologous stem cells collected in very early remission from acute non-lymphoblastic leukaemia produce prompt but incomplete haemopoietic reconstitution after high dose melphalan or supralethal chemoradiotherapy. Br J Haematol. 1985;61:739–45.
23. Kessinger A, Armitage JO, Landmark JD, et al. Reconstitution of human hematopoietic function with autologous cryopreserved circulating stem cells. Exp Hematol. 1986; 14:192–6.
24. Korbling M, Dorken B, Ho AD, et al. Autologous transplantation of blood-derived hemopoietic stem cells after myeloablative therapy in a patient with Burkitt's lymphoma. Blood 1986;67:529–32.
25. Kessinger A, Armitage JO, Landmark JD, et al. Autologous peripheral hematopoietic stem cell transplantation restores hematopoietic function following marrow ablative therapy. Blood 1988;71:723–7.
26. Gianni AM, Siena S, Bregni M, et al. Granulocyte-macrophage colony-stimulating factor to harvest circulating haemopoietic stem cells for autotransplantation. Lancet 1989; 2:580–5.
27. Civin CI, Strauss LC, Brovall C, et al. Antigenic analysis of hematopoiesis. III. A hematopoietic progenitor cell surface antigen defined by a monoclonal antibody raised against KG-1a cells. J Immunol. 1984;133:157–65.
28. Vogl DT, Stadtmauer EA. High-dose chemotherapy and autologous hematopoietic stem cell transplantation for metastatic breast cancer: a therapy whose time has passed. Bone Marrow Transplant. 2006;37:985–7.
29. Philip T, Guglielmi C, Hagenbeek A, et al. Autologous bone marrow transplantation as compared with salvage chemotherapy in relapses of chemotherapy-sensitive non-Hodgkin's lymphoma. N Engl J Med. 1995;333:1540–5.
30. Yuen AR, Rosenberg SA, Hoppe RT, et al. Comparison between conventional salvage therapy and high-dose therapy with autografting for recurrent or refractory Hodgkin's disease. Blood 1997;89:814–22.
31. Schmitz N, Pfistner B, Sextro M, et al. Aggressive conventional chemotherapy compared with high-dose chemotherapy with autologous haemopoietic stem-cell transplantation for relapsed chemosensitive Hodgkin's disease: a randomised trial. Lancet 2002;359: 2065–71.
32. Attal M, Harousseau JL, Stoppa AM, et al. A prospective, randomized trial of autologous bone marrow transplantation and chemotherapy in multiple myeloma. Intergroupe Français du Myélome. N Engl J Med. 1996;335:91–7.
33. Child JA, Morgan GJ, Davies FE, et al. High-dose chemotherapy with hematopoietic stem-cell rescue for multiple myeloma. N Engl J Med. 2003;348:1875–83.
34. Palumbo A, Bringhen S, Petrucci MT, et al. Intermediate-dose melphalan improves survival of myeloma patients aged 50 to 70: results of a randomized controlled trial. Blood 2004;104:3052–7.
35. Dreyling M, Lenz G, Hoster E, et al. Early consolidation by myeloablative radiochemotherapy followed by autologous stem cell transplantation in first remission significantly prolongs progression-free survival in mantle-cell lymphoma: results of a prospective randomized trial of the European MCL Network. Blood 2005;105:2677–84.
36. Schouten HC, Qian W, Kvaloy S, et al. High-dose therapy improves progression-free survival and survival in relapsed follicular non-Hodgkin's lymphoma: results from the randomized European CUP trial. J Clin Oncol. 2003;21:3918–27.
37. Gribben JG, Zahrieh D, Stephans K, et al. Autologous and allogeneic stem cell transplantations for poor-risk chronic lymphocytic leukemia. Blood 2005;106: 4389–96.
38. Breems DA, Löwenberg B. Autologous stem cell transplatation in the treatment of adults with acute myeloid leukaemia. Br J Haematol 2005;130:825–33.
39. Nathan PC, Sung L, Crump M, et al. Consolidation therapy with autologous bone marrow transplantation in adults with acute myeloid leukemia: a meta-analysis. J Natl Cancer Inst. 2004;96:38–45.

40. Gratwohl A, Passweg J, Bocelli-Tyndall C, et al. Autologous hematopoietic stem cell transplantation for autoimmune diseases. Bone Marrow Transplant. 2005;35:869–79.
41. Chute JP. Stem cell homing. Curr Opin Hematol. 2006;13:399–406.
42. Majolino I, Pearce R, Taghipour G, et al. Peripheral-blood stem-cell transplantation versus autologous bone marrow transplantation in Hodgkin's and non-Hodgkin's lymphomas: A new matched-pair analysis of the European Group for Blood and Marrow Transplantation Registry Data—Lymphoma Working Party of the European Group for Blood and Marrow Transplantation. J Clin Oncol. 1997;15:509–17.
43. Mills W, Chopra R, McMillan A, et al. BEAM chemotherapy and autologous bone marrow transplantation for patients with relapsed or refractory non-Hodgkin's lymphoma. J Clin Oncol. 1995;13:588–95.
44. Wheeler C, Strawderman M, Ayash L, et al. Prognostic factors for treatment outcome in autotransplantation of intermediate-grade and high-grade non-Hodgkin's lymphoma with cyclophosphamide, carmustine, and etoposide. J Clin Oncol. 1993;11: 1085–91.
45. Philip T, Armitage JO, Spitzer G, et al. High-dose therapy and autologous bone marrow transplantation after failure of conventional chemotherapy in adults with intermediate-grade or high-grade non-Hodgkin's lymphoma. N Engl J Med. 1987;316:1493–8.
46. Horning SJ, Chao NJ, Negrin RS, et al. High-dose therapy and autologous hematopoietic progenitor cell transplantation for recurrent or refractory Hodgkin's disease: analysis of the Stanford University results and prognostic indices. Blood 1997;89:801–13.
47. Schot BW, Zijlstra JM, Sluiter WJ, et al. Early FDG-PET assessment in combination with clinical risk scores determines prognosis in recurring lymphoma. Blood 2007; 109:486–91.
48. Olivieri AA, Santini GG, Patti CC, et al. Upfront high-dose sequential therapy (HDS) versus VACOP-B with or without HDS in aggressive non-Hodgkin's lymphoma: long-term results by the NHLCSG. Ann Oncol. 2005;16:1941–8.
49. Vellenga E, van Putten WL, van 't Veer MB, et al. Rituximab improves the treatment results of DHAP-VIM-DHAP and ASCT in relapsed/progressive aggressive CD20+ NHL: a prospective randomized HOVON trial. Blood 2008;111:537–43.
50. Andersen NS, Pedersen L, Elonen E, et al. Primary treatment with autologous stem cell transplantation in mantle cell lymphoma: outcome related to remission pretransplant. Eur J Haematol. 2003;71:73–80.
51. Vandenberghe E, Ruiz de Elvira C, Loberiza FR, et al. Outcome of autologous transplantation for mantle cell lymphoma: a study by the European Blood and Bone Marrow Transplant and Autologous Blood and Marrow Transplant Registries. Br J Haematol. 2003;120:793–800.
52. Lenz G, Dreyling M, Schiegnitz E, et al. Myeloablative radiochemotherapy followed by autologous stem cell transplantation in first remission prolongs progression-free survival in follicular lymphoma: results of a prospective, randomized trial of the German Low-Grade Lymphoma Study Group. Blood 2004;104:2667–74.
53. Rohatiner AZ, Nadler L, Davies AJ, et al. Myeloablative therapy with autologous bone marrow transplantation for follicular lymphoma at the time of second or subsequent remission: long-term follow-up. J Clin Oncol. 2007;25:2554–9.
54. Forstpointner R, Unterhalt M, Dreyling M, et al. Maintenance therapy with rituximab leads to a significant prolongation of response duration after salvage therapy with a combination of rituximab, fludarabine, cyclophosphamide, and mitoxantrone (R-FCM) in patients with recurring and refractory follicular and mantle cell lymphomas: results of a prospective randomized study of the German Low Grade Lymphoma Study Group (GLSG). Blood 2006;108:4003–8.
55. Desikan R, Barlogie B, Sawyer J, et al. Results of high-dose therapy for 1000 patients with multiple myeloma: durable complete remissions and superior survival in the absence of chromosome 13 abnormalities. Blood 2000;95:4008–10.

56. Gertz MA, Lacy MQ, Dispenzieri A, et al. Clinical implications of t(11;14)(q13;q32), t(4;14)(p16.3;q32), and -17p13 in myeloma patients treated with high-dose therapy. Blood 2005;106:2837–40.
57. Attal M, Harousseau JL, Facon T, et al. Single versus double autologous stem-cell transplantation for multiple myeloma. N Engl J Med. 2003;349:2495–502.
58. Yanada M, Matsuo K, Emi N, et al. Efficacy of allogeneic hematopoietic stem cell transplantation depends on cytogenetic risk for acute myeloid leukemia in first disease remission: a metaanalysis. Cancer 2005;103:1652–8.
59. Suciu S, Mandelli F, de Witte T, et al. Allogeneic compared with autologous stem cell transplantation in the treatment of patients younger than 46 years with acute myeloid leukemia (AML) in first complete remission (CR1): an intention-to-treat analysis of the EORTC/GIMEMAAML-10 trial. Blood 2003;102:1232–40.
60. Slovak ML, Kopecky KJ, Cassileth PA, et al. Karyotypic analysis predicts outcome of preremission and postremission therapy in adult acute myeloid leukemia: a Southwest Oncology Group/Eastern Cooperative Oncology Group study. Blood 2000;96:4075–83.
61. Burnett AK, Goldstone AH, Stevens RM, et al. Randomised comparison of addition of autologous bone-marrow transplantation to intensive chemotherapy for acute myeloid leukaemia in first remission: results of MRC AML 10 trial. UK Medical Research Council Adult and Children's Leukaemia Working Parties. Lancet 1998;351:700–8.
62. Specchia G, Pastore D, Mestice A, et al. Early and long-term engraftment after autologous peripheral stem cell transplantation in acute myeloid leukemia patients. Acta Haematol. 2006;116:229–37.
63. Bensinger WI, Longin K, Appelbaum F, et al. Peripheral blood stem cells (PBSCs) collected after recombinant granulocyte colony stimulating factor (rhG-CSF): an analysis of factors correlating with the tempo of engraftment after transplantation. Br J Haematol. 1994;87:825–31.
64. Perry AR, Peniket AJ, Watts MJ, et al. Peripheral blood stem cell versus autologous bone marrow transplantation for Hodgkin's disease: equivalent survival outcome in a single-centre matched-pair analysis. Br J Haematol. 1999;105:280–7.
65. Kottaridis PD, Peggs K, Schmitz N, et al. Survival and freedom from progression in autotransplant lymphoma patients is independent of stem cell source: further follow-up from the original randomised study to assess engraftment. Leuk Lymphoma. 2002; 43:531–6.
66. Vose JM, Sharp G, Chan WC, et al. Autologous transplantation for aggressive non-Hodgkin's lymphoma: results of a randomized trial evaluating graft source and minimal residual disease. J Clin Oncol. 2002;20:2344–52.
67. Richman CM, Weiner RS, Yankee RA. Increase in circulating stem cells following chemotherapy in man. Blood 1976;47:1031–9.
68. Nowrousian MR, Waschke S, Bojko P, et al. Impact of chemotherapy regimen and hematopoietic growth factor on mobilization and collection of peripheral blood stem cells in cancer patients. Ann Oncol. 2003;14:i29–36.
69. Koç ON, Gerson SL, Cooper BW, et al. Randomized cross-over trial of progenitor-cell mobilization: high-dose cyclophosphamide plus granulocyte colony-stimulating factor (G-CSF) versus granulocyte-macrophage colony-stimulating factor plus G-CSF. J Clin Oncol. 2000;18:1824–30.
70. Cashen AF, Nervi B, DiPersio J. AMD3100: CXCR4 antagonist and rapid stem cell-mobilizing agent. Future Oncol. 2007;3:19–27.
71. Stiff PJ. Management strategies for the hard-to-mobilize patient. Bone Marrow Transplant. 1999;23 Suppl 2:S29–33.
72. Facon T, Harousseau J-L, Maloisel F, et al. Stem cell factor in combination with filgrastim after chemotherapy improves peripheral blood progenitor cell yield and reduces apheresis requirements in multiple myeloma patients: a randomized, controlled trial. Blood 1999;94:1218–25.

73. Shpall EJ, Wheeler CA, Turner SA, et al. A randomized phase 3 study of peripheral blood progenitor cell mobilization with stem cell factor and filgrastim in high-risk breast cancer patients. Blood 1999;93:2491–501.
74. da Silva MG, Pimentel P, Carvalhais A, et al. Ancestim (recombinant human stem cell factor, SCF) in association with filgrastim does not enhance chemotherapy and/or growth factor-induced peripheral blood progenitor cell (PBPC) mobilization in patients with a prior insufficient PBPC collection. Bone Marrow Transplant. 2004;34:683–91.
75. Kroschinsky F, Kittner T, Mauersberger S, et al. Pelvic magnetic resonance imaging after bone marrow harvest—a retrospective study in 50 unrelated marrow donors. Bone Marrow Transplant. 2005;35:667–73.
76. Lemoli RM, de Vivo A, Damiani D, et al. Autologous transplantation of granulocyte colony-stimulating factor-primed bone marrow is effective in supporting myeloablative chemotherapy in patients with hematologic malignancies and poor peripheral blood stem cell mobilization. Blood 2003;102:1595–600.
77. Seshadri T, Al-Farsi K, Stakiw J, et al. Short and long term efficacy of autologous bone marrow cells to support intensive chemotherapy in patients failing peripheral blood stem cell mobilization. Blood 2007;110:(abstract #2999).
78. Reddy RL. Mobilization and collection of peripheral blood progenitor cells for transplantation. Transfus Apher Sci. 2005;32:63–72.
79. Basquiera AL, Abichain P, Damonte JC, et al. The number of CD34(+) cells in peripheral blood as a predictor of the CD34(+) yield in patients going to autologous stem cell transplantation. J Clin Apheresis. 2006;21:92–5.
80. Armitage S, Hargreaves R, Samson D, et al. CD34 counts to predict the adequate collection of peripheral blood progenitor cells. Bone Marrow Transplant. 1997;20: 587–91.
81. Berz D, McCormack EM, Winer ES, et al. Cryopreservation of hematopoietic stem cells. Am J Hematol. 2007;82:463–72.
82. Rivadeneyra-Espínoza L, Pérez-Romano B, González-Flores A, et al. Instrument- and protocol-dependent variation in the enumeration of CD34+ cells by flow cytometry. Transfusion 2006;46:530–6.
83. Jansen J, Thompson JM, Dugan MJ, et al. Peripheral blood progenitor cell transplantation. Ther Apheresis. 2002;6:5–14.
84. Sumikuma T, Shimazaki C, Inaba T, et al. CD34+/CD90+ cells infused best predict late haematopoietic reconstitution following autologous peripheral blood stem cell transplantation. Br J Haematol. 2002;117:238–44.
85. Millar BC, Millar JL, Shepherd V, Blackwell P, Porter H, Cunningham D, Judson I, Treleaven J, Powles RL, Catovsky D. The importance of CD34+/CD33 cells in platelet engraftment after intensive therapy for cancer patients given peripheral blood stem cell rescue. Bone Marrow Transplant. 1998;22:469–75.
86. Rowley SD, Feng Z, Chen L, et al. A randomized phase III clinical trial of autologous blood stem cell transplantation comparing cryopreservation using dimethylsulfoxide vs dimethylsulfoxide with hydroxyethylstarch. Bone Marrow Transplant. 2003;31: 1043–51.
87. Klein MA, Kadidlo D, McCullough J, et al. Microbial contamination of hematopoietic stem cell products: incidence and clinical sequelae. Biol Blood Marrow Transplant. 2006;12:1142–9.
88. Kelly M, Roy DC, Labbe AC, et al. What is the clinical significance of infusing hematopoietic cell grafts contaminated with bacteria? Bone MarrowTransplant. 2006;38:183–8.
89. Kamble R, Pant S, Selby GB, et al. Microbial contamination of hematopoietic progenitor cell grafts-incidence, clinical outcome, and cost-effectiveness: an analysis of 735 grafts. Transfusion 2005;45:874–8.
90. FDA 21 CFR parts 16 a: Current good tissue practice for human cell, tissue and cellular and tissue-based products establishments; inspections and enforcement; final rule. Fed Regist. 2004;69:Docket No. 1997 N–484P.

91. Wannesson L, Panzarella T, Mikhael J, et al. Feasibility and safety of autotransplants with noncryopreserved marrow or peripheral blood stem cells: a systematic review. Ann Oncol. 2007;18:623–32.
92. Brenner MK RD, Moen RC, Krance RA, Heslop HE, Mirro J, Anderson WF, Ihle JN. Gene marking and autologous bone marrow transplantation. Ann NY Acad Sci. 1994;31:204–14.
93. Jacobsen E, Freedman A. B-cell purging in autologous stem-cell transplantation for non-Hodgkin lymphoma. Lancet Oncol. 2004;5:711–7.
94. Gianni AM, Magni M, Martelli M, et al. Long-term remission in mantle cell lymphoma following high-dose sequential chemotherapy and in vivo rituximab-purged stem cell autografting (R-HDS regimen). Blood 2003;102:749–55.
95. Corradini P, Ladetto M, Zallio F, et al. Long-term follow-up of indolent lymphoma patients treated with high-dose sequential chemotherapy and autografting: evidence that durable molecular and clinical remission frequently can be attained only in follicular subtypes. J Clin Oncol. 2004;22:1460–8.
96. Schilder RJ, Johnson S, Gallo J, et al. Phase I trial of multiple cycles of high-dose chemotherapy supported by autologous peripheral-blood stem cells. J Clin Oncol. 1999; 17:2198–207.
97. Norton L, Day R. Potential innovations in scheduling of cancer chemotherapy. In: DeVita VT, Hellman S, Rosenberg SA, editors. Important advances in oncology. Philadelphia: Lippincott; 1991. p. 57–72.
98. Josting A, Sieniawski M, Glossmann JP, et al. High-dose sequential chemotherapy followed by autologous stem cell transplantation in relapsed and refractory aggressive non-Hodgkin's lymphoma: results of a multicenter phase II study. Ann Oncol. 2005; 16:1359–65.
99. Caballero MD, Rubio V, Rifon J, et al. BEAM chemotherapy followed by autologous stem cell support in lymphoma patients: analysis of efficacy, toxicity and prognostic factors. Bone Marrow Transplant. 1997;20:451–8.
100. Moreau P, Facon T, Attal M, et al. Comparison of 200 mg/m^2 melphalan and 8 Gy total body irradiation plus 140 mg/m^2 melphalan as conditioning regimens for peripheral blood stem cell transplantation in patients with newly diagnosed multiple myeloma: final analysis of the Intergroupe Francophone du Myelome 9502 randomized trial. Blood 2002;99:731–5.
101. Kuruvilla J, Nagy T, Pintilie M, et al. Similar response rates and superior early progression-free survival with gemcitabine, dexamethasone, and cisplatin salvage therapy compared with carmustine, etoposide, cytarabine, and melphalan salvage therapy prior to autologous stem cell transplantation for recurrent or refractory Hodgkin lymphoma. Cancer 2006;106:353–60.
102. Mollee P, Gupta V, Song K, et al. Long-term outcome after intensive therapy with etoposide, melphalan, total body irradiation and autotransplant for acute myeloid leukemia. Bone Marrow Transplant. 2004;33:1201–8.
103. Santos GW, Tutschka PJ, Brookmeyer R, et al. Marrow transplantation for acute nonlymphocytic leukemia after treatment with busulfan and cyclophosphamide. N Engl J Med. 1983;309:1347–53.
104. Socie G, Clift RA, Blaise D, et al. Busulfan plus cyclophosphamide compared with total-body irradiation plus cyclophosphamide before marrow transplantation for myeloid leukemia: long-term follow-up of 4 randomized studies. Blood 2001;98:3569–74.
105. Clift RA, Buckner CD, Thomas ED, et al. Marrow transplantation for chronic myeloid leukemia: a randomized study comparing cyclophosphamide and total body irradiation with busulfan and cyclophosphamide. Blood 1994;84:2036–43.
106. Stockerl-Goldstein KE, Horning SJ, Negrin RS, et al. Influence of preparatory regimen and source of hematopoietic cells on outcome of autotransplantation for non-Hodgkin's lymphoma. Biol Blood Marrow Transplant. 1996;2:76–85.
107. Caballero MD, Pérez-Simón JA, Iriondo A, et al. High-dose therapy in diffuse large cell lymphoma: results and prognostic factors in 452 patients from the GEL-TAMO Spanish Cooperative Group. Ann Oncol. 2003;14:140–51.

108. Lefrère F, Delmer A, Suzan F, et al. Sequential chemotherapy by CHOP and DHAP regimens followed by high-dose therapy with stem cell transplantation induces a high rate of complete response and improves event-free survival in mantle cell lymphoma: a prospective study. Leukemia 2002;16:587–93.
109. Ferry C, Socié G. Busulfan-cyclophosphamide versus total body irradiation-cyclophosphamide as preparative regimen before allogeneic hematopoietic stem cell transplantation for acute myeloid leukemia: what have we learned? Exp Hematol. 2003;31:1182–6.
110. Zenz T, Ritgen M, Dreger P, et al. Autologous graft-versus-host disease-like syndrome after an alemtuzumab-containing conditioning regimen and autologous stem cell transplantation for chronic lymphocytic leukemia. Blood 2006;108:2127–30.
111. McDonnell AM, Lenz KL. Palifermin: role in the prevention of chemotherapy- and radiation-induced mucositis. Ann Pharmacother. 2007;41:86–94.
112. Dreger P, Rieger M, Seyfarth B, et al. Rituximab-augmented myeloablation for first-line autologous stem cell transplantation for mantle cell lymphoma: effects on molecular response and clinical outcome. Haematologica 2007;92:42–9.
113. Nademanee A, Forman S, Molina A, et al. A phase 1/2 trial of high-dose yttrium-90-ibritumomab tiuxetan in combination with high-dose etoposide and cyclophosphamide followed by autologous stem cell transplantation in patients with poor-risk or relapsed non-Hodgkin lymphoma. Blood 2005;106:2896–902.
114. Vose JM, Bierman PJ, Enke C, et al. Phase I trial of iodine-131 tositumomab with high-dose chemotherapy and autologous stem-cell transplantation for relapsed non-hodgkin's lymphoma. J Clin Oncol. 2005;23:461–7.
115. Strother D, Ashley D, Kellie SJ, et al. Feasibility of four consecutive high-dose chemotherapy cycles with stem-cell rescue for patients with newly diagnosed medulloblastoma or supratentorial primitive neuroectodermal tumor after craniospinal radiotherapy: results of a collaborative study. J Clin Oncol. 2001;19:2696–704.
116. George RE, Li S, Medeiros-Nancarrow C, et al. High-risk neuroblastoma treated with tandem autologous peripheral-blood stem cell-supported transplantation: long-term survival update. J Clin Oncol. 2006;24:2891–6.
117. Einhorn LH, Williams SD, Chamness A, et al. High-dose chemotherapy and stem-cell rescue for metastatic germ-cell tumors. N Engl J Med. 2007;357:340–8.
118. Haioun C, Mounier N, Quesnel B, et al. Tandem autotransplant as first-line consolidative treatment in poor-risk aggressive lymphoma: a pilot study of 36 patients. Ann Oncol. 2001;12:1749–55.
119. Ahmed T, Rashid K, Waheed F, et al. Long-term survival of patients with resistant lymphoma treated with tandem stem cell transplant. Leuk Lymphoma. 2005;46:405–14.
120. Rizzo JD, Wingard JR, Tichelli A, et al. Recommended screening and preventive practices for long-term survivors after hematopoietic cell transplantation: joint recommendations of the European Group for Blood and Marrow Transplantation, the Center for International Blood and Marrow Transplant Research, and the American Society of Blood and Marrow Transplantation. Biol Blood Marrow Transplant. 2006;12:138–51.
121. Schimmer AD, Mah K, Bordeleau L, et al. Decreased bone mineral density is common after autologous blood or marrow transplantation. Bone Marrow Transplant. 2001;28:387–91.
122. Díez-Campelo M, Pérez-Simón JA, González-Porras JR, et al. Quality of life assessment in patients undergoing reduced intensity conditioning allogeneic as compared to autologous transplantation: results of a prospective study. Bone Marrow Transplant. 2004;34:729–38.
123. Metayer C, Curtis RE, Vose J, et al. Myelodysplastic syndrome and acute myeloid leukemia after autotransplantation for lymphoma: a multicenter case-control study. Blood 2003;101:2015–23.
124. Hake CR, Graubert TA, Fenske TS. Does autologous transplantation directly increase the risk of secondary leukemia in lymphoma patients? Bone Marrow Transplant. 2007;39:59–70.

125. Jantunen E, Itälä M, Siitonen T, et al. Late non-relapse mortality among adult autologous stem cell transplant recipients: a nation-wide analysis of 1,482 patients transplanted in 1990-2003. Eur J Haematol. 2006;77:114–9.
126. Brugger W, Hirsch J, Grunebach F, et al. Rituximab consolidation after high-dose chemotherapy and autologous blood stem cell transplantation in follicular and mantle cell lymphoma: a prospective, multicenter phase II study. Ann Oncol. 2004;15:1691–8.
127. Maloney DG, Molina AJ, Sahebi F, et al. Allografting with nonmyeloablative conditioning following cytoreductive autografts for the treatment of patients with multiple myeloma. Blood 2003;102:3447–54.
128. Bruno B, Rotta M, Patriarca F, et al. A comparison of allografting with autografting for newly diagnosed myeloma. N Engl J Med. 2007;356:1110–20.
129. Spielberger R, Stiff P, Bensinger W, et al. Palifermin for oral mucositis after intensive therapy for hematologic cancers. N Engl J Med. 2004;351:2590–8.
130. Jantunen E, Salonen J, Juvonen E, et al. Invasive fungal infections in autologous stem cell transplant recipients: a nation-wide study of 1188 transplanted patients. Eur J Haematol. 2004;73:174–8.
131. Spitzer TR. Engraftment syndrome following hematopoietic stem cell transplantation. Bone Marrow Transplant. 2001;27:893–8.
132. Jantunen E, Itala M, Lehtinen T, et al. Early treatment-related mortality in adult autologous stem cell transplant recipients: a nation-wide survey of 1482 transplanted patients. Eur J Haematol. 2006;76:245–50.
133. Ljungman P, Engelhard D, de la Cámara R, et al. Vaccination of stem cell transplant recipients: recommendations of the Infectious Diseases Working Party of the EBMT. Bone Marrow Transplant. 2005;35:737–46.
134. Somali M, Mpatakoias V, Avramides A, et al. Function of the hypothalamic-pituitary-gonadal axis in long-term survivors of hematopoietic stem cell transplantation for hematological diseases. Gynecol Endocrinol. 2005;21:18–26.
135. Schimmer AD, Quatermain M, Imrie K, et al. Ovarian function after autologous bone marrow transplantation. J Clin Oncol. 1998;16:2359–63.
136. Brice P, Haioun C, André M, et al. Pregnancies after high-dose chemotherapy and autologous stem cell transplantation in aggressive lymphomas. Blood 2002;100:736.
137. Schimmer AD, Ali V, Stewart AK, et al. Male sexual function after autologous blood or marrow transplantation. Biol Blood Marrow Transplant. 2001;7:279–83.
138. Mihelic R, Kaufman JL, Lonial S. Maintenance therapy in multiple myeloma. Leukemia 2007.
139. Attal M, Harousseau J-L, Leyvraz S, et al. Maintenance therapy with thalidomide improves survival in patients with multiple myeloma. Blood 2006;108:3289–94.
140. Dhedin N, Dombret H, Thomas X, et al: Autologous stem cell transplantation in adults with acute lymphoblastic leukemia in first complete remission: analysis of the LALA-85, -87 and -94 trials. Leukemia 2005;20:336–44
141. Moore HCF, Green SJ, Gralow JR, et al. Intensive dose-dense compared with high-dose adjuvant chemotherapy for high-risk operable breast cancer: Southwest Oncology Group/Intergroup study 9623. J Clin Oncol. 2007;25:1677–82.
142. Peters WP, Rosner GL, Vredenburgh JJ, et al. Prospective, randomized comparison of high-dose chemotherapy with stem-cell support versus intermediate-dose chemotherapy after surgery and adjuvant chemotherapy in women with high-risk primary breast cancer: a report of CALGB 9082, SWOG 9114, and NCIC MA-13. J Clin Oncol. 2005;23: 2191–200
143. Schmid P, Schippinger W, Nitsch T, et al. Up-front tandem high-dose chemotherapy compared with standard chemotherapy with doxorubicin and paclitaxel in metastatic breast cancer: results of a randomized trial. J Clin Oncol. 2005;23:432–40.
144. Einhorn LH, Williams SD, Chamness A, et al. High-dose chemotherapy and stem-cell rescue for metastatic germ-cell tumors. N Engl J Med. 2007;357:340–8.

Chapter 3
Natural Killer Cell Activity and Killer Immunoglobulin-Like Receptors in Hematopoietic Stem Cell Transplantation

Loredana Ruggeri, Shuhong Zhang, and Sherif S. Farag

3.1 Introduction

Natural killer (NK) cells are important effector cells of the innate immune system and are known to have potent cytotoxic activity against a variety of cancer cells. Until recently, however, the potential beneficial role of NK cell activity in allogeneic hematopoietic stem cell transplantation (HSCT) has remained poorly defined and largely overshadowed by immune reactions mediated by other effector cells. In most allogeneic transplants, where close histocompatibility matching of donor and recipient has been the goal, T-lymphocyte mediated immune reactions have been the focus of most attention. For example, the graft-versus-leukemia (GvL) effect following allogeneic HSCT and donor lymphocyte infusion for relapsed leukemia has highlighted the significant curative potential of these immune effector cells, even in chemotherapy-resistant malignancies. The GvL effect, however, is mediated largely by alloreactive T lymphocytes recognizing minor or major histocompatibility (MHC) antigens shared by both neoplastic and normal cells, and in the majority of cases, therefore, lacks specificity with the potential for widespread host tissue damage and severe graft-versus-host disease (GvHD) in many patients [1, 2]. NK cell activity, at best, has been considered to have a secondary role in these reactions. Indeed, specific depletion of T lymphocytes from donor stem cells is known to completely abrogate GvHD, although at the expense of also eliminating the GvL effect with increased relapse [1]. Over the past decade, data from haplotype-mismatched allogeneic HSCT at the University of Perugia has confirmed an important role for NK cells in mediating potent GvL effects without GvHD under specific transplant conditions. At the same time, understanding of NK cell receptor biology and the means by which NK cells recognize and lyse leukemic cells has paved the way for investigating novel ways of better harnessing the therapeutic effect of these cells. This chapter will review the aspects of NK cell

L. Ruggeri (✉)
University of Perugia, Perugia, Italy
e-mail: loredana.ruggeri@unipg.it

M.R. Bishop (ed.), *Hematopoietic Stem Cell Transplantation*,
Cancer Treatment and Research 144, DOI 10.1007/978-0-387-78580-6_3,

receptor biology important to the transplant physician and the clinical role of NK cell activity in HSCT.

3.2 Human NK Cells: Biology and Recognition of Target Cells

Human NK cells are innate immune effector cells that comprise approximately 10–15% of all peripheral blood lymphocytes and are characterized phenotypically as $CD56^{+}CD3^{-}$ cells. Based on the surface expression of CD56, humans NK cells can be subdivided into two subsets with distinct and phenotypic and functional properties [3]. In peripheral blood, approximately 90% of NK cells are $CD56^{dim}$ and express high levels of the $Fc\gamma$ receptor III (CD16) that binds the Fc portion of IgG. The $CD56^{dim}$ NK cells are functionally cytotoxic and capable of antibody-dependent cellular cytotoxicity. The remaining subpopulation is $CD56^{bright}$ and $CD16^{dim}$, and has predominantly a regulatory role through the secretion of immunoregulatory cytokines following monokine stimulation [4]. In addition, $CD56^{bright}$ NK cells constitutively express the high affinity interleukin-2 (IL-2) receptor (IL-2R$\alpha\beta\gamma$) and expand in vitro and in vivo in response to low concentrations of IL-2 [5, 6], while resting $CD56^{dim}$ NK cells express only the intermediate affinity IL-2 receptor (IL-2R$\beta\gamma$), and proliferate weakly in response to IL-2 concentrations [6, 7]. While $CD56^{dim}$ NK cells are more naturally cytotoxic against NK-sensitive targets and respond to IL-2 with increased cytotoxicity compared to $CD56^{bright}$ NK cells [8], following treatment with IL-2 in vitro and in vivo, however, $CD56^{bright}$ and $CD56^{dim}$ NK cells show similar levels of cytotoxicity [5, 9]. Based on these early observations, a novel therapeutic dosing schedule of low-dose IL-2 with intermediate-dose bolus IL-2 has been developed with good patient tolerability [10]. Finally, as discussed below $CD56^{bright}$ and $CD56^{dim}$ NK cell subsets also differ in their pattern of expression of NK cell receptors important in mediating killing of target cells, which might also account for the observed differences in cytotoxic capacity.

The mechanism by which an NK cell recognizes a target cell with subsequent activation or inhibition of killing differs significantly from those used by T and B lymphocytes. Unlike the latter, NK cells do not rearrange genes encoding receptors for specific antigen recognition but express a unique class of receptors, NK cell receptors (NKR), which exist in both activating and inhibitory forms that recognize major histocompatibility complex (MHC) class I or class I-like molecules on target cells. Recognition of target cells is normally mediated predominantly by paired inhibitory and activating NKR, as well as various adhesion and costimulatory molecules [11, 12]. Table 3.1 lists the important inhibitory and activating NKR together with their known ligands. Ultimately, cytotoxicity is a function of a balance of inhibitory and triggering signals through these receptors.

Table 3.1 Human NK cell receptors and their ligands

	Inhibitory		Activating	
	Receptor	Ligand	Receptor	Ligand
Killer Ig-like receptors (KIR)	KIR2DL1	Group 2 HLA-C alleles	KIR2DS1	Group 2 HLA-C alleles
	KIR2DL2	Group 1 HLA-C alleles	KIR2DS2	Unknown
	KIR2DL3		KIR2DS4	Unknown
	KIR3DL1	HLA-Bw4	KIR2DS5	Unknown
	KIR3DL2	HLA-A3, -A11	KIR3DS1	Unknown
	KIR2DL5	unknown	KIR2DL4[a]	HLA-G
	KIR3DL7	unknown		
Heterodimeric C-type lectin receptors	CD94/ NKG2A (-B)	HLA-E	CD94/ NKG2C	HLA-E
			CD94/ NKG2E	Unknown
Natural cytotoxicity receptors (NCR)			NKp30	Unknown
			NKp46	Unknown
			NKp44	Unknown
C-type lectin			NKG2D	MICA, MICB ULBP-1, -2, -3
Other receptors and coreceptors			ILT-1 (LIR-1)	Unknown
			DNAM-1	nectin-2; nectin-5
			FcγRIII (CD16)	Fc of IgG
			CD2	CD58 (LFA-3)
			LFA-1	ICAM-1
			2B4	CD48
			NKp80	Unknown
			CD69	Unknown
			CD40 Ligand	CD40

[a] Although KIR2DL4 has a long cytoplasmic tail and ITIM motifs, it is functionally an activating KIR which mediates NK cell secretion of interferon-γ without inducing cytotoxicity

3.2.1 Killer Immunoglobulin-Like Receptors

The killer immunoglobulin (Ig)-like receptors (KIR) exist as paired activating and inhibitory receptors and are the best recognized superfamily of NKR in the context of allogeneic HSCT. Early studies noted an inverse correlation between surface HLA class I molecule expression on target cells and susceptibility to NK cell-mediated lysis, suggesting that HLA molecules protect self cells lysis by NK cells. Conversely, lack of expression of self HLA molecules on target cells resulted in the susceptibility to lysis ("missing self" recognition) [13–17]. It is now known that inhibitory KIR play an important role in recognition of self HLA molecules, protecting against NK cell autoreactivity.

Structurally, KIR are characterized by either two Ig-like (KIR2D) or three Ig-like (KIR3D) extracellular domains that specifically recognize groups of HLA class I molecules. Further, KIR are classified according to the length of their cytoplasmic tails; long (KIR2DL and KIR3DL) and short (KIR2DS and KIR3DS) cytoplasmic tails determine their functional properties. The long tail KIR mediate an inhibitory signal due to the presence of immunoreceptor tyrosine-based inhibition motifs (ITIM) in their cytoplasmic domains, while the short tail receptors are associated with activating signals due to their association with adaptor proteins bearing immunoreceptor tyrosine-based activating motifs (ITAM).

Human NK cells discriminate between allelic forms of HLA molecules predominantly via inhibitory KIR [18–22]. Importantly, there is not a KIR for each specific MHC class I molecule, but sets of KIR recognize epitopes shared by a group of MHC class I molecules. In addition, many HLA-A and HLA-B alleles have no cognate KIR, indicating that the KIR repertoire is not all inclusive for human classical class I allotypes [23]. Whereas KIR exist that are specific for a number of MHC class I molecules, HLA-C is the predominant class I isotype involved in the inhibitory regulation of human NK cells. A single inhibitory KIR, KIR2DL1, recognizes an epitope shared by alleles of the group 1 HLA-C allotypes characterized by Asn at position 77 and Lys at position 80 in the $\alpha1$ helix of the MHC molecule [24, 25]. On the other hand, KIR2DL2 and KIR2DL3 recognize an epitope shared by alleles of the group 2 HLA-C allotypes characterized by Ser77 and Asn80 (Table 3.2) [26]. Other inhibitory KIR recognize epitopes shared by of HLA-Bw4 alleles (KIR3DL1) [27, 28] and epitopes shared by HLA-A3 and -A11 (KIR3DL2) [29], respectively. For many HLA-A and -B alleles, therefore, no corresponding KIR exist. Furthermore, although previously thought to recognize the same ligands as their inhibitory counterparts, further study has indicated that this is not the case and the ligands for the activating KIR, with the exception of KIR2DS1, remain undefined [26, 30].

The KIR repertoire of an individual's NK cells is not dependent on HLA type, but is determined by the KIR genotype. While NK cells are tolerant to autologous cells expressing self-MHC class I molecules, the genes encoding HLA and KIR are inherited independently. The *KIR* genes are located in the leukocyte receptor cluster on chromosome 19p13.4 [31]. Two broad human KIR haplotypes, A and B, have been defined based on the distribution and number of activating and inhibitory *KIR* genes [22, 32]. While all A and B haplotypes contain several inhibitory KIR, group A haplotypes contain fewer expressed *KIR* genes, with only *KIR2DS4* and *KIR2DL4* as activating receptor genes, while the group B haplotypes contain diverse combinations of activating *KIR* genes [32, 33]. In addition, individual *KIR* genes are polymorphic, so that *KIR* haplotypes that are identical by gene content may differ significantly at the allele level. Thus, *KIR* gene content, allelic polymorphism, and the combination of maternal and paternal haplotypes contribute to significant diversity in *KIR* genotype. As discussed below, KIR haplotypes as well as individual KIR may play important roles in determining the outcome of HSCT.

Table 3.2 List of group 1 and group 2 HLA-C and HLA-Bw4 alleles

Group 1 HLA-C alleles	Group 2 HLA-C alleles	HLA-Bw4 alleles
Cw1 (all)[a]	Cw2 (all)	B5 (all)
Cw3 (all except C*0307, C*0310 and C*0315)	C*0307	B13 (all)
Cw7 (all except C*0707 and C*0709)	C*0315	B17 (all)
Cw8 (all)	Cw4 (all)	B27 (all)
Cw12 (all except C*1205, C*12041, C*12042)	Cw5 (all)	B37 (all)
Cw13 (all)	Cw6 (all)	B38 (all)
Cw14 (all, except C*1404)	C*0707	B44 (all)
C*1507	C*0709	B47 (all)
Cw16 (all except C*1602)	C*1205	B49 (all)
	C*12041	B51 (all)
	C*12042	B52 (all)
	Cw15 (all except C*1507)	B53 (all)
	C*1602	B57 (all)
	Cw17 (all)	B58 (all)
	Cw18 (all)	B59 (all)
		B63 (all)
		B77 (all)
		B*1513, B*1516, B*1517, B*1523, B*1524

Note: C*0310 (Ser77, Lys80) behaves as if it belonged to Group 1 and to Group 2 HLA-C [24]. In other words, C*0310 blocks NK cells expressing any HLA-C-specific receptor; it does not block clones expressing the Bw4 receptor. C*1404 (Asn77, Asn80) is the opposite. It does not belong to Group 1 or to Group 2 HLA-C [24]. In other words, it does not block NK cells expressing HLA-C specific receptors. So, expression of C*1404 may be ignored in a patient because it is as if the patient did not express HLA-C alleles at all. Of course one has to consider the other allele. C*1207 (Gly77, Asn80) cannot be assigned to either group based on its amino acid sequence, and still needs to be tested functionally

[a] all = all molecular types within a serologically-defined group of alleles

The expression of *KIR* genes on human NK cells occurs in a clonal manner [16]. Studies on NK cell clones generated from normal individuals have shown that one to eight different receptors from the inhibitory or activating *KIR* present on a given genotype are expressed on individual NK cells [34]. Although the mechanism regulating KIR expression is not fully understood, the process appears to be largely stochastic and involves variable DNA silencing of *KIR* genes by DNA methylation [35, 36]. It is important to note that the possession of a *KIR* gene does not mean that it is expressed on NK cells [37, 38]. For example, in a study of normal allogeneic blood stem donors, 7% of 68 individuals in whom the *KIR2DL1* gene was present and in 15% of 67 in whom *KIR3DL1* was present, the corresponding receptor was not expressed on the surface on NK cells [39]. Furthermore, while in all individuals tested one or both allelic forms of *KIR2DL2/KIR2DL3* were present, *KIR2DL3* was preferentially expressed with transcripts of *KIR2DL2* not transcribed in 42% of cases [39]. Finally, while *KIR2DL4* is constitutively expressed in all NK cells at the transcriptional level, cell surface expression appears to be quite variable [34, 40, 41]. These studies suggest, therefore, that in investigating the clinical significance of KIR in the setting of HSCT, *KIR* genotyping alone will not be optimal.

3.2.2 CD94/NKG2 Heterodimeric C-Type Lectin Receptors

The heterodimeric C-type lectin receptors share a common subunit, CD94, linked to distinct glycoproteins encoded by the *NKG2* gene family. While the CD94 subunit lacks a cytoplasmic domain for intrinsic signal transduction, the extracellular and cytoplasmic domains of the NKG2 molecules determine the functional specificity of the receptor [42]. The CD94/NKG2 family of receptors is considerably less diverse than KIR. Only a single receptor of this family, CD94/NKG2A (and its splice variant NKG2B), is inhibitory and possesses a long intracytoplasmic tail containing ITIM that mediate inhibitory signals. The other heterodimers of this family, CD94/NKG2C and CD94/NKG2E (and its splice variant NKG2H), are activating receptors and have only short cytoplasmic tails that associate with adaptor proteins bearing ITAM. Both activating and inhibitory receptors recognize HLA-E, loaded with leader peptides derived from the signal sequences of classic class I MHC molecules HLA-A, -B and -C [43, 44], and in effect sense overall MHC class I expression target cells. The *CD94* and *NKG2* genes are all closely linked on chromosome 12p12.3-p13.1, and are much less complex [45, 46].

During development of the NK cell repertoire in an individual, the HLA class I genotype imposes selection by dictating which KIR are to be used as inhibitory receptors for self HLA class I and the frequencies of NK cells expressing a given KIR. NK cells that do not express an inhibitory KIR for self HLA class I express the CD94/NKG2A (or B) inhibitory receptor complex, which fills in the gaps in the KIR repertoire. The significance of the existence of paired inhibitory and activating receptors for MHC class I remains unclear. Under normal conditions, the signals mediated by the inhibitory KIR and CD94/NKG2 receptors override those from the activating counterparts, likely due to the lower affinity of the activating receptors to their ligands compared to that of the inhibitory receptors [47, 48]. However, only a minority of NK cells express both activating and inhibitory isoforms recognizing the same HLA allotypes [21, 34]. More commonly, NK cell clones expressing an activating receptor coexpress at least one inhibitory receptor specific for a different HLA class I allele, which can be either a KIR or CD94/NKG2 (because the individual's HLA selects the self tolerant repertoire). The MHC class I-specific activating receptors may function to detect altered class I expression on cells. It should be noted that despite the modulating effect of HLA class I genotype, the NK cell receptor repertoire is still primarily determined by differential expression of *KIR* and *NKG2* genes.

3.2.3 Non-MHC Class I Specific Activating Receptors

While NK cell activation can be mediated by activating KIR and CD94/NKG2 receptors, other activating receptors exist and are likely to play a more important role in mediating NK cell cytotoxicity. The best characterized activating receptors are the natural cytotoxicity receptors (NCR; NKp46, NKp30, and NKp44) [49–51], for which ligands are not known, and NKG2D [52, 53], which recognize non-MHC class I molecules of two distinct families, the polymorphic MHC class I chain-related (MIC) peptides, MICA and MICB, and the human cytomegalovirus UL16 binding proteins (ULBP-1, -2 and -3), on target cells [53–55]. The ligands of NKG2D are either absent or expressed only in low density on normal tissues, but are induced or upregulated on target cells following stress and neoplastic transformation. Variable expression of NKG2D ligands has been demonstrated on a number of different malignant cell types [10, 56, 57]. Both the NCR and NKG2D are known to play an important role in mediating NK cell-mediated lysis of a variety of tumor cells [56, 58–60]. In addition, a number of activating receptors with no apparent specificity for MHC class I molecules has been reported, although many act as coactivators rather than direct stimulators of NK cell function [52]. Activating coreceptors include FcγRIII (CD16), CD2, 2B4, NKp80, CD69, LFA-1, CD40 ligand, and DNAM-1 (CD226), although their relative importance in interacting with NCR and NKG2D is uncertain. While the expression of activating ligands on tumor cells is known to be important for activating NK cells, and likely contributes an important role in NK cell-mediated GvL effects, the effect of activating receptors and ligand expression on leukemic cells on transplant outcomes has not been investigated.

3.3 NK Cell Alloreactivity in Hematopoietic Stem Cell Transplantation: Mismatching of KIR Ligands

The great diversity of KIR expression ensures generation of alloreactive NK cells between individuals who are mismatched for MHC class I allele groups. Therefore, the NK cells from any given individual will be alloreactive toward cells from others who lack their KIR ligands and will be tolerant of cells from individuals

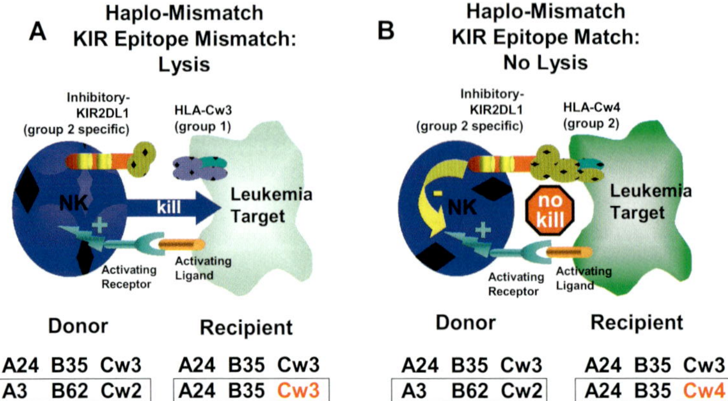

Fig. 3.1 KIR-ligand mismatching in haplotype-mismatched stem cell transplantation predicting NK cell alloreactivity in the GvH direction. (**a**) In this example, donor and recipient are HLA haplotype-mismatched and are KIR-epitope mismatched at the HLA-C locus. The donor NK cell clones expressing KIR2DL1 recognize and are inhibited by an epitope shared by the group 2 HLA-C alleles (HLA-Cw2, 4, 5 and 6). The recipient's leukemic blasts express HLA-Cw3, a member of the group 1 HLA-C alleles, and are therefore not recognized by the donor's KIR2DL1, and activation of donor NK cell occurs with leukemic cell lysis. (**b**) Here, donor and recipient are haplotype-mismatched, but express HLA-C alleles of the same supertype group 2 (HLA-Cw2, 4, 5 and 6). Therefore, donor NK cell clones expressing the inhibitory KIR2DL1 recognize a "self-epitope" (HLA-Cw4) on the recipient's cells with inhibition of lysis of leukemic blasts. KIR epitope mismatching exerts another level of graft alloreactivity and a potent graft-versus-leukemia effect [61]

who have the same or additional KIR ligands. In HSCT, this KIR ligand mismatching between donor and recipient occurs only in HLA class I-mismatched transplants. Figure 3.1 illustrates how KIR ligand mismatching exerts a GvL effect by alloreactive NK cells in T-cell depleted haplotype-mismatched transplantation, where most clinical data has been generated (see below). Following transplantation, NK cell clones developing from transplanted donor $CD34^+$ cells will not be inhibited by recipient cells that fail to express appropriate KIR ligands (i.e., appropriate HLA-class I). In this context, a GvL effect is observed despite T-cell depletion when donor-recipient pairs are selected for KIR ligand mismatches in the graft-versus-host (GvH) direction because leukemic cells of host origin fail to express the inhibitory epitopes. In Fig. 3.1, the donor and recipient are haplotype-mismatched. However, only in panel 1A, are the donor and recipient also KIR ligand mismatched in the GvH direction. In this case where the donor expresses both groups 1 and 2 HLA-C alleles (i.e., a Cw3 and a Cw2, respectively), newly developing donor-derived NK cells in the recipient will express at least one inhibitory KIR recognizing either the group 1 (e.g., KIR2DL2) or group 2 (e.g., KIR2DL1) alleles, but not necessarily both. As the recipient only expresses an HLA-C group 1 allele (homozygous for Cw3), some donor derived NK cell clones that express only KIR2DL1 will not engage

Table 3.3 Donor and recipient combinations for alloreactivity in the GvH direction

Recipient HLA type	HLA type of NK alloreactive donor[a]
Group 1 HLA-C, group 2 HLA-C, HLA-Bw4	No NK alloreactive donor
Group 1 HLA-C, group 2 HLA-C	HLA-Bw4
Group 1 HLA-C, HLA-Bw4	Group 2 HLA-C
Group 2 HLA-C, HLA-Bw4	Group 1 HLA-C
Group 1 HLA-C	Group 2 HLA-C and/or HLA-Bw4
Group 2 HLA-C	Group 1 HLA-C and/or HLA-Bw4

Note: HLA-A3/A11 mismatch is rarely, if ever, found alone. In studies at the University of Perugia, mismatch was always only in conjunction with HLA-C group mismatches [62]

[a] In each recipient/donor combination the donor has an NK repertoire which contains NK cells that are specifically blocked by the allele group(s) indicated in the donor column. These NK cells will be alloreactive because the corresponding recipient does not express this allele group

inhibitory ligands on the recipient's leukemic cells and therefore will be alloreactive in the GvH direction. In Fig. 3.1b, as the recipient's target cells are heterozygous for groups 1 and 2 HLA-C alleles (i.e., Cw2/Cw4), they will inhibit all donor-derived NK cell clones that express either KIR2DL1 or KIR2DL2/3 and no NK cell alloreactivity will be observed despite the observed HLA-C mismatch.

Therefore, individuals who express group 2 HLA-C alleles and possess NK cells that express the specific KIR for group 2 HLA-C alleles (KIR2DL1) are alloreactive against cells from individuals who do not express group 2 HLA-C alleles. Individuals who express group 1 HLA-C alleles possess NK cells with the specific KIR for group 1 HLA-C alleles (KIR2DL2 and/or KIR2DL3) and are alloreactive against cells from individuals who do not express group 1 HLA-C alleles. Likewise, HLA-Bw4 positive individuals expressing the Bw4-specific KIR3DL1 receptor may possess NK cells that are alloreactive against Bw4-negative cells (Table 3.3). In most cases, therefore, alloreactive donors may be inferred from high-resolution Class I HLA-typing of donor and recipient. However, it should be noted that uncommonly, expected KIR expression may not occur. For example, in some individuals allelic variants may not allow full receptor expression at the cell membrane [63]. In a study screening 198 individuals at the University of Perugia, while it was observed that 100% of donors expressed KIR2DL2/3 as expected, 3% lacked KIR2DL1 and 6% lacked KIR3DL1, indicating that in some situations, KIR genotyping of donors will show whether the donor possesses the KIR gene, ensure NK alloreactions, and improve the accuracy of NK alloreactive donor identification [62].

3.4 Preclinical Data Supporting the Role of NK Cell Alloreactivity in Haploidentical Transplantation

As in the human, a fine balance between inhibitory and activating signals regulates NK cell killing in mice [64]. The "hybrid resistance" transplantation model illustrated that NK cell alloreactions in the host-versus-graft (HvG) direction used inhibitory Ly49 molecules which bind primarily MHC class I ligands to mediate rejection of bone marrow grafts and to recognize allogeneic lympho-hematopoietic cells in vivo [65]. As the hybrid recipient mouse tolerated skin and organ allografts, NK cell alloreactivity appeared to be restricted to lympho-hematopoietic targets [65–69]. When the hybrid resistance partners were reversed, the in vivo effects of NK cell alloreactivity held true in the GvH direction. In F1 H-2d/b→parent H-2b transplantations donor T cells were tolerant of recipient MHC. Donor NK cells that did not express the H-2b-specific Ly49C/I inhibitory receptor but bore H-2d-specific Ly49A/G2 receptors, are activated to kill recipient targets [64].

In murine haploidentical transplant models alloreactive NK cells homed to all lympho-hematopoietic sites and ablated recipient-type lympho-hematopoietic cells within 48 h [70]. Lack of NK cell-mediated attack on normal tissues indicates that healthy organ tissues, unlike lympho-hematopoietic cells, did not express ligands at a sufficient level to engage activating NK cell receptors and so alloreactive NK cells did not cause GvHD. Killing of recipient T lymphocytes was associated with engraftment of the MHC-mismatched bone marrow. Killing of recipient dendritic cells, which initiate GvHD by presenting host alloantigens to donor T cells, prevented T-cell-mediated GvHD despite the mice receiving mismatched bone marrow grafts containing up to 30 times the lethal dose of allogeneic T cells [70]. Finally, alloreactive NK cells hastened immune reconstitution by promoting brisk recovery of donor B- and T-cell precursors, which matured correctly, and of donor dendritic cells that are crucial in protecting mice from infectious challenges [69]. Furthermore, transfer of NK cells into non-obese diabetic (NOD)-SCID mice eradicated transplanted human AML provided that the NK cells were alloreactive.

3.5 Clinical Significance of NK Cell Activity in Haplotype-Mismatched Hematopoietic Stem Cell Transplantation

Although transplantation from HLA-identical siblings is the treatment of choice, 75% of patients do not have such a brother or sister. Consequently, other sources of hematopoietic stem cells today include HLA-matched unrelated volunteers, unrelated umbilical cord blood units, and full-haplotype mismatched (haploidentical) family members. Nearly every patient has a family member (parent, child, sibling, cousin, aunt, uncle), who is identical for one HLA haplotype (haploidentical) and fully mismatched for the other, and who could immediately serve as donor. Until the early 1990s, transplantation across the HLA barrier was unsuccessful because T-cell mediated alloreactions in the HvG direction caused rejection and in the GvH direction caused fatal GvHD because alloreactive donor T cells recognize HLA antigens on recipient. Extensive ex vivo T-cell depletion of bone marrow to a maximum of $2–4 \times 10^4$

T cells/kg body weight prevents acute and chronic GvHD without any post-transplant immunosuppressive prophylaxis in patients with severe combined immunodeficiency (SCID) who received transplants from haploidentical family members [71]. However, several clinical trials demonstrated that when tested in leukemia patients, haploidentical T-cell depleted bone marrow transplantation was associated with a high incidence of rejection because the balance between competing recipient and donor T cells shifted in favor of the unopposed HvG reaction [72].

In acute leukemia patients, rejection and lethal GvHD after haploidentical transplantation were successfully overcome by means of a highly immunosuppressive and myeloablative conditioning regimen and a "megadose" allograft of extensively T-cell depleted, granulocyte-colony-stimulating factor (G-CSF) mobilized peripheral blood progenitor cells. Primary sustained engraftment was achieved in over 90% of 17 end-stage patients and acute (>grade I) GVHD occurred in under 10% [73]. In over 175 adult patients with high-risk acute myeloid (AML) or lymphoblastic (ALL) leukemia, haploidentical transplants were associated with full donor type engraftment in over 95% of patients, rapid hematopoietic recovery and ≤10% grade II–IV acute GvHD without post-transplant immune suppression as prophylaxis [73, 74]. Event-free survival approached 50% when patients were transplanted in any remission, but dropped to approximately 10% when they were transplanted in chemoresistant relapse. Besides relapse, the main cause of death was a 35% transplant-related mortality, which was largely infectious [74–76]. Since haploidentical transplants rely for their success on extensive T-cell depletion, T-cell alloreactivity plays a minimal role in engraftment and the GvL effect, but NK cell alloreactivity is triggered and has been associated with beneficial effects [61, 77, 78].

Following T-cell depleted haploidentical HSCT, NK cell recovery occurs early, within 4 weeks after transplantation with donor-derived alloreactive NK cell clones detectable in the recipient's blood for up to 4 months [77]. However, in spite of this short duration during which alloreactive NK cell clones are detectable, a remarkable GvL effect is observed in patients with high-risk AML. In an early report of 57 AML patients at high risk of relapse, donor-versus-recipient NK cell alloreactivity reduced the risk of leukemia relapse, improved engraftment and protected against GvHD. An updated analysis of 112 haploidentical transplants for high-risk AML performed at the Perugia Bone Marrow Transplant Centre provided definitive evidence that transplantation from NK alloreactive donors controlled AML relapse and improved event-free survival. It was associated with a significantly lower relapse rate in patients transplanted in CR (3% versus 47%, $P < 0.003$) (Fig. 3.2), better event-free survival in patients transplanted in relapse (34% versus 6%, $P = 0.04$) and in remission (67% versus 18%, $P = 0.02$), and reduced risk of relapse or death (relative risk versus non-NK-alloreactive donor, 0.48; 95% CI, 0.29–0.78; $P < 0.001$). For AML patients in any remission who received transplants from non-NK-alloreactive donors the probability of event-free survival was 18% compared with 67% when grafts derived from NK-alloreactive donors ($P = 0.02$) (Fig. 3.2). In multivariate

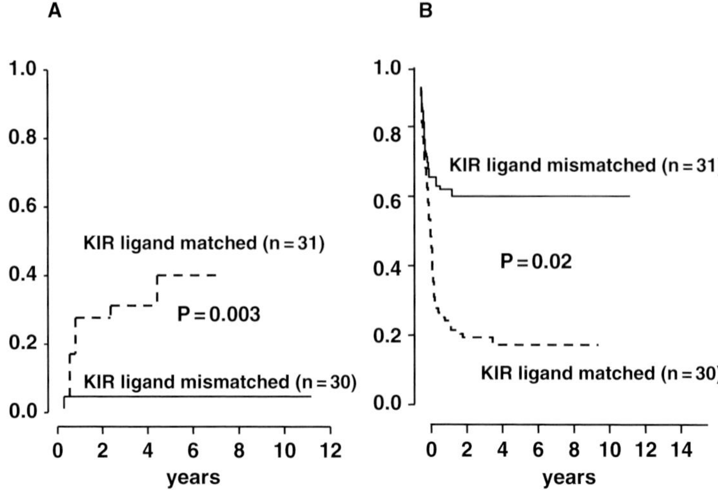

Fig. 3.2 Transplantation from haploidentical NK alloreactive donors controls AML relapse and improves survival in patients transplanted in any remission. (**a**) Relapse in patients transplanted in remission from NK alloreactive versus non-NK alloreactive donors. (**b**) Survival in patients transplanted in any remission from NK alloreactive versus non-NK alloreactive donors

analysis, transplantation from an NK-alloreactive donor was a strong independent factor predicting survival (transplantation from NK-alloreactive versus non-NK alloreactive donor: hazard ratio = 0.44, 95% confidence interval: 0.25–0.77, $P = 0.004$) [62]. This probability of surviving event-free is particularly striking, as it is in the range of best survival rates after transplantation from unrelated donors and cord blood units. The lack of NK alloreactive donors may be considered as a contraindication to transplantation for patients in chemoresistant relapse as very few survive.

It should be noted that alloreactive donors, as defined by KIR ligand mismatching in the GvH direction, are likely to be found for only up to approximately 70% of patients with haplotype-mismatched family members as about 30% of the population are resistant to alloreactive NK killing due to the expression by target cells of inhibitory HLA class I alleles (KIR ligands) from all subgroups with the ability to inhibit all donor NK cell clones [79–81]. More recently, another algorithm known as the "missing ligand" model, has been proposed to identify alloreactive donors. The missing ligand model includes (1) KIR ligand-matched transplants from donors possessing an "extra" KIR for which neither donor nor recipient has an HLA ligand and (2) all KIR ligand mismatched transplants. This is a frequent combination because the majority of individuals possess a full complement of the three inhibitory KIR for group 1 and 2 HLA-C and for HLA-Bw4 alleles, while many possess only one or two KIR ligands in their HLA type. Such donors are hypothesized to possess potentially autoreactive KIR-bearing NK cells in an anergic/regulated state which, upon transfer into the recipient, become activated and exert a GvL effect. Self-tolerant NK cells that do not express inhibitory receptors for self-MHC molecules have been described [82–87], and no studies are available to demonstrate anergic NK cells acquire effector function after transplant. Studies in haploidentical transplants in children with acute leukemia, as well as in matched related sibling and in unrelated donor transplants for AML, have reported a better outcome for KIR ligand-matched transplants from donors possessing an "extra" KIR for which neither donor nor recipient has an HLA ligand [39, 88, 89]. However, in the series of haploidentical and matched sibling transplants performed at the Perugia Transplant Centre, when outcomes of transplants from KIR ligand-matched donors expressing a KIR gene for which neither donor nor recipient had an HLA ligand (i.e., according to the missing ligand model) were analyzed, no informative results emerged [62].

3.5.1 Donor Activating KIR in Haploidentical Transplantation

The role of activating KIR in allogeneic HSCT has been less well studied. Activating KIR show allelic polymorphism in specific genes and show extensive variation in gene number and content, leading to heterogeneity in the general population and different ethnic groups [90]. As noted above, KIR genes segregate in haplotypes. Group A haplotypes bear the main inhibitory KIR genes and the KIR2DS4 activating KIR gene, which, however, encodes for a non-functional protein in approximately 2/3 of individuals. Group B haplotypes carry, besides inhibitory KIR genes, various combinations of activating KIR genes (KIR2DS1-2-3-5 and KIR3DS1). Approximately one in four individuals are homozygous for A haplotypes, while three out of four are either heterozygous or homozygous for B haplotypes and, thus, carry activating KIR genes. In retrospective analyses, transplantation from donors carrying activating KIR genes generally adversely affects transplantation outcomes after matched sibling, unrelated, and partially T-cell depleted haploidentical transplants, mainly through an increased incidence of acute GvHD [91–95]. As NK cells do not themselves cause GvHD, it is likely that activating KIR on T cells might facilitate excess T-cell alloreactivity, which consequently triggers GvHD. This would not be expected to occur following extensively T-cell depleted haploidentical transplants. In fact, an analysis of haploidentical transplantations performed at Perugia, transplantation from NK-alloreactive donors who carry activating KIR genes (group B haplotype) did not cause GvHD, but was associated with less infectious mortality and better survival when transplanted from an NK-alloreactive donor.

3.6 Clinical Significance of NK Cell Activity in Unrelated Donor Hematopoietic Stem Cell Transplantation

The observation of the importance of NK cell alloreactivity with KIR ligand mismatching in haploidentical transplantation has stimulated investigation of the clinical impact of NK cells in unrelated donor transplants with HLA class I mismatches. The role of NK cell alloreactivity in unrelated donor transplantation, however, remains poorly defined at present with mixed and conflicting results reported.

In some reports, KIR ligand mismatching is associated with positive effects on different clinical endpoints following transplantation. For example, in a study of patients with ALL, AML, chronic myelogenous leukemia (CML), and myelodysplastic syndromes (MDS) undergoing unmanipulated bone marrow transplantation from unrelated donors where in vivo T-cell depletion was effected using anti-thymocyte globulin (ATG), KIR ligand incompatibility in the GvH direction was associated with improved outcome [96]. At 4.5 years patients with KIR ligand incompatibility ($n = 20$) had higher probability of overall survival (87% versus 48%, $P = 0.006$) and disease-free survival (87% versus 39%, $P = 0.007$) compared with those without KIR ligand incompatibility ($n = 110$). The improved outcome was related to a significant reduction in transplant-related mortality and relapse in patients receiving KIR ligand mismatched grafts. In a larger retrospective analysis of 374 patients with myeloid leukemias, KIR ligand incompatibility in the GvH direction was associated with a significant reduction in 5-year risk of leukemic relapse compared to HLA-identical and HLA class I disparate, KIR ligand matched transplants (5% versus 22% and 18%, respectively; $P < 0.04$) [97]. Unlike the former study, however, an increased incidence of graft failure was observed in patients receiving KIR ligand mismatched transplantation. Furthermore, KIR ligand incompatibility was not associated with any beneficial effect on the important endpoints of transplantation-related mortality, and overall or event-free survival. In a similar analysis restricted to 236 patients with CML, KIR ligand mismatching was associated with a decreased risk of molecular relapse after transplantation, although no improvement in overall survival was observed [98]. Finally, KIR ligand mismatching was also associated with a reduction in the risk of relapse of multiple myeloma, although this did not translate to a long-term survival benefit [99].

In other studies, however, KIR-ligand mismatching was associated with either no significant effect on important clinical endpoints [100–102]. In a large registry analysis involving over 1500 patients with myeloid malignancies, KIR ligand incompatibility was not associated with any beneficial effect on leukemia relapse, incidence of GvHD, disease-free survival, or overall survival [102]. On the other hand, adverse effects on relapse, treatment-related mortality, or survival were associated with KIR ligand incompatibility in three reported studies [103–105]. In 118 patients with myeloid malignancies, patients receiving KIR ligand mismatched transplants ($n = 15$) had a higher risk of relapse compared to those receiving fully matched or HLA-mismatched, KIR ligand matched transplants [103]. In an additional report, an increased risk of infection that translated to higher treatment-related mortality and worse overall survival was observed in patients receiving KIR ligand mismatched transplants from unrelated donors [104].

Beyond KIR ligand mismatching, two studies have reported mixed effects of NK cell alloreactivity in unrelated donor transplantation when the "missing ligand" algorithm is used to define alloreactive donors (see above). In an analysis of 1770 patients undergoing myeloablative T-cell-replete transplantation from HLA-matched or mismatched unrelated donors for the treatment of myeloid and lymphoid leukemias, absence of HLA-C group 2 or HLA-Bw4 KIR ligands in the recipient was associated with significantly lower risks of relapse in patients only receiving HLA-mismatched unrelated donor transplants [106]. In a larger analysis of 2026 transplants facilitated by the National Marrow Donor Program, the absence of one or more KIR ligands in the recipient versus the presence of all ligands was protective against relapse in patients with early myeloid leukemia, which was independent of HLA matching and T-cell depletion, although no effect was observed on survival [107]. On the other hand, in patients with late chronic phase CML, missing a KIR ligand independently predicted a greater risk of developing grade III–IV acute GvHD [107].

While it remains to be determined which is the better model for investigating KIR mismatching in the setting of unrelated donor transplantation, more complex relationships have also been reported indicating that NK cell activity in transplantation is likely significantly more complicated that previously thought. Recently, an analysis of 108 CML patients undergoing unrelated donor transplantation has suggested that specific group C expression of the recipient and donor may an important determinant of transplant outcome beyond KIR ligand mismatching [108]. Patients homozygous for group 1 HLA-C alleles (C1/C1) had significantly improved survival compared to patients who were heterozygous (C1/C2) or homozygous for group 2 HLA C alleles (C2/C2) [108]. In contrast, presence of C1 ligands in the donor was associated with significantly reduced patient survival. The investigators hypothesized that the differential roles of the two HLA-C ligands may be explained by the observation that NK cell reconstitution and KIR expression after transplantation appeared to be sequential, where C1-specific KIR2DL2/3 NK cells reconstituted earlier and at higher frequency than the C2-specific KIR2DL1 NK cells [108]. Finally, the donor KIR haplotype also appears to be important as donors with KIR haplotype A or with low numbers of activating KIR genes reduced the leukemia relapse and improved disease-free survival in leukemia patients undergoing transplantation [105].

In summary, while it is difficult to draw definitive conclusions regarding the specific role of NK cell activity and KIR in unrelated donor transplantation from the mixed observations of reported studies, it may be at least concluded that NK cells appear to play a more complex role in determining the outcome of transplantation than previously expected from the results of KIR ligand mismatching in the haploidentical setting. Differences in sample size, transplantation techniques, and methods of determining alloreactivity across reported studies have confounded conclusions. It is likely, however, that the transplant conditions are important factors in modulating the effect of NK cells on transplant outcome. In this respect, none of the studies of unrelated donor transplantation analyzing the effect of NK cell alloreactivity have included patients transplanted using the same conditions as those haploidentical transplants in which KIR ligand incompatibility was shown to have a beneficial effect, namely extensive T-cell depletion, high stem cell dose, and absence of post-transplant pharmacological immunosuppression. It has been demonstrated, for example, that T-cell alloreactivity dominates over NK cell alloreactivity in minimally T-cell depleted HLA-nonidentical transplantations [91, 101]. Furthermore, the presence of significant numbers of T cells in the graft may affect NK cell receptor acquisition after transplantation [109]. A comparison of NK cell receptor expression of baseline recipient and donor-derived engrafting NK cells at 100 days after unrelated donor transplantation showed diminished reconstitution of KIR expression with increased expression of the activating receptor NKG2D in T-replete transplantations compared with T-cell depleted transplantations [109]. This was also associated with a higher proportion of engrafted NK cells secreting interferon-γ in response to interleukin (IL)-12 and IL-18 [109]. Thus any beneficial effect of KIR ligand mismatching in unrelated donor transplantation, analogous to that seen in haploidentical stem cell transplantation, may be masked by effects of alloreactive T cells and post-transplantation immune suppression. Until the role of KIR ligand mismatching is better defined in the context of unrelated donor transplantation, there is currently no indication to base the choice of a mismatched unrelated donor on KIR ligand mismatching or KIR genotype profile.

3.7 Conclusions

Over the past decade, we have gained significantly improved understanding of NK cell receptor biology and the mechanisms by which NK cells recognize and kill leukemic target cells. It is now appreciated that NK cell responses are a result of competing signals mediated through inhibitory and activating receptors. In parallel with this has developed a better appreciation of the importance of NK cell activity in HSCT. Of the numerous NK cell receptors described, KIR receptors have been most extensively studied in the context of hematopoietic stem cell transplantation. The recognition of the ability of NK cells to exert a potent GvL effect against myeloid malignancies by mismatching donor and recipient KIR ligands in the GvH direction, in the absence of T cells, has allowed the safer application of haplotype-mismatched transplantation to patients who would otherwise have no curative option for their disease. While the complexity of NK cell alloreactivity in the setting of unrelated donor transplantation is becoming better appreciated, clinical trials investigating transplantation under conditions similar to haploidentical transplants where the beneficial effects of KIR ligand mismatching have been observed are required before the choice of unrelated donor can be based on knowledge of NK cell biology.

The near future should see innovations in the application of NK cell receptor biology to the design of clinical trials in HSCT. Pre-clinical models show that NK cell alloreactivity can enhance engraftment following reduced-intensity regimens. Furthermore, by killing host dendritic cells, alloreactive NK cells used as part of the preparative regimen may permit the infusion of greater numbers of T cells in the graft, which can protect against post-transplant opportunistic infections. Finally, the development of monoclonal antibodies against KIR and other inhibitory NK cells receptors to break tolerance of NK cells to HLA-matched targets will permit the design of clinical trials that can investigate harnessing the anti-leukemic effect of NK cells in both autologous and HLA-matched HSCT. Over the forthcoming decade, it is expected that translation of our improved knowledge of NK cell biology and receptors will lead to advancements in the outcome of HSCT.

References

1. Horowitz MM, Gale RP, Sondel PM, et al. Graft-versus-leukemia reactions after bone marrow transplantation. Blood 1990;75:555–62.
2. Collins RH Jr, Shpilberg O, Drobyski WR, et al. Donor leukocyte infusions in 140 patients with relapsed malignancy after allogeneic bone marrow transplantation. J Clin Oncol. 1997;15:433–44.
3. Cooper MA, Fehniger TA, Caligiuri MA. The biology of human natural killer-cell subsets. Trends Immunol. 2001;22:633–40.
4. Cooper MA, Fehniger TA, Turner SC, et al. Human natural killer cells: a unique innate immunoregulatory role for the CD56(bright) subset. Blood 2001;97:3146–51.
5. Caligiuri MA, Zmuidzinas A, Manley TJ, Levine H, Smith KA, Ritz J. Functional consequences of interleukin 2 receptor expression on resting human lymphocytes. Identification of a novel natural killer cell subset with high affinity receptors. J Exp Med. 1990;171:1509–26.
6. Baume DM, Robertson MJ, Levine H, Manley TJ, Schow PW, Ritz J. Differential responses to interleukin 2 define functionally distinct subsets of human natural killer cells. Eur J Immunol. 1992;22:1–6.
7. Caligiuri MA, Murray C, Robertson MJ, et al. Selective modulation of human natural killer cells in vivo after prolonged infusion of low dose recombinant interleukin 2. J Clin Invest. 1993;91:123–32.
8. Nagler A, Lanier LL, Cwirla S, Phillips JH. Comparative studies of human FcRIII-positive and negative natural killer cells. J Immunol. 1989;143:3183–91.
9. Nagler A, Lanier LL, Phillips JH. Constitutive expression of high affinity interleukin 2 receptors on human CD16-natural killer cells in vivo. J Exp Med. 1990;171:1527–33.
10. Farag SS, George SL, Lee EJ, et al. Postremission therapy with low-dose interleukin 2 with or without intermediate pulse dose interleukin 2 therapy is well tolerated in elderly

patients with acute myeloid leukemia: Cancer and Leukemia Group B study 9420. Clin Cancer Res. 2002;8:2812–9.
11. Lanier LL. Activating and inhibitory NK cell receptors. Adv Exp Med Biol. 1998;452:13–8.
12. Bakker AB, Wu J, Phillips JH, Lanier LL. NK cell activation: distinct stimulatory pathways counterbalancing inhibitory signals. Hum Immunol. 2000;61:18–27.
13. Ljunggren HG, Karre K. In search of the "missing self": MHC molecules and NK cell recognition. Immunol Today. 1990;11:237–44.
14. Moretta A, Bottino C, Pende D, et al. Identification of four subsets of human CD3-CD16+ natural killer (NK) cells by the expression of clonally distributed functional surface molecules: correlation between subset assignment of NK clones and ability to mediate specific alloantigen recognition. J Exp Med. 1990;172:1589–98.
15. Moretta L, Ciccone E, Moretta A, Hoglund P, Ohlen C, Karre K. Allorecognition by NK cells: nonself or no self? Immunol Today. 1992;13:300–6.
16. Ciccone E, Pende D, Viale O, et al. Evidence of a natural killer (NK) cell repertoire for (allo) antigen recognition: definition of five distinct NK-determined allospecificities in humans. J Exp Med. 1992;175:709–18.
17. Colonna M, Brooks EG, Falco M, Ferrara GB, Strominger JL. Generation of allospecific natural killer cells by stimulation across a polymorphism of HLA-C. Science 1993;260:1121–4.
18. Moretta A, Vitale M, Bottino C, et al. P58 molecules as putative receptors for major histocompatibility complex (MHC) class I molecules in human natural killer (NK) cells. Anti-p58 antibodies reconstitute lysis of MHC class I-protected cells in NK clones displaying different specificities. J Exp Med. 1993;178:597–604.
19. Colonna M, Samaridis J. Cloning of immunoglobulin-superfamily members associated with HLA-C and HLA-B recognition by human natural killer cells. [comment]. Science 1995;268:405–8.
20. Long EO. Regulation of immune responses through inhibitory receptors. Annu Rev Immunol. 1999;17:875–904.
21. Uhrberg M, Valiante NM, Shum BP, et al. Human diversity in killer cell inhibitory receptor genes. Immunity 1997;7:753–63.
22. Vilches C, Parham P. KIR: diverse, rapidly evolving receptors of innate and adaptive immunity. Annu Rev Immunol. 2002;20:217–51.
23. Lanier LL. NK cell receptors. Annu Rev Immunol. 1998;16:359–93.
24. Biassoni R, Falco M, Cambiaggi A, et al. Amino acid substitutions can influence the natural killer (NK)-mediated recognition of HLA-C molecules. Role of serine-77 and lysine-80 in the target cell protection from lysis mediated by "group 2" or "group 1" NK clones. J Exp Med. 1995;182:605–9.
25. Mandelboim O, Reyburn HT, Vales-Gomez M, et al. Protection from lysis by natural killer cells of group 1 and 2 specificity is mediated by residue 80 in human histocompatibility leukocyte antigen C alleles and also occurs with empty major histocompatibility complex molecules. J Exp Med. 1996;184:913–22.
26. Winter CC, Gumperz JE, Parham P, Long EO, Wagtmann N. Direct binding and functional transfer of NK cell inhibitory receptors reveal novel patterns of HLA-C allotype recognition. J Immunol. 1998;161:571–7.
27. Rojo S, Wagtmann N, Long EO. Binding of a soluble p70 killer cell inhibitory receptor to HLA-B*5101: requirement for all three p70 immunoglobulin domains. Eur J Immunol. 1997;27:568–71.
28. Gumperz JE, Barber LD, Valiante NM, et al. Conserved and variable residues within the Bw4 motif of HLA-B make separable contributions to recognition by the NKB1 killer cell-inhibitory receptor. J Immunol. 1997;158:5237–41.
29. Dohring C, Scheidegger D, Samaridis J, Cella M, Colonna M. A human killer inhibitory receptor specific for HLA-A1,2. J Immunol. 1996;156:3098–101.

30. Saulquin X, Gastinel LN, Vivier E. Crystal structure of the human natural killer cell activiating receptor KIR2DS2 (CD158j). J Exp Med. 2003;197:933–8.
31. Wilson MJ, Torkar M, Trowsdale J. Genomic organization of a human killer cell inhibitory receptor gene. Tissue Antigens. 1997;49:574–9.
32. Shilling HG, Guethlein LA, Cheng NW, et al. Allelic polymorphism synergizes with variable gene content to individualize human KIR genotype. J Immunol. 2002;168:2307–15.
33. Uhrberg M, Parham P, Wernet P. Definition of gene content for nine common group B haplotypes of the Caucasoid population: KIR haplotypes contain between seven and eleven KIR genes. Immunogenetics 2002;54:221–9.
34. Valiante NM, Uhrberg M, Shilling HG, et al. Functionally and structurally distinct NK cell receptor repertoires in the peripheral blood of two human donors. Immunity 1997;7:739–51.
35. Santourlidis S, Trompeter HI, Weinhold S, et al. Crucial role of DNA methylation in determination of clonally distributed killer cell Ig-like receptor expression patterns in NK cells. J Immunol. 2002;169:4253–61.
36. Chan HW, Kurago ZB, Stewart CA, et al. DNA methylation maintains allele-specific KIR gene expression in human natural killer cells. J Exp Med. 2003;197:245–55.
37. Torkar M, Norgate Z, Colonna M, Trowsdale J, Wilson MJ. Isotypic variation of novel immunoglobulin-like transcript/killer cell inhibitory receptor loci in the leukocyte receptor complex.. Eur J Immunol. 1998;28:3959–67.
38. Long EO, Barber DF, Burshtyn DN, et al. Inhibition of natural killer cell activation signals by killer cell immunoglobulin-like receptors (CD158). Immunol Rev. 2001;181:223–33.
39. Leung W, Iyengar R, Triplett B, et al. Comparison of killer Ig-like receptor genotyping and phenotyping for selection of allogeneic blood stem cell donors. J Immunol. 2005; 174:6540–5.
40. Rajagopalan S, Long EO. A human histocompatibility leukocyte antigen (HLA)-G-specific receptor expressed on all natural killer cells. J Exp Med. 1999;189:1093–100.
41. Goodridge JP, Witt CS, Christiansen FT, Warren HS. KIR2DL4 (CD158d) genotype influences expression and function in NK cells. J Immunol. 2003;171:1768–74.
42. Chang C, Rodriguez A, Carretero M, Lopez-Botet M, Phillips JH, Lanier LL. Molecular characterization of human CD94: a type II membrane glycoprotein related to the C-type lectin superfamily. Eur J Immunol. 1995;25:2433–7.
43. Braud VM, Allan DS, O'Callaghan CA, et al. HLA-E binds to natural killer cell receptors CD94/NKG2A, B and C. Nature 1998;391:795–9.
44. Borrego F, Ulbrecht M, Weiss EH, Coligan JE, Brooks AG. Recognition of human histocompatibility leukocyte antigen (HLA)-E complexed with HLA class I signal sequence-derived peptides by CD94/NKG2 confers protection from natural killer cell-mediated lysis. J Exp Med. 1998;187:813–8.
45. Glienke J, Sobanov Y, Brostjan C, et al. The genomic organization of NKG2C, E, F, and D receptor genes in the human natural killer gene complex. Immunogenetics 1998; 48:163–73.
46. Sobanov Y, Glienke J, Brostjan C, Lehrach H, Francis F, Hofer E. Linkage of the NKG2 and CD94 receptor genes to D12S77 in the human natural killer gene complex. Immunogenetics 1999;49:99–105.
47. Vales-Gomez M, Reyburn HT, Mandelboim M, Strominger JL. Kinetics of interaction of HLA-C ligands with natural killer cell inhibitory receptors. Immunity 1998;9:337–44.
48. Vales-Gomez M, Reyburn HT, Erskine RA, Lopez-Botet M, Strominger JL. Kinetics and peptide dependency of the binding of the inhibitory NK receptor CD94/NKG2-A and the activating receptor CD94/NKG2-C to HLA-E. Embo J. 1999;18:4250–60.
49. Pende D, Parolini S, Pessino A, et al. Identification and molecular characterization of NKp30, a novel triggering receptor involved in natural cytotoxicity mediated by human natural killer cells. J Exp Med. 1999;190:1505–16.

50. Sivori S, Vitale M, Morelli L, et al. p46, a novel natural killer cell-specific surface molecule that mediates cell activation. J Exp Med. 1997;186:1129–36.
51. Vitale M, Bottino C, Sivori S, et al. NKp44, a novel triggering surface molecule specifically expressed by activated natural killer cells, is involved in non-major histocompatibility complex-restricted tumor cell lysis. J Exp Med. 1998;187:2065–72.
52. Moretta A, Bottino C, Vitale M, et al. Activating receptors and coreceptors involved in human natural killer cell-mediated cytolysis. Annu Rev Immunol. 2001;19:197–223.
53. Bauer S, Groh V, Wu J, et al. Activation of NK cells and T cells by NKG2D, a receptor for stress-inducible MICA. [comment]. Science 1999;285:727–9.
54. Bahram S. MIC genes: from genetics to biology. Adv Immunol. 2000;76:1–60.
55. Sutherland CL, Chalupny NJ, Schooley K, VandenBos T, Kubin M, Cosman D. UL16-binding proteins, novel MHC class I-related proteins, bind to NKG2D and activate multiple signaling pathways in primary NK cells. J Immunol. 2002;168:671–9.
56. Pende D, Cantoni C, Rivera P, et al. Role of NKG2D in tumor cell lysis mediated by human NK cells: cooperation with natural cytotoxicity receptors and capability of recognizing tumors of nonepithelial origin. Eur J Immunol. 2001;31:1076–86.
57. Groh V, Rhinehart R, Randolph-Habecker J, Topp MS, Riddell SR, Spies T. Costimulation of CD8alphabeta T cells by NKG2D via engagement by MIC induced on virus-infected cells. Nat Immunol. 2001;2:255–60.
58. Groh V, Rhinehart R, Secrist H, Bauer S, Grabstein KH, Spies T. Broad tumor-associated expression and recognition by tumor-derived gamma delta T cells of MICA and MICB. Proc Natl Acad Sci USA. 1999;96:6879–84.
59. Cantoni C, Bottino C, Vitale M, et al. NKp44, a triggering receptor involved in tumor cell lysis by activated human natural killer cells, is a novel member of the immunoglobulin superfamily. J Exp Med. 1999;189:787–96.
60. Pessino A, Sivori S, Bottino C, et al. Molecular cloning of NKp46: a novel member of the immunoglobulin superfamily involved in triggering of natural cytotoxicity. J Exp Med. 1998;188:953–60.
61. Farag SS, Fehniger TA, Ruggeri L, Velardi A, Caligiuri MA. Natural killer cell receptors: new biology and insights into the graft-versus-leukemia effect. Blood 2002;100:1935–47.
62. Ruggeri L, Mancusi A, Capanni M, et al. Donor natural killer cell allorecognition of missing self in haploidentical hematopoietic transplantation for acute myeloid leukemia: challenging its predictive value. Blood 2007;110:433–40.
63. Pando MJ, Gardiner CM, Gleimer M, McQueen KL, Parham P. The protein made from a common allele of KIR3DL1 (3DL*004) is poorly expressed at cell surfaces due to substitution at position 86 in Ig domain 0 and 182 in Ig domain 1. J Immunol. 2003;171:6640–7.
64. Ortaldo JR, Young HA. Mouse Ly49 NK receptors: balancing activation and inhibition. Mol Immunol. 2005;42:445–50.
65. Cudkowicz G, Bennett M. Peculiar immunobiology of bone marrow allografts. II. Rejection of parental grafts by resistant F 1 hybrid mice. J Exp Med. 1971;134:1513–28.
66. Murphy WJ, Kumar V, Bennett M. Rejection of bone marrow allografts by mice with severe combined immune deficiency (SCID). Evidence that natural killer cells can mediate the specificity of marrow graft rejection. J Exp Med. 1987;165:1212–7.
67. Yu YY, George T, Dorfman JR, Roland J, Kumar V, Bennett M. The role of Ly49A and 5E6(Ly49C) molecules in hybrid resistance mediated by murine natural killer cells against normal T cell blasts. Immunity 1996;4:67–76.
68. Ogasawara K, Benjamin J, Takaki R, Phillips JH, Lanier LL. Function of NKG2D in natural killer cell-mediated rejection of mouse bone marrow grafts. Nat Immunol. 2005;6:938–45.
69. Ruggeri L, Perruccio K, Montagnoli C, Romani L, Velardi A. NK cell conditioning to T cell replete mismatched BMT confers immediate responsiveness to infectious challenges. Bone Marrow Transplant. 2004;33:S18.

70. Ruggeri L, Capanni M, Urbani E, et al. Effectiveness of donor natural killer call alloreactivity in mismatched hematopoietic transplants. Science 2002;295:2097–3100.
71. O'Reilly RJ, Keever CA, Small TN, Brochstein J. The use of HLA-non-identical T-depleted marrow transplants for correction of severe combined immunodeficiency disease. Immunodefic Rev. 1989;1:273–309.
72. Reisner Y, Martelli M. Stem cell escalation enables HLA-disparate hematopoietic transplants in leukemia patients. Immunol Today. 1999;20:343–7.
73. Aversa F, Tabilio A, Terenzi A, et al. Successful engraftment of T-cell-depleted haploidentical "three-loci" incompatible transplants in leukemia patients by addition of recombinant human granulocyte colony-stimulating factor-mobilized peripheral blood progenitor cells to bone marrow inoculum. Blood 1994;84: 3948–55.
74. Aversa F, Tabilio A, Velardi A, et al. Treatment of high-risk acute leukemia with T-cell-depleted stem cells from related donors with one fully mismatched HLA haplotype. N Engl J Med. 1998;339:1186–93.
75. Aversa F, Velardi A, Tabilio A, Reisner Y, Martelli MF. Haploidentical stem cell transplantation in leukemia. Blood Rev. 2001;15:111–9.
76. Aversa F, Terenzi A, Tabilio A, et al. Full haplotype-mismatched hematopoietic stem-cell transplantation: a phase II study in patients with acute leukemia at high risk of relapse. J Clin Oncol. 2005;23:3447–54.
77. Ruggeri L, Capanni M, Casucci M, et al. Role of natural killer cell alloreactivity in HLA-mismatched hematopoietic stem cell transplantation. Blood 1999;94:333–9.
78. Velardi A, Ruggeri L, Alessandro, Moretta A, Moretta L. NK cells: a lesson from mismatched hematopoietic transplantation. Trends Immunol. 2002;23:438–44.
79. Caligiuri MA, Velardi A, Scheinberg DA, Borrello IM. Immunotherpeutic approaches for hematological malignancies. In: Hematology 2004, ASH Education Program Book. Washington: American Society of Hematology; 2004. p. 337–53.
80. Ruggeri L, Mancusi A, Capanni M, Martelli MF, Velardi A. Exploitation of alloreactive NK cells in adoptive immunotherapy of cancer. Curr Opin Immunol. 2005;17:211–7.
81. Velardi A, Moretta A. Role of natural killer cell alloreactivity in hematopoietic stem cell transplantation. In: Atkinson K, Fibbe W, Champlin R, Ljungman L, Ritz J, Brenner MK, editors. Clinical Bone Marrow and Blood Stem Cell Transplantation. Cambridge University Press; 2004. p. 247–61.
82. Salcedo M, Andersson M, Lemieux S, Van Kaer L, Chambers BJ, Ljunggren HG. Fine tuning of natural killer cell specificity and maintenance of self tolerance in MHC class I-deficient mice. Eur J Immunol. 1998;28:1315–21.
83. Johansson MH, Bieberich C, Jay G, Karre K, Hoglund P. Natural killer cell tolerance in mice with mosaic expression of major histocompatibility complex class I transgene. J Exp Med. 1997;186:353–64.
84. Raulet DH. Interplay of natural killer cells and their receptors with the adaptive immune response. Nat Immunol. 2004;5:996–1002.
85. Raulet DH, Vance RE, McMahon CW. Regulation of the natural killer cell receptor repertoire. Annu Rev Immunol. 2001;19:291–330.
86. Fernandez NC, Treiner E, Vance RE, Jamieson AM, Lemieux S, Raulet DH. A subset of natural killer cells achieves self-tolerance without expressing inhibitory receptors specific for self-MHC molecules. Blood 2005;105:4416–23.
87. Kim S, Poursine-Laurent J, Truscott SM, et al. Licensing of natural killer cells by host major histocompatibility complex class I molecules. Nature 2005;436:709–13.
88. Leung W, Iyengar R, Turner V, et al. Determinants of antileukemia effects of allogeneic NK cells. J Immunol. 2004;172:644–50.
89. Hsu KC, Keever-Taylor CA, Wilton A, et al. Improved outcome in HLA-identical sibling hematopoietic stem-cell transplantation for acute myelogenous leukemia predicted by KIR and HLA genotypes. Blood 2005;105:4878–84.

90. Parham P. MHC class I molecules and KIRs in human history, health and survival. Nat Rev Immunol. 2005;5:201–14.
91. Bishara A, De Santis D, Witt CC, et al. The beneficial role of inhibitory KIR genes of HLA class I NK epitopes in haploidentically mismatched stem cell allografts may be masked by residual donor-alloreactive T cells causing GVHD. Tissue Antigens. 2004;63:204–11.
92. Gagne K, Brizard G, Gueglio B, et al. Relevance of KIR gene polymorphisms in bone marrow transplantation outcome. Hum Immunol. 2002;63:271–80.
93. De Santis D, Bishara A, Witt CS, et al. Natural killer cell HLA-C epitopes and killer cell immunoglobulin-like receptors both influence outcome of mismatched unrelated donor bone marrow transplants. Tissue Antigens. 2005;65:519–28.
94. Sun JY, Gaidulis L, Dagis A, et al. Killer Ig-like receptor (KIR) compatibility plays a role in the prevalence of acute GVHD in unrelated hematopoietic cell transplants for AML. Bone Marrow Transplant. 2005;36:525–30.
95. Verheyden S, Schots R, Duquet W, Demanet C. A defined donor activating natural killer cell receptor genotype protects against leukemic relapse after related HLA-identical hematopoietic stem cell transplantation. Leukemia 2005;19:1446–51.
96. Geibel S, Locatelli F, Maccario R, et al. Survival advantage with KIR ligand incompatibility in unrelated donor transplantation. Blood 2003;102:814–9.
97. Beelen DW, Ottinger HD, Ferencik S, et al. Genotypic inhibitory killer immunoglobulin-like receptor ligand incompatibility enhances the long-term antileukemic effect of unmodified allogeneic hematopoietic stem cell transplantation in patients with myeloid leukemias. Blood 2005;105:2594–600.
98. Elmaagacli AH, Ottinger H, Koldehoff M, et al. Reduced risk for molecular disease in patients with chronic myeloid leukemia after transplantation from a KIR-mismatched donor. Transplantation 2005;79:1741–7.
99. Kroger N, Shaw B, Iacobelli S, et al. Comparison between antithymocyte globulin and alemtuzumab and the possible impact of KIR-ligand mismatch after dose-reduced conditioning and unrelated stem cell transplantation in patients with multiple myeloma. Br J Haematol. 2005;129:631–43.
100. Davies SM, Ruggieri L, DeFor T, et al. Evaluation of KIR ligand incompatibility in mismatched unrelated donor hematopoietic transplants. Killer immunoglobulin-like receptor. Blood 2002;100:3825–7.
101. Lowe EJ, Turner V, Handgretinger R, et al. T-cell alloreactivity dominates natural killer cell alloreactivity in minimally T-cell-depleted HLA-non-identical paediatric bone marrow transplantation. Br J Haematol. 2003;123:323–6.
102. Farag SS, Bacigalupo A, Eapen M, et al. The effect of KIR ligand incompatibility on the outcome of unrelated donor transplantation: a report from the center for international blood and marrow transplant research, the European blood and marrow transplant registry, and the Dutch registry. Biol Blood Marrow Transplant. 2006;12:876–84.
103. Bornhauser M, Schwerdtfeger R, Martin H, Frank KH, Theuser C, Ehninger G. Role of KIR ligand incompatibility in hematopoietic stem cell transplantation using unrelated donors. Blood 2004;103:2860–1; author reply 2862.
104. Schaffer M, Malmberg KJ, Ringden O, Ljunggren HG, Remberger M. Increased infection-related mortality in KIR-ligand-mismatched unrelated allogeneic hematopoietic stem-cell transplantation. Transplantation 2004;78:1081–5.
105. Kroger N, Binder T, Zabelina T, et al. Low number of donor activating killer immunoglobulin-like receptors (KIR) genes but not KIR-ligand mismatch prevents relapse and improves disease-free survival in leukemia patients after in vivo T-cell depleted unrelated stem cell transplantation. Transplantation 2006;82:1024–30.
106. Hsu KC, Gooley T, Malkki M, et al. KIR ligands and prediction of relapse after unrelated donor hematopoietic cell transplantation for hematologic malignancy. Biol Blood Marrow Transplant. 2006;12:828–36.

107. Miller JS, Cooley S, Parham P, et al. Missing KIR ligands are associated with less relapse and increased graft-versus-host disease (GVHD) following unrelated donor allogeneic HCT. Blood 2007;109:5058–61.
108. Fischer JC, Ottinger H, Ferencik S, et al. Relevance of C1 and C2 epitopes for hemopoietic stem cell transplantation: role for sequential acquisition of HLA-C-specific inhibitory killer Ig-like receptor. J Immunol. 2007;178:3918–23.
109. Cooley S, McCullar V, Wangen R, et al. KIR reconstitution is altered by T cells in the graft and correlates with clinical outcomes after unrelated donor transplantation. Blood 2005;106:4370–6.

Chapter 4
Advancement and Clinical Implications of HLA Typing in Allogeneic Hematopoietic Stem Cell Transplantation

Lee Ann Baxter-Lowe and Carolyn Katovich Hurley

4.1 Introduction

One of the best established risk factors for hematopoietic stem cell transplantation (HSCT) is human leukocyte antigen (HLA) disparity between the recipient and donor. HLA disparity has been associated with graft failure, delayed immune reconstitution, graft-versus-host disease (GvHD), and mortality. These undesirable effects can be offset somewhat by reduced relapse rates in patients with hematological malignancies. This chapter reviews current understanding of HLA biology and its clinical implications.

Several relatively recent advances have dramatically changed this field. Perhaps the most important of these is development of DNA-based HLA typing, which has made it possible to define HLA disparities at an amino acid level. Advances in HLA typing have been complemented by improved matching algorithms utilized by unrelated donor registries. There have also been breakthroughs in the understanding of the molecular mechanisms of allorecognition. For decades, research and clinical medicine have focused on allorecognition involving interactions between T-cell receptors (TCR) and their HLA ligands. A relatively new and major discovery is that HLA molecules are also ligands for several other receptors, including inhibitory receptors expressed on natural killer (NK) cells and some T lymphocytes. Under certain conditions, these receptors can mediate alloimmune responses, substantially influencing transplantation outcomes. In addition, new transplant procedures, particularly those which use alternative graft sources, alter the effects of HLA disparity.

L.A. Baxter-Lowe (✉)
Department of Surgery, University of California, San Francisco, San Francisco, CA, USA
e-mail: LeeAnn.BaxterLowe@ucsfmedctr.org

M.R. Bishop (ed.), *Hematopoietic Stem Cell Transplantation*, Cancer Treatment and Research 144, DOI 10.1007/978-0-387-78580-6_4,

4.2 HLA Structure and Function

4.2.1 HLA Structure

The established transplantation antigens are divided into two major classes: Class I (HLA-A, -B, and -C) and Class II (HLA-DR, -DQ, and -DP). HLA Class I and Class II molecules are heterodimers with similar three-dimensional structures. All of these molecules contain an antigen-binding cleft which is occupied by a peptide. The bound peptides can be derived from the degradation of either normal cellular proteins or abnormal proteins from pathogens or other foreign proteins encountered by the cell. The peptides bound to HLA Class I molecules are typically 8–10 amino acids long and derived from inside the cell [1, 2], while peptides bound to HLA Class II molecules are much longer (usually > 20 amino acids) and derived from outside the cell [3, 4]. The amino acids in the HLA molecule that line the binding cleft determine the characteristics of peptides that are preferentially bound to each molecule [5]. The characteristics of the peptides bound to various HLA molecules are catalogued by the NIH (http://www-bimas.cit.nih.gov/molbio/hla_bind/hla_motif_search_info.html).

4.2.2 HLA Functions

The HLA Class I-peptide complexes are ligands for TCR on $CD8^{+}$ T cells while the HLA Class II complexes are ligands for TCR on $CD4^{+}$ cells [6]. The recognition of HLA-peptide complexes by T lymphocytes leads to adaptive immune responses to nonself. The HLA Class I molecules play an additional role; they are ligands for killer immunoglobulin-like receptors (KIR), which are inhibitory receptors expressed on NK cells and a subset of T lymphocytes [7]. Loss of HLA on the surface of abnormal cells causes the loss of the KIR-mediated inhibitory signal in these lymphocytes, which shifts the balance of receptor signals from tolerance toward activation and target cell killing.

4.2.3 HLA Expression

Another difference between HLA Class I and Class II molecules is their cell surface expression [8]. HLA Class I molecules are expressed by all nucleated cells with the highest levels on hematopoietic cells. HLA Class II molecules are constitutively expressed by a subset of cells in the immune system (e.g., specialized antigen presenting cells), and their expression can be induced on many other cells. HLA expression can be increased by certain cytokines and reduced by some pathogens and tumors.

4.3 Allorecognition

HLA molecules are potent alloantigens, molecules that stimulate an immune response against cells from other humans. Alloimmune responses can occur after transplantation, pregnancy, or transfusion. T lymphocytes play a central role in responses to alloantigens, but the actions of NK cells and B lymphocytes can also be very important [9, 10].

4.3.1 T Lymphocytes

In healthy individuals, tolerance to self is maintained through inactivation of autoreactive T lymphocytes in the thymus, as well as through peripheral tolerance mechanisms [9]. T lymphocytes that respond to self antigens are eliminated during development in the thymus. The surviving T lymphocytes are specific for pathogenic peptides bound to self HLA molecules. Thus, recovery of this selection process is important for immune reconstitution following HSCT. Lymphocytes that have been selected to recognize pathogenic peptides bound to self HLA molecules can become activated by non-self HLA molecules [11]. Thus, these T lymphocytes can play a major role in graft rejection and GvHD.

There are three mechanisms for allorecognition by T lymphocytes: direct, indirect and semi-direct. Direct allorecognition involves recognition of foreign HLA molecules displayed on the surface of non-self cells (Fig. 4.1). For direct allorecognition, the majority of T lymphocytes are sensitive to differences in the peptides bound to the HLA molecules [12–15].

Indirect HLA allorecognition occurs when T lymphocytes recognize foreign peptides presented by self HLA molecules. Some of these peptides can be derived from foreign HLA molecules. Since foreign peptides are generally derived from outside the cell, the indirect pathway is dominated by $CD4^+$ T lymphocytes responding to foreign peptides bound to HLA Class II molecules.

Semi-direct HLA allorecognition results from intercellular transfer of HLA molecules. After solid organ transplantation, HLA molecules from the donor can be transferred to immune cells of the recipient. T lymphocytes can recognize the intact donor HLA molecules that have been transferred to the plasma membrane of the recipient's immune cells [16–19]. Hypothetically, the semi-direct pathway could play a role in HSCT, but this has not yet been established.

4.3.2 Minor Histocompatibility Antigens

Minor histocompatibility antigens result from differences among individuals in protein expression (e.g., products of the Y chromosome), genetic polymorphism that changes the protein sequence, or differences in protein processing [20].

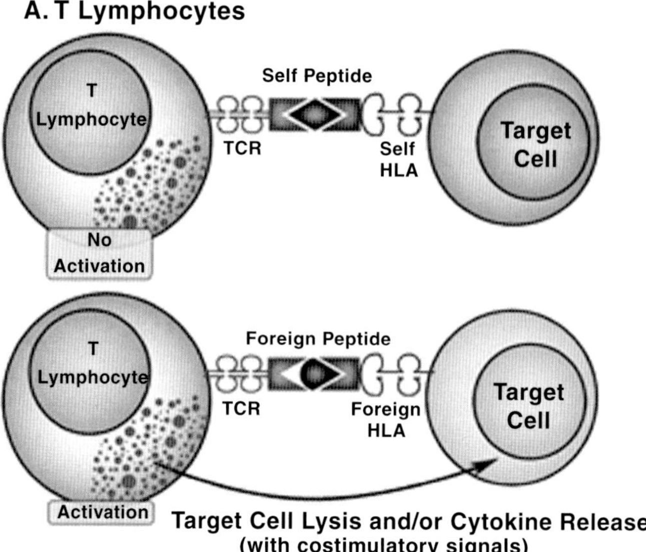

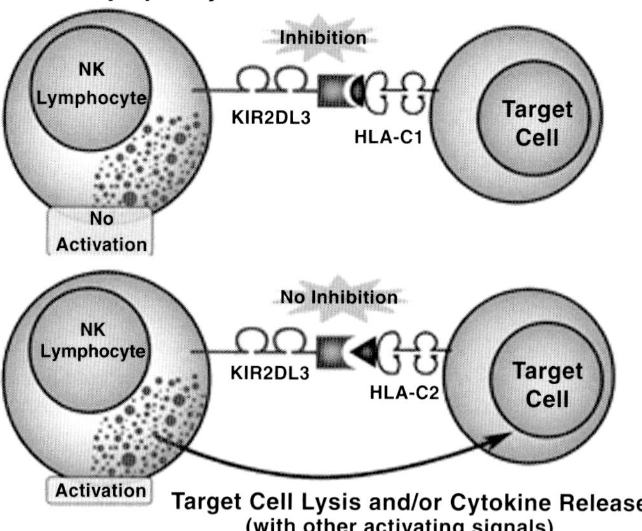

Fig. 4.1 (**a**) T lymphocytes are not activated by self HLA molecules with self peptides in the binding cleft (*top*) but can be activated if the peptide or the HLA molecule is foreign. (**b**) KIR interactions with their HLA ligands provide inhibitory signals (*top*).If the HLA ligand is not present, the balance of receptor signals is shifted from tolerance toward activation and target cell killing

After HSCT, HLA molecules can present peptides from nonself-derived minor histocompatibility antigens, which can elicit clinically significant immune responses. Responses against minor histocompatibility antigens are usually easier to manage than those against major histocompatibility antigens (i.e., HLA) and in some cases can give rise to beneficial anti-tumor effects. Thus, the minor antigens can serve as targets for immunotherapy for cancer.

4.3.3 NK Cells

Several recent investigations have established that allogeneic responses mediated by NK cells can play an important role in clinical transplantation through potent graft-versus-tumor (GvT) effects and perhaps involvement in GvHD [21–24]. The role and functions of NK cells are also described in Chap. 3. NK cells express a combination of inhibiting and activating receptors which maintain tolerance to healthy cells and cause responses against diseased and allogeneic cells [25]. Inhibitory receptors, which are members of the killer cell immunoglobulin (Ig)-like receptor (KIR) family with specificity for specific HLA ligands, play an important role in allorecognition.

Nearly all individuals have genes encoding inhibitory KIR specific for HLA-C molecules with Ser77, Asn80 (referred to as the C1 group), HLA-C molecules with Asn77, Lys80 (referred to as the C2 group), and Bw4, an epitope in many HLA-B molecules that is created by amino acids 77–83. To ensure self-tolerance, most NK lymphocytes have undergone a tolerization process that is influenced by self-HLA molecules and prevents reactivity to their own cells [26]. After transplantation or adoptive transfer of NK cells, NK cells may kill recipient cells if they do not express the requisite KIR ligand (Fig. 4.1).

4.3.4 B Lymphocytes

B lymphocytes can play a major role in graft rejection and have recently been implicated in GvHD. B lymphocytes can make alloantibodies against any foreign molecule, including HLA and other alloantigens. If a transplant recipient has preexisting antibodies against donor alloantigens, the risk for graft rejection is substantially increased [27, 28]. Antibody responses to H-Y minor histocompatibility antigens have recently been correlated with chronic GvHD as well as disease remission after HSCT [29]. This discovery has created interest in the possibility that H-Y and other alloantigens may provide useful targets for cancer immunotherapy mediated by B lymphocytes.

4.4 HLA Genetics

4.4.1 Major Histocompatibility Complex

One of the hallmarks of HLA proteins is their diversity, which is generated by multiple genes and extensive polymorphism for each gene (Fig. 4.2). HLA genes are located in the major histocompatibility complex (MHC) on chromosome 6p21.3 (high resolution map available at http://www.nature.com/nrg/journal/v5/n12/poster/MHCmap/index.html). The extended MHC complex spans 7.6 Mb and contains more than 400 genes [30]. The HLA Class I cluster contains nine expressed genes which include the classical HLA Class I genes (HLA-A, -B, and -C) as well as non-classical Class I genes (HLA-E, -F, -G, HFE) and Class I-like genes (MICA and MICB). The Class II HLA cluster contains the classical Class II HLA genes (HLA-DR, -DQ, and -DP) and non-classical Class II HLA genes (HLA-DM and -DO).

The role of the classical HLA genes in transplantation is well established, but other MHC encoded proteins may also influence allogeneic transplants. For example, proteins involved in loading peptides into HLA binding clefts, serving as ligands for receptors on NK lymphocytes or mediating cellular reactivity, may influence an individual's risk for immunological complications after transplantation [31–33].

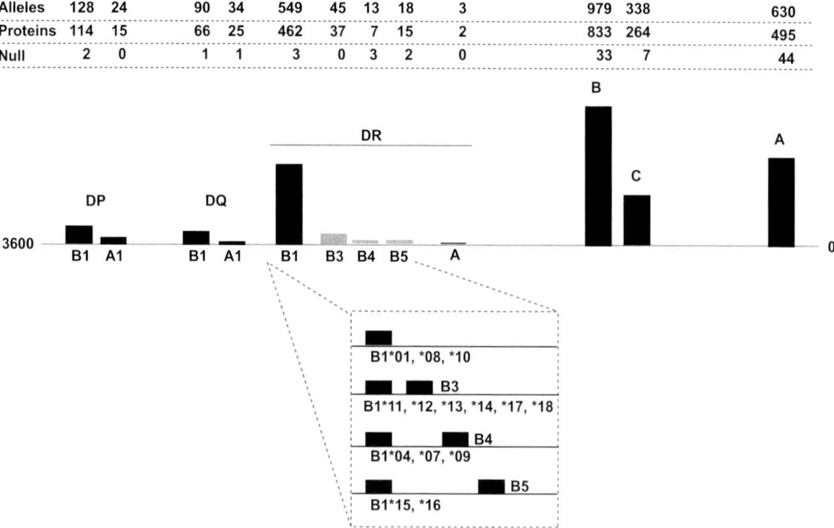

Fig. 4.2 The bars indicating each of the HLA genes are proportional to the number of known HLA alleles for each locus. The number of alleles, unique proteins, and null alleles is indicated above each locus. HLA-DRB3, -DRB4, and DRB5 loci are present on certain haplotypes as shown in the inset

4.4.2 HLA Diversity

HLA-A, -B, and -C loci are extremely polymorphic with hundreds of alleles already known for each locus (Fig. 4.2) and more being discovered every year. Comprehensive analysis of chromosome 6 has identified HLA-B as the most polymorphic gene in the human genome [34].

HLA-DRA, -DRB1, DQA1, DQB1, DPA1, and DPB1 genes are present in every haplotype (the set of HLA genes inherited on each chromosome), and diversity is generated by polymorphism as well as the variable presence of additional genes (DRB3, DRB4, and DRB5, Fig. 4.2). Each haplotype contains pairs of A and B genes for each HLA Class II locus. The products of the pairs form Class II heterodimers. For the HLA-DR locus, the HLA-DRA gene is relatively non-polymorphic but diversity is generated by differences in the number of HLA-DRB genes. One HLA-DRB1 gene is always present and some haplotypes have one additional HLA-DRB gene (HLA-DRB3, -DRB4, or -DRB5).

For HLA-DQ and -DP, the A and B genes are both polymorphic (Fig. 4.2). Each haplotype contains a combination of alleles that encodes compatible alpha and beta chains to produce a functional protein. For these loci, diversity can be generated by alternative heterodimers of alpha and beta chains that are encoded on different copies of chromosome 6 (i.e., trans association). Thus, each genome has the potential to generate four different HLA-DQ and -DP proteins. The relevance of the trans heterodimers in transplantation has not been evaluated.

4.4.3 HLA Nomenclature

The WHO Nomenclature Committee for Factors of the HLA System names each HLA allele; names consist of the locus followed by an asterisk and a unique number consisting of four to eight digits (Table 4.1). The current list of alleles and nomenclature is available at http://www.ebi.ac.uk/imgt/hla/nomenclature/index.html. To aid in exchange of HLA typing data, the U.S. unrelated donor registry, the National Marrow Donor Program (NMDP), has established a system of allele codes that is used by registries world wide [35].

4.4.4 HLA Allele Frequencies and Linkage Disequilibrium

HLA alleles are present in the population at different frequencies, and these frequencies vary among racial and ethnic groups [36–38]. Some alleles are unique to a particular race or ethnic group. Certain alleles are very rare and have been observed only once. Each haplotype contains multiple HLA loci (at a minimum HLA-A, -B, -C, DRA, DRB1, DQA1, DQB1, DPA1, and DPB1). Certain combinations of HLA alleles are observed in the same haplotype much

Table 4.1 HLA nomenclature

Designation	Examples	Comments
Differences in digits 1,2	A*0101, A*0201	Two digit designation describes an allele group which often corresponds to serologic specificity; alleles with differences in digits 1,2 differ in both nucleotide and protein sequence
Differences in digits 3,4	A*0101, A*0102	Designates order of discovery; alleles differ in both nucleotide and protein sequence
Differences in digits 5, 6	A*010101, A*010102	Alleles differ in nucleotide but not protein sequence
Differences in digits 7, 8	A*01010101, A*01010102	Alleles differ for nucleotides outside of protein-encoding exons
Addition of single letter	A*01010102 N	Designates abnormal expression: N indicates the allele is not expressed; the meaning of other suffixes can be found at http://www.ebi.ac.uk/imgt/hla/nomenclature/suffixes.html
Addition of multiple letters to 2 digit assignment	A*01AB, A*02AMAY	Letter codes assigned by the NMDP to indicate alternative alleles beginning with the two digits indicated; the individual tested carries one of these; http://bioinformatics.nmdp.org/HLA/Allele_Codes/Allele_Code_Lists/index.html
Only first two digits listed	A*01, A*02	Indicates that the allele family is present but the typing has not identified which allele in the family is present

more frequently than expected if alleles were randomly distributed [37, 38]. The frequency of the patient's alleles and their haplotypes impacts the likelihood of finding an HLA matched unrelated donor [39].

4.5 HLA Typing

4.5.1 Typing Methods

Advances in HLA typing have transformed our ability to detect HLA disparity and enabled clinical investigation of the relevance of HLA disparity between donor and recipient. HLA types were historically determined using serological reagents which define groups of HLA alleles corresponding to allele families. After the polymerase chain reaction (PCR) technique became available, numerous DNA-based typing methods were developed, including hybridization with sequence-specific oligonucleotide probes (SSO), amplification with sequence-specific primers (SSP), and automated sequencing-based typing (SBT).

For SSO typing, a segment of the target HLA gene is amplified by PCR and hybridized with a panel of oligonucleotide probes that detect key polymorphic sequences which distinguish specific HLA alleles. The pattern of positive and negative hybridization with the probes is used to assign HLA alleles that are potentially present in the individual (i.e., an HLA "type"). SSP typing takes advantage of the specificity of the PCR to amplify segments of alleles based upon the presence of key polymorphic sequences located in one or both primers. The presence or absence of PCR products from a panel of primer pairs is used to assign HLA types. For SBT, automated nucleotide sequencing is used to determine the sequence of an amplified segment of DNA. The sequence is compared with a library of known sequences to assign an HLA type.

Routine use of DNA-based typing has improved the accuracy of HLA typing [40], revealed HLA disparity between donors and recipients that could not be detected by the conventional serological methods [41, 42], and led to the discovery of an unexpectedly large number of HLA alleles [43]. Although there have been dramatic improvements in HLA typing, limitations remain. Much of an allele's sequence is not typically interrogated, and presence of a relatively small number of polymorphisms can be used to assign types.

Another limitation is that typing data are often consistent with multiple alternative genotypes (i.e., combinations of HLA alleles), often referred to as ambiguities (http://www.ebi.ac.uk/imgt/hla/ambig.html). This circumstance is becoming more frequent as the number of known alleles continues to increase [44]. Although it is feasible to resolve all alleles, this is expensive and requires considerable expertise. One approach to address this limitation has been to exclude putative rare alleles based upon their low likelihood [45].

4.5.2 Typing Nomenclature

Types determined using serological methods are assigned numbers corresponding to specificities that have been defined by the WHO Nomenclature Committee for Factors of the HLA system (e.g., A1, A2). Types determined by DNA-based typing methods are based upon the nomenclature for HLA alleles (Table 4.1).

4.5.3 Typing Resolution

Dramatic differences between the ability of conventional serological typing and DNA-based typing to detect HLA disparity have led to a variety of terms to describe the level of typing resolution used to detect HLA differences. When

DNA-based typing is used to approximate serological types or specificities, it is referred to as typing that is low resolution or antigen level. High resolution or allele-level typing is used to describe types that identify a single allele or one common allele with a small number of rare alleles.

4.6 HLA Matching

There are several factors to consider in evaluation of HLA matching. One component is the HLA loci that are being considered in the evaluation. When allogeneic bone marrow transplantation began, the HLA-A, -B, and -DR types were evaluated for HLA matching. Since most individuals have two different alleles at each locus, a total of six types were compared. If all of the types were matched, the recipient and donor were considered to be a 6/6 HLA match for the HLA-A, -B, and -DR loci. If one of the types was mismatched, the donor-recipient pair was described as a 5/6 HLA match. Today, several additional loci may also be considered: HLA-C, -DQA1, -DQB1, -DPA1, and -DPB1. If all of these loci are evaluated, a perfect match would be 16/16.

Another factor is the level of resolution of the match. If the types that are compared are high resolution types, HLA matching is described as a "high resolution" match or an "allele level" match. If one or both types are low resolution or serological specificities, the matching is described as a "low resolution," "antigen," or "serological" match. If high resolution level typing is available, mismatching of the first two digits is referred to as a "low resolution," "antigen," or "serological" mismatch. If the first two digits are matched, but the second two digits are different, the mismatch is often referred to as "high resolution" or "allele level" mismatch.

If a donor or recipient is homozygous for a type that is present in the other member of the pair and the other member of the pair is heterozygous (e.g., donor is HLA-A*02,A*02 and recipient is HLA-A*02,A*24), the mismatch is described as directional or as having a vector. In this example, alloreactivity is directed against the recipient (i.e., host) and it is described as the graft-versus-host (GvH) direction or GvH vector. If the situation is reversed (e.g., donor is HLA-A*02,A*24 and recipient is HLA-A*02,A*02), the directionality is called host-versus-graft (HvG) or rejection direction because the "foreign HLA type" is only present in the donor.

The minimal HLA matching requirements are influenced by multiple factors including the graft characteristics (e.g., source and graft manipulation), transplant protocol (e.g., immunosuppressive regimen) and patient factors (e.g., diagnosis, disease stage, and age). One of the few variables that physicians can modify is donor selection. When allogeneic HSCT began, all donors were living related individuals. Since most patients lacked a well matched family donor, registries of volunteer donors were developed to locate unrelated donors who are well matched for HLA [39]. Although there are now more than 12 million donors listed in world-wide registries, some patients are still unable to locate a suitably matched donor, or transplantation urgency precludes the lengthy search process.

These limitations have motivated development of umbilical cord blood as an alternative graft source. In the 10 years after the first cord blood transplant involving an unrelated donor [46], 47 cord blood banks have been established [47]. Two major advantages of cord blood grafts are less stringent requirements for HLA matching and rapid availability of the graft. Availability of numerous options for allografts has led to development of algorithms to customize donor searches to achieve optimal outcomes for each patient [48].

4.7 Related Donors

4.7.1 Genetics

Each person inherits one haplotype from his or her mother (maternal haplotype) and one haplotype from his or her father (paternal haplotype). Since cross-over events within the MHC are infrequent, within a family, individuals inheriting the same MHC haplotypes carry identical alleles at the HLA loci as well as at all of the other genes located within the MHC [49]. Inheritance of MHC haplotypes is Mendelian, and HLA alleles are codominant. The likelihood that two siblings will share two, one, or no haplotypes is 25%, 50%, and 25%, respectively. If siblings have inherited the same two haplotypes, they are often called a "2-haplotype match." Sharing of only one haplotype is referred to as "haplotype matched" or "haploidentical." The extent of HLA matching from the non-share haplotypes is variable.

4.7.2 Transplant Outcomes

The best outcomes have been consistently observed for HLA identical siblings (2-haplotype match), but this donor is not available for the majority of recipients. For leukemia patients, early studies showed that transplantation from partially HLA-matched related donors can be successful, but it is associated with delayed engraftment, neutropenia, graft rejection, and acute GvHD [50]. A recent large retrospective study from China did not detect statistically significant differences between outcomes of transplantation from HLA identical siblings and HLA mismatched family members, but for every endpoint, there was a trend for better outcomes using HLA-identical sibling donors [51]. In another recent study of children with congenital diseases, survival was 80% if donors were HLA-identical siblings with reductions in survival when HLA disparity increased [52].

Since nearly all patients who might benefit from transplantation have a haplo-identical donor, there have been many attempts to overcome the histocompatibility barriers posed by HLA mismatches on the non-shared haplotype. Early experience with haplo-identical donors who had several HLA mismatches was associated with high rates of rejection, GvHD, and relapse [28, 50, 53–55]. Successful transplantation was reported for patients with severe combined immunodeficiency syndrome (SCID) who received transplants from haplo-identical donors after T lymphocytes were depleted from the graft [56]. However, when T-cell depleted grafts from haplo-identical donors were initially attempted for patients with malignant diseases, there were many problems including high rates of graft failure and relapse.

The engraftment and GvHD barriers observed for haplo-identical transplants were overcome by the use of grafts depleted of T lymphocytes with megadoses of $CD34^+$ cells [57]. Recently Ruggeri et al. reported that this approach produced exceptional outcomes for AML patients transplanted from haplo-identical donors [58]. It is believed that this success is attributable to elimination of tumor cells by alloreactive NK cells [24]. This benefit has not been observed in patients transplanted for ALL, because these tumor cells are resistant to killing by NK cells [23].

4.7.3 Tolerance to Non-Inherited Maternal Antigens

Contact between a mother and fetus in utero can result in fetal tolerance to the non-inherited maternal HLA antigens [59]. The importance of this mechanism in blood and marrow transplantation remains controversial, perhaps because the transplant procedure influences non-inherited maternal HLA antigen effects [60, 61].

4.7.4 HLA Typing Recommendations

Typing of the candidate recipient and family members is used to identify potential family donors, to confirm HLA assignments in the patient, and to establish HLA haplotypes for use in an unrelated donor search. Low resolution HLA typing is often sufficient to determine haplotypes within the family. However, if the same low resolution HLA type is present in multiple haplotypes or if parent samples are not available, higher resolution typing may be required to determine HLA identity.

Among related donors, an HLA-matched sibling who has inherited the same MHC haplotypes is the donor of choice. Related donors who are partially HLA-mismatched can be acceptable.

4.8 Unrelated Donors

4.8.1 HLA Typing

Unrelated individuals who are matched for low resolution HLA types often have HLA disparity uncovered by high resolution typing. For example, a retrospective study of transplants facilitated by the NMDP showed that 29% of pairs who were 6/6 HLA matched (HLA-A, -B, and -DRB1) using low resolution HLA typing had at least one allele-level mismatch at one of these loci, and 92% had at least one allele mismatch when eight HLA loci were considered [42]. Today, high resolution typing is generally accepted as requisite for transplantation involving unrelated donors. Serologic testing may be useful to confirm HLA expression because DNA typing may not detect mutations that prevent expression of an allele [62]. Cellular assays such as a measure of cytotoxic T-lymphocyte precursors (CTLp) directed to HLA-mismatched antigens or the mixed lymphocyte culture (MLC) are not routinely used to assess compatibility [63, 64].

4.8.2 Transplant Outcomes

Although many studies have shown that transplantation from unrelated donors can have acceptable outcomes using donors who are not HLA identical [52, 65–69], a single HLA mismatch can reduce survival [66, 70–74]. HLA disparity is generally detrimental, but it is important to remember that transplantation from an HLA-mismatched donor is often a superior option to non-transplant alternatives.

Recent research has focused on identifying HLA mismatches that should be avoided and determining the other factors that influence the impact of HLA disparity. Investigating these questions is challenging because HLA mismatches in transplanted populations are diverse in both number and characteristics. The situation is exacerbated by a large number of confounding variables. This chapter reviews the reports that best address these challenges by having large sample sizes or homogeneous patient populations.

4.8.3 Comparison of HLA Loci

Several large studies have been designed to determine if the specific HLA locus influences the effect of HLA disparity. A recent report on 3,857 patients, who were transplanted under the auspices of the NMDP, confirmed previous studies showing that the best outcomes were observed for donor-recipient pairs that are matched at an allele level at HLA-A, -B, -C, and DRB1 [71]. HLA-A, -B, -C, and DRB1 disparity reduced survival; there was a 9–10% decrement in survival for each allele mismatch at these loci. Mismatches at HLA-B or -C appeared to be better tolerated than mismatches at HLA-A and -DRB1 although the number of mismatched pairs in some of these subsets was small. In this investigation, survival was not affected by HLA-DQ or -DP disparity, suggesting that HLA-DQ and -DP mismatches may be acceptable.

A smaller retrospective study of Japanese patients ($n = 1298$) transplanted from unrelated donors who were HLA-A, -B and -DR serologically matched reported that high resolution mismatches at HLA-A and/or -B were associated with mortality. The Japanese study did not detect adverse effects of HLA-C or -DRB1 disparity. HLA-DP was not considered in this investigation because a prior study did not detect any effects of HLA-DP disparity [75].

In a single center study of 948 patients who were transplanted for CML, Petersdorf et al. concluded that HLA-C mismatches should be avoided and that HLA-DQ disparity may be deleterious when combined with other HLA mismatches [74]. In this investigation, the total number of HLA mismatches was a significant risk factor for mortality. However, the effects of a single mismatch were detected only in low-risk patients.

Although none of these large studies detected a relationship between HLA-DP disparity and survival, the NMDP study and several small studies with less heterogeneous patient populations suggest that HLA-DP may play a role in GvHD and/or GvT effects [71, 76, 77]. Other studies have suggested that the impact of HLA-DP disparity is affected by mismatching of particular residues within the molecule [78–80]. The latter observation is consistent with the hypothesis that there are deleterious and permissive HLA mismatches.

Several factors may contribute to the differences observed in studies investigating locus-specific effects including differences in the numbers of subjects, the characteristics of the HLA mismatches, the methods used for comparing the effects of mismatches and other transplant variables such as type of disease, disease stage, and race. At this time, there are no well-accepted guidelines for a preferred locus of an HLA mismatch.

4.8.4 Number of HLA Mismatches

Several investigations have observed decremental effects of multiple HLA mismatches. The NMDP study showed 9–10% decrement in survival for each HLA-A, -B, -C, or -DRB1 mismatch [71]. A recent retrospective study of 334 transplants performed in France reported that a single mismatch was associated with a significant decrement in survival (HR = 1.41, CI 1.1–2.0, $p = 0.046$), and multiple mismatches were more deleterious (HR = 1.91, CI 1.26–2.91, $p = 0.003$) [81]. This situation makes it difficult to investigate the effects of particular HLA disparities or loci because all of the above studies have included patients who have received allografts from donors with HLA disparities at multiple HLA loci.

4.8.5 Molecular Characteristics of HLA Mismatches

Several reports have suggested that there may be differences between antigen and allele-level mismatches [70, 82]. This is appealing because antigen disparities have more mismatched amino acids than allele-level mismatches, and these additional differences could increase the number of targets for allorecognition. However, this possibility was not confirmed by Lee et al., which is the largest study to date that addressed this question [71].

The number of mismatched amino acids may not be as important as the characteristics of the amino acids involved in the mismatch. Analysis of data from the International Histocompatibility Workshop showed that the combinations of alleles involved in HLA-A*02 mismatches observed in Japanese were very different from those observed in Caucasians [83]. In Japanese patients, the most frequent mismatch was HLA-A*0201 and HLA-A*0206, and this mismatch was deleterious. In contrast, the most common HLA-A*02 mismatch in Caucasians was HLA-A*0201 with HLA-A*0205, and an adverse relationship between this mismatch and transplantation outcomes was not detected. Observations such as these, along with a large body of data from experimental models, have stimulated efforts to develop systems to rank HLA mismatches based upon amino acid differences rather than HLA types. One approach proposed a matching score (dissimilarity index) that is based on the similarity of mismatched amino acids [84]. However, this particular model has not been supported by clinical or in vitro studies [85, 86].

Another approach has been to compare each mismatched amino acid with transplantation outcomes [87]. Kawase et al. identified 15 allele mismatch combinations and 6 amino acid substitution positions that were statistically associated with severe acute GvHD. These observations require independent confirmation or other supporting data because large numbers of comparisons were made to detect this small number of relationships, and there are many confounding variables [88].

4.8.6 Limitations and Non-HLA Factors to Consider

Although there is a large body of evidence showing that HLA matching is beneficial, several patient factors including diagnosis, disease stage, cytomegalovirus status, and age are as predictive of patient survival as HLA matching [71]. Physicians can influence the stage of disease by performing transplantation earlier, but the other factors cannot be changed. Delaying transplantation in order to search for an HLA identical donor may be deleterious to the patient. For example, Petersdorf et al. showed that the benefit of HLA matching was lost when CML patients had more advanced disease [74]. Another limitation is that the majority of patients in the above studies received T-cell replete bone marrow after myeloablative conditioning. The conclusions from these investigations may not be valid for transplantation procedures using reduced intensity conditioning regimens or alternative graft sources [89].

4.8.7 Recommendations for Unrelated Donor Typing

Since allele-level HLA disparity can influence transplantation outcomes, a minimum of high resolution HLA-A, -B, -C, and HLA-DQ typing of recipients and donors is now generally recommended [90, 91] and some groups require HLA-DQ typing [92]. In addition, there is agreement that HLA-DRB3, -DRB4, DRB5 and -DPB1 may be useful if multiple alternative donors well-matched at HLA-A, -B, -C, -DRB1 are available. These recommendations do not imply that donors and recipients must be HLA-A, -B, -C, and DRB1 matched at an allele level. Instead, high resolution types can be used to select the best HLA-matched donor among several candidates and to ensure that transplantation is not performed when there are unacceptable levels of HLA disparity. Patients who will undergo HLA-mismatched transplantation should be assessed for the presence of antibodies directed to the mismatched HLA antigens [27, 28].

The selection of donors is facilitated by algorithms such as the NMDP's HapLogic^{SM}, which uses allele and haplotype frequencies to predict high resolution matching when complete high resolution typing is not available for a donor. Information on the greater than 12 million donors and cord blood units around the world is provided by Bone Marrow Donors Worldwide. Typing of several potential donors identified through a registry search is recommended because, following further HLA typing, some donors will not be matched at the allele level for key loci or will not be willing or available for donation.

4.9 Umbilical Cord Blood Transplantation

Early reports on transplantation of cord blood, which focused on feasibility, demonstrated that HLA disparity is tolerated [93]. Many of the early reports on cord blood transplantation from unrelated donors were based upon low resolution typing for HLA-A and -B and low or high resolution typing for HLA-DRB1. Using this level of typing, the benefit of HLA matching became apparent only when large numbers of transplants were examined [94–97]. Subsequent reports detected an interaction between cell dose and HLA matching [98, 99]. In these and other preliminary reports, the impact of HLA disparity is increased when the cell dose is low.

Since low cell dose has been associated with less favorable outcomes, most of the cord blood recipients have been children. Nevertheless, cord blood transplantation can be successful in adults [100, 101] (also refer to Chap. 10). Success in larger patients has been increased by transplantation of two cord blood units [102, 103]. When two cord blood units are transplanted, only one of the cord blood units usually survives beyond 100 days. The surviving unit is not necessarily the best HLA match, and controversy remains regarding the characteristics that are associated with long-term engraftment [103, 104].

The majority of the cord blood transplantation literature uses HLA typing that is often low resolution, usually limited to the HLA-A, -B, and DRB1 loci. When typing of additional loci and/or higher resolution typing has been performed for several relatively small studies, additional HLA disparity has been detected [105–107]. Much larger patient populations must be studied to clarify the clinical significance of HLA disparity in cord blood transplantation.

4.9.1 HLA Typing for Umbilical Cord Blood Transplantation

There are currently no clear guidelines for HLA typing requirements for cord blood transplantation. The majority of the literature is based upon low resolution typing for HLA-A and B along with HLA-DRB1 typed at variable levels of resolution. It will be challenging to establish guidelines because HLA disparity can be well tolerated and the effects of HLA disparity are influenced by cell dose [98, 99]. A recent editorial from the NMDP recommends high resolution HLA-A, -B, -C, DRB1, and DQB1 assignments for confirmatory typing of cord blood units [47]. However, the requirement for releasing a unit for transplantation is a minimum of 5/6 matching for low resolution HLA-A and -B and high resolution HLA-DRB1 types. Typing for HLA-C and DQ was primarily recommended to facilitate retrospective analysis.

4.10 Additional Factors in Donor Selection for Hematopoietic Stem Cell Transplantation

4.10.1 Killer Cell Immunoglobulin-Like Receptors

Models of KIR recognition of missing HLA ligands in a transplant setting have become more complex as the understanding of KIR has advanced. The ligand incompatibility model used by Ruggeri [24] predicted KIR reactivity based on recipient HLA types. Alloreactive NK cells were isolated from recipients lacking a C1, C2, and/or Bw4 ligand. The targets for NK cell killing were thought to be tumor cells and cellular mediators of GvHD. Later studies refined the model to include consideration of expression of KIR on donor NK cells because many KIR genes are absent or not expressed in certain individuals [108]. The lack of

KIR expression would abrogate the effects described by Ruggeri. Further refinement of the model has considered the impact of donor HLA on subsequent NK function in the recipient. These effects may occur in the context of both HLA matched and mismatched donors. Finally, studies have suggested that NK cells are dysfunctional at 100 days post-transplantation, and the NK activity is difficult to predict [109, 110]. Although it is appealing to try to take advantage of the potentially beneficial aspects of HLA-KIR interaction, data from the large studies described above suggest that deliberate mismatching of HLA to get a KIR effect may be detrimental. KIR may be more effectively used in adoptive transfer of NK cells to target relapse [111].

4.10.2 Other Genes

Other genetic factors that might impact transplantation outcome are being evaluated, but there is no clear understanding yet of their importance in donor selection or outcome [112–114].

Acknowledgments The authors thank Shauna O'Donnell and Ronen Kaley for their assistance with the figures and formatting.

References

1. Bjorkman PJ, Saper MA, Samraoui B, Bennett WS, Strominger JL, Wiley DC. Structure of the human class I histocompatibility antigen, HLA-A2. Nature 1987;329:506–12.
2. Bjorkman PJ, Saper MA, Samraoui B, et al. The foreign antigen binding site and T cell recognition regions of class I histocompatibility antigens. Nature 1987;329:512–8.
3. Brown JH, Jardetzky TS, Gorga JC, et al. Three-dimensional structure of the human class II histocompatibility antigen HLA-DR1. Nature 1993;364:33–9.
4. Stern LJ, Brown JH, Jardetzky TS, et al. Crystal structure of the human class II MHC protein HLA-DR1 complexed with an influenza virus peptide. Nature 1994;368:215–21.
5. Madden DR. The three-dimensional structure of peptide-MHC complexes. Annu Rev Immunol. 1995;13:587–622.
6. Rudolph MG, Stanfield RL, Wilson IA. How TCRs bind MHCs, peptides, and coreceptors. Annu Rev Immunol. 2006;24:419–66.
7. Parham P. MHC class I molecules and KIRs in human history, health and survival. Nat Rev Immunol. 2005;5:201–14.
8. van den Elsen PJ, Holling TM, Kuipers HF, van der Stoep N. Transcriptional regulation of antigen presentation. Curr Opin Immunol. 2004;16:67–75.
9. Singh NJ, Schwartz RH. Primer: mechanisms of immunologic tolerance. Nat Clin Pract Rheumatol. 2006;2:44–52.
10. Parham P. Taking license with natural killer cell maturation and repertoire development. Immunol Rev. 2006;214:155–60.
11. Burrows SR, Khanna R, Burrows JM, Moss DJ. An alloresponse in humans is dominated by cytotoxic T lymphocytes (CTL) cross-reactive with a single Epstein-Barr virus CTL epitope: implications for graft-versus-host disease. J Exp Med. 1994;179:1155–61.
12. Whitelegg AM, Oosten LE, Jordan S, et al. Investigation of peptide involvement in T cell allorecognition using recombinant HLA class I multimers. J Immunol. 2005;175:1706–14.

13. Smith PA, Brunmark A, Jackson MR, Potter TA. Peptide-independent recognition by alloreactive cytotoxic T lymphocytes (CTL). J Exp Med. 1997;185:1023–33.
14. Weber DA, Terrell NK, Zhang Y, et al. Requirement for peptide in alloreactive CD4+ T cell recognition of class II MHC molecules. J Immunol. 1995;154:5153–64.
15. Eckels DD, Gorski J, Rothbard J, Lamb JR. Peptide-mediated modulation of T-cell allorecognition. Proc Natl Acad Sci USA. 1988;85:8191–5.
16. Game DS, Rogers NJ, Lechler RI. Acquisition of HLA-DR and costimulatory molecules by T cells from allogeneic antigen presenting cells. Am J Transplant. 2005;5:1614–25.
17. Harshyne LA, Watkins SC, Gambotto A, Barratt-Boyes SM. Dendritic cells acquire antigens from live cells for cross-presentation to CTL. J Immunol. 2001;166:3717–23.
18. Herrera OB, Golshayan D, Tibbott R, et al. A novel pathway of alloantigen presentation by dendritic cells. J Immunol. 2004;173:4828–37.
19. Morelli AE, Larregina AT, Shufesky WJ, et al. Endocytosis, intracellular sorting, and processing of exosomes by dendritic cells. Blood 2004;104:3257–66.
20. Hambach L, Spierings E, Goulmy E. Risk assessment in haematopoietic stem cell transplantation: minor histocompatibility antigens. Best Pract Res Clin Haematol. 2007;20:171–87.
21. Witt CS, Christiansen FT. The relevance of natural killer cell human leucocyte antigen epitopes and killer cell immunoglobulin-like receptors in bone marrow transplantation. Vox Sang. 2006;90:10–20.
22. Hsu KC, Gooley T, Malkki M, et al. KIR ligands and prediction of relapse after unrelated donor hematopoietic cell transplantation for hematologic malignancy. Biol Blood Marrow Transplant. 2006;12:828–36.
23. Ruggeri L, Capanni M, Casucci M, et al. Role of natural killer cell alloreactivity in HLA-mismatched hematopoietic stem cell transplantation. Blood 1999;94:333–9.
24. Ruggeri L, Mancusi A, Capanni M, et al. Donor natural killer cell allorecognition of missing self in haploidentical hematopoietic transplantation for acute myeloid leukemia: challenging its predictive value. Blood 2007;110:433–40.
25. Bottino C, Moretta L, Pende D, Vitale M, Moretta A. Learning how to discriminate between friends and enemies, a lesson from Natural Killer cells. Mol Immunol. 2004;41:569–75.
26. Yokoyama WM, Kim S. How do natural killer cells find self to achieve tolerance? Immunity 2006;24:249–57.
27. Ottinger HD, Rebmann V, Pfeiffer KA, et al. Positive serum crossmatch as predictor for graft failure in HLA-mismatched allogeneic blood stem cell transplantation. Transplantation 2002;73:1280–5.
28. Anasetti C, Amos D, Beatty PG, et al. Effect of HLA compatibility on engraftment of bone marrow transplants in patients with leukemia or lymphoma. N Engl J Med. 1989;320:197–204.
29. Miklos DB, Kim HT, Miller KH, et al. Antibody responses to H-Y minor histocompatibility antigens correlate with chronic graft-versus-host disease and disease remission. Blood 2005;105:2973–8.
30. Horton R, Wilming L, Rand V, et al. Gene map of the extended human MHC. Nat Rev Genet. 2004;5:889–99.
31. Wright CA, Kozik P, Zacharias M, Springer S. Tapasin and other chaperones: models of the MHC class I loading complex. Biol Chem. 2004;385:763–78.
32. Busch R, Rinderknecht CH, Roh S, et al. Achieving stability through editing and chaperoning: regulation of MHC class II peptide binding and expression. Immunol Rev. 2005;207:242–60.
33. Kitcharoen K, Witt CS, Romphruk AV, Christiansen FT, Leelayuwat C. MICA, MICB, and MHC beta block matching in bone marrow transplantation: relevance to transplantation outcome. Hum Immunol. 2006;67:238–46.

34. Mungall AJ, Palmer SA, Sims SK, et al. The DNA sequence and analysis of human chromosome 6. Nature 2003;425:805–11.
35. Bochtler W, Maiers M, Oudshoorn M, et al. World Marrow Donor Association guidelines for use of HLA nomenclature and its validation in the data exchange among hematopoietic stem cell donor registries and cord blood banks. Bone Marrow Transplant. 2007;39:737–41.
36. Cao K, Hollenbach J, Shi X, Shi W, Chopek M, Fernandez-Vina MA. Analysis of the frequencies of HLA-A, B, and C alleles and haplotypes in the five major ethnic groups of the United States reveals high levels of diversity in these loci and contrasting distribution patterns in these populations. Hum Immunol. 2001;62:1009–30.
37. Maiers M, Gragert L, Klitz W. High-resolution HLA alleles and haplotypes in the United States population. Hum Immunol. 2007;68:779–88.
38. Mori M, Beatty PG, Graves M, Boucher KM, Milford EL. HLA gene and haplotype frequencies in the North American population: the National Marrow Donor Program Donor Registry. Transplantation 1997;64:1017–27.
39. Hurley CK, Fernandez-Vina M, Setterholm M. Maximizing optimal hematopoietic stem cell donor selection from registries of unrelated adult volunteers. Tissue Antigens. 2003;61:415–24.
40. Noreen HJ, Yu N, Setterholm M, et al. Validation of DNA-based HLA-A and HLA-B testing of volunteers for a bone marrow registry through parallel testing with serology. Tissue Antigens. 2001;57:221–9.
41. Hurley CK, Baxter-Lowe LA, Begovich AB, et al. The extent of HLA class II allele level disparity in unrelated bone marrow transplantation: analysis of 1259 National Marrow Donor Program donor-recipient pairs. Bone Marrow Transplant. 2000;25:385–93.
42. Hurley CK, Fernandez-Vina M, Hildebrand WH, et al. A high degree of HLA disparity arises from limited allelic diversity: analysis of 1775 unrelated bone marrow transplant donor-recipient pairs. Hum Immunol. 2007;68:30–40.
43. Marsh SG, Albert ED, Bodmer WF, et al. Nomenclature for factors of the HLA system, 2004. Int J Immunogenet. 2005;32:107–59.
44. Voorter CE, Mulkers E, Liebelt P, Sleyster E, van den Berg-Loonen EM. Reanalysis of sequence-based HLA-A, -B and -Cw typings: how ambiguous is today's SBT typing tomorrow. Tissue Antigens. 2007;70:383–9.
45. Cano P, Klitz W, Mack SJ, et al. Common and well-documented HLA alleles: report of the Ad-Hoc Committee of the American Society for Histocompatiblity and Immunogenetics. Hum Immunol. 2007;68:392–417.
46. Kurtzberg J, Laughlin M, Graham ML, et al. Placental blood as a source of hematopoietic stem cells for transplantation into unrelated recipients. N Engl J Med. 1996;335:157–66.
47. Kamani N, Spellman S, Hurley CK, et al. State of the art review: HLA matching and outcome of unrelated donor umbilical cord blood transplants. Biol Blood Marrow Transplant. 2008;14:1–6.
48. Barker JN, Krepski TP, DeFor TE, Davies SM, Wagner JE, Weisdorf DJ. Searching for unrelated donor hematopoietic stem cells: availability and speed of umbilical cord blood versus bone marrow. Biol Blood Marrow Transplant. 2002;8:257–60.
49. Miretti MM, Walsh EC, Ke X, et al. A high-resolution linkage-disequilibrium map of the human major histocompatibility complex and first generation of tag single-nucleotide polymorphisms. Am J Hum Genet. 2005;76:634–46.
50. Beatty PG, Clift RA, Mickelson EM, et al. Marrow transplantation from related donors other than HLA-identical siblings. N Engl J Med. 1985;313:765–71.
51. Lu DP, Dong L, Wu T, et al. Conditioning including antithymocyte globulin followed by unmanipulated HLA-mismatched/haploidentical blood and marrow transplantation can achieve comparable outcomes with HLA-identical sibling transplantation. Blood 2006;107:3065–73.

52. Caillat-Zucman S, Le Deist F, Haddad E, et al. Impact of HLA matching on outcome of hematopoietic stem cell transplantation in children with inherited diseases: a single-center comparative analysis of genoidentical, haploidentical or unrelated donors. Bone Marrow Transplant. 2004;33:1089–95.
53. Anasetti C, Beatty PG, Storb R, et al. Effect of HLA incompatibility on graft-versus-host disease, relapse, and survival after marrow transplantation for patients with leukemia or lymphoma. Hum Immunol. 1990;29:79–91.
54. Kernan NA, Flomenberg N, Dupont B, O'Reilly RJ. Graft rejection in recipients of T-cell-depleted HLA-nonidentical marrow transplants for leukemia. Identification of host-derived antidonor allocytotoxic T lymphocytes. Transplantation 1987;43:842–7.
55. Soiffer RJ, Mauch P, Tarbell NJ, et al. Total lymphoid irradiation to prevent graft rejection in recipients of HLA non-identical T cell-depleted allogeneic marrow. Bone Marrow Transplant. 1991;7:23–33.
56. Buckley RH, Schiff SE, Schiff RI, et al. Hematopoietic stem-cell transplantation for the treatment of severe combined immunodeficiency. N Engl J Med. 1999;340:508–16.
57. Aversa F, Tabilio A, Terenzi A, et al. Successful engraftment of T-cell-depleted haploidentical "three-loci" incompatible transplants in leukemia patients by addition of recombinant human granulocyte colony-stimulating factor-mobilized peripheral blood progenitor cells to bone marrow inoculum. Blood 1994;84:3948–55.
58. Ruggeri L, Capanni M, Urbani E, et al. Effectiveness of donor natural killer cell alloreactivity in mismatched hematopoietic transplants. Science 2002;295:2097–100.
59. van den Boogaardt DE, van Rood JJ, Roelen DL, Claas FH. The influence of inherited and noninherited parental antigens on outcome after transplantation. Transpl Int. 2006;19:360–71.
60. van Rood JJ, Loberiza FR Jr, Zhang MJ, et al. Effect of tolerance to noninherited maternal antigens on the occurrence of graft-versus-host disease after bone marrow transplantation from a parent or an HLA-haploidentical sibling. Blood 2002;99:1572–7.
61. Yoshihara T, Okada K, Kobayashi M, et al. Outcome of non-T-cell-depleted HLA-haploidentical hematopoietic stem cell transplantation from family donors in children and adolescents. Int J Hematol. 2007;85:246–55.
62. Oudshoorn M, Horn PA, Tilanus M, Yu N. Typing of potential and selected donors for transplant: methodology and resolution. Tissue Antigens. 2007;69 Suppl 1:10–2.
63. Mickelson EM, Bartsch GE, Hansen JA, Dupont B. The MLC assay as a test for HLA-D region compatibility between patients and unrelated donors: results of a national marrow donor program involving multiple centers. Tissue Antigens. 1993;42:465–72.
64. Oudshoorn M, Doxiadis, II, van den Berg-Loonen PM, Voorter CE, Verduyn W, Claas FH. Functional versus structural matching: can the CTLp test be replaced by HLA allele typing? Hum Immunol. 2002;63:176–84.
65. Gaziev D, Galimberti M, Lucarelli G, et al. Bone marrow transplantation from alternative donors for thalassemia: HLA-phenotypically identical relative and HLA-nonidentical sibling or parent transplants. Bone Marrow Transplant. 2000;25:815–21.
66. Drobyski WR, Klein J, Flomenberg N, et al. Superior survival associated with transplantation of matched unrelated versus one-antigen-mismatched unrelated or highly human leukocyte antigen-disparate haploidentical family donor marrow grafts for the treatment of hematologic malignancies: establishing a treatment algorithm for recipients of alternative donor grafts. Blood 2002;99:806–14.
67. Bunin N, Aplenc R, Leahey A, et al. Outcomes of transplantation with partial T-cell depletion of matched or mismatched unrelated or partially matched related donor bone marrow in children and adolescents with leukemias. Bone Marrow Transplant. 2005;35:151–8.
68. Mielcarek M, Storer BE, Sandmaier BM, et al. Comparable outcomes after nonmyeloablative hematopoietic cell transplantation with unrelated and related donors. Biol Blood Marrow Transplant. 2007;13:1499–507.

69. Petersdorf E, Bardy P, Cambon-Thomsen A, et al. 14th International HLA and Immunogenetics Workshop: report on hematopoietic cell transplantation. Tissue Antigens. 2007;69 Suppl 1:17–24.
70. Flomenberg N, Baxter-Lowe LA, Confer D, et al. Impact of HLA class I and class II high-resolution matching on outcomes of unrelated donor bone marrow transplantation: HLA-C mismatching is associated with a strong adverse effect on transplantation outcome. Blood 2004;104:1923–30.
71. Lee SJ, Klein J, Haagenson M, et al. High-resolution donor-recipient HLA matching contributes to the success of unrelated donor marrow transplantation. Blood 2007;110:4576–83.
72. Morishima Y, Sasazuki T, Inoko H, et al. The clinical significance of human leukocyte antigen (HLA) allele compatibility in patients receiving a marrow transplant from serologically HLA-A, HLA-B, and HLA-DR matched unrelated donors. Blood 2002;99:4200–6.
73. Morishima Y, Yabe T, Matsuo K, et al. Effects of HLA allele and killer immunoglobulin-like receptor ligand matching on clinical outcome in leukemia patients undergoing transplantation with T-cell-replete marrow from an unrelated donor. Biol Blood Marrow Transplant. 2007;13:315–28.
74. Petersdorf EW, Anasetti C, Martin PJ, et al. Limits of HLA mismatching in unrelated hematopoietic cell transplantation. Blood 2004;104:2976–80.
75. Sasazuki T, Juji T, Morishima Y, et al. Effect of matching of class I HLA alleles on clinical outcome after transplantation of hematopoietic stem cells from an unrelated donor. Japan Marrow Donor Program. N Engl J Med. 1998;339:1177–85.
76. Shaw BE, Gooley TA, Malkki M, et al. The importance of HLA-DPB1 in unrelated donor hematopoietic cell transplantation. Blood 2007;110:4560–6.
77. Gallardo D, Brunet S, Torres A, et al. Hla-DPB1 mismatch in HLA-A-B-DRB1 identical sibling donor stem cell transplantation and acute graft-versus-host disease. Transplantation 2004;77:1107–10.
78. Zino E, Vago L, Di Terlizzi S, et al. Frequency and targeted detection of HLA-DPB1 T cell epitope disparities relevant in unrelated hematopoietic stem cell transplantation. Biol Blood Marrow Transplant. 2007;13:1031–40.
79. Fleischhauer K, Locatelli F, Zecca M, et al. Graft rejection after unrelated donor hematopoietic stem cell transplantation for thalassemia is associated with nonpermissive HLA-DPB1 disparity in host-versus-graft direction. Blood 2006;107:2984–92.
80. Zino E, Frumento G, Marktel S, et al. A T-cell epitope encoded by a subset of HLA-DPB1 alleles determines nonpermissive mismatches for hematologic stem cell transplantation. Blood 2004;103:1417–24.
81. Loiseau P, Busson M, Balere ML, et al. HLA Association with hematopoietic stem cell transplantation outcome: the number of mismatches at HLA-A, -B, -C, -DRB1, or -DQB1 is strongly associated with overall survival. Biol Blood Marrow Transplant. 2007;13:965–74.
82. Petersdorf EW, Hansen JA, Martin PJ, et al. Major-histocompatibility-complex class I alleles and antigens in hematopoietic-cell transplantation. N Engl J Med. 20 2001;345:1794–800.
83. Morishima Y, Kawase T, Malkki M, Petersdorf EW. Effect of HLA-A2 allele disparity on clinical outcome in hematopoietic cell transplantation from unrelated donors. Tissue Antigens. 2007;69 Suppl 1:31–5.
84. Elsner HA, DeLuca D, Strub J, Blasczyk R. HistoCheck: rating of HLA class I and II mismatches by an internet-based software tool. Bone Marrow Transplant. 2004;33:165–9.
85. Heemskerk MB, Doxiadis, II, Roelen DL, Claas FH, Oudshoorn M. The HistoCheck algorithm does not predict T-cell alloreactivity in vitro. Bone Marrow Transplant. 2005;36:927–8.

86. Shaw BE, Barber LD, Madrigal JA, Cleaver S, Marsh SG. Scoring for HLA matching? A clinical test of HistoCheck. Bone Marrow Transplant. 2004;34:367–8;author reply 369.
87. Kawase T, Morishima Y, Matsuo K, et al. High-risk HLA allele mismatch combinations responsible for severe acute graft-versus-host disease and implication for its molecular mechanism. Blood 2007;110:2235–41.
88. Halloran PF, Reeve J, Kaplan B. Lies, damn lies, and statistics: the perils of the P value. Am J Transplant. 2006;6:10–1.
89. Urbano-Ispizua A. Risk assessment in haematopoietic stem cell transplantation: stem cell source. Best Pract Res Clin Haematol. 2007;20:265–80.
90. Hurley CK, Baxter Lowe LA, Logan B, et al. National Marrow Donor Program HLA-matching guidelines for unrelated marrow transplants. Biol Blood Marrow Transplant. 2003;9:610–5.
91. Ottinger HD, Muller CR, Goldmann SF, et al. Second German consensus on immuno-genetic donor search for allotransplantation of hematopoietic stem cells. Ann Hematol. 2001;80:706–14.
92. Horn PA, Elsner HA, Blasczyk R. Tissue typing for hematopoietic cell transplantation: HLA-DQB1 typing should be included. Pediatr Transplant. 2006;1:753–4.
93. Wagner JE, Rosenthal J, Sweetman R, et al. Successful transplantation of HLA-matched and HLA-mismatched umbilical cord blood from unrelated donors: analysis of engraftment and acute graft-versus-host disease. Blood 1996;88:795–802.
94. Rubinstein P, Carrier C, Scaradavou A, et al. Outcomes among 562 recipients of placental-blood transplants from unrelated donors. N Engl J Med. 1998;339:1565–77.
95. Gluckman E, Rocha V, Boyer-Chammard A, et al. Outcome of cord-blood transplantation from related and unrelated donors. Eurocord Transplant Group and the European Blood and Marrow Transplantation Group. N Engl J Med. 1997;337:373–81.
96. Gluckman E, Rocha V, Arcese W, et al. Factors associated with outcomes of unrelated cord blood transplant: guidelines for donor choice. Exp Hematol. 2004;32:397–407.
97. Wagner JE, Barker JN, DeFor TE, et al. Transplantation of unrelated donor umbilical cord blood in 102 patients with malignant and nonmalignant diseases: influence of CD34 cell dose and HLA disparity on treatment-related mortality and survival. Blood 2002;100:1611–8.
98. Eapen M, Rubinstein P, Zhang MJ, et al. Outcomes of transplantation of unrelated donor umbilical cord blood and bone marrow in children with acute leukaemia: a comparison study. Lancet 2007;369:1947–54.
99. Gluckman E, Rocha V. Donor selection for unrelated cord blood transplants. Curr Opin Immunol. 2006;18:565–70.
100. Laughlin MJ, Eapen M, Rubinstein P, et al. Outcomes after transplantation of cord blood or bone marrow from unrelated donors in adults with leukemia. N Engl J Med. 2004;351:2265–75.
101. Rocha V, Labopin M, Sanz G, et al. Transplants of umbilical-cord blood or bone marrow from unrelated donors in adults with acute leukemia. N Engl J Med. 2004;351:2276–85.
102. Ballen KK, Spitzer TR, Yeap BY, et al. Double unrelated reduced-intensity umbilical cord blood transplantation in adults. Biol Blood Marrow Transplant. 2007;13:82–9.
103. Brunstein CG, Barker JN, Weisdorf DJ, et al. Umbilical cord blood transplantation after nonmyeloablative conditioning: impact on transplantation outcomes in 110 adults with hematologic disease. Blood 2007;110:3064–70.
104. Haspel RL, Kao G, Yeap BY, et al. Preinfusion variables predict the predominant unit in the setting of reduced-intensity double cord blood transplantation. Bone Marrow Transplant. 2008;41:523–9.
105. Cornetta K, Laughlin M, Carter S, et al. Umbilical cord blood transplantation in adults: results of the prospective Cord Blood Transplantation (COBLT). Biol Blood Marrow Transplant. 2005;11:149–60.

106. Kogler G, Enczmann J, Rocha V, Gluckman E, Wernet P. High-resolution HLA typing by sequencing for HLA-A, -B, -C, -DR, -DQ in 122 unrelated cord blood/patient pair transplants hardly improves long-term clinical outcome. Bone Marrow Transplant. 2005;36:1033–41.
107. Ohnuma K, Isoyama K, Ikuta K, et al. The influence of HLA genotyping compatibility on clinical outcome after cord blood transplantation from unrelated donors. J Hematother Stem Cell Res. 2000;9:541–50.
108. Dupont B, Hsu KC. Inhibitory killer Ig-like receptor genes and human leukocyte antigen class I ligands in haematopoietic stem cell transplantation. Curr Opin Immunol. 2004;16:634–43.
109. Cooley S, McCullar V, Wangen R, et al. KIR reconstitution is altered by T cells in the graft and correlates with clinical outcomes after unrelated donor transplantation. Blood 2005;106:4370–6.
110. Miller JS, Cooley S, Parham P, et al. Missing KIR ligands are associated with less relapse and increased graft-versus-host disease (GVHD) following unrelated donor allogeneic HCT. Blood 2007;109:5058–61.
111. Miller JS, Soignier Y, Panoskaltsis-Mortari A, et al. Successful adoptive transfer and in vivo expansion of human haploidentical NK cells in patients with cancer. Blood 2005;105:3051–7.
112. Petersdorf EW, Malkki M, Gooley TA, Martin PJ, Guo Z. MHC haplotype matching for unrelated hematopoietic cell transplantation. PLoS Med. Jan 2007;4:e8.
113. Dickinson AM, Harrold JL, Cullup H. Haematopoietic stem cell transplantation: can our genes predict clinical outcome? Expert Rev Mol Med. 2007;9:1–19.
114. Dickinson AM, Middleton PG. Beyond the HLA typing age: genetic polymorphisms predicting transplant outcome. Blood Rev. Nov 2005;19:333–40.

Chapter 5
Immunogenomics and Proteomics in Hematopoietic Stem Cell Transplantation: Predicting Post-Hematopoietic Stem Cell Transplant Complications

Eva M. Weissinger and Anne M. Dickinson

5.1 Introduction

Since its early success in the 1950s, hematopoietic stem cell transplantation (HSCT) has continued to be carried out exponentially worldwide rising to over 7,000 transplants alone across Europe in 2007. HSCT is the major curative therapy for leukemia, lymphoma and other hematological diseases such as aplastic anemia and congenital immunodeficiency diseases such as severe combined immunodeficiency [1, 2]. In recent years it has also been used to down-regulate autoimmune diseases with success in juvenile rheumatoid arthritis and systemic lupus erythematosus [3, 4]. Allogeneic HSCT, however, still has a 40–50% risk of morbidity and mortality, largely due to complications that arise post-transplant, such as infection and graft-versus-host disease (GvHD). Matching between recipient and donor at human leukocyte antigen (HLA) loci is imperative to reduce GvHD, and among patients receiving transplants from matched unrelated donors (MUD), mismatches at either HLA Class I or Class II result in increased risk of GvHD, graft failure and overall survival [5].

Over the last 20 years, therefore, in vitro methods of predicting GvHD have been developed. Originally the mixed lymphocyte reaction (MLR) was used to identify responder lymphocytes in HLA-mismatched patient/donor pairs. The results, however, were too insensitive to correlate with GvHD responses post-transplant [6, 7]. Modifications of the MLR, utilizing limiting dilution techniques, diluting responder cells against a standard number of recipient lymphocytes and measuring either cytotoxic T lymphocyte precursor (CTLp) frequencies using tritiated thymidine uptake or helper T lymphocyte precursor (HTLp) responses measuring interleukin-2 (IL-2) production, were used and results assessed against post-transplant GvHD outcome [8–12]. Although CTLp frequencies correlated with both degree of HLA-mismatch and GvHD in the MUD transplant

E.M. Weissinger (✉)
Hannover Medical School, Department of Hematology, Hemostasis, Oncology and Stem Cell Transplantation, Carl-Neuberg-Str.1, 30625 Hannover, Germany
e-mail: mischak-weissinger.eva@mh-hannover.de

M.R. Bishop (ed.), *Hematopoietic Stem Cell Transplantation*,
Cancer Treatment and Research 144, DOI 10.1007/978-0-387-78580-6_5,

setting, they were too insensitive to detect minor histocompatibility antigen mismatches of HLA-matched sibling transplants and, therefore, the CTLp results did not correlate with GvHD. Several reports suggested that HTLp frequencies may correlate with GvHD in HLA-matched sibling transplants but results were inconsistent [11–15]. With the advent of high resolution HLA typing, CTLp and HTLp frequencies analysis has largely been made redundant. However, sensitive CTLp functional assays are still used to detect one amino acid differences between peptide sequences within the HLA antigen binding groove and are useful to assess "permissible" mismatches. A recent review by Claas et al. [16] summarizes the usefulness of measuring cellular and humoral immune responses for donor selection, and recent work suggests that for cytotoxic immune responses HLA mismatches with few amino acid differences appear immunogenic while HLA mismatches with many amino acid differences may be less or non-immunogenic [17]. These findings suggest that the HLA-Matchmaker algorithm, which takes into account differences in HLA triplet peptides, may not be a good predictor of response in HSCT [18].

Despite this important area of research, functional assays to predict HSCT outcome have largely been superseded by advanced DNA typing techniques based on DNA sequence polymorphisms including polymerase chain reaction (PCR), sequence specific primers (SSP) amplification, sequence specific oligonucleotide probes (SSOP), and heteroduplex analyses as reviewed by Little et al. [19].

Several alternative methods for predicting transplant outcomes, especially GvHD, have been published and utilized in a number of transplant centers. These methods have included modification of the MLR [20, 21], measurement of cytokines or other molecules either in the MLR supernatant, HTLp assay supernatants, e.g., interleukin 4 (IL-4) or serum levels of cytokines in the patient post-transplant [22–25].

One alternative method that was described by Vogelsang et al. used an in vitro skin explant assay for predicting GvHD in HLA-matched siblings [26]. The results from our laboratory have consistently verified the usefulness of the assay, which involves an MLR followed by incubation of donor MLR responder cells with patient skin pretransplant. The grade of histopathological damage in the skin (grades I–IV) parallels that seen in patients with clinical GvHD and, importantly, correlates with systemic and not just skin GvHD. The ability of the assay to predict GvHD pretransplant depends on the degree of prophylaxis given to the patient and type of transplant [27]. The assay can predict presence or absence of GvHD in 80% of HLA-matched sibling transplant patients when prophylaxis is cyclosporine alone [28, 29], but it is reduced to 50–60%, if patients are given cyclosporine plus methotrexate [27], or in the case of MUD transplants if the stem cell grafts are T-cell depleted [30]. Nevertheless, the assay has been used extensively to investigate the immunobiology of GvHD [28, 31–33] and has been shown to correlate with degree of HLA mismatch and minor histocompatibility mismatch in the way of female-to-male transplants [34].

The fact that some of the skin explant results could not fully predict outcome in HLA-matched sibling transplants together with the work of Holler and colleagues led researchers to investigate the role of non-HLA cytokine genes in HLA-matched sibling patient and donor pairs. Holler et al. had shown that pretransplant production by peripheral blood mononuclear cells of tumour necrosis factor alpha (TNFα) and interleukin-10 (IL-10) by peripheral blood mononuclear cells correlated with GvHD outcome; patients with high levels of TNFα during the conditioning period and low levels of IL-10 developed more severe GvHD [35]. At about the same time, Middleton et al. [36] demonstrated that patient or donor cytokine gene polymorphisms on *IL-10* and *TNF*α genes, which were associated with levels of production of these cytokines, correlated with transplant outcome. These initial results were studied in a heterogeneous cohort of HLA-matched siblings given either cyclosporine alone [36] or cyclosporine plus methotrexate [37] as GvHD prophylaxis. Since these analyses, a plethora of information has been reported on the numerous cytokine genes and other genes of molecules associated with both the immunopathology of GvHD, infection and innate immunity.

This chapter will therefore summarize the most recent results of these studies and usefulness to the clinician. In addition, methods of predicting post-transplant complications have been further developed by use of proteomics and this chapter will provide an overview on the use of these new technologies and the most recent results.

5.2 Cytokine Involvement in Graft-Versus-Host Disease

Graft-versus-host disease has been described as consisting of three phases involving an initial pretransplant phase giving rise to target organ (skin, gut, or liver) tissue damage caused by total body irradiation, cytotoxic drug therapy and release of pro-inflammatory cytokines such as TNFα and interleukin-1 (IL-1) with concomitant up regulation of molecules on target tissues such as HLA and adhesion molecules. The conditioning regimens may modulate this initial release with reduced conditioning regimens reducing this first phase of cytokine storm, causing less damage by release of lower levels of cytokines. Studies in animals and man [38] have shown that this initial release of cytokines can aid in predicting the severity of GvHD post-transplant. After this first phase, the incoming donor T cells recognizing target tissue as foreign by their over expression of HLA Class I and II molecules and adhesion molecules (e.g., ICAM) initiate the second phase of target cell damage via further release of T-cell cytokines such as interferon gamma (IFNγ). Host antigen presenting cells are involved in this second phase and exacerbate the effect of the T cells. The third phase or effector phase of the "cytokine storm" involves cellular cytopathic damage due to the direct action of T cells. In this regard, subsets of T cells, including T regulatory cells, may play a role in regulating the GvHD response. In recent years, in order to try to more fully understand the mechanisms of GvHD and to try to predict patient and donor responses, the genetics of cytokine and cytokine receptors and other molecules involved in the immune

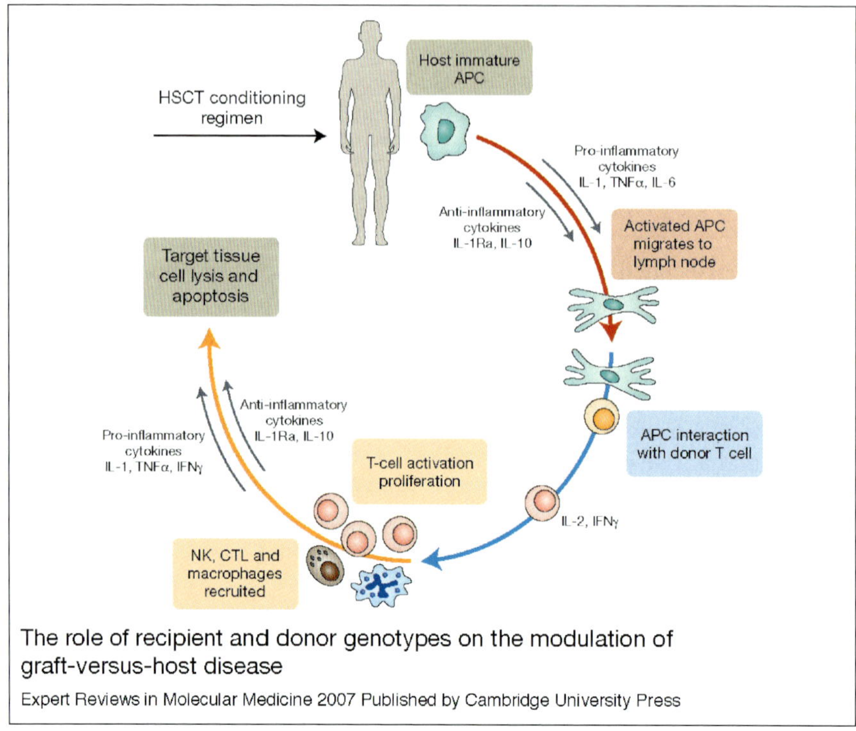

Fig. 5.1 Published with permission from Expert Reviews in Molecular Medicine 2007 (published by Cambridge University Press) and modified with permission from Cullup and Stark [48] (©2005 Taylor and Francis). The initial stage of the cytokine storm involves the effect of the conditioning regimen on the host tissues; activating antigen presenting cells (APCs), release of inflammatory cytokines, (e.g., IL-1, TNFα, IL-6) and initial damage to target tissues. This is influenced by the recipient genotype, producing levels of pro- and anti-inflammatory genotypes depending on the type of SNP or microsatellite polymorphism within the recipient genome. The activated APCs migrate to the lymph node and interaction in Phase two of the cytokine storm with incoming donor T cells. Via activation of T cells further cytokines are produced, e.g., IL-2, IFNγ, which are influenced by the donor genotype. During Phase three of the cytokine storm more cytokines are produced and the target tissues of GvHD undergo apoptosis and cellular damage. This phase is influenced by levels of both pro- and anti-inflammatory cytokines and genotypes f patient and donor

response of transplantation have been studied (See Figs. 5.1 and 5.2). Single nucleotide polymorphisms (SNPs) or microsatellites, with the regulatory sequences of genes encoding these molecules give rise to higher or lower in vitro or serum levels of these proteins. The majority of SNPs or microsatellites studied in the HSCT setting have also been investigated in disease-association studies including solid organ transplantation [39–40] and autoimmune diseases such as systemic lupus erythematosus (SLE) [41–45], juvenile chronic arthritis [46], and insulin dependent diabetes mellitus [47].

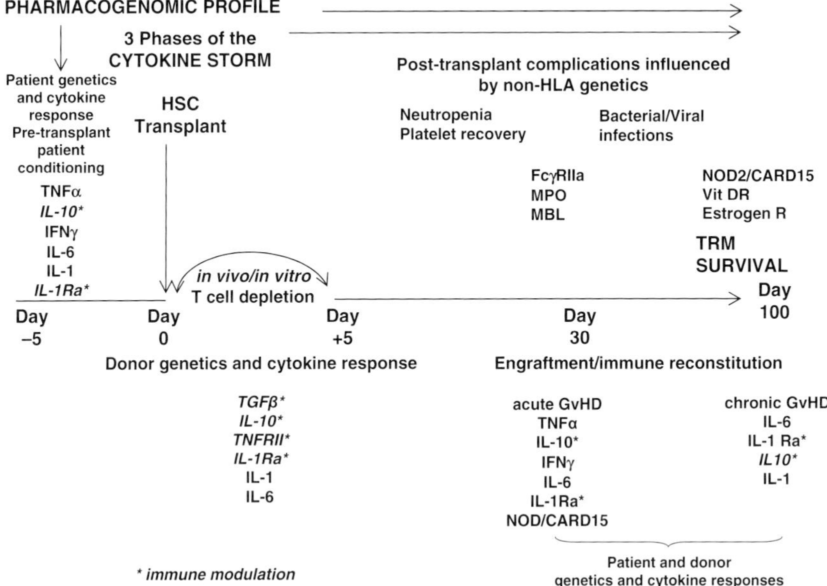

Fig. 5.2 Hematopoietic stem cell transplant schema; potential role of patient and donor, non-HLA genotypes. Pretransplant conditioning, either myeloablative or nonmyeloablative, influences the amount of cytokine release as well as patient genotype. In vitro or in vivo T cell depletion procedures as well as standard immunosuppression and GvHD prophylaxis protocols may alter the effect of patient or donor genotype at the time of transplant and during the engraftment and immune constitution phase. Ensuing post-therapy transplant complications including neutropenia, platelet engraftment, bacterial or viral infections have also been shown to be influenced by patient or donor genotype. Acute and chronic GvHD has been shown to be influenced by non-HLA genetics as has survival and transplant-related mortality (TRM). The pharmacogenomic profile of the patient or donor which may influence response to both the pretransplant conditioning drug regimens and well as post-transplant immunosuppression and GvHD prophylaxis drugs may also influence outcome and survival

The majority of the studies in the HSCT setting have been carried out in heterogeneous (relative to diagnosis, transplant type and condition regimens) HLA-matched sibling HSCT cohorts, although an increasing number of MUD transplants have started to be investigated. Results of patient and donor non-HLA genetics (including pro- and anti-inflammatory cytokines, cytokine receptors, and genes of other immune response molecules) have been correlated with respect to transplant outcome, including acute GvHD, chronic GvHD, transplant-related mortality, (TRM) overall survival, relapse, and infection. It is important to appreciate that of course correlation of patient non-HLA genotype may reflect all phases of the cytokine storm, whereas donor genotype reflects only phases two and three. In most studies both patient and donor genotypes are examined for associations with HSCT outcome [49].

5.2.1 Cytokine Genes

5.2.1.1 Tumour Necrosis Factor Alpha

Polymorphic genes located within the major histocompatibility complex (MHC) on chromosome 6 such as tumour necrosis factor alpha *(TNFA)*, lymphotoxin and the heat-shock proteins (e.g., *Hsp*), within the Class III region of the MHC complex, will be identical between patient and donor HLA-matched siblings. However in both the HLA-matched sibling and MUD transplant setting, genotypes of other genes, including those of cytokines not situated on chromosome 6, such as *IL-1* and *IL-6* genes, will differ between patient and donor.

TNFA polymorphisms are in linkage disequilibrium with HLA class I and class II genotypes, and since certain HLA genotypes are known to influence GvHD development, association with *TNFA* genotype may be secondary to or interact with the HLA associations [49, 50]. TNFα plays a central role in the pathogenesis of GvHD. It is a pro-inflammatory cytokine induced and produced by monocytes and macrophages during the initial phase of the cytokine storm, and it up regulates adhesion and MHC molecule expression on target organs as well as directly induce cell death [51].

The role of *TNFA* polymorphisms (SNPs and microsatellites), has been investigated in a number of studies with respect to HSCT outcome. *TNF-308* within the promoter region of the gene, reported to give rise to higher levels of TNFα in vitro and in vivo [52, 53], has been associated with GvHD, but results have been inconsistent. Some reports have demonstrated a positive association with acute GvHD [54, 55], but the majority of the larger studies found no association [36, 52, 56–59]. *TNFA –308*, along with the *TNFB* +1069 polymorphism, has been linked to toxic complications post-transplant [60].

Patients carrying the A allele of *TNFA* +488 have been shown to develop significantly higher grades of acute GvHD than +488A-negative patients, and the A allele was also associated with chronic GvHD and early death [56].

Of the microsatellite polymorphisms within *TNFA* (*TNFa*, *TNFb*, *TNFc*, *TNFd,* and *TNFe)* [61–63], *TNFd3* and *TNFa2* alleles are associated with high TNFα production, and the *TNFa6* allele with lower production [39, 64]. The *TNFd3* homozygous genotype has been associated with increased incidence of acute GvHD and early death [36, 37], and the *TNFd4* allele with development of moderate to severe acute GvHD [52]. In MUD transplantation, TNFα serum levels and patients homozygous for the *TNFd*3 or *TNFd*4 alleles have correlated with GvHD. Patients with these genotypes have significantly higher TNFα levels during conditioning and more frequently develop acute GvHD [65]. In addition to *TNFd*, the presence of the *d*4 allele in conjunction with the *TNFA* 1031C allele in either recipients or donors significantly increased the incidence of TRM [66]. *TNFa*5, an allele associated with the *TNFd*4/1031C haplotype, has been linked to increased TRM, and the *TNFd* microsatellite has been associated with survival. A decrease in survival rates however, has been reported for patients carrying *TNF d*3/*d*3, *d*4, and *d*5, compared to TNFd1/d2d3 genotypes [67].

In the MUD HSCT setting, possession of the *TNFA**2 allele SNP in the donor has been associated with severe (grade III–IV) acute GvHD. Strong linkage disequilibrium between the *TNFA* –308, –238 SNPs and extended HLA haplotypes exists and the *TNFA* –308/238 AG haplotype is also associated with significantly delayed neutrophil engraftment [50, 54].

TNFA –863 (C/A) and –857 (C/T) polymorphisms in donors and/or recipients correlate with a higher incidence of GvHD and a lower rate of relapse. When the analysis was carried out with HLA A-, HLA B-, and DRB1-matched pairs, the association with relapse, due to linkage disequilibrium, was not observed [68].

5.2.1.2 Tumour Necrosis Factor Receptor II

The mechanism of action of TNFα is mediated by the TNF superfamily receptors (TNFRSF) 1 and receptor 2. Tumor necrosis factor receptor II (TNFRII) gene mediates many of the functions of TNFα such as induction of nuclear factor κB (NF κB), cytokine production, cytotoxic responses, and proliferation of T and B cells [69–71]. TNFRSF2 is present on endothelial and hematopoietic cells, and via TNFα binding, induces apoptosis of CD8^{+} cells [70]. The *TNFRSF1B* gene is located on chromosome 1 at position 1p36 and an SNP(M/R) occurs within exon 6 at codon 196. The 196R TNFRII allele has been shown to upregulate IL-6 production, potentially aiding in the development of autoimmune B cells in some disease states [72]. It is therefore of relevance that patients undergoing HLA-matched sibling transplants homozygous for the R allele, have shown to have an increased incidence of extensive chronic GvHD [72, 73]. The R allele also associates with lower soluble TNFRSF2 levels in the serum and, therefore, comparatively higher TNF levels compared with the M allele [74]. MUD transplants patients receiving a transplant from *TNFRSF1B*–196R-positive donors have a higher incidence of severe GvHD and a lower rate of relapse than patients transplanted from 196 M homozygous donors [68].

5.2.1.3 Interleukin-10

Interleukin-10 (IL-10) inhibits T-cell proliferative responses and suppresses production of pro-inflammatory cytokines including TNFα, IL-1, IL-6, IL-12 and IFNγ. Several studies have suggested a role of IL-10 in inducing tolerance post-transplant. In a mouse model of GvHD, high levels of IL-10 were associated with exacerbation of GvHD, and low levels were protective. Holler et al. have shown that high pretransplant levels of IL-10 in patients' serum were protective of GvHD. Similar contrasting results have been reported on the role of IL-10 SNPs and microsatellites in controlling IL-10 production. The IL-10 gene lies on chromosome 1 (1q31-32) and contains several microsatellites and five SNPs that resolve into three haplotypes representing high l(GCC), intermediate (ATA), and low (ACC) producers of IL-10 [73]. Other reports, however, have shown that the GCC or –1082 G allele is associated with decreased production of IL-10 [75], and the –592A allele linked with the TC-ATA haplotype is associated with higher levels of IL-10 [76]. This latter haplotype has been associated with protection of GvHD in two large HLA-matched sibling cohorts [59].

Initial studies, in small but relatively homogeneous HLA-matched sibling transplants treated with cyclosporine alone or cyclosporine plus methotrexate, showed that ACC haplotype and the longer *IL10* –1064 $(CA)_n$ microsatellite (>12) alleles associated with the development of severe (grade III–IV) acute GvHD [36, 37]. The increasing number of CA short tandem repeats, which control IL-10 production, equating to decreased levels of IL-10 possession of ATA/ATA in the recipient genotype, has been shown to decrease the risk of acute GvHD in a large cohort of HLA-matched sibling transplants [59], and a study of peripheral blood stem cell transplants has demonstrated that the presence of *IL10* haplotypes (ACC/ACC vs ATA/ATC vs ATA/ATA) increased the incidence of chronic GvHD. Individuals possessing the ATA haplotype required longer immunosuppression and were more susceptible to invasive pulmonary aspergillosis [77, 78].

5.2.1.4 Interferon Gamma

Interferon gamma (IFNγ) is a pleiotropic regulatory cytokine with potent pro-inflammatory actions that are important in cellular anti-tumor and immune surveillance [79]. The first intron of the *IFNG* gene on chromosome 12q14-15 possesses a $(CA)_n$ microsatellite polymorphism with short tandem repeats. Pravica et al. showed that 12 CA repeats (allele 2) was associated with T (thymine) at position +874 and a greater level of in vitro IFNγ production by peripheral blood mononuclear cells than allele 3 [or 13 CA repeats; or A (adenine) at position +874] [80, 81]. The difference in this nucleotide sequence appears to affect the binding of nuclear factor-kappa B (NF-κB) and cytokine production [82]. In HLA-matched sibling transplants an association between recipient 3/3 homozygosity and an increased risk of acute GvHD has been reported [83]. Other studies have also shown an association between the possession in the patient, of the 3/3 genotype, i.e., lower IFNγ production, or lack of the 2/2 genotype, and acute or chronic GvHD [84, 85]. One explanation why lower IFNγ genotypes may be associated with GvHD incidence and severity may be due to IFNγ having a negative feedback regulatory role, as seen in some murine models, where weekly injections of IFNγ in a murine model of subacute GvHD prevented the condition and increased survival. In contrast, mice receiving stem cells from IFNγ-knockout donors developed accelerated lethal GvHD [86]. Another explanation may be the role of IFNγ in anti-viral surveillance since the presence of the IFNγ 3/3 genotype in the recipient has been associated with increased risk of Epstein-Barr virus reactions post-sibling or MUD HSCT [87].

5.2.1.5 Interleukin-1 Family

During conditioning, leakage of bacterial lipopolysaccharide (LPS) after damage to the gut endothelial cells initiates release of interleukin-1 (IL-1) and TNFα by monocytes and macroaphges. The IL-1 family consists of 10 structural members. The IL-1α and IL-1β genes (*IL1A* and *IL1B*) are agonists, and the IL-1 receptor (IL-1 Ra; gene IL-1RN) is a specific receptor antagonist, down regulating the production of IL-1, which is reviewed by Cullup and Stark [48]. Binding of IL-1 to its receptor leads to induction of a wide range of genes and other molecules that play a role in the inflammatory response such as cytokines (i.e., IL-6), chemokines, nitric oxide synthase, and type 2 cyclooxygenase.

The associations of polymorphisms in *IL1A*, *IL1B,* and *IL1RN* with HSCT outcomes have been investigated in HLA-matched sibling transplants and one small study of paediatric MUD transplants [48]. Possession of allele 2 in the donor genotype of the *IL1RN* variable number tandem repeat (VNTR), which down regulates IL-1 production, has correlated with less-severe acute GvHD. Possession of the same allele in the recipient genotype associated with acute GvHD [57, 88], and possession of allele 2 of the *IL1A* gene in the donor (either the VNTR or –889 polymorphism) has been associated with chronic GvHD [89].

5.2.1.6 Interleukin-6

Interleukin-6 (IL-6) is a pro-inflammatory cytokine produced by many cell types, including keratinocytes, monocytes, macrophages, and dendritic cells. In the presence of IL-2, IL-6 induces cytotoxic T cells and synergies with IL-13 to promote cell differentiation including B cell maturation.

The *IL6* gene is located on chromosome 7p21 and contains both microsatellites and SNPs [90, 91]. A G/C (guanine/cytosine) SNP is in the promoter region at position –174, and the G allele of this SNP correlates with higher serum IL-6 levels [46]. Several studies have also found the G allele associated with both acute GvHD and chronic GvHD following HLA-matched sibling transplants [49, 58, 83, 92].

5.2.1.7 Transforming Growth Factor Beta

Transforming Growth Factor β (TGFβ) is a pleiotropic cytokine with immunoregulatory properties. The two SNPs that exist within its gene on chromosome 19, at positions –800 (G/A) and –509 (C/T), associate with variations in plasma TGFβ concentration. The TT genotype at position –509 is associated with higher TGFβ production [93, 94]. A significant association between this high expression phenotype and severe GvHD has been reported, but no association was found with other HSCT outcomes [94, 95].

Polymorphisms at codons 10 and 25 of *TGFB*, result in amino acid substitutions (Leu/Pro and Arg/Pro respectively) and a link between possession of donor *TGFB* codon 10 polymorphism and the development of acute GvHD has been reported in a pediatric HSCT cohort [96]. The high-producer G/G genotype is also linked with the development of severe acute GvHD following both sibling and MUD transplants [95].

5.2.1.8 Other Cytokine Genes

Other cytokine genes and polymorphisms associated with HSCT outcome include IL-2, IL-7 and IL-18. They have to date only been studied in MUD transplant cohorts. The high producer IL-2 polymorphism, the G allele of a T/G SNP within the *IL2* gene promoter region at position −330, associates with an increased risk for acute GvHD [97], whereas polymorphisms within the IL-7 receptor genes and IL-18 genes have been associated with TRM and survival [98, 99].

5.2.2 Chemokines and Chemokine Receptors

The relationship between chemokines, their receptors, chemotaxis, and the inflammatory responses may also be influenced by genetic polymorphisms. One report has demonstrated that a *CCR5* gene deletion mutation (Δ32) resulted in loss of chemokine receptor function and protection from acute GvHD [100]. Another *CCR5* gene polymorphism (−2554 G/T in the promoter) has been linked to cytomegalovirus (CMV) infection, the virus [101] evading immune attack by T cells since homing to the site of inflammation is impaired.

5.2.3 Innate Immunity

Pathogen recognition receptors (PRRs) are molecules that recognize pathogens and activate the immune response. These include the transmembrane receptors, the toll-like receptors (TLR), and intracellular receptors such as the nucleotide-binding oligomerization domain (NOD) proteins. Antigen presenting cells (APCs) have ligands for different TLRs [102–104]. A few studies have investigated TLR genotype (TLR1, TLR4, and TLR6) and infection including invasive aspergillosis or bacteraemia [105, 106].

The NOD-like receptors are associated with inflammatory bowel disease, and there are three SNPs in *NOD2/CARD15* (nucleotide-binding oligomerization domains containing 2/caspase recruitment domain family number 15), SNP8, SNP12, and SNP13, which are involved in defective NF-κB responses. Several studies have now shown an association with these SNPs and sibling and MUD HSCT outcome. Presence of two or more *NOD2/CARD15* variants in either both the patient and donor genotype or either genotype has been shown to be associated with more severe GvHD and increased TRM [107]. In an HLA-matched sibling cohort [108] gastrointestinal decontamination before transplantation alleviated the genetic risk of the NOD mutation. Possession of *NOD2/CARD15* SNPs in T-cell depleted transplants was associated with lower disease-free survival [109]. In additional studies the NOD mutations have been associated with a severe complication of HSCT, bronchiolitis obliterans. These results illustrate the importance of the altered immune response associated with *NOD* gene variants and demonstrate how the type of immunomodulation (e.g., bacterial decontamination) or type of immunosuppression (e.g., T-cell depletion) may modulate the genetic risk.

A number of molecules responsible for interacting with pathogens such as mannose-binding lectin (MBL), which binds a range of pathogens, and myeloperoxidase (MPO), which opsonizes them, have a number of SNPs within their regulatory genes. The incidence of severe bacterial infections has been associated post-transplant with the myeloperoxidase gene (*MPO*) SNPs, while SNPs in the promoter region of *MBL* affect serum MBL levels with low MBL levels being associated with an elevated risk of infection in immunocompromised individuals. Although results have not been confirmed [57], *MBL2* mutations in the recipient and/or donor genotype have been associated with risk of major infection following HSCT [110]. Other genotypes that have been studied with respect to infectious episodes include the *Fcγ RIIa*-R 131 genotype and *FcRIIIb* HNA-1a/HNA-1b [57, 111], which are present in the genes encoding Fcγ receptor present on Langerhan cells, dendritic cells, endothelial cells, and leukemic cells.

5.2.4 Other Polymorphisms Studied for Association with HSCT Outcome

The restriction fragment length polymorphisms (RFLPs) within intron 8 of the vitamin D receptor (*VDR*) and intron 1 of the estrogen receptor (*ESR*) genes were found to correlate with acute GvHD and lower overall survival [112, 113]. The *FAS* –670 G allele has been correlated with infection and chronic GvHD [56], and the *HSPA1L* SNP has been linked to toxic complications in two independent transplant cohorts [114, 115]. An increasing interest is also being developed in the potential use of pharmacogenomics in HSCT with polymorphisms within genes encoding for some of the enzymes associated with some of the more commonly used drugs in HSCT, such as methotrexate, being more intensively studied. In this regard, an SNP (C677T) within the gene encoding methylenetetrahydrofolate reductase (*MTHFR*), an enzyme involved in methotrexate metabolism, has recently been associated with HSCT outcome in a number of studies, but results have been inconsistent [116–121].

5.3 Predicting Outcome Using Proteomics and Non-HLA Genetics and Application to the Clinic

Owing to the heterogeneity of the patient cohorts across HSCT centers, studies using either non-HLA genetics or proteomics to determine outcomes are fraught with potential difficulties that may only be overcome by stratification of HSCT protocols across transplant centers and studies of more homogeneous patient populations. It has, for example, been shown in a number of studies that the same SNP has been associated with acute rather than chronic GvHD and survival depending on the transplant cohort under study. In addition there have been a number of negative associations in one cohort and not in another. Negative associations for example, have included the *TNFd* microsatellite, with many studies demonstrating no association at all with either GvHD or outcome [36, 49, 52, 57–59, 66]. Other negative associations include those for *IL1B* –511, *IL1RN* –9261, *IL6* –174, *IL10* –592A/C and −1082 A/G, *TNFA* −308, *IL4R* −1902 and −3223, *IL1RN* VNTR86 intron 2, and *IL2* genotypes [59, 67]. All HSCT genotypic analysis must take into account clinical risk factors, such as age, female-to-male transplants, CMV status of patient and donor, stage of disease at transplant, and time of diagnosis to transplant. The type of conditioning and GvHD prophylaxis protocols all may influence the immunobiology of the transplant and the impact of non-HLA genetics. In addition other biomarkers such as those identified from proteomics assays may also be influenced by the type of transplant protocol. Several clinical risk factors have been included in risk models for assessment of the outcome of HSCT [58, 122–125].

Algorithms for survival and GvHD outcome are being developed. One clinical model for predicting mortality of patients with GvHD uses parameters such as bilirubin levels, treatment with steroids, and performance score [126]. A clinical model for overall survival for chronic myelogenous leukemia uses clinical factors to devise a risk score that can be applied to the clinic [123].

These clinical risk assessments may potentially be improved by the addition of non-HLA genotypes. For example if HLA typing for patient and donor reveals after multivariate statistics two or three non-HLA genotypes which influence outcome, these could be added to a known clinical assessment to develop an individualized scoring system for patients, allowing the clinician to assess, pretransplant, the best therapy and clinical protocol. In addition this type of risk analysis could also include biomarkers, which may include cell surface marker characteristics, e.g., those of dendritic cells and/or serum factors or proteins identified by proteomic screening of tissue culture supernatant or body fluids.

5.4 Overview of Proteome Research

Proteome analysis is a newly evolving field gaining rapidly in importance for application in clinical research as well as in the diagnosis of a variety of diseases. About 35,000 genes code for more than a million different proteins, thus underlining the possibilities for diagnosis based on proteomic research, but also highlighting the potential problems associated with using proteins for diagnostic purposes. The vast number of proteins and peptides that are expressed in cells, cellular compartments, or excreted in body fluids (e.g., plasma, serum, urine) makes the detection, separation and identification of particular peptides or proteins (important for particular diseases or changes within the body) particularly challenging. Historically, the analysis of body fluids has a longstanding reputation for detecting changes in the health status of individuals. The introduction of electrophoresis in the early 1950s allowed separation and detection of potentially distinct proteins [127] in urine. In 1975, O'Farrell described the separation of proteins of *Escherichia coli* by two-dimensional gel electrophoresis, [128] performing proteomics for the first time. Nowadays, with modern mass spectrometers for the analysis of proteins and peptides as well as the development of sophisticated bioinformatics to evaluate and compare the vast amount of information generated, the era of proteomics has started with profound hope for the future of diagnostics, following in the footsteps of "genomics."

5.4.1 *Basic Considerations*

Several key aspects have to be taken into account when performing clinical proteomic analysis. These have recently been reviewed in detail [129]. Among these, a well defined clinical question is essential, together with assessment of reproducibility/comparability of the analysis (including pre-analytical parameters), application of appropriate statistics, and validation of the results in a blinded cohort, are the most important factors for consideration.

The proteins in a complex sample cannot be analyzed without prior preparation in mass spectrometry (MS). Different modes of separation can be applied to complex samples, and are summarized together with MS approaches below. All modern MS techniques currently require appropriate sample preparation, as well as fractionation/separation steps prior to the MS analysis (Fig. 5.3). Separation of the proteins and peptides within one sample is most commonly performed by gel electrophoresis (two dimensional, 2DE) or by liquid chromatography (LC) or capillary electrophoresis (CE). Mass spectrometry has been vigorously developed over the past decades, and a vast number of instruments and technology platforms are currently available. A mass spectrometer consists of an ion source (ionization), a mass analyzer that measures the mass-to-charge ratio (m/z) of the ionized analytes, and a detector that registers the number of

Sample Preparation	• removal of salts and confounding materials • enrichment for protein and peptides
Separation	• (2D)-gel electrophoresis • HPLC-fractionation • (capillary) electrophoresis
Ionization	• Matrix Assisted Laser Desorption Ionization (MALDI) • Electrospray Ionization (ESI)
Mass Spectrometry	• Iontrap • time of flight (Q-TOF, TOF/TOF) • quadrupole mass spectrometer • Fourier transform ion cyclotron resonance
Data evaluation	• Statistics • Bioinformatics

Fig. 5.3 Summary of steps common in all proteomic techniques: Sample preparation: Once the proper sample is chosen (blood, urine, other) the sample has to be prepared for the analysis. Ideally, a crude unprocessed sample should be analyzed, in order to avoid artifacts, such as loss of analytes (peptides) or biases arising from sample preparation. The presence of large molecules, e.g., albumin, immunoglobulin and others, hamper this direct approach and will interfere with the detection of smaller, less abundant proteins and peptides. Thus preparation of the samples is necessary, but should be limited to a few steps, such as removal of large molecules and enrichment for proteins and peptides. Separation: the high complexity of biological samples also calls for a separation step, prior to MS-analysis. Gel electrophoreses (one or two dimensions), fractionation using High Performance Liquid Chromatography (HPLC) and capillary electrophoresis are most commonly used to separate analytes according to their size, isoelectric point and charge, respectively prior to analysis in the MS. A mass spectrometer consists of an ion source (ionization) in combination with mass analyzers, which measure the m/z ratio and detectors registering the number of ions at each m/z value (mass spectrometry) yielding to the signal intensity. Ionization: Electrospray ionization (ESI) and matrix-assisted laser desorption/ ionization (MALDI) are the two techniques most commonly used to volatize and ionize the proteins or peptides for mass spectrometry. ESI ionizes the analytes out of a solution and is therefore readily coupled to liquid-based (for example, chromatographic like high performance liquid chromatography; HPLC) or electrophoretic, like capillary electrophoresis (CE) separation tools. MALDI sublimates and ionizes the samples out of a dry, crystalline matrix via laser pulses. MALDI-MS is normally used to analyze relatively simple peptide mixtures, whereas integrated liquid-chromatography ESI-MS systems (LC-MS) are preferred for the analysis of complex samples. Mass spectrometry: Essentially four different types of mass analyzers are used in proteomics; these are the ion trap, time-of-flight (TOF), quadrupole (Q) and Fourier transform ion cyclotron resonance (FT-ICR) analyzers, which can either stand alone or are combined in tandem in order to combine different benefits of instruments. Data evaluation: most proteomic studies in a clinical setting showed that not a single marker, but rather a pattern of different biomarkers may be more useful for differential diagnosis of diseases. Thus, statistic analysis and applications of tools like support vector machines (SVM [130]) become increasingly important for clinically oriented proteomic analysis

ions at each m/z value (mass spectrometry). The ion sources most frequently used are electrospray ionization (ESI) based ionizers and matrix assisted laser desorption/ionization (MALDI). ESI is capable of ionizing in liquid phase and readily combined with LC or CE for separation. This technology platform is used for highly complex samples. MALDI ionizes the sample on a dry, crystalline surface and is most commonly used for less complex samples. Both ionizers can be combined with the mass analyzers described in the following part. The mass analyzer is central to the technology, and its key parameters are sensitivity, resolution, and mass accuracy. Although there are several mass analyzers available, here we focus on those essentially used in proteomic screening approaches. In general four mass analyzers are currently in use for proteomic screening: ion-trap, time-of-flight (TOF), quadrupole (Q), and Fourier transform-ion cyclotron resonance (FT-ICR) instruments or their combinations (e.g., hybrid instruments such as Q-TOF, combining quadrupole and time-of-flight). Ion trap analyzers capture ions for a certain time interval, and these are then subjected to MS. In time of flight (mainly reflector TOF) analyzers, the ions are accelerated to high kinetic energy and are separated along a flight tube as a result of their different velocities. The reflector compensates for slight differences in kinetic energy. TOF are most commonly used today in preclinical and clinical proteomics approaches. Quadrupole analyzers select by time-varying electric fields between four rods, which permit a stable trajectory only for ions of a particular desired m/z. The Fourier transform ion cyclotron resonance (FT-ICR) analyzers are ion traps, but they do so with the help of strong magnetic fields in a high vacuum. FT-ICR have particularly high sensitivity, mass accuracy, resolution and wide dynamic ranges, but the expense and the operational complexity currently limit the application in proteomic research. To obtain sequence information as well as information on post-translational modifications (PTMs), sequential use of these techniques, termed tandem mass spectrometry (MS/MS), is employed. In general, the first MS instrument serves as a mass filter, permitting only ions with the mass of interest ("parent ions"), and the second MS instrument analyzes the fragmentation products ("daughter ions"), which may be generated by collision with other molecules (collision-induced dissociation) or transfer of electrons (electron transfer dissociation). Frequently, individual advantages of the different mass spectrometers are combined (e.g., the precision of quadrupoles and the high accuracy of the measurements of mass with TOF in a Q-TOF instrument). The choice of the technology platform used will strongly depend on the choice of sample and vice versa. Clinical proteomics can be seen as a comparative analysis of multidimensional datasets, which is further complicated by biological variability. It cannot be overemphasized that any experiment must include assessment of all variable parameters in order to accurately evaluate the data. Furthermore, appropriate use of the correct statistical methods (e.g., adjustment for multiple variables) is of the outmost importance. Common steps required for proteomic screening are shown in Fig. 5.3.

Four different MS based technology platforms are currently predominantly used for proteomic analysis associated with clinical application and are briefly described below. The first two approaches, two dimensional gel electrophoresis followed by MS (2DE-MS) and liquid chromatography fractionation followed by MS (LC-MS), appear less well suited for routine clinical application mostly due to their running time. However these techniques play an important role in the further processing of information obtained via high throughput proteomic techniques, especially when used with tandem-MS for sequencing defined biomarkers. Consequently, biomarkers identified with these technologies have to be subsequently transferred to another platform to validate them for clinical use. The latter two, Surface enhance laser desorption ionization (SELDI)-MS, and capillary electrophoresis coupled on line to an ESI-TOF (CE-MS) are in principal applicable to clinical use.

5.4.1.1 Two-Dimensional Gel Electrophoresis Followed by Mass Spectrometry (2DE-MS)

The two-dimensional gel electrophoresis (2DE) method reported by O'Farrell in 1975 [128], laid the foundation for what we understand today as proteomics. Proteins are first separated by electrofocusing (proteins migrate to their isoelectric point in a pH gradient) and then in a perpendicular dimension by sodium dodecyl sulfate polyacrylamide gel electrophoresis (SDS-PAGE), proteins migrate based on their molecular mass. This procedure enables the separation of >1,000 unidentified proteins, which can be visualised using different staining or labeling procedures. However, proteins are not identified yet. A major advancement in the identification of proteins was achieved with the implementation of MS. The first step in the process of identifying proteins in the 2DE spots by MS is a proteolytic in-gel digestion (e.g., by exposing the excised spot to trypsin) [131, 132] followed by extraction of the proteolytic fragments from the gel. Masses of at least three proteolytic fragments are needed for identification of a protein from a database of proteins. The identity of a match can be subsequently verified by tandem MS (MS/MS) sequencing or by other techniques, such as western blotting (if a specific antibody is available). Limitations of the 2DE approach include low reproducibility, the considerable time for the analysis, and the difficulty of automating the process. Recently, the concept of two-dimensional differential in-gel electrophoresis (2D-DIGE) has been introduced to reduce gel-to-gel variability. Briefly, two samples are differentially labeled with fluorescent dyes (Cy3 and Cy5), and the two samples are then resolved simultaneously within the same 2DE gel (Fig. 5.4). While the comparison of two samples with 2D-DIGE has been satisfactory [133], the comparison of several different experiments remains challenging. In addition post-translational modifications cannot be identified by use of this technique, since the excised spots are subjected to tryptic digestion prior to MS/MS analyses for sequence information. Furthermore, the technique is generally limited to proteins >10 kDa. Nevertheless,

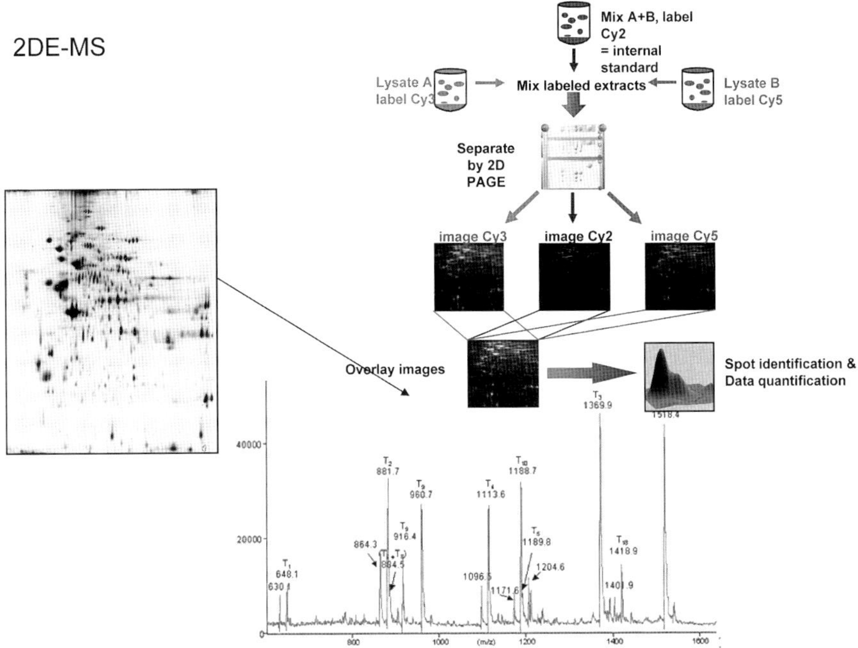

Fig. 5.4 Two-dimensional gel electrophoresis coupled mass spectrometry (2-DE-MS). (**a**) Proteins in samples from different individuals are separated in two dimensions according to the isoelectric point and molecular weight. The resulting 2D-gels are stained and compared. (**b**) Protein spots that appear to differ between the two gels are excised, digested with trypsin, and the resulting peptides analyzed using mass spectrometry. (**c**) Derivatization of the samples before analysis using different fluorescent dyes allows the analysis of two different samples in the same gel

2DE-MS still appears to be the method of choice for the comparative analysis of unmodified medium size or large proteins in the discovery phase of biomarker definition.

5.4.1.2 Liquid Chromatography Coupled to Mass Spectrometry

Liquid chromatography (LC) provides a powerful fractionation method compatible with virtually any mass spectrometer [134, 135]. LC-columns can separate large amounts of analytes with high resolution [135]. Therefore, if the sensitivity of detection is a consideration, LC is an excellent choice. Sequential separation using different principles (e.g., ion-exchange followed by reversed phase chromatography) in two independent steps provides a multidimensional fractionation that can generate vast amounts of information. Multidimensional protein identification technology (MudPIT, Fig. 5.5) [136–138] or a 2D liquid-phase fractionation

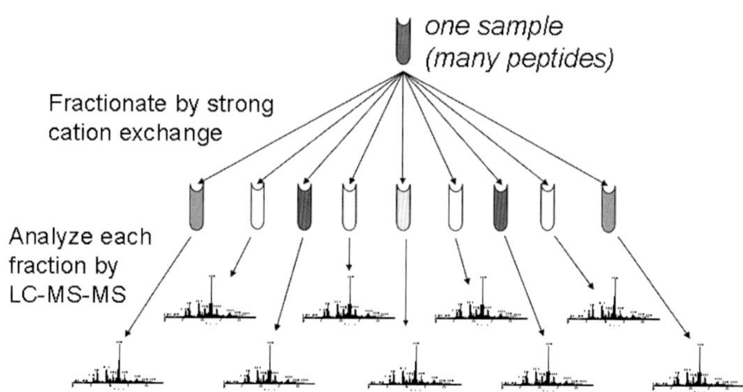

Fig. 5.5 Multidimensional liquid chromatography coupled mass spectrometry (LC-MS). Proteins are digested and fractionated in first dimension, utilizing cation- or anion-exchange chromatography. Each of these individual fractions is subsequently analyzed in depth, e.g., by reversed phase LC coupled to MS/MS instruments

approach [139] are well suited for in-depth analysis of body fluids such as urine. Limitations include difficulties with comparative analysis in part due to the variability in multidimensional separations, and the substantial time required for analysis of a single sample (generally days). Furthermore, the method suffers from its sensitivity to interfering compounds (e.g., lipids or detergents, large molecules that may precipitate and/or adsorb to the column) [140].

5.4.1.3 Surface-Enhanced Laser Desorption Ionization Mass Spectrometry

Surface-enhanced laser desorption ionization mass spectrometry (SELDI-MS) is an MS-based approach for the proteomic analysis of body fluids that has frequently been used in multiple clinically relevant investigations since it provides a simple and user-friendly solution to several obstacles of proteome analysis [141–143]. SELDI reduces the complexity of samples by fractionation based on selective interactions of polypeptides with different immobilized matrices, like reverse-phase or ion-exchange materials, ligands, etc. Due to the selectivity and the limited capacity of the active surface, only a small fraction of the polypeptides in a sample binds to the surface of the SELDI chip, facilitating the subsequent MS analysis of the originally highly complex samples (Fig. 5.6). Numerous reports on biomarkers for a variety of diseases have been published using this strategy [144–147]. However, the utility of the SELDI-MS approach has subsequently been heavily debated [148–150].

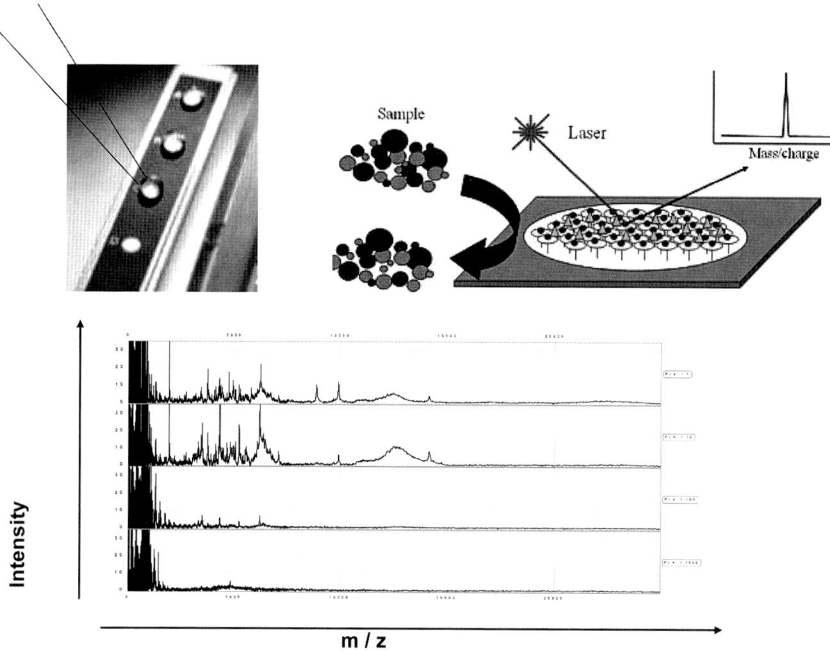

Fig. 5.6 Surface-enhanced laser desorption ionization mass spectrometry (SELDI-MS). The sample is deposited on the active chip surface (*upper left*). After several washing steps, only a few proteins stay bound to the surface; these are subsequently analyzed using low-resolution mass spectrometry. The lower panel shows a typical SELDI-MS spectrum from urine (reprinted with permission from Neuhoff et al. [152])

Problems include low resolution of the spectrometer, which have been addressed by the use of more appropriate units, such as MALDI-TOF instruments, as recently described [151].

5.4.1.4 Capillary Electrophoresis Coupled with Mass Spectrometry

Capillary electrophoresis coupled with mass spectrometry (CE-MS) is based on capillary electrophoresis (CE), instead of LC, as a fractionation device coupled to a mass spectrometer. CE separates proteins based on migration in the electrical field (300–500 V/cm) with high resolution. CE-MS has the advantage of providing fast and robust separation at high resolution (Fig. 5.7a, b) [153], is compatible with most buffers and analytes [154], and it provides a stable constant flow, thereby avoiding gradients in the buffer that may otherwise hamper detection by MS [155]. As LC, CE can be interfaced with most mass spectrometers, and technical considerations that must be taken into account for such coupling have been reviewed [140, 154, 156]. Limitations include that it is difficult to apply CE for the analysis of high-molecular-weight proteins. This is

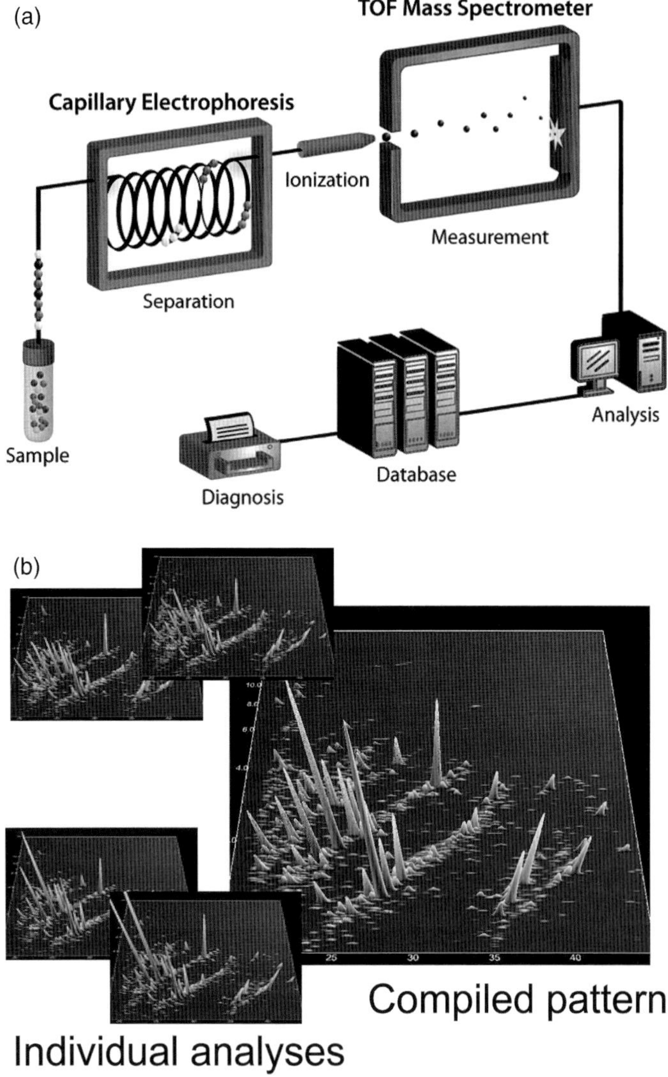

Fig. 5.7 **(a)** Schematic drawing of the on-line coupling of capillary electrophoresis to the mass spectrometer (CE-MS). Capillary electrophoresis separates polypeptides according to their charge and size. After the electrophoretic separation, the polypeptides are ionized on-line by the application of high voltage and analyzed in the mass spectrometer (ESI-TOF). The combination of the two instruments yields a mass spectrogram of mass per charge plotted against migration time. Subsequently, specialized software solutions allow automated data interpretation. **(b)** Urine samples of different individuals are analyzed by CE-MS (**a**). The small panels on the left in (**b**) are data sets obtained from samples from healthy volunteers. Proteins are displayed as peaks defined by migration time, molecular weight, and signal amplitude (*colour coded*). (*Right*) Data can be compiled to generate a typical pattern. The migration time (in min) and the mass (in kD, on a logarithmic scale) are indicated

due to the acidity of the buffer generally used for CE-MS analysis, which results in precipitation of larger proteins. Another limitation of CE is the relatively small sample volume that can be loaded onto the capillary (less than 1 μl), leading to a lower sensitivity of detection in comparison to LC. Improved methods of ionization by micro- or nano-ion spray and improvements in the detection limits of mass spectrometers enabling detection in the low- or sub-femtomol range [157–159] eliminated this problem to a large degree. For MS/MS sequencing, the limited amount of sample that can be loaded represents a significant obstacle. However, CE-MS data can be matched to LC-MS/MS data, using migration time as a second identifying parameter [160]. A combination of CE-MS analysis enabling higher throughput and consequently data of higher statistical quality with LC-MS/MS for subsequent sequencing of the potential biomarkers may be a promising approach for biomarker discovery.

Success is dependent on the choice of sample for any research or diagnostic study. Two basic sources of material are available for proteomic studies: body fluids (e.g., urine and blood) and tissue. While examination of tissue may theoretically be advantageous, several issues like ease of accessibility and high variability due to different cell types have greatly hindered progress in this field. As outlined recently, investigation of tissue may lead to the discovery of biomarkers that can subsequently be detected in body fluids [161]. Since such approaches currently are in their infancy, we will not further elaborate on them.

In contrast to polypeptides in tissues and most types of cells, the polypeptides in body fluids are relatively easily accessible and changes within the circulating peptides/proteins can theoretically be readily detected. Comprehensive profiling of peptides and proteins in body fluids such as plasma or urine has advantages over the analysis of proteins and peptides expressed in particular cells or tissues. Among various body fluids, urine and blood derived fluids (plasma, serum) are the most extensively investigated. While blood-derived samples appear certainly as the first choice, more in depth investigation has revealed several, yet unresolved problems. Activation of proteases and consequently generation of an array of proteolytic breakdown products is often associated already with the collection [162]. Standardization of collection protocols and storage is therefore necessary, since different pre-analytical handling and activation of proteases appear to be major causes for a lack of comparability between different centers. Further, the enormous dynamic range of proteins of 10^{12} appears to be yet another major obstacle [161, 163].

On the other hand, urine appears to be an especially attractive source of information [164]. One of the first attempts to define the urinary proteome was published by Spahr, Davis et al. [165, 166] Using liquid chromatography mass spectrometry (LC-MS) tryptic peptides of pooled urine samples were analyzed and 124 proteins were identified. While this study did not attempt to define any urinary biomarkers for a disease, it clearly highlighted the amount of information in the urinary proteome and also indicated a possible approach toward its mining. More recently, Adachi et al. identified more than 1,500 proteins (or their fragments) in the urine of healthy individuals, further underlining the complexity of the human urinary proteome [167].

There are several advantages of urine testing compared to blood (serum or plasma):

(1) Urine can be obtained in large quantities by non-invasive procedures. Consequently, ample material is available for analysis, assessment of reproducibility, and for optimization of analytical protocols. In addition, repeated sampling from the same individual is simple, facilitating longitudinal studies.

(2) Urine generally contains proteins and peptides of lower molecular mass (<30 kDa) that are highly soluble. Higher molecular weight proteins are removed by the physiological function of the kidney. Higher molecular-weight compounds can be removed by ultrafiltration without substantial loss of information, easing the analysis. If the ultrafiltration step is performed in the presence of a detergent and a chaotropic agent (e.g., urea and SDS), protein-protein interactions (and consequently irreproducible loss of analyte) are avoided [168]. These features facilitate analysis of such polypeptides in their natural state, without any need for additional manipulation (e.g., tryptic digests).

(3) Urinary polypeptides are stable and generally do not undergo significant proteolysis within several hours after the collection. Urine stored for up to 3 days at 4°C or up to 6 h at room temperature by two independent groups was shown to be stable in its composition [147, 169]. In contrast, blood collection is associated with free activation of proteases and consequently generation of an array of proteolytic breakdown products [162]. Nonetheless, standardization of the collection protocol and storage of the samples is of utmost importance if the information is to be used/ validated as a diagnostic test.

5.4.2 Proteomics in Hematopoietic Stem Cell Transplantation

The outcome of HSCT is influenced by the occurrence of opportunistic infections and GvHD, both adding to morbidity and mortality after HSCT together with recurrence of the malignant disease [122, 170]. Screening for the occurrence of complications after HSCT in an unbiased manner is a desirable goal, and proteomic analyses may help toward the identification of biomarkers associated with particular complications, such as acute GvHD or concomitant infectious episodes. GvHD is still a major cause of morbidity and mortality after HSCT, developing in about 35–70% of the patients and requiring immunosuppressive therapy in more than 35% [171]. To date, the diagnosis of acute GvHD is mainly based on clinical features, such as skin rash, gastrointestinal complications, or elevation of liver enzymes, and is verified with tissue biopsies and histopathological examination. Several single markers have been described to be elevated during infection or inflammation after allogeneic HSCT or specific for acute GvHD [32, 172, 173]. Although these studies are interesting and show promising results, it is unlikely that one single marker will be increased or decreased on more than one occasion, thus making differential diagnosis of similar diseases difficult. Proteomic screening allows the analysis of an enormous number of proteins and peptides and thus enables a profiling and pattern generation for specific diseases and recognition of yet unknown proteins and potential key players in the development of post-transplant complications. The simultaneous monitoring of more than one protein or peptide within a sample holds greater promise for the differential diagnosis of diseases, including acute GvHD.

Recently, the application of proteomic tools allowing screening for differentially expressed or excreted proteins in body fluids is gaining importance in the field of haematology [174, 175]. While the data on proteomic screening after HSCT are still limited, some results have been published and will be briefly be described below. CE-MS has been applied over the past 4–5 years to a number of clinical samples in order to establish proteomic screening as an additional diagnostic tool for a variety of diseases, but also for early detection of the development of acute GvHD. CE-MS allows the simultaneous analysis of more than a thousand different proteins and peptides in one sample within a short time period [164, 176]. In CE-MS, proteins and peptides are identified via their specific m/z ratio, the migration time in the capillary electrophoresis, as well as the signal intensity, which gives a measure of the relative abundance of the peptides [177]. The method allows compilation of data generated from different samples as well as patients and thus allows the generation of proteomic patterns specific for different pathological conditions (Fig. 5.6, lower panel). The specific patterns may also be modulated during disease progression or response to therapy and thus may add to current diagnostic and follow up criteria [178]. Support vector machine (SVM) based model prediction [130] allows the best possible separation of disease groups and controls.

CE-MS has recently been applied to generate proteomic patterns for the early diagnosis of acute GvHD [179, 180]. Screening of urine samples collected and analyzed at the time of GvHD development yielded 170 polypeptides differentially excreted in samples from patients with or without acute GvHD. From these peptides 31 were chosen to form a tentative acute GvHD-specific pattern. Application of this pattern to 599 blinded samples from 141 patients enabled diagnosis of acute GvHD grade II or more, even prior to clinical diagnosis with a sensitivity of 83.1% [95% CI 731–879] and a specificity of 75.6% [95% CI 716–794]. To date, this study is the first to correlate proteomic data with the clinical diagnosis of acute GvHD using a blinded, prospectively collected, multicenter approach. Other groups have investigated the changes induced by GvHD by application of different proteomic approaches and technology platforms. Wang and colleagues applied an intact-protein based quantitative analysis on plasma samples derived prior to any signs of acute GvHD (between engraftment and day + 21 after HSCT) or collected within 24 h of acute GvHD diagnosis [181]. After removal of the most abundant proteins by immunodepletion, samples were labeled with fluorescence dye (Cy5 or Cy3) prior to liquid isoelectric focusing and subsequent fractionation with reversed phase HPLC. The third dimension was SDS-PAGE. In this paper 75 differentially expressed candidate peptides and proteins were described that could be indicative for acute GvHD development. Tryptic digestions of differentially expressed bands and subsequent MS/MS analysis and database search yielded the identification of 48 proteins, including HLA-Class I, T cell receptor beta, integrin-alpha and vitronectin, all increased in expression in samples collected at diagnosis of acute GvHD. It will be interesting to see whether the proteins and peptides described in this study can be correlated to the onset of GvHD in a prospective manner. Two other papers describe the application of SELDI-MS to either serum collected from patients with and without GvHD after allogeneic HSCT [182] or saliva collected from patients at different time points after HSCT [183].

Srinivasan and colleagues [182] collected serum from 34 patients prior to HSCT and at different time points after HSCT, with 22 samples obtained at the onset of acute GvHD symptoms. They described differentially expressed molecules which could be identified according to their mass/charge ratio, allowing correct classification of GvHD samples from non-GvHD samples. Prospective evaluation of the SELDI-data has yet to be shown. Although the data appear encouraging both the technology used, as well as the stability of the body fluid chosen, are currently under debate [149, 184–186]. Imanguli and colleagues collected saliva from 41 patients undergoing HSCT, comparing samples collected pretransplant to those collected 1, 2 or 6 month after HSCT. Thirty peaks (m/z values) were identified in the SELDI-spectra, which were generated using two different SELDI-chips. Further analysis was performed by pooling samples of 24 patients collected prior to HSCT or 1 month after HSCT respectively and separating the proteins using 2DE-DIGE and subsequent MS/MS for sequence analysis. In the 2DE-DIGE, 13 differentially analyzed spots were detected between months 1 and 4 post-transplant. Four of these were identified by MALDI-MS/MS sequencing, as lactoferrin, cystatin, albumin and salivary amylase. To date, results using the techniques hold promise in aiding early diagnosis of complications developing post-HSCT. Further comparative studies will be necessary to evaluate the impact of the current results and published data. Ongoing research includes the generation of data for early diagnosis, prediction of the development or severity of chronic GvHD. The first results of potential biomarkers were recently published by Imanguli and colleagues. The predictive value of the proteomics patterns specific for acute GvHD is currently under investigation using the results to pre-emptively treat acute GvHD.

In summary, we can conclude that proteomic screening of patient samples for the development of complications after HSCT may add current forms of diagnosis, especially in combination with clinical data and information on donor and recipient genetic disparities. The analysis of genetic differences between donor and recipient pairs, either for predicting GvHD, infectious complications and or survival and the subsequent potential prognostic risk models, will also be very useful methods of applying results from proteomic screening to particular high risk patient groups.

Acknowledgements and Funding The authors thank the peer reviewers for helpful suggestions and discussion. Funding for current research on non-HLA gene polymorphisms and support to J.H., H.C. (Australia) is via European Commission grants TRANSNET (MCRTN-CT-2004-512253) TRANSMODULATE (MCOIF-CT-2004-509939) and STEMDIAGNOSTICS (LSHB-CT-2007-037703), the Leukaemia Research Fund, and the Tyneside Leukaemia Research Association. Funding for current research on proteomics applied to clinical diagnostics is provided by the "Deutsche Jose Carreras Leukämie Stiftung" (DJCLS R05/08) to EMW and the German research foundation (DFG Mi 681/4-1).

References

1. Antoine C, Muller S, Cant A, et al. Long-term survival and transplantation of haemopoietic stem cells for immunodeficiencies: report of the European experience 1968–99. Lancet 2003;361:553–60.
2. Schrezenmeier H, Bacigalupo A. Aplastic anemia—pathophysiology and treatment. Cambridge: Cambridge University Press; 2000.
3. Gratwohl A, Passweg J, Gerber I, Tyndall A. Stem cell transplantation for autoimmune diseases. Best Pract Res Clin Haematol. 2001;14:755–76.
4. Tyndall A, Gratwohl A. Haemopoietic stem and progenitor cells in the treatment of severe autoimmune diseases. Ann Rheum Dis. 1996;55:149–51.
5. Petersdorf EW, Anasetti C, Martin PJ, Hansen JA. Tissue typing in support of unrelated hematopoietic cell transplantation. Tissue Antigens 2003;61:1–11.
6. DeGast GC, Mickelson EM, Beatty PG, et al. Mixed leukocyte culture reactivity and graft-versus-host disease in HLA-identical marrow transplantation for leukemia. Bone Marrow Transplant. 1992;9:87–90.
7. Mickelson EM, Anasetti C, Yoon Choo S, et al. Role of the mixed lymphocyte culture reaction in predicting acute graft-versus-host disease after marrow transplants from haploidentical and unrelated donors. Transplant Proc. 1993;25:1239–40.
8. Kaminski E. Cell-based histocompatibility testing. In: Bidwell G, Navarette C, editors. Histocompatibility testing. London: Imperial College Press; 1999:307–45.
9. Kaminski E, Hows J, Man S, et al. Prediction of graft versus host disease by frequency analysis of cytotoxic T cells after unrelated donor bone marrow transplantation. Transplantation 1989;48:608–13.
10. Theobald M, Nierle T, Bunjes D, Arnold R, Heimpel H. Host-specific interleukin-2-secreting donor T-cell precursors as predictors of acute graft-versus-host disease in bone marrow transplantation between HLA-identical siblings. N Engl J Med. 1992;327:1613–7.
11. Schwarer AP, Jiang YZ, Brookes PA, et al. Frequency of anti-recipient alloreactive helper T-cell precursors in donor blood and graft-versus-host disease after HLA-identical sibling bone-marrow transplantation. Lancet 1993;341:203–5.
12. Roosnek E, Hogendijk S, Zawadynski S, et al. The frequency of pretransplant donor cytotoxic T cell precursors with anti-host specificity predicts survival of patients transplanted with bone marrow from donors other than HLA-identical siblings. Transplantation 1993;56:691–6.

13. Dickinson AM, Sviland L, Wang XN, et al. Predicting graft-versus-host disease in HLA-identical bone marrow transplant: a comparison of T-cell frequency analysis and a human skin explant model. Transplantation 1998;66:857–63.
14. Fussell ST, Donnellan M, Cooley MA, Farrell C. Cytotoxic T lymphocyte precursor frequency does not correlate with either the incidence or severity of graft-versus-host disease after matched unrelated donor bone marrow transplantation. Transplantation 1994;57:673–6.
15. Freidel A-C, Michallet M, Gebuhrer L, et al. Study of HTLp in adult patients receiving bone marrow transplantation from HLA geno-identical sibs. Hum Immunol. 1996;47:84 (Abstract).
16. Claas FH, Roelen DL, Mulder A, Doxiadis, II, Oudshoorn M, Heemskerk M. Differential immunogenicity of HLA class I alloantigens for the humoral versus the cellular immune response: "towards tailor-made HLA mismatching." Hum Immunol. 2006;67:424–9.
17. Heemskerk MB, Roelen DL, Dankers MK, et al. Allogeneic MHC class I molecules with numerous sequence differences do not elicit a CTL response. Hum Immunol. 2005;66:969–76.
18. Dankers MK, Heemskerk MB, Duquesnoy RJ, et al. HLAMatchmaker algorithm is not a suitable tool to predict the alloreactive cytotoxic T-lymphocyte response in vitro. Transplantation 2004;78:165–7.
19. Little AM, Marsh SG, Madrigal JA. Current methodologies of human leukocyte antigen typing utilized for bone marrow donor selection. Curr Opin Hematol. 1998;5:419–28.
20. Bishara A, Brautbar C, Nagler A, et al. Prediction by a modified mixed leukocyte reaction assay of graft-versus-host disease and graft rejection after allogeneic bone marrow transplantation. Transplantation 1994;57:1474–9.
21. Tanaka J, Imamura M, Kasai M, et al. Cytokine gene expression in the mixed lymphocyte culture in allogenic bone marrow transplants as a predictive method for transplantation-related complications. Br J Haematol. 1994;87:415–8.
22. Miyamoto T, Akashi K, Hayashi S, et al. Serum concentration of the soluble interleukin-2 receptor for monitoring acute graft-versus-host disease. Bone Marrow Transplant. 1996;17:185–90.
23. Puppo F, Brenci S, Ghio M, et al. Serum HLA class I antigen levels in allogeneic bone marrow transplantation: a possible marker of acute GVHD. Bone Marrow Transplant. 1996;17:753–8.
24. Westhoff U, Doxiadis I, Beelen DW, Schaefer UW, Grosse-Wilde H. Soluble HLA class I concentrations and GVHD after allogeneic marrow transplantation. Transplantation 1989;48:891–3.
25. Liem LM, van Houwelingen HC, Goulmy E. Serum cytokine levels after HLA-identical bone marrow transplantation. Transplantation 1998;66:863–71.
26. Vogelsang GB, Hess AD, Berkman AW, et al. An in vitro predictive test for graft versus host disease in patients with genotypic HLA-identical bone marrow transplants. N Engl J Med. 1985;313:645–50.
27. Dickinson AM, Hromadníková I, Sviland L, et al. Use of a skin explant model for predicting GvHD in HLA-matched bone marrow transplants—effect of GvHD prophylaxis. Bone Marrow Transplant. 1999;24:857–63.
28. Dickinson AM, Sviland L, Jackson G, et al. Cytokine involvement in predicting clinical graft versus host disease (GvHD) in allogeneic bone marrow transplant recipients. Bone Marrow Transplant. 1994;13:65–70.
29. Sviland L, Dickinson AM, Carey PJ, Pearson ADJ, Proctor SJ. An in vitro predictive test for clinical graft versus host disease, correlation with clinical GvHD stage in allogeneic bone marrow transplant recipients. Bone Marrow Transplant. 1990;5:105–9.

30. Wang XN, Collin M, Sviland L, et al. Skin explant model of human graft-versus-host disease: Prediction of clinical outcome and correlation with biological risk factors. Biol Blood Marrow Transplant. 2006;12:152–9.
31. Dickinson AM, Sviland L, Dunn J, Carey P, Proctor SJ. Demonstration of direct involvement of cytokines in graft-versus-host reactions using an *in vitro* human skin explant model. Bone Marrow Transplant. 1991;7:209–16.
32. Jarvis M, Marzolini M, Wang XN, Jackson G, Sviland L, Dickinson AM. Heat shock protein 70: correlation of expression with degree of graft-versus-host response and clinical graft-versus-host disease. Transplantation 2003;76:849–53.
33. Jarvis M, Schulz U, Dickinson AM, et al. The detection of apoptosis in a human in vitro skin explant assay for graft versus host reactions. J Clin Pathol. 2002;55:127–32.
34. Dickinson AM, Wang XN, Sviland L, et al. In situ dissection of the graft-versus-host activities of cytotoxic T cells specific for minor histocompatibility antigens. Nat Med. 2002;8:410–4.
35. Holler E, Roncarolo MG, Hintermeier-Knabe R, et al. Prognostic significance of increased IL-10 production in patients prior to allogeneic bone marrow transplantation. Bone Marrow Transplant. 2000;25:237–41.
36. Middleton PG, Taylor PRA, Jackson G, Proctor SJ, Dickinson AM. Cytokine Gene polymorphisms associating with severe acute graft-versus-host disease in HLA-identical sibling transplants. Blood 1998;92:3943–8.
37. Cavet J, Middleton PG, Segall M, Noreen H, Davies SM, Dickinson AM. Recipient tumor necrosis factor-alpha and interleukin-10 gene polymorphisms associate with early mortality and acute graft-versus-host disease severity in HLA-matched sibling bone marrow transplants. Blood 1999;94:3941–6.
38. Shlomchik WD. Graft-versus-host disease. Nat Rev Immunol. 2007;7:340–52.
39. Turner D, Grant SC, Yonan N, et al. Cytokine gene polymorphism and heart transplant rejection. Transplantation 1997;64:776–9.
40. Turner DM, Grant SC, Lamb WR, et al. A genetic marker of high TNF-alpha production in heart transplant recipients. Transplantation 1995;60:1113–7.
41. Sankaran D, Asderakis A, Ashraf S, et al. Cytokine gene polymorphisms predict acute graft rejection following renal transplantation. Kidney Int. 1999;56:281–8.
42. Kim TG, Kim HY, Lee SH, et al. Systemic lupus erythematosus with nephritis is strongly associated with the TNFB*2 homozygote in the Korean population. Hum Immunol. 1996;46:10–7.
43. Sullivan KE, Wooten C, Schmekpeper BJ, Goldman D, Petri MA. A promoter polymorphism of tumor necrosis factor alpha associated with systemic lupus erythematosus in African–Americans. Arthritis Rheum. 1997;40:2207–11.
44. Fong KY, Howe HS, Tin SK, Boey ML, Feng PH. Polymorphism of the regulatory region of tumour necrosis factor alpha gene in patients with systemic lupus erythematosus. Ann Acad Med Singapore. 1996;25:22–30.
45. Eskdale J, Wordsworth P, Bowman S, Field M, Gallagher G. Association between polymorphisms at the human IL-10 locus and systemic lupus erythematosus. Tissue Antigens. 1997;49:635–7.
46. Fishman D, Faulds G, Jeffery R, et al. The effect of novel polymorphisms in the interleukin-6 (IL-6) gene on IL-6 transcription and plasma IL-6 levels, and an association with systemic-onset juvenile chronic arthritis. J Clin Invest. 1998;102:1369–76.
47. Awata T, Matsumoto C, Urakami T, Hagura R, Amemiya S, Kanazawa Y. Association of polymorphisms in the interferon gamma gene with IDDM. Diabetologia. 1994;37:1159–62.
48. Cullup H, Stark G. Interleukin-1 polymorphisms and Graft versus Host Disease. Leuk Lymphoma. 2005;46:517–23.
49. Mullighan CG, Bardy PG. Advances in the genomics of allogeneic haemopoietic stem cell transplantation. Drug Dev Res. 2004;62:273–92.

50. Shaw BE, Maldonado H, Madrigal JA, et al. Polymorphisms in the TNFA gene promoter region show evidence of strong linkage disequilibrium with HLA and are associated with delayed neutrophil engraftment in unrelated donor hematopoietic stem cell transplantation. Tissue Antigens. 2004;63:401–11.
51. Lichtman AH, Krenger W, Ferrara JLM. Cytokine Networks. In: Ferrara JLM, Deeg HJ, Burakoff SJ, eds. Graft-vs-Host Disease. New York: Marcel Dekker, Inc; 1996. p. 179–218.
52. Nordlander A, Uzunel M, Mattsson J, Remberger M. The TNFd4 allele is correlated to moderate-to-severe acute graft-versus-host disease after allogeneic stem cell transplantation. Br J Haematol. 2002;119:1133–336.
53. Wilson AG, Symons JA, McDowell TL, McDevitt HO, Duff GW. Effects of a polymorphism in the human tumor necrosis factor alpha promoter on transcriptional activation. Proc Natl Acad Sci USA. 1997;94:3195–9.
54. Takahashi H, Furukawa T, Hashimoto S, et al. Contribution of TNF-alpha and IL-10 gene polymorphisms to graft-versus-host disease following allo-hematopoietic stem cell transplantation. Bone Marrow Transplant. 2000;26:1317–23.
55. Wang J, Pan K, Li D, Lu D. [The relationship between donor TNFalpha—308 (G/A) genotype and recipient acute GVHD in allo-BMT]. Zhonghua Xue Ye Xue Za Zhi. 2002;23:397–9.
56. Mullighan C, Heatley S, Doherty K, et al. Non-HLA immunogenetic polymorphisms and the risk of complications after allogeneic hemopoietic stem-cell transplantation. Transplantation 2004;77:587–96.
57. Rocha V, Franco RF, Porcher R, et al. Host defence and inflammatory gene polymorphisms are associated with outcomes after HLA-identical sibling bone marrow transplant. Blood 2002;100:3908–18.
58. Socié G, Loiseau P, Tamouza R, et al. Both genetic and clinical factors predict the development of graft-versus-host disease after allogeneic hematopoietic stem cell transplantation. Transplantation 2001;72:699–706.
59. Lin MT, Storer B, Martin PJ, et al. Relation of an interleukin-10 promoter polymorphism to graft-versus-host disease and survival after hematopoietic-cell transplantation. N Engl J Med. 2003;349:2201–10.
60. Bogunia-Kubik K, Polak M, Lange A. TNF polymorphisms are associated with toxic but not with aGVHD complications in the recipients of allogeneic sibling haematopoietic stem cell transplantation. Bone Marrow Transplant. 2003;32:617–22.
61. Nedospasov SA, Udalova IA, Kuprash DV, Turetskaya RL. DNA sequence polymorphism at the human tumor necrosis factor (TNF) locus. Numerous TNF/lymphotoxin alleles tagged by two closely linked microsatellites in the upstream region of the lymphotoxin (TNF-beta) gene. J Immunol. 1991;147:1053–9.
62. Udalova IA, Nedospasov SA, Webb GC, Chaplin DD, Turetskaya RL. Highly informative typing of the human TNF locus using six adjacent polymorphic markers. Genomics 1993;16:180–6.
63. Holzinger I, de Baey A, Messer G, Kick G, Zwierzina H, Weiss EH. Cloning and genomic characterization of LST1: a new gene in the human TNF region. Immunogenetics 1995;42:315–22.
64. Pociot F, Molvig J, Wogensen L, et al. A tumour necrosis factor beta gene polymorphism in relation to monokine secretion and insulin-dependent diabetes mellitus. Scand J Immunol. 1991;33:37–49.
65. Remberger M, Jaksch M, Uzunel M, Mattsson J. Serum levels of cytokines correlate to donor chimerism and acute graft-vs.-host disease after haematopoietic stem cell transplantation. Eur J Haematol. 2003;70:384–91.
66. Keen LJ, DeFor TE, Bidwell JL, Davies SM, Bradley BA, Hows JM. Interleukin-10 and tumor necrosis factor alpha region haplotypes predict transplant-related mortality after unrelated donor stem cell transplantation. Blood 2004;103:3599–602.

67. Bettens F, Passweg J, Gratwohl A, et al. Association of TNFd and IL-10 polymorphisms with mortality in unrelated hematopoietic stem cell transplantation. Transplantation 2006;81:1261–7.
68. Ishikawa Y, Kashiwase K, Akaza K, et al. Polymorphisms in TNFA and TNFR2 affect outcome of unrelated bone marrow transplantation. Bone Marrow Transplant. 2002;29:569–75.
69. Barbara JA, Smith WB, Gamble JR, et al. Dissociation of TNF-alpha cytotoxic and proinflammatory activities by p55 receptor- and p75 receptor-selective TNF-alpha mutants. EMBO J. 1994;13:843–50.
70. Zheng L, Fisher G, Miller RE, Peschon J, Lynch DH, Lenardo MJ. Induction of apoptosis in mature T cells by tumour necrosis factor. Nature 1995;377:348–51.
71. MacEwan DJ. TNF receptor subtype signalling: differences and cellular consequences. Cell Signal. 2002;14:477–92.
72. Morita C, Horiuchi T, Tsukamoto H, et al. Association of tumor necrosis factor receptor type II polymorphism 196R with Systemic lupus erythematosus in the Japanese: molecular and functional analysis. Arthritis Rheum. 2001;44:2819–27.
73. Edwards-Smith CJ, Jonsson JR, Purdie DM, Bansal A, Shorthouse C, Powell EE. Interleukin-10 promoter polymorphism predicts initial response of chronic hepatitis C to interferon alfa. Hepatology 1999;30:526–30.
74. Stark GL, Dickinson AM, Jackson GH, Taylor PR, Proctor SJ, Middleton PG. Tumour necrosis factor receptor type II 196 M/R genotype correlates with circulating soluble receptor levels in normal subjects and with graft-versus-host disease after sibling allogeneic bone marrow transplantation. Transplantation 2003;76:1742–9.
75. Keijsers V, Verweij C, Westendorp RGJ, Breedveld FC, Huizinga TWJ. IL10 polymorphisms in relation to production and rheumatoid arthritis. Arthritis Rheum. 1997;40:S179 (Abstract).
76. Gibson AW, Edberg JC, Wu J, Westendorp RG, Huizinga TW, Kimberly RP. Novel single nucleotide polymorphisms in the distal IL-10 promoter affect IL-10 production and enhance the risk of systemic lupus erythematosus. J Immunol. 2001;166:3915–22.
77. Kim DH, Lee NY, Sohn SK, et al. IL-10 promoter gene polymorphism associated with the occurrence of chronic GVHD and its clinical course during systemic immunosuppressive treatment for chronic GVHD after allogeneic peripheral blood stem cell transplantation. Transplantation 2005;79:1615–22.
78. Seo KW, Kim DH, Sohn SK, et al. Protective role of interleukin-10 promoter gene polymorphism in the pathogenesis of invasive pulmonary aspergillosis after allogeneic stem cell transplantation. Bone Marrow Transplant. 2005;36:1089–95.
79. Yang YG, Wang H, Asavaroengchai W, Dey BR. Role of Interferon-gamma in GvHD and GvL. Cell Mol Immunol. 2005;2:323–9.
80. Pravica V, Asderakis A, Perrey C, Hajeer A, Sinnott PJ, Hutchinson IV. In vitro production of IFN-gamma correlates with CA repeat polymorphism in the human IFN-gamma gene. Eur J Immunogenet. 1999;26:1–3.
81. Pravica V, Perrey C, Stevens A, Lee JH, Hutchinson IV. A single nucleotide polymorphism in the first intron of the human IFN-gamma gene: absolute correlation with a polymorphic CA microsatellite marker of high IFN-gamma production. Hum Immunol. 2000;61:863–6.
82. Sica A, Tan TH, Rice N, Kretzschmar M, Ghosh P, Young HA. The c-rel protooncogene product c-Rel but not NF-kappa B binds to the intronic region of the human interferon-gamma gene at a site related to an interferon-stimulable response element. Proc Natl Acad Sci USA. 1992;89:1740–4.
83. Cavet J, Dickinson AM, Norden J, Taylor PR, Jackson GH, Middleton PG. Interferon-gamma and interleukin-6 gene polymorphisms associate with graft-versus-host disease in HLA-matched sibling bone marrow transplantation. Blood 2001;98:1594–600.

84. Bogunia-Kubik K, Mlynarczewska A, Wysoczanska B, Lange A. Recipient interferon-gamma 3/3 genotype contributes to the development of chronic graft-versus-host disease after allogeneic hematopoietic stem cell transplantation. Haematologica 2005;90:425–6.
85. Mlynarczewska A, Wysoczanska B, Karabon L, Bogunia-Kubik K, Lange A. Lack of IFN-gamma 2/2 homozygous genotype independently of recipient age and intensity of conditioning regimen influences the risk of aGVHD manifestation after HLA-matched sibling haematopoietic stem cell transplantation. Bone Marrow Transplant. 2004;34:339–44.
86. Brok HP, Heidt PJ, van der Meide PH, Zurcher C, Vossen JM. Interferon-gamma prevents graft-versus-host disease after allogeneic bone marrow transplantation in mice. J Immunol. 1993;151:6451–9.
87. Bogunia-Kubik K, Mlynarczewska A, Jaskula E, Lange A. The presence of IFNG 3/3 genotype in the recipient associates with increased risk for Epstein-Barr virus reactivation after allogeneic haematopoietic stem cell transplantation. Br J Haematol. 2006;132:326–32.
88. Cullup H, Dickinson AM, Jackson GH, Taylor PRA, Cavet J, Middleton PG. Donor interleukin-1 receptor antagonist genotype associated with acute graft-versus-host disease in human leukocyte antigen-matched sibling allogeneic transplants. Br J Haematol. 2001;113:807–13.
89. Cullup H, Dickinson AM, Cavet J, Jackson GH, Middleton PG. Polymorphisms of IL-1alpha constitute independent risk factors for chronic graft versus host disease following allogeneic bone marrow transplantation. Br J Haematol. 2003;122:778–87.
90. Terry CF, Loukaci V, Green FR. Cooperative influence of genetic polymorphisms on interleukin 6 transcriptional regulation. J Biol Chem. 2000;275:18138–44.
91. Ferrari SL, Ahn-Luong L, Garnero P, Humphries SE, Greenspan SL. Two promoter polymorphisms regulating interleukin-6 gene expression are associated with circulating levels of C-reactive protein and markers of bone resorption in postmenopausal women. J Clin Endocrinol Metab. 2003;88:255–9.
92. Karabon L, Wysoczanska B, Bogunia-Kubik K, Suchnicki K, Lange A. IL-6 and IL-10 promoter gene polymorphisms of patients and donors of allogeneic sibling hematopoietic stem cell transplants associate with the risk of acute graft-versus-host disease. Hum Immunol. 2005;66:700–10.
93. Banovic T, MacDonald KP, Morris ES, et al. TGF-beta in allogeneic stem cell transplantation: friend or foe? Blood 2005;106:2206–14.
94. Grainger DJ, Heathcote K, Chiano M, et al. Genetic control of the circulating concentration of transforming growth factor type beta 1. Hum Mol Genet. 1999;8:93–7.
95. Leffell MS, Vogelsang GB, Lucas DP, Delaney NL, Zachary AA. Association between TGF-beta expression and severe GVHD in allogeneic bone marrow transplantation. Transplant Proc. 2001;33:485–6.
96. Hattori H, Matsuzaki A, Suminoe A, et al. Polymorphisms of transforming growth factor-beta1 and transforming growth factor-beta1 type II receptor genes are associated with acute graft-versus-host disease in children with HLA-matched sibling bone marrow transplantation. Bone Marrow Transplant. 2002;30:665–71.
97. MacMillan ML, Radloff GA, Kiffmeyer WR, DeFor TE, Weisdorf DJ, Davies SM. High-producer interleukin-2 genotype increases risk for acute graft-versus-host disease after unrelated donor bone marrow transplantation. Transplantation 2003;76:1758–62.
98. Shamim Z, Ryder LP, Heilmann C, et al. Genetic polymorphisms in the genes encoding human interleukin-7 receptor-alpha: prognostic significance in allogeneic stem cell transplantation. Bone Marrow Transplant. 2006;37:485–91.
99. Cardoso SM, DeFor TE, Tilley LA, Bidwell JL, Weisdorf DJ, MacMillan ML. Patient interleukin-18 GCG haplotype associates with improved survival and decreased transplant-related mortality after unrelated-donor bone marrow transplantation. Br J Haematol. 2004;126:704–10.

100. Bogunia-Kubik K, Duda D, Suchnicki K, Lange A. CCR5 deletion mutation and its association with the risk of developing acute graft-versus-host disease after allogeneic hematopoietic stem cell transplantation. Haematologica 2006;91:1628–34.
101. Loeffler J, Steffens M, Arlt EM, et al. Polymorphisms in the genes encoding chemokine receptor 5, interleukin-10, and monocyte chemoattractant protein 1 contribute to cytomegalovirus reactivation and disease after allogeneic stem cell transplantation. J Clin Micriobiol. 2006;44:1847–50.
102. Xu D, Liu H, Komai-Koma M. Direct and indirect role of Toll-like receptors in T cell mediated immunity. Cell Mol Immunol. 2004;1:239–46.
103. Kaisho T, Akira S. Pleiotropic function of Toll-like receptors. Microbes Infect. 2004;6:1388–94.
104. Kaisho T, Akira S. Regulation of dendritic cell function through toll-like receptors. Curr Mol Med. 2003;3:759–71.
105. Lorenz E, Schwartz DA, Martin PJ, et al. Association of TLR4 mutations and the risk for acute GVHD after HLA-matched-sibling hematopoietic stem cell transplantation. Biol Blood Marrow Transplant. 2001;7:384–7.
106. Kesh S, Mensah NY, Peterlongo P, et al. TLR1 and TLR6 polymorphisms are associated with susceptibility to invasive aspergillosis after allogeneic stem cell transplantation. Ann NY Acad Sci. 2005;1062:95–103.
107. Holler E, Rogler G, Herfarth H, et al. Both donor and recipient NOD2/CARD15 mutations associate with transplant-related mortality and GvHD following allogeneic stem cell transplantation. Blood 2004;104:889–94.
108. Holler E, Rogler G, Brenmoehl J, et al. Prognostic significance of NOD2/CARD15 variants in HLA-identical sibling hematopoietic stem cell transplantation: Effect on long term outcome is confirmed in 2 independent cohorts and may be modulated by the type of gastrointestinal decontamination. Blood 2006;107:4189–93.
109. Granell M, Urbano-Ispizua A, Arostegui JI, et al. Effect of NOD2/CARD15 variants in T-cell depleted allogeneic stem cell transplantation. Haematologica 2007;91:1372–6.
110. Mullighan CG, Heatley S, Doherty K, et al. Mannose-binding lectin gene polymorphisms are associated with major infection following allogeneic hemopoietic stem cell transplantation. Blood 2002;99:3524–9.
111. van der Straaten HM, Fijnheer R, Nieuwenhuis HK, van de Winkel JG, Verdonck LF. The FcgammaRIIa-polymorphic site as a potential target for acute graft-versus-host disease in allogeneic stem cell transplantation. Biol Blood Marrow Transplant. 2005;11:206–12.
112. Middleton PG, Cullup H, Cavet J, Jackson GH, Taylor PRA, Dickinson AM. Oestrogen receptor alpha gene polymorphism associates with occurrence of graft-versus-host disease and reduced survival in HLA-matched sib-allo BMT. Bone Marrow Transplant. 2003;32:41–7.
113. Middleton PG, Cullup H, Dickinson AM, et al. Vitamin D receptor gene polymorphism associates with graft-versus-host disease and survival in HLA-matched sibling allogeneic bone marrow transplantation. Bone Marrow Transplant. 2002;30:223–8.
114. Bogunia-Kubik K, Lange A. HSP70-hom gene polymorphism in allogeneic hematopoietic stem-cell transplant recipients correlates with the development of acute graft-versus-host disease. Transplantation 2005;79:815–20.
115. Bogunia-Kubik K, Uklejewska A, Dickinson AM, Jarvis M, Lange A. *HSP70-hom* gene polymorphism as a prognostic marker of graft-versus-host disease. Transplantation 2006;82:1116–7 (Letter).
116. Robien K, Ulrich CM, Bigler J, et al. Methylenetetrahydrofolate reductase genotype affects risk of relapse after hematopoietic cell transplantation for chronic myelogenous leukemia. Clin Cancer Res. 2004;10:7592–8.
117. Ulrich CM, Yasui Y, Storb R, et al. Pharmacogenetics of methotrexate: toxicity among marrow transplantation patients varies with the methylenetetrahydrofolate reductase C677T polymorphism. Blood 2001;98:231–4.

118. Rocha V, Porcher R, Filion A, et al. Association of Pharmacogenes polymorphisms with toxicities and GvHD after HLA-identical sibling bone marrow transplantation. Blood 2003;102:241a (Abstract 848).
119. Kalayoglu-Besisik S, Caliskan Y, Sargin D, Gurses N, Ozbek U. Methylenetetrahydrofolate reductase C677T polymorphism and toxicity in allogeneic hematopoietic cell transplantation. Transplantation 2003;76:1775–7.
120. Murphy N, Diviney M, Szer J, et al. Donor methylenetetrahydrofolate reductase genotype is associated with graft-versus-host disease in hematopoietic stem cell transplant patients treated with methotrexate. Bone Marrow Transplant. 2006;37:773–9.
121. Kim I, Lee K-H, Kim JH, et al. Polymorphisms of the methylenetetrahydrofolate reductase gene and clinical outcomes in HLA-matched sibling allogeneic hematopoietic stem cell transplantation. Ann Hematol. 2007;86:41–8.
122. Gratwohl A, Brand R, Apperley J, et al. Graft-versus-host disease and outcome in HLA-identical sibling transplantations for chronic myeloid leukemia. Blood 2002;100:3877–86.
123. Gratwohl A, Hermans J, Goldman JM, et al. Risk assessment for patients with chronic myeloid leukaemia before allogeneic blood or marrow transplantation. Chronic Leukemia Working Party of the European Group for Blood and Marrow Transplantation. Lancet 1998;352:1087–92.
124. Weisdorf D, Hakke R, Blazar B, et al. Risk factors for acute graft-versus-host disease in histocompatible donor bone marrow transplantation. Transplantation 1991;51:1197–203.
125. Niederwieser D, Pepe M, Storb R, Witherspoon R, Longton G, Sullivan K. Factors predicting chronic graft-versus-host disease and survival after marrow transplantation for aplastic anemia. Bone Marrow Transplant. 1989;4:151–6.
126. Leisenring WM, Martin PJ, Petersdorf EW, et al. An acute graft-versus-host disease activity index to predict survival after hematopoietic cell transplantation with myeloablative conditioning regimens. Blood 2006;108:749–55.
127. Seitz W, Zimmer E, Alberti PE. [Paper-electrophoretic studies on proteins in urine of normal and sick individuals.]. Z Klin Med. 1953;152:196–201.
128. O'Farrell PH. High resolution two-dimensional electrophoresis of proteins. J Biol Chem. 1975;250:4007–21.
129. Mischak H, Apweiler R, Banks RE, et al. Clinical proteomics: a need to define the field and to begin to set adequate standards. Proteomics Clin Appl. 2007;1:148–56.
130. Kapetanovic IM, Rosenfeld S, Izmirlian G. Overview of commonly used bioinformatics methods and their applications. Ann NY Acad Sci. 2004;1020:10–21.
131. Henzel WJ, Billeci TM, Stults JT, Wong SC, Grimley C, Watanabe C. Identifying proteins from two-dimensional gels by molecular mass searching of peptide fragments in protein sequence databases. Proc Natl Acad Sci USA. 1993;90:5011–5.
132. Henzel WJ, Watanabe C, Stults JT. Protein identification: the origins of peptide mass fingerprinting. J Am Soc Mass Spectrom. 2003;14:931–42.
133. Wu TL. Two-dimensional difference gel electrophoresis. Methods Mol Biol. 2006;328:71–95.
134. Issaq HJ. The role of separation science in proteomics research. Electrophoresis 2001;22:3629–38.
135. Issaq HJ, Conrads TP, Janini GM, Veenstra TD. Methods for fractionation, separation and profiling of proteins and peptides. Electrophoresis 2002;23:3048–61.
136. Chen EI, Hewel J, Felding-Habermann B, Yates JR, 3rd. Large scale protein profiling by combination of protein fractionation and multidimensional protein identification technology (MudPIT). Mol Cell Proteomics. 2006;5:53–6.
137. Cagney G, Park S, Chung C, et al. Human tissue profiling with multidimensional protein identification technology. J Proteome Res. 2005;4:1757–67.
138. Kislinger T, Gramolini AO, MacLennan DH, Emili A. Multidimensional protein identification technology (MudPIT): technical overview of a profiling method optimized for

the comprehensive proteomic investigation of normal and diseased heart tissue. J Am Soc Mass Spectrom. 2005;16:1207–20.
139. Soldi M, Sarto C, Valsecchi C, et al. Proteome profile of human urine with two-dimensional liquid phase fractionation. Proteomics 2005;5:2641–7.
140. Kolch W, Neususs C, Pelzing M, Mischak H. Capillary electrophoresis-mass spectrometry as a powerful tool in clinical diagnosis and biomarker discovery. Mass Spectrom Rev. 2005;24:959–77.
141. Yip TT, Lomas L. SELDI ProteinChip array in oncoproteomic research. Technol Cancer Res Treat. 2002;1:273–80.
142. von Eggeling F, Junker K, Fiedle W, et al. Mass spectrometry meets chip technology: a new proteomic tool in cancer research? Electrophoresis 2001;22:2898–902.
143. Weinberger SR, Viner RI, Ho P. Tagless extraction-retentate chromatography: a new global protein digestion strategy for monitoring differential protein expression. Electrophoresis 2002;23:3182–92.
144. Tang N, Tornatore P, Weinberger SR. Current developments in SELDI affinity technology. Mass Spectrom Rev. 2004;23:34–44.
145. Petricoin EF, Ardekani AM, Hitt BA, et al. Use of proteomic patterns in serum to identify ovarian cancer. Lancet 2002;359:572–7.
146. Rosenblatt KP, Bryant-Greenwood P, Killian JK, et al. Serum proteomics in cancer diagnosis and management. Annu Rev Med. 2004;55:97–112.
147. Schaub S, Wilkins J, Weiler T, Sangster K, Rush D, Nickerson P. Urine protein profiling with surface-enhanced laser-desorption/ionization time-of-flight mass spectrometry. Kidney Int. 2004;65:323–32.
148. Kolch W, Mischak H, Chalmers MJ, Pitt A, Marshall AG. Clinical proteomics: a question of technology. Rapid Commun Mass Spectrom. 2004;18:2365–6.
149. Check E. Proteomics and cancer: running before we can walk? Nature 2004;429:496–7.
150. Baggerly KA, Morris JS, Coombes KR. Reproducibility of SELDI-TOF protein patterns in serum: comparing datasets from different experiments. Bioinformatics 2004;20:777–85.
151. Orvisky E, Drake SK, Martin BM, et al. Enrichment of low molecular weight fraction of serum for MS analysis of peptides associated with hepatocellular carcinoma. Proteomics 2006;6:2895–902.
152. Neuhoff N, Kaiser T, Wittke S, et al. Mass spectrometry for the detection of differentially expressed proteins: a comparison of surface-enhanced laser desorption/ionization and capillary electrophoresis/mass spectrometry. Rapid Commun Mass Spectrom. 2004;18:149–56.
153. Johannesson N, Wetterhall M, Markides KE, Bergquist J. Monomer surface modifications for rapid peptide analysis by capillary electrophoresis and capillary electrochromatography coupled to electrospray ionization-mass spectrometry. Electrophoresis 2004;25:809–16.
154. Hernandez-Borges J, Neususs C, Cifuentes A, Pelzing M. On-line capillary electrophoresis-mass spectrometry for the analysis of biomolecules. Electrophoresis 2004;25:2257–81.
155. Neususs C, Pelzing M, Macht M. A robust approach for the analysis of peptides in the low femtomole range by capillary electrophoresis-tandem mass spectrometry. Electrophoresis 2002;23:3149–59.
156. Schmitt-Kopplin P, Englmann M. Capillary electrophoresis—mass spectrometry: survey on developments and applications 2003–2004. Electrophoresis 2005;26:1209–20.
157. Sassi AP, Andel F, 3rd, Bitter HM, et al. An automated, sheathless capillary electrophoresis-mass spectrometry platform for discovery of biomarkers in human serum. Electrophoresis 2005;26:1500–12.
158. Klampfl CW. Recent advances in the application of capillary electrophoresis with mass spectrometric detection. Electrophoresis 2006;27:3–34.

159. Ullsten S, Danielsson R, Backstrom D, Sjoberg P, Bergquist J. Urine profiling using capillary electrophoresis-mass spectrometry and multivariate data analysis. J Chromatogr A. 2006;1117:87–93.
160. Zurbig P, Renfrow MB, Schiffer E, et al. Biomarker discovery by CE-MS enables sequence analysis via MS/MS with platform-independent separation. Electrophoresis 2006;27:2111–25.
161. Lescuyer P, Hochstrasser D, Rabilloud T. How Shall We Use the Proteomics Toolbox for Biomarker Discovery? J Proteome Res. 2007;6:3371–6.
162. Omenn GS, States DJ, Adamski M, et al. Overview of the HUPO Plasma Proteome Project: results from the pilot phase with 35 collaborating laboratories and multiple analytical groups, generating a core dataset of 3020 proteins and a publicly-available database. Proteomics 2005;5:3226–45.
163. Anderson NL, Anderson NG. The human plasma proteome: history, character, and diagnostic prospects. Mol Cell Proteomics. 2002;1:845–67.
164. Fliser D, Novak J, Thongboonkerd V, et al. Advances in urinary proteome analysis and biomarker discovery. J Am Soc Nephrol. 2007;18:1057–71.
165. Davis MT, Spahr CS, McGinley MD, et al. Towards defining the urinary proteome using liquid chromatography-tandem mass spectrometry. II. Limitations of complex mixture analyses. Proteomics 2001;1:108–17.
166. Spahr CS, Davis MT, McGinley MD, et al. Towards defining the urinary proteome using liquid chromatography-tandem mass spectrometry. I. Profiling an unfractionated tryptic digest. Proteomics 2001;1:93–107.
167. Adachi J, Kumar C, Zhang Y, Olsen JV, Mann M. The human urinary proteome contains more than 1500 proteins, including a large proportion of membrane proteins. Genome Biol. 2006;7:R80.
168. Theodorescu D, Fliser D, Wittke S, et al. Pilot study of capillary electrophoresis coupled to mass spectrometry as a tool to define potential prostate cancer biomarkers in urine. Electrophoresis 2005;26:2797–808.
169. Theodorescu D, Wittke S, Ross MM, et al. Discovery and validation of new protein biomarkers for urothelial cancer: a prospective analysis. Lancet Oncol. 2006;7:230–40.
170. Copelan EA. Hematopoietic stem-cell transplantation. N Engl J Med. 2006;354:1813–26.
171. Kolb HJ, Schmid C, Barrett AJ, Schendel DJ. Graft-versus-leukemia reactions in allogeneic chimeras. Blood 2004;103:767–76.
172. Hambach L, Eder M, Dammann E, et al. Diagnostic value of procalcitonin serum levels in comparison with C-reactive protein in allogeneic stem cell transplantation. Haematologica 2002;87:643–51.
173. Seidel C, Ringden O, Remberger M. Increased levels of syndecan-1 in serum during acute graft-versus-host disease. Transplantation 2003;76:423–6.
174. Cristea IM, Gaskell SJ, Whetton AD. Proteomics techniques and their application to hematology. Blood 2004;103:3624–34.
175. Weissinger EM, Mischak H, Ganser A, Hertenstein B. Value of proteomics applied to the follow-up in stem cell transplantation. Ann Hematol. 2006;85:205–11.
176. Weissinger EM, Hertenstein B, Mischak H, Ganser A. Online coupling of capillary electrophoresis with mass spectrometry for the identification of biomarkers for clinical diagnosis. Expert Rev Proteomics. 2005;2:639–47.
177. Kaiser T, Wittke S, Just I, et al. Capillary electrophoresis coupled to mass spectrometer for automated and robust polypeptide determination in body fluids for clinical use. Electrophoresis 2004;25:2044–55.
178. Weissinger EM, Wittke S, Kaiser T, et al. Proteomic patterns established with capillary electrophoresis and mass spectrometry for diagnostic purposes. Kidney Int. 2004;65:2426–34.
179. Kaiser T, Kamal H, Rank A, et al. Proteomics applied to the clinical follow-up of patients after allogeneic hematopoietic stem cell transplantation. Blood 2004;104:340–9.

180. Weissinger EM, Schiffer E, Hertenstein B, et al. Proteomic patterns predict acute graft-versus-host disease after allogeneic hematopoietic stem cell transplantation. Blood 2007;109:5511–9.
181. Wang H, Clouthier SG, Galchev V, et al. Intact-protein-based high-resolution three-dimensional quantitative analysis system for proteome profiling of biological fluids. Mol Cell Proteomics. 2005;4:618–25.
182. Srinivasan R, Daniels J, Fusaro V, et al. Accurate diagnosis of acute graft-versus-host disease using serum proteomic pattern analysis. Exp Hematol. 2006;34:796–801.
183. Imanguli MM, Atkinson JC, Harvey KE, et al. Changes in salivary proteome following allogeneic hematopoietic stem cell transplantation. Exp Hematol. 2007;35:184–92.
184. Hsieh SY, Chen RK, Pan YH, Lee HL. Systematical evaluation of the effects of sample collection procedures on low-molecular-weight serum/plasma proteome profiling. Proteomics 2006;6:3189–98.
185. Rai AJ, Gelfand CA, Haywood BC, et al. HUPO Plasma Proteome Project specimen collection and handling: towards the standardization of parameters for plasma proteome samples. Proteomics 2005;5:3262–77.
186. Rai AJ, Vitzthum F. Effects of preanalytical variables on peptide and protein measurements in human serum and plasma: implications for clinical proteomics. Expert Rev Proteomics. 2006;3:409–26.

Chapter 6
Clinical Implications of Immune Reconstitution Following Hematopoietic Stem Cell Transplantation

Karl S. Peggs, Aviva C. Krauss and Crystal L. Mackall

6.1 Introduction

Allogeneic hematopoietic stem cell transplantation (HSCT) seeks to transfer a fully functional lymphohematopoietic system from donor to recipient. Hematopoietic function typically normalizes within weeks of the transplant, whereas immune function remains abnormal for months to years, resulting in substantial infection-related morbidity and mortality [1]. Furthermore, the success of HSCT often depends upon the reconstituting immune system's ability to eradicate minimal residual neoplastic disease. Thus, improving the effectiveness of allogeneic HSCT is intimately linked to the development of new approaches to enhance immune reconstitution. Substantial progress has been made in understanding the biology of immune reconstitution, and new therapies designed to improve immune reconstitution are now emerging. Recent scientific progress has provided a clearer understanding of lymphopenia-induced changes in immune physiology, which in turn provides new therapeutic approaches for inducing antitumor immunity following HSCT. A more precise understanding of the progenitor populations required for efficient thymic reconstitution has now been gleaned, raising the possibility that thymic progenitor cell based therapies could be used to hasten immune recovery. Potent new immunorestoratives have also been identified, providing new pharmacologic agents that could enhance immune reconstitution. This chapter will review fundamental concepts of immune reconstitution following HSCT, emphasizing recent scientific and clinical observations, and then discuss opportunities for clinical progress in this arena, both for enhancing global immune reconstitution and for directing immune responses following HSCT to diminish infectious risk and enhance graft-versus-tumor (GvT) effects. The discussion focuses primarily on allogeneic

K.S. Peggs (✉)
Royal Free and University College London Medical Schools, London, United Kingdom
e-mail: k.peggs@ucl.ac.uk

M.R. Bishop (ed.), *Hematopoietic Stem Cell Transplantation*,
Cancer Treatment and Research 144, DOI 10.1007/978-0-387-78580-6_6,

HSCT, but studies in lymphopenic hosts following intensive chemotherapy or autologous transplant that have enlightened the field will also be reviewed.

6.2 Immune Reconstitution Following HSCT

6.2.1 Principles of T and B Cell Regeneration

Reconstitution of lymphocytes (NK cells, T cells and B cells) depends firstly on successful engraftment of lymphoid stem cells, from which they all derive. The consistent, early and complete recovery of NK cells following dose-intensive chemotherapy, autologous HSCT, and allogeneic HSCT [2, 3] provides clear evidence of the vitality of the lymphoid stem cell in these settings. Indeed, rapid reconstitution of NK cells, as compared to T and B-cell populations is one factor fueling enthusiasm for selecting donors based upon NK KIR mismatch, an area reviewed in Chap. 3. Unlike NK cells however, regeneration of lymphoid stem cell derived T and B cells requires expansion and selection within intricate microenvironments, in the thymus and bone marrow respectively. These microenvironments are highly susceptible to damage by drugs, irradiation, graft-versus-host disease (GvHD), and age (thymus only), which fundamentally limits regeneration of T and B cells from lymphoid stem cells following HSCT. Moreover, since generation of memory B cells requires CD4$^+$ T cell help, reconstitution of humoral immunity is highly dependent upon effective CD4$^+$ regeneration. Thus, damage to the thymic and marrow microenvironments is one fundamental factor limiting the pace of immune reconstitution in most patients undergoing HSCT.

6.2.2 Immunobiology of Homeostatic Peripheral Expansion

T cells can also regenerate via homeostatic peripheral expansion (HPE), an alternate, thymic-independent pathway of reconstitution, which is theoretically inferior but can provide a remarkably effective layer of immunity for many years following HSCT. HPE represents mitotic expansion of residual mature T cells, usually contained within the stem cell graft. It results from quantitative and qualitative changes in T-cell physiology induced by lymphopenia, and is characterized by augmented T-cell reactivity to cognate antigens (quantitative effect) and the development of proliferative responses to low affinity self antigens (qualitative effect). Interleukin-7 (IL-7) is necessary for HPE of naïve T cells, and MHC Class I and Class II are necessary for HPE of naïve CD4$^+$ and CD8$^+$ T cells respectively. Supraphysiologic levels of IL-7 are present in the serum and tissues of lymphopenic hosts, and the increased availability of IL-7 provides a primary stimulus for driving HPE of naïve T cells and memory CD4$^+$ T cells during lymphopenia. HPE of CD8$^+$ memory T cells during lymphopenia may be driven by IL-15 and/or IL-7.

For reasons that remain unclear, HPE of CD8$^+$ T cells is much more efficient than HPE of CD4$^+$ T cells, resulting in chronically reduced CD4$^+$ T-cell numbers and inverted CD4/CD8 ratios for months to years following HSCT in hosts with limited thymic function. CD4$^+$ T-cell number and function is highly dependent upon thymic-dependent T-cell regeneration, which occurs in only a fraction of adults undergoing HSCT, even with prolonged follow-up [4], and the T-cell repertoire generated via HPE is limited in diversity and prone to skewing [5], whereas thymic-dependent immune reconstitution generates a diverse T-cell repertoire [6]. Recent clinical studies have confirmed that these differences are clinically significant, since patients who experience thymic-dependent immune reconstitution have a more effective response to vaccination [7] and CD4$^+$ T-cell counts post-transplant are predictive of infectious complications [1]. Thus, it is tempting to minimize the importance of HPE; CD4$^+$ T-cell numbers remain suboptimal, inverted CD4/CD8 ratios are the rule, and HPE generated T cell receptor (TCR) repertoires are prone to skewing. However, despite its limitations, HPE provides substantial immunocompetence, illustrated by the fact that patients who receive transplants with profoundly T-cell depleted allografts experience more infectious complications and a greater likelihood of tumor recurrence than those receiving T-cell replete grafts [8]. Recent basic and clinical studies have also demonstrated that lymphopenia induced alterations in immune physiology that give rise to HPE are exploitable for therapeutic gain, especially when targeting tumor antigens (see below). Thus, HPE represents an important and potentially exploitable pathway of immune reconstitution following HSCT.

6.2.2.1 Homeostatic Peripheral Expansion of Regulatory T Cells

The "rediscovery" of suppressor T-cell populations by Sakaguchi and colleagues in the mid 1990s augured the rebirth of an entire field. CD4$^+$CD25$^+$Foxp3$^+$ regulatory T cells (T^{regs}) are essential mediators of self-tolerance [9–11]. Although their mechanism(s) of action is not yet fully understood, they regulate CD4$^+$ and CD8$^+$ T-cell activity in a cell extrinsic manner, and their depletion can enhance T-cell responses to pathogens [12, 13], self-antigens [11], and tumors [14]. In the context of allogeneic HSCT, the suppressive activity of Foxp3$^+$T^{regs} may be either desirable (inhibition of GvHD) or detrimental (fostering immune privilege in tumors), fueling interest in developing approaches to interfere with Foxp3$^+$ T^{reg} number or function for therapeutic benefit. Recent studies have investigated the relative contribution of thymic-dependent versus thymic-independent pathways of T^{reg} generation during primary T-cell development and following lymphopenia inducing insults. While primary T^{reg} development is thymic-dependent and the repertoire of the thymic-derived CD4$^+$CD25$^+$Foxp3$^+$ subset is heavily skewed toward self-antigens, T^{regs} can also be generated peripherally following antigenic stimulation, where they undergo more rapid turnover compared to CD4$^+$Foxp3$^+$ cells in unperturbed hosts, and they undergo substantial HPE in lymphopenic hosts, resulting in proportional increases in T^{reg} frequency in humans and mice during lymphopenia [15]. Recent evidence has suggested that both $CD25^+$ and $CD25^-$ subsets can give rise to $CD4^+Foxp3^+$ cells since this subset can be rapidly regenerated in lymphopenic humans and mice following administration of T-cell inocula depleted of $CD25^+$ cells [16]. Thus, $CD4^+Foxp3^+$ cells are ably supported by HPE.

The importance of T^{reg} depletion in supporting or enhancing homeostatic peripheral expansion of non-regulatory populations has been a matter of some discussion, especially since self antigens are primary drivers of T-cell expansion during lymphopenia. While hosts treated with adoptive transfer of cytolytic T cells (CTL) in the context of transplant or chemotherapy induced lymphopenia have a diminished T^{reg}/Teffector ratios which can enhance expansion of the adoptively transferred CTL [17], it is important to realize that lymphopenic hosts who do not receive large numbers of adoptively transferred CTL tend to have increased rather than decreased frequencies of T^{reg} populations [15] (reviewed in [18]). In the setting of allogeneic HSCT, brisk T^{reg} regeneration may have functional significance since donor $CD4^+Foxp3^+$ T-cell counts are inversely associated with risk of GvHD following HLA-identical sibling HSCT [19]), and adoptive transfer of T^{reg} populations can prevent GvHD in murine models [20, 21]. Clinical studies have begun using T^{reg} as GvHD prophylactics with the hope that GvT activity will be preserved [22], but the risk of suppression of anti-tumor responses remains an unknown variable. Other points of relevance regarding T^{regs} and immune reconstitution following allogeneic HSCT relate to differential effects of immunosuppressants on this subset. Whereas calcineurin inhibitors profoundly inhibit T^{reg} expansion [23], likely via inhibition of IL-2 signaling, rapamycin and its analogs spare T^{regs} allowing unfettered expansion of this subset following allogeneic HSCT. Whether the beneficial effects of an expanded T^{reg} subset on limiting GvHD outweigh a potential negative impact on tumor recurrence will require more study and will likely vary with the individual setting.

6.2.2.2 Homeostatic Peripheral Expansion of B Cells

B-cell reconstitution requires a microenvironment in the bone marrow capable of sustaining expansion and selection of early B-cell progenitors (comprehensively reviewed in [24]). In addition, recent evidence has shown that like T cells, mature B cells undergo HPE in response to open B-cell niches in the periphery of hosts with B-cell lymphopenia. Studies using CFSE (carboxyfluorescein succinimidyl ester)-labeled $B220^+$ splenocytes were the first to demonstrate that mature B cells can proliferate in untreated recipient mice [25], and subsequent work demonstrated that B-cell proliferation increases in the setting of B-cell deficiency [26–28]. Recently, van Zelm et al. [29] developed an elegant method using kappa-deleting recombination excision circles (KRECs) to measure the proliferative history of B-cells, an approach similar to the sjTREC (T cell receptor excision circles)/cjTREC analysis that has been used to assess T-cell replication history [30–32]. In both human and mouse B cells, V(D)J recombination is followed by rearrangement of the *Jk*-*Ck* intron recombination sequence to the kappa-deleting element. Comparing the ratio of the coding joint, housed permanently in the B-cell genome after this excision and thus stable with cell division, to that of the signal joint that has been removed from the genome, sits on the KREC, and is thus diluted out with each subsequent round of mitosis, can give an estimate of the degree of peripheral B-cell proliferation (Fig. 6.1). Such KREC based studies confirmed that mature B-cell proliferation occurs in vivo and contributes to B-cell reconstitution. Questions remain regarding the role of B-cell receptor (BCR) signaling in this process. If B-cell HPE is antigen-independent, as has been proposed [28, 29], or if it represents augmented proliferation to low affinity B-cell antigens, as has been observed for T-cell HPE, then this pathway would play an important role in maintaining B-cell repertoire diversity in response to B-cell depletion. However, if BCR signaling plays a central role in this process, then the B-cell repertoire generated would be predicted to be highly skewed. Future studies are needed to more carefully measure the repertoire diversity generated as a result of B-cell HPE in vivo.

6.2.3 Clinical Studies of T and B Cell Immune Reconstitution Following HSCT

Regimen-specific and host-specific factors impact immune recovery in the individual case: the intensity of the conditioning regimen, stem cell source, recipient age, dose of mature T cells contained in the graft, and the presence or absence of GvHD. The autologous setting, being most consistent in terms of donor cell source (PBSC), absence of T-cell depletion and absence of GvHD, has provided an opportunity to explore the critical role of age in immune reconstitution. Whereas thymic-dependent immune reconstitution occurs reliably within 6–12 months after intensive chemotherapy in individuals less than 15 years of age, thymic dependent recovery does not occur during this time period in older patients [35]. Recent long-term follow-up of a similar cohort (median age at treatment = 15 years; range, 7–34) treated with dose-intensive, lymphodepleting chemotherapy demonstrated full immune recovery in all patients evaluated at a median of 17.3 years (range 2.9–32.6) following completion of therapy [36]. Another recent study evaluating women 31–64 years of age treated with autologous HSCT following an alkylator-based preparative regimen for breast cancer demonstrated limited and inconsistent immune recovery during 2 years of follow-up [4]. Interestingly, with each advancing decade of patient age between 30 and 60, a decreasing percentage of patients (60% of patients in their 30s, 23% in their 40s and 0% >50 years of age) showed evidence for thymic-dependent $CD4^+$ immune reconstitution as measured by recovery of naïve $CD4^+$ subsets, TREC levels, and thymic regrowth by CT scanning. Thus, age is a fundamental factor limiting the capacity for the thymic microenvironment to support T-cell regeneration. For individuals that experience T-cell depletion within the first three decades of life, one can reasonably

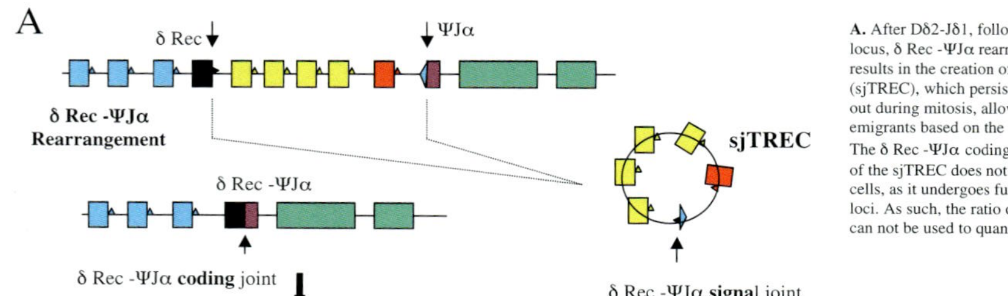

A. After Dδ2-Jδ1, followed by Vδ2-Dδ2, rearrangement of the TCR locus, δ Rec -ΨJα rearrangement, as outlined in this schematic, results in the creation of a signal joint T-cell Receptor Excision Circle (sjTREC), which persists stably in the mature T-cell, and is diluted out during mitosis, allowing for quantification of recent thymic emigrants based on the concentration of TRECs in peripheral blood. The δ Rec -ΨJα coding joint that is created as a result of the excision of the sjTREC does not remain on the genome in the majority of T-cells, as it undergoes further rearrangement with fusion of the Vα-Jα loci. As such, the ratio of sjTRECs to coding joints on the genome can not be used to quantify T-cell proliferation.

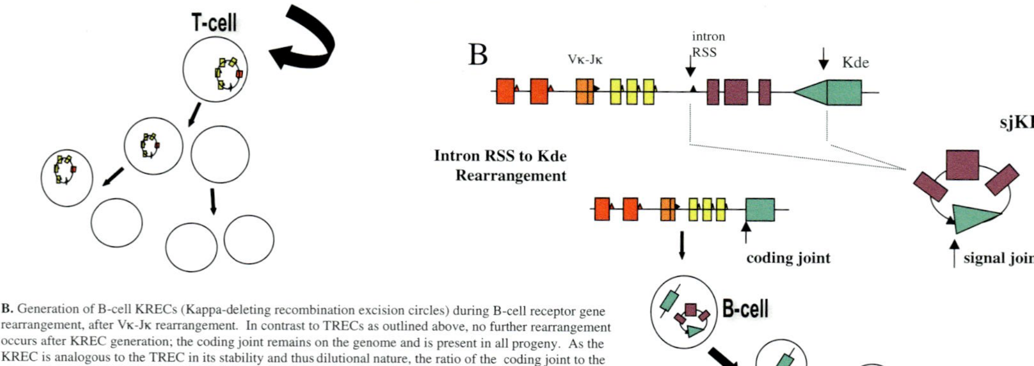

B. Generation of B-cell KRECs (Kappa-deleting recombination excision circles) during B-cell receptor gene rearrangement, after Vκ-Jκ rearrangement. In contrast to TRECs as outlined above, no further rearrangement occurs after KREC generation; the coding joint remains on the genome and is present in all progeny. As the KREC is analogous to the TREC in its stability and thus dilutional nature, the ratio of the coding joint to the signal joint (present on the KREC) increases with each cell division, allowing for quantification of B-cell replication. RSS- recombination signal sequence

Adapted from van Zelm et al J Exp med 2007, Ribeiro et al Immunological Reviews 2007, Geenen et al Journal of Endocrinology 2003, Poulin et al J Exp Med 1999, Douek et al Nature 1998

conclude that thymic-dependent T-cell regeneration and full immune reconstitution will eventually occur if further thymotoxic insults are avoided. However, it remains unclear whether full immune reconstitution can be assured in all patients who sustain profound T-cell depletion at later ages.

In the allogeneic transplant arena, the "spectrum" of transplant with regard to pattern and extent of immune reconstitution spans two extremes. At one extreme would be an infant diagnosed "early" with severe combined immunodeficiency (SCID), who receives HSCT with no conditioning regimen. In this setting, thymus-dependent immune reconstitution is the dominant pathway and robust immune reconstitution is typically observed within 6 months [37]. At the opposite end of the spectrum is a patient >50 years of age, who receives a fully ablative, irradiation-containing conditioning regimen and who develops GvHD. The combined effects of an irradiation based conditioning regimen [38], advanced age and GvHD [39, 40] all contribute to a damaged thymic microenvironment, rendering the patient essentially entirely dependent upon HPE for immune reconstitution. This pattern is associated with chronically inverted CD4/CD8 ratios, suboptimal $CD4^+$ T-cell number and function, limited TCR repertoire diversity, and impaired humoral immunity for years following HSCT. While most clinical settings of HSCT fall somewhere between these two extremes, most HSCT recipients show impaired immune function for at least 2 years following HSCT [3, 41].

Because multiple factors collude in the clinical setting of HSCT to diminish thymopoiesis, immune reconstitution in this setting depends heavily on HPE of mature T cells infused with the graft [42]. Importantly, however, multiple factors influence the capacity for HPE to provide immune competence following HSCT. The T-cell dose administered is critically important, as evidenced by

Fig. 6.1 KRECs as a measure of mature B-cell homeostasis: Schematic comparison and contrast to TRECs. A. After Dδ2-Jδ1, followed by Vδ2-Dδ2, rearrangement of the TCR locus, δ Rec -ΨJα rearrangement, as outlined in this schematic, results in the creation of a signal joint T-cell Receptor Excision Circle (sjTREC), which persists stably in the mature T-cell, and is diluted out during mitosis, allowing for quantification of recent thymic emigrants based on the concentration of TRECs in peripheral blood. The δ Rec -ΨJα coding joint that is created as a result of the excision of the sjTREC does not remain on the genome in the majority of T cells, as it undergoes further rearrangement with fusion of the Vα-Jα loci. As such, the ratio of sjTRECs to coding joints on the genome can not be used to quantify T-cell proliferation. B. Generation of B-cell KRECs (Kappa-deleting recombination excision circles) during B-cell receptor gene rearrangement, after Vα-Jα rearrangement. In contrast to TRECs as outlined above, no further rearrangement occurs after KREC generation; the coding joint remains on the genome and is present in all progeny. As the KREC is analogous to the TREC in its stability and thus dilutional nature, the ratio of the coding joint to the signal joint (present on the KREC) increases with each cell division, allowing for quantification of B-cell replication. RSS- recombination signal sequence. Adapted from van Zelm et al.[29], Ribeiro et al. [33], Geenen et al. [34], Poulin et al. [31], Douek et al. [30]

the inefficient immune reconstitution observed following the use of T-cell depleted allografts [43]. Some studies have also shown more rapid early immune reconstitution following PBSC in comparison to bone marrow (BM) grafts [44–47], raising the possibility that this reflects enhanced HPE due to higher numbers of mature T cells in PBSC vs. BM grafts. GvHD also profoundly inhibits HPE, at least in part via a cell extrinsic process, since cells transferred from mice with GvHD into normal hosts regain their proliferative capacity and conversely, T cells from normal hosts lose their proliferative capacity when adoptively transferred into a mouse with GVHD. These results suggest that GvHD may damage an as yet poorly defined "HPE microenvironemental niche" that results in diminished HPE in the setting of GvHD [48, 49].

With regard to B-cell regeneration, naïve B-cell numbers can potentially be restored within several months of completion of HSCT [50, 51]; however, B-cell lymphopoiesis is exquisitely susceptible to GvHD. In both mouse and human studies, diminished or absent naïve B-cell recovery is a highly sensitive indicator of GvHD [52, 53]. Moreover, naïve B-cell recovery does not necessarily mean that full humoral immune competence will follow, since the generation of memory B cells requires $CD4^+$ T-cell help via IL-2 and CD40L for class switching. Thus, while there is no evidence for an age-dependent decline in the function of the "bursal equivalent," age-dependent declines in thymic function indirectly impair B-cell recovery by limiting $CD4^+$ T-cell regeneration.

6.2.3.1 Immune Reconstitution Following "Alternative Transplants"

Changes in transplantation practices over recent years have led to a dramatic rise in the number of "nonmyeloablative" and reduced-intensity conditioning (RIC) allogeneic HSCT (reviewed in Chap. 9), as well as an increase in the use of cord blood as an alternative graft source. In both cases there may be clinically relevant differences in immune reconstitution. Considering the clear evidence for radiation-induced thymic damage [38], some have postulated that radiation-free and/or reduced-intensity approaches may cause less toxicity to the thymus, potentially leading to better immune reconstitution. Attempts have been made to compare immune reconstitution following RIC vs. that following conventional full intensity ("myeloablative") allogeneic HSCT; however, these have been limited to non-randomized studies. Contradictory findings have been reported to date, likely related to confounding effects of many factors already known to influence immune reconstitution, which cannot be matched in such studies (e.g., agents used for GvHD prophylaxis, GvHD incidence, patient and donor age, etc). In addition, individual RIC regimens vary considerably in their myelo- and lympho-ablative potential, and studies have generally failed to include sufficient patient numbers to power the statistically meaningful multivariate analyses that might help to definitively unravel these issues. Despite these caveats, early data suggest that RIC regimens may in fact allow more robust thymic-dependent immune reconstitution, and this issue should be more carefully addressed in future studies.

Reduction in conditioning intensity can also allow persistence of valuable elements of host immunity in the early post-transplant period, complementing the reconstituting donor immune system. This appears particularly pertinent to plasma cells, which are now known to be long lived [54]. Recipient plasma cells can persist for months following HSCT, especially following RIC, and provide a major source of neutralizing antibody for containing infection. Thus, recipient plasma cell derived IgG provides an important level of defense for infections for which immune memory is already established within the recipient at the time of transplant. It is important to note, however, that "normal" levels of circulating IgG in the early post-transplant period, derived from recipient plasma cells, cannot be equated with humoral "immunocompetence" as it relates to responding to new infection. For T-cell dependent antigens, such protection requires reconstitution of both new naive B cells and a broad $CD4^+$ T-cell repertoire to mediate effective memory B-cell generation, both of which are limited in aging hosts and/or hosts with GvHD [55]. Moreover, persistence of recipient plasma cells and their resultant IgG may be disadvantageous in some settings. For example, anti-donor isohemagglutinins can cause prolonged red cell transfusion dependence and even pure red cell aplasia following major-ABO mismatched reduced intensity transplants [56], and similar considerations may apply for transplants performed for autoimmune disorders. Persistence of recipient T-cell immunity may also provide some level of protection against infections, and this is likely to be more evident with regimens that result in early mixed chimerism. Indeed, recipient cytomegalovirus (CMV)-specific T-cell responses, either alone or in combination with donor responses, appeared protective in mixed chimeras following T-cell depleted transplantation [57].

Cord blood offers a number of potential advantages over other graft sources, including less stringent requirements for HLA-matching, but may also result in impaired immune reconstitution, especially in adult recipients. Indeed, cord blood recipients typically experience prolonged $CD4^+$ and $CD8^+$ T-cell depletion [58], with the effect on CD8 T cells being more pronounced than that observed using other graft sources [59, 60]. The reasons for impaired immune reconstitution following cord blood transplant have not been entirely delineated, but potentially relate to three factors. First, cord blood grafts typically contain approximately 50-fold fewer T cells than PBSC grafts, and about one-fifth of the number of T cells as marrow grafts [61], raising the possibility that the number (and as a result, the TCR repertoire) of T cells transferred may be insufficient to sustain effective HPE. Animal models have demonstrated a clear threshold below which T-cell inocula are simply quantitatively insufficient to restore immune competence [42]. Secondly, T cells contained in cord grafts contain mainly naïve T cells, lacking antigen-specific memory, as compared to mixed populations in other graft sources. The extent to which this qualitative change in T-cell content affects immune reconstitution remains unclear. Animal models demonstrate that naïve T cells contribute to HPE [5, 62], and in fact are central to this process since expansion of the broad repertoire contained within the naïve cell population in response to self antigens is critical for maintaining repertoire diversity. Recent clinical studies also demonstrated that naïve T cells contribute to antigen-specific anti-herpes virus responses early post-transplant (detectable from day 29 for herpes simplex virus, day 44 for cytomegalovirus, and day 94 for Varicella zoster virus in one study), although such responses develop in less than half of evaluated patients [63]. Thus, whilst there is clear evidence that naïve T cells can contribute to immune reconstitution via HPE, it remains possible that the pace and extent of immune reconstitution from a graft composed essentially entirely of naïve elements is less efficient than that generated from a mixed population.

Finally, a third potential cause for the diminished rate of immune reconstitution following cord blood transplantation could relate to the limited number of hematopoietic stem cells provided, raising the possibility that pre-thymic lymphpoid progenitor numbers may be limiting. Although cord blood $CD34^+$ cells appear more potent on a cell-per-cell basis for generating T cells ex vivo as compared to $CD34^+$ cells derived from adult bone marrow [64], the numbers of $CD34^+$ cells provided in cord blood grafts are typically 1–2 logs less than those contained in marrow or blood grafts [65]. Recipients of cord blood grafts show substantial differences between children and adults with regard to the degree of thymic-dependent immune reconstitution observed with children showing robust thymic-dependent recovery [66, 67] and adults showing largely absent thymic-dependent recovery [58]. Whether this reflects the already described age dependent differences in the resiliency of the thymic microenvironment or whether the limiting effect of age on thymopoiesis is magnified in the cord graft setting as a result of limiting numbers of prethymic progenitors cannot be determined by the clinical results currently available, but warrants further investigation.

6.3 Augmenting and Directing Immune Reconstitution

6.3.1 Thymopoiesis

6.3.1.1 Common Progenitors Re-Defined

Substantial recent progress has been made in identifying cellular subsets responsible for thymic seeding and ultimately, thymic-dependent T-cell regeneration. Classic models evoked segregation of hematopoietic stem cell (HSC) differentiation along two mutually exclusive pathways, the myelo-erythroid and lymphoid lineages respectively, and emphasized a common lymphoid progenitor (CLP) in murine bone marrow that expressed IL7Rα [68]. Based upon this model, studies sought to enhance immune reconstitution via cotransplantation of purified CLPs with purified HSCs. While the addition of CLPs to HSCs augmented early immune reconstitution (including T, B and NK lineages) and enhanced resistance in a murine model of cytomegalovirus (CMV) without increasing GvHD [69], beyond day 14 post-transplant the beneficial effects were mainly limited to the B-cell lineage, raising the possibility that CLPs may not efficiently give rise to

T cells in the long term. Subsequently, Allman et al. demonstrated directly that thymopoiesis derived from CLPs is inefficient when compared to that derived from an alternative IL7Rα– progenitor, termed the early T-lineage progenitor (ETP) [70]. ETPs reside in the thymus but derive from a multipotent marrow population termed MPPs that efficiently seed the thymus, and ultimately give rise to ETPs. MPPs retain the capacity to generate both NK and T cells, but early upon settling in the thymic microenvironment, Notch1 signaling via the Delta-like 1 (DL1) ligand induces T cell lineage commitment, differentiation to ETPs and commitment to the T-cell program [71] (Fig. 6.2).

Recent studies have defined the phenotype and growth requirements of MPPs and ETPs (reviewed in [72]), and as a result, several groups are developing approaches to expand MPPs and ETPs ex vivo and/or in vivo, in an attempt to enhance thymic-dependent T-cell regeneration. Notch1-based culture systems have enabled ex vivo expansion of committed T and NK cell progenitors by coculturing HSCs with immobilized DL1-hIgG fusion protein ($DL1^{ext\text{-}IgG}$ [73]) or OP9 bone marrow stromal cells expressing DL1 [74, 75]. In a murine model of allogeneic HSCT, cotransplantation of HSC and precursors expanded with the OP9-DL1 system enhanced thymic engraftment and cellularity, increased circulating donor T-cell numbers, and resulted in more rapid conversion to full donor chimerism [76]. NK cell reconstitution was also enhanced, resistance to *Listeria monocytogenes* was improved, and there was a suggestion that GvT activity might also be enhanced without an increase in GvHD. Thus, advances in our understanding of prethymic and early thymic subsets have provided possibilities for new approaches to expand these subsets in vivo and ex vivo. Importantly however, while CLPs, MPPs and ETPs have been clearly defined in the mouse, much less is known regarding the biology of similar subsets in humans. A $CD34^{+}CD38^{-}CD7^{+}$ human progenitor population lacking IL-7Rα expression has been identified in cord blood, but the phenotype of the critical marrow and thymic T-cell progenitors remain to be clearly defined in the human system [77]. It is imperative that the human counterpart of murine subsets be defined, both in the marrow and the thymus, in order for clinical applications to derive from these impressive fundamental insights.

6.3.1.2 Cytokines

Flt3 ligand is an important growth factor for early hematopoietic progenitors and the lymphoid progenitors described above including MPPs, ETPs and early thymic subsets [71]. Not surprisingly therefore, treatment of animals with pharmacologic doses of flt3 ligand enhances immune reconstitution with evidence for more robust thymopoiesis and improved immune competence as measured by skin graft rejection [78]. Interestingly, however, flt3 ligand therapy also augments HPE, perhaps as a result of dendritic cell expansion, which provides a greater availability of Class II to support HPE of $CD4^{+}$ T cells. Thus, flt3 ligand therapy increases both thymic-dependent and thymic-independent immune

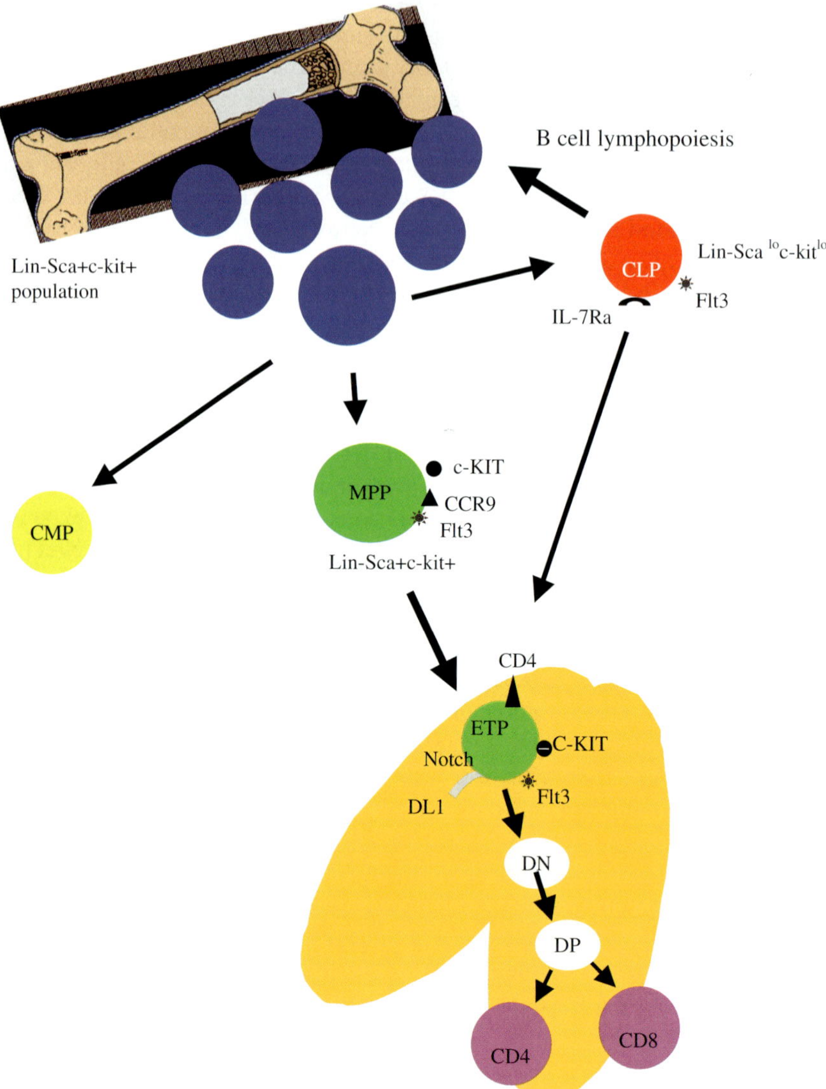

Fig. 6.2 Classical model of T-cell development described the common lymphoid progenitor (CLP) as the universal intermediary between bone marrow hematopoietic stem cell (HSC) precursors and early thymocytes, but new models describe an alternate route of T-cell development, with the multipotential progenitor (MPP) as a more efficient T-cell precursor with an enhanced capacity to seed the thymus, differentiate into ETPs and undergo robust T cell differentiation

reconstitution in mice, and future studies are warranted to investigate whether these effects can be translated into the clinical setting.

IL-7 is another cytokine with impressive immunorestorative effects when administered in pharmacologic doses. Despite the absence of IL7Rα on MPPs and ETPs, IL-7 remains an essential growth factor for expansion and survival of early triple negative thymocytes, and an essential role for IL-7 in thymopoiesis is illustrated by the profound lymphopenia observed in IL-7$-/-$ mice [79] and humans with severe combined immunodeficiency, in whom T-cell deficiency is attributed to a loss of IL-7 signaling [80]. These studies, combined with evidence that radiation induced damage to the thymic epithelium is associated with diminished IL-7 production [38], lend credence to the notion that pharmacologic dosing of IL-7 could enhance thymopoiesis. In animal studies conducted thus far, IL-7 potently augments immune restoration following HSCT [81–84], but it remains unclear whether IL-7 therapy augments thymic output. IL-7 potently augments HPE of mature T cells, with a predilection for augmenting HPE of naïve T cells, which results in enhanced thymic-dependent progeny in both mice and primates [84, 85]; however, this is not typically associated with thymic enlargement and has generally been associated with diminished TREC numbers [86]. Thus, current models hold that IL-7 potently enhances immune reconstitution following stem cell transplantation in both mice and primates, but most, if not all of this effect, occurs as a result of enhanced homeostatic peripheral expansion.

The issues regarding the relative roles for enhanced thymopoiesis versus enhanced peripheral expansion in response to both cytokines that could be used to enhance immune reconstitution is of more than academic interest. In the setting of allogeneic HSCT, agents which augment homeostatic peripheral expansion are also prone to augment GvHD, and mouse studies have clearly shown that pharmacologic dosing of both IL-7 [87] and flt3 ligand [88] aggravate GvHD. Such results do not rule out the possibility that these agents could be useful in the context of allogeneic HSCT, but they emphasize that early clinical studies should focus upon the T-cell depleted or cord blood settings where immune incompetence is a significant problem and where GvHD is less likely to occur [89]. The same considerations apply to IL-15, which in preclinical models specifically enhances peripheral expansion of $CD8^+$ T cells but has the potential to aggravate GvHD [90, 91].

6.3.1.3 Targeting the Thymic Microenvironment

Successful thymic-dependent immune reconstitution requires that cells contained in the marrow graft efficiently initiate the elaborate thymic differentiation process by seeding available thymic niches [92, 93]. Reciprocal interactions between thymic epithelium and developing thymocytes are critical throughout this process [94, 95]. However, conditioning therapies and GvHD damage thymic epithelium cells (TECs) in HSCT recipients and diminish the ability of the thymus to sustain de novo generation of T cells following HSCT [96].

Keratinocyte growth factor (KGF), a member of the acidic fibroblast growth factor family, is an epithelial cell specific growth factor [97] that exerts protective effects on and can enhance thympoiesis post transplant in murine models [98]. In an acute GvHD model, KGF treated mice showed normal thymic architecture, in contrast to the disorganized, disrupted thymic epithelium present in untreated mice with GVHD [99]. KGF can also protect from steroid, radiation-induced, and age associated thymic damage in mouse models [100], raising the possibility that KGF's thymopoietic effects could be effective in several clinical settings associated with thymic insufficiency. Subsequent work has demonstrated that KGF induces TEC proliferation through expression of Wnt and BMP family members [101] and that KGF's thymopoietic effects are mediated primarily via IL-7 [102]. Thus, KGF represents a new class of immunorestorative, which mediates its effect primarily on stromal and epithelial populations within lymphoid tissues rather than on the lymphocytes themselves. One potential advantage to the use of KGF in the setting of allogeneic HSCT over the cytokine approaches discussed above, is that KGF does not augment homeostatic peripheral expansion and thus it does not appear to augment GvHD.

6.3.2 Homeostatic Peripheral Expansion

6.3.2.1 Virus-Specific T Cells Revisited: the Path to Tumor-Specific Immunotherapies?

It has long been known that HPE occurring in lymphopenic hosts enhances expansion and survival of adoptively transferred T cells. Following myeloablative and lympho-ablative regimens, the specific physiologic changes that drive HPE include removal of cytokine sinks resulting in elevated levels of IL-7 and potentially other homeostatic cytokines, diminished absolute numbers of suppressors (T^{reg}, myeloid suppressor cells), and potentially activation of antigen presenting cells as a result of lipopolysaccharide (LPS) leakage across a gut that is damaged by a cytotoxic conditioning regimen [17, 103–105]. Thus, the post-transplant setting provides and optimal milieu for the development of adoptive cell therapy. In this regard, significant progress has have been made in targeting viral infections. Advances in culture techniques have allowed rapid generation of polyclonal products including both $CD4^+$ and $CD8^+$ virus-specific elements, which when transferred into lymphopenic hosts induce impressive in vivo expansion and persistence and an apparent reduction in viral reactivation [106, 107]. While CMV has been the major focus, the rise of adenovirus as an important pathogen has provided a further target for adoptive cellular therapy [108]. To obviate the need for preparation of specific T-cell lines for each virus in every eligible individual, some groups have pursued genetic modification of antigen-presenting cell lines using viral vectors to allow presentation of epitopes of multiple viruses. Resulting bi- or tri-specific T-cell lines expand multiple discrete virus-specific populations and provide clinically measurable antiviral activity following transfer [109]. Selection of virus specific T-cells directly from donors has become feasible with the development of cytokine-capture and HLA-multimer technologies [110, 111], and when precursor frequencies are high enough, ex vivo expansion can sometimes be avoided altogether, which may be advantageous for more widespread application [108, 112]. The relative merits of each approach have yet to be carefully compared and the field is now ready for randomized studies to more formally assess the true benefits of adoptive cellular therapies to prevent or treat viral infections. Furthermore, many challenges remain. Generation of primary immune responses ex vivo remains technically demanding, limiting these approaches to those with sero-positive donors and posing significant challenges for generating such products from cord blood. In addition, the bias of cord blood T cells toward Th2/Tc2 function forms a further barrier to generation of virus-specific T cells. Despite these considerations, progress has been made in producing CMV-specific IFNγ- and TNFα-producing CD4$^+$ (Th1) and CD8$^+$ (Tc1) T cells from cord blood products [113].

The immunogenicity of exogenous viral antigens and the relatively restricted and reproducible range of immunodominant antigens targeted by antiviral immune responses have aided the development of cellular therapies to target viral infection. Unfortunately, targeting human cancers presents a more difficult challenge. Unmanipulated donor lymphocyte infusions (DLI) are highly effective in preventing recurrence and in inducing remission of chronic myelogenous leukemia following HSCT. However, augmenting the effectiveness of DLI and expanding this success to other leukemias and solid tumors has remained a challenge. Recently, several groups have attempted to exploit the physiologic changes which drive HPE to improve the effectiveness of immunotherapies directed toward solid tumors [114]. This is appealing since a cardinal feature of HPE is enhanced T-cell proliferation in response to low-affinity self antigens, which when combined with the heightened susceptibility to skewing, can permit the generation of T-cell repertoires capable of mediating potent immune responses toward tumor antigens, which are known to represent weak, self antigens. In melanoma, combining adoptive cellular therapy with lymphodepletion and IL-2 has resulted in significant response rates providing proof-of-principle for this approach [115]. The lack of well-defined tumor-specific targets and the limitations of attempting to target multiple HLA alleles, however, have hampered wider application tumor-specific adoptive cellular therapies in HSCT. As a result, many groups have worked to generate ex vivo culture techniques that do not require specific knowledge of antigenic targets [116] and to optimize TCR gene transfer techniques to re-direct T-cell specificities [117, 118] or engineer T cells with antibody binding receptors that are not subject to HLA restriction. The use of therapeutic vaccines in vivo, either in isolation or in combination with adoptive cellular therapies [119, 120], is another important component to emerging T-cell-based immunotherapies targeting minimal residual neoplastic disease post-transplant. Finally, approaches that aim to interfere with T cell intrinsic immune regulatory checkpoints (monoclonal antibodies to CTLA-4 for $CD4^+$ and PD1 for $CD8^+$ T cells) could potentially enhance the effectiveness of tumor-specific vaccination during lymphopenia, and may not enhance GvHD, since costimulatory pathways are thought not to be important in HPE [121].

6.3.2.2 Enhancing "Global" Immune Reconstitution with Allo-Depleted T Cells

Rebuilding global immunity following allogeneic HSCT by piecemeal application of antigen-specific therapies becomes increasingly impractical as the number of desirable specificities increases. Given that increasing the dose of unselected DLI eventually results in an unacceptable rate of GvHD due to the presence of alloreactive T cells, selective depletion of alloreactive specificities is another attractive approach for providing optimal doses of T cells without initiating GvHD. A number of small phase 1/2 studies [122–124] have demonstrated clinical feasibility of ex vivo selective allodepletion using an anti-CD25 immunotoxin following allo-stimulation. This approach generates products which retain anti-pathogen and even anti-tumor T-cell specificities but are depleted of alloreactive T cells [125, 126], and proof-of-principle for the ability to separate GvT from GvH-specific $CD4^+$ T cells was elegantly demonstrated by sequencing the TCR of selectively depleted T cell clones and comparing these to those of clones subsequently elicited by leukemia of the same stimulator [127]. One important issue for the use of CD25 targeting to deplete alloreactive T cells also is that the approach is predicted to deplete the infused graft of $CD4^+CD25^+Foxp3^+$ regulatory T cells. Theoretically, GvT activity could be enhanced but could also increase the risk of exacerbating GvHD. Interestingly, preliminary results thus far have not observed excessive rates of GvHD, even in early clinical studies of allodepletion in the haploidentical transplant setting [122, 123]. This may reflect the rapid regeneration of $CD4^+Foxp3^+$ T cells from a $CD4^+CD25lo/-$ subset [128], or of expansion of inducible T^{reg} from $CD4^+Foxp3^+$ T cells. Future studies are needed to more fully assess the capacity for allodepleted grafts to mediate substantial GvT in the absence of GvHD.

6.4 Summary

The evolution of understanding regarding key issues involved in immune reconstitution should allow movement from indirect supportive care of immuno-incompetence following HSCT to proactive measures designed to enhance reconstitution in this setting. Future clinical studies using lymphoid progenitors, thymoprotective agents and immunostimulatory cytokines are needed to test the clinical utility of these approaches and agents which have had promising results in preclinical models. Importantly, while solid pre-clinical supporting data exist for many agents and approaches, clinical application must proceed carefully, with particular attention to issues that may depend critically on timing and dose. Allogeneic HSCT presents a challenging arena for the application of immune based therapies because of the need to respect the delicate balance between GvHD, GvT responses, rejection and reconstitution of specific immunity against pathogens. Armed with our current and rapidly evolving knowledge, it is hopes that the coming years will witness the evolutionary development of clinical practice in this arena.

References

1. Storek J, Gooley T, Witherspoon RP, Sullivan KM, Storb R. Infectious morbidity in long-term survivors of allogeneic marrow transplantation is associated with low CD4 T cell counts. Am J Hematol. 1997;54:131–8.
2. Anderson KC, Ritz J, Takvorian T, Coral F, Daley H, Gorgone BC, et al. Hematologic engraftment and immune reconstitution posttransplantation with anti-B1 purged autologous bone marrow. Blood 1987;69:597–604.
3. Storek J, Dawson MA, Storer B, Stevens-Ayers T, Maloney DG, Marr KA, et al. Immune reconstitution after allogeneic marrow transplantation compared with blood stem cell transplantation. Blood 2001;97:3380–9.
4. Hakim FT, Memon SA, Cepeda R, Jones EC, Chow CK, Kasten-Sportes C, et al. Age-dependent incidence, time course, and consequences of thymic renewal in adults. J Clin Invest. 2005;115:930–9.
5. Mackall CL, Bare CV, Granger LA, Sharrow SO, Titus JA, Gress RE. Thymic-independent T cell regeneration occurs via antigen-driven expansion of peripheral T cells resulting in a repertoire that is limited in diversity and prone to skewing. J Immunol. 1996;156:4609–16.
6. Dumont-Girard F, Roux E, van Lier RA, Hale G, Helg C, Chapuis B, et al. Reconstitution of the T-cell compartment after bone marrow transplantation: restoration of the repertoire by thymic emigrants. Blood 1998;92:4464–71.
7. Weinberg K, Annett G, Kashyap A, Lenarsky C, Forman SJ, Parkman R. The effect of thymic function on immunocompetence following bone marrow transplantation. Biol Blood Marrow Transplant. 1995;1:18–23.
8. Kalwak K, Moson I, Cwian J, Gorczynska E, Toporski J, Turkiewicz D, et al. A prospective analysis of immune recovery in children following allogeneic transplantation of T-cell-depleted or non-T-cell-depleted hematopoietic cells from HLA-disparate family donors. Transplant Proc. 2003;35:1551–5.
9. Fontenot JD, Gavin MA, Rudensky AY. Foxp3 programs the development and function of CD4+CD25+ regulatory T cells. Nat Immunol. 2003;4:330–6.
10. Hori S, Nomura T, Sakaguchi S. Control of regulatory T cell development by the transcription factor Foxp3. Science 2003;299:1057–61.
11. Kim JM, Rasmussen JP, Rudensky AY. Regulatory T cells prevent catastrophic autoimmunity throughout the lifespan of mice. Nat Immunol. 2007;8:191–7.
12. Belkaid Y, Piccirillo CA, Mendez S, Shevach EM, Sacks DL. CD4+CD25+ regulatory T cells control Leishmania major persistence and immunity. Nature 2002;420:502–7.
13. Mendez S, Reckling SK, Piccirillo CA, Sacks D, Belkaid Y. Role for CD4(+) CD25(+) regulatory T cells in reactivation of persistent leishmaniasis and control of concomitant immunity. J Exp Med. 2004;200:201–10.
14. Onizuka S, Tawara I, Shimizu J, Sakaguchi S, Fujita T, Nakayama E. Tumor rejection by in vivo administration of anti-CD25 (interleukin-2 receptor alpha) monoclonal antibody. Cancer Res. 1999;59:3128–33.

15. Zhang H, Chua KS, Guimond M, Kapoor V, Brown MV, Fleisher TA, et al. Lymphopenia and interleukin-2 therapy alter homeostasis of CD4+CD25+ regulatory T cells. Nat Med. 2005;11:1238–43.
16. Powell DJ Jr, de Vries CR, Allen T, Ahmadzadeh M, Rosenberg SA. Inability to mediate prolonged reduction of regulatory T Cells after transfer of autologous CD25-depleted PBMC and interleukin-2 after lymphodepleting chemotherapy. J Immunother (1997). 2007;30:438–47.
17. Antony PA, Piccirillo CA, Akpinarli A, Finkelstein SE, Speiss PJ, Surman DR, et al. CD8+ T cell immunity against a tumor/self-antigen is augmented by CD4+ T helper cells and hindered by naturally occurring T regulatory cells. J Immunol. 2005; 174:2591–601.
18. Krupica T Jr, Fry TJ, Mackall CL. Autoimmunity during lymphopenia: a two-hit model. Clin Immunol. 2006;120:121–8.
19. Rezvani K, Mielke S, Ahmadzadeh M, Kilical Y, Savani BN, Zeilah J, et al. High donor FOXP3–positive regulatory T-cell (Treg) content is associated with a low risk of GVHD following HLA-matched allogeneic SCT. Blood 2006;108:1291–7.
20. Hoffmann P, Ermann J, Edinger M, Fathman CG, Strober S. Donor-type CD4(+)CD25(+) regulatory T cells suppress lethal acute graft-versus-host disease after allogeneic bone marrow transplantation. J Exp Med. 2002;196:389–99.
21. Nguyen VH, Shashidhar S, Chang DS, Ho L, Kambham N, Bachmann M, et al. The impact of regulatory T cells on T cell immunity following hematopoeitic cell transplantation. Blood 2007;111:945–53.
22. Edinger M, Hoffmann P, Ermann J, Drago K, Fathman CG, Strober S, et al. CD4+CD25+ regulatory T cells preserve graft-versus-tumor activity while inhibiting graft-versus-host disease after bone marrow transplantation. Nat Med. 2003;9:1144–50.
23. Zeiser R, Nguyen VH, Beilhack A, Buess M, Schulz S, Baker J, et al. Inhibition of CD4+CD25+ regulatory T-cell function by calcineurin-dependent interleukin-2 production. Blood 2006;108:390–9.
24. LeBien TW. Fates of human B-cell precursors. Blood 2000;96:9–23.
25. Lyons AB, Parish CR. Determination of lymphocyte division by flow cytometry. J Immunol Methods. 1994;171:131–7.
26. Agenes F, Freitas AA. Transfer of small resting B cells into immunodeficient hosts results in the selection of a self-renewing activated B cell population. J Exp Med. 1999;189:319–30.
27. Agenes F, Rosado MM, Freitas AA. Independent homeostatic regulation of B cell compartments. Eur J Immunol. 1997;27:1801–7.
28. Cabatingan MS, Schmidt MR, Sen R, Woodland RT. Naive B lymphocytes undergo homeostatic proliferation in response to B cell deficit. J Immunol. 2002;169:6795–805.
29. van Zelm MC, Szczepanski T, van der Burg M, van Dongen JJ. Replication history of B lymphocytes reveals homeostatic proliferation and extensive antigen-induced B cell expansion. J Exp Med. 2007;204:645–55.
30. Douek DC, McFarland RD, Keiser PH, Gage EA, Massey JM, Haynes BF, et al. Changes in thymic function with age and during the treatment of HIV infection. Nature 1998;396:690–5.
31. Poulin JF, Viswanathan MN, Harris JM, Komanduri KV, Wieder E, Ringuette N, et al. Direct evidence for thymic function in adult humans. J Exp Med. 1999;190:479–86.
32. Takeshita S, Toda M, Yamagishi H. Excision products of the T cell receptor gene support a progressive rearrangement model of the alpha/delta locus. Embo J. 1989;8:3261–70.
33. Ribeiro RM, Perelson AS. Determining thymic output quantitatively: using models to interpret experimental T-cell receptor excision circle (TREC) data. Immunol Rev. 2007;216:21–34.
34. Geenen V, Poulin JF, Dion ML, Martens H, Castermans E, Hansenne I, et al. Quantification of T cell receptor rearrangement excision circles to estimate thymic function: an important new tool for endocrine-immune physiology. J Endocrinol. 2003;176:305–11.

35. Mackall CL, Fleisher TA, Brown MR, Andrich MP, Chen CC, Feuerstein IM, et al. Age, thymopoiesis, and CD4+ T-lymphocyte regeneration after intensive chemotherapy. N Engl J Med. 1995;332:143–9.
36. Shand JC, Mansky PJ, Brown MV, Fleisher TA, Mackall CL. Adolescents and young adults successfully restore lymphocyte homeostasis after intensive T-cell depleting therapy for cancer. Br J Haematol. 2006;135:270–1.
37. Buckley RH, Schiff SE, Schiff RI, Roberts JL, Markert ML, Peters W, et al. Haploidentical bone marrow stem cell transplantation in human severe combined immunodeficiency. Semin Hematol. 1993;30 Suppl 4:92–101; discussion 2–4.
38. Chung B, Barbara-Burnham L, Barsky L, Weinberg K. Radiosensitivity of thymic interleukin-7 production and thymopoiesis after bone marrow transplantation. Blood 2001;98:1601–6.
39. Desbarats J, Lapp WS. Thymic selection and thymic major histocompatibility complex class II expression are abnormal in mice undergoing graft-versus-host reactions. J Exp Med. 1993;178:805–14.
40. Storek J, Joseph A, Dawson MA, Douek DC, Storer B, Maloney DG. Factors influencing T-lymphopoiesis after allogeneic hematopoietic cell transplantation. Transplantation 2002;73:1154–8.
41. Atkinson K, Hansen JA, Storb R, Goehle S, Goldstein G, Thomas ED. T-cell subpopulations identified by monoclonal antibodies after human marrow transplantation. I. Helper-inducer and cytotoxic-suppressor subsets. Blood 1982;59:1292–8.
42. Fry TJ, Christensen BL, Komschlies KL, Gress RE, Mackall CL. Interleukin-7 restores immunity in athymic T-cell-depleted hosts. Blood 2001;97:1525–33.
43. Daley JP, Rozans MK, Smith BR, Burakoff SJ, Rappeport JM, Miller RA. Retarded recovery of functional T cell frequencies in T cell-depleted bone marrow transplant recipients. Blood 1987;70:960–4.
44. Dey BR, Shaffer J, Yee AJ, McAfee S, Caron M, Power K, et al. Comparison of outcomes after transplantation of peripheral blood stem cells versus bone marrow following an identical nonmyeloablative conditioning regimen. Bone Marrow Transplant. 2007;40:19–27.
45. Koehl U, Bochennek K, Zimmermann SY, Lehrnbecher T, Sorensen J, Esser R, et al. Immune recovery in children undergoing allogeneic stem cell transplantation: absolute CD8+ CD3+ count reconstitution is associated with survival. Bone Marrow Transplant. 2007;39:269–78.
46. Powles R, Mehta J, Kulkarni S, Treleaven J, Millar B, Marsden J, et al. Allogeneic blood and bone-marrow stem-cell transplantation in haematological malignant diseases: a randomised trial. Lancet 2000;355:1231–7.
47. Roberts MM, To LB, Gillis D, Mundy J, Rawling C, Ng K, et al. Immune reconstitution following peripheral blood stem cell transplantation, autologous bone marrow transplantation and allogeneic bone marrow transplantation. Bone Marrow Transplant. 1993;12:469–75.
48. Dulude G, Roy DC, Perreault C. The effect of graft-versus-host disease on T cell production and homeostasis. J Exp Med. 1999;189:1329–42.
49. Gorski J, Chen X, Gendelman M, Yassai M, Krueger A, Tivol E, et al. Homeostatic expansion and repertoire regeneration of donor T cells during graft versus host disease is constrained by the host environment. Blood 2007;109:5502–10.
50. Small TN, Keever CA, Weiner-Fedus S, Heller G, O'Reilly RJ, Flomenberg N. B-cell differentiation following autologous, conventional, or T-cell depleted bone marrow transplantation: a recapitulation of normal B-cell ontogeny. Blood 1990;76:1647–56.
51. Storek J, Witherspoon RP, Storb R. Reconstitution of membrane IgD- (mIgD-) B cells after marrow transplantation lags behind the reconstitution of mIgD+ B cells. Blood 1997;89:350–1.

52. Hakim FT, Sharrow SO, Payne S, Shearer GM. Repopulation of host lymphohematopoietic systems by donor cells during graft-versus-host reaction in unirradiated adult F1 mice injected with parental lymphocytes. J Immunol. 1991;146:2108–15.
53. Storek J, Wells D, Dawson MA, Storer B, Maloney DG. Factors influencing B lymphopoiesis after allogeneic hematopoietic cell transplantation. Blood 2001;98:489–91.
54. Manz RA, Thiel A, Radbruch A. Lifetime of plasma cells in the bone marrow. Nature 1997;388:133–4.
55. Isaacs JD, Thiel A. Stem cell transplantation for autoimmune disorders. Immune reconstitution. Best Pract Res Clin Haematol. 2004;17:345–58.
56. Bolan CD, Leitman SF, Griffith LM, Wesley RA, Procter JL, Stroncek DF, et al. Delayed donor red cell chimerism and pure red cell aplasia following major ABO-incompatible nonmyeloablative hematopoietic stem cell transplantation. Blood 2001;98:1687–94.
57. Chalandon Y, Degermann S, Villard J, Arlettaz L, Kaiser L, Vischer S, et al. Pretransplantation CMV-specific T cells protect recipients of T-cell-depleted grafts against CMV-related complications. Blood 2006;107:389–96.
58. Komanduri KV, St John LS, de Lima M, McMannis J, Rosinski S, McNiece I, et al. Delayed immune reconstitution after cord blood transplantation is characterized by impaired thymopoiesis and late memory T cell skewing. Blood 2007;110:4543–51.
59. Niehues T, Rocha V, Filipovich AH, Chan KW, Porcher R, Michel G, et al. Factors affecting lymphocyte subset reconstitution after either related or unrelated cord blood transplantation in children—a Eurocord analysis. Br J Haematol. 2001;114:42–8.
60. Thomson BG, Robertson KA, Gowan D, Heilman D, Broxmeyer HE, Emanuel D, et al. Analysis of engraftment, graft-versus-host disease, and immune recovery following unrelated donor cord blood transplantation. Blood 2000;96:2703–11.
61. Theilgaard-Monch K, Raaschou-Jensen K, Palm H, Schjodt K, Heilmann C, Vindelov L, et al. Flow cytometric assessment of lymphocyte subsets, lymphoid progenitors, and hematopoietic stem cells in allogeneic stem cell grafts. Bone Marrow Transplant. 2001;28:1073–82.
62. Goldrath AW, Bevan MJ. Low-affinity ligands for the TCR drive proliferation of mature CD8+ T cells in lymphopenic hosts. Immunity 1999;11:183–90.
63. Cohen G, Carter SL, Weinberg KI, Masinsin B, Guinan E, Kurtzberg J, et al. Antigen-specific T-lymphocyte function after cord blood transplantation. Biol Blood Marrow Transplant. 2006;12:1335–42.
64. Robin C, Bennaceur-Griscelli A, Louache F, Vainchenker W, Coulombel L. Identification of human T-lymphoid progenitor cells in CD34+ CD38low and CD34+ CD38+ subsets of human cord blood and bone marrow cells using NOD-SCID fetal thymus organ cultures. Br J Haematol. 1999;104:809–19.
65. Wagner JE, Barker JN, DeFor TE, Baker KS, Blazar BR, Eide C, et al. Transplantation of unrelated donor umbilical cord blood in 102 patients with malignant and nonmalignant diseases: influence of CD34 cell dose and HLA disparity on treatment-related mortality and survival. Blood 2002;100:1611–8.
66. Moretta A, Maccario R, Fagioli F, Giraldi E, Busca A, Montagna D, et al. Analysis of immune reconstitution in children undergoing cord blood transplantation. Exp Hematol. 2001;29:371–9.
67. Talvensaari K, Clave E, Douay C, Rabian C, Garderet L, Busson M, et al. A broad T-cell repertoire diversity and an efficient thymic function indicate a favorable long-term immune reconstitution after cord blood stem cell transplantation. Blood 2002;99:1458–64.
68. Kondo M, Weissman IL, Akashi K. Identification of clonogenic common lymphoid progenitors in mouse bone marrow. Cell 1997;91:661–72.
69. Arber C, BitMansour A, Sparer TE, Higgins JP, Mocarski ES, Weissman IL, et al. Common lymphoid progenitors rapidly engraft and protect against lethal murine

cytomegalovirus infection after hematopoietic stem cell transplantation. Blood 2003;102:421–8.
70. Allman D, Sambandam A, Kim S, Miller JP, Pagan A, Well D, et al. Thymopoiesis independent of common lymphoid progenitors. Nat Immunol. 2003;4:168–74.
71. Sambandam A, Maillard I, Zediak VP, Xu L, Gerstein RM, Aster JC, et al. Notch signaling controls the generation and differentiation of early T lineage progenitors. Nat Immunol. 2005;6:663–70.
72. Bhandoola A, Sambandam A. From stem cell to T cell: one route or many? Nat Rev Immunol. 2006;6:117–26.
73. Ohishi K, Varnum-Finney B, Bernstein ID. Delta-1 enhances marrow and thymus repopulating ability of human CD34(+)CD38(–) cord blood cells. J Clin Invest. 2002;110:1165–74.
74. Schmitt TM, de Pooter RF, Gronski MA, Cho SK, Ohashi PS, Zuniga-Pflucker JC. Induction of T cell development and establishment of T cell competence from embryonic stem cells differentiated in vitro. Nat Immunol. 2004;5:410–7.
75. Schmitt TM, Zuniga-Pflucker JC. Induction of T cell development from hematopoietic progenitor cells by delta-like-1 in vitro. Immunity 2002;17:749–56.
76. Zakrzewski JL, Kochman AA, Lu SX, Terwey TH, Kim TD, Hubbard VM, et al. Adoptive transfer of T-cell precursors enhances T-cell reconstitution after allogeneic hematopoietic stem cell transplantation. Nat Med. 2006;12:1039–47.
77. Hao QL, Zhu J, Price MA, Payne KJ, Barsky LW, Crooks GM. Identification of a novel, human multilymphoid progenitor in cord blood. Blood 2001;97:3683–90.
78. Fry TJ, Sinha M, Milliron M, Chu YW, Kapoor V, Gress RE, et al. Flt3 ligand enhances thymic-dependent and thymic-independent immune reconstitution. Blood 2004;104:2794–800.
79. von Freeden-Jeffry U, Vieira P, Lucian LA, McNeil T, Burdach SE, Murray R. Lymphopenia in interleukin (IL)-7 gene-deleted mice identifies IL-7 as a nonredundant cytokine. J Exp Med. 1995;181:1519–26.
80. Plum J, De Smedt M, Leclercq G, Verhasselt B, Vandekerckhove B. Interleukin-7 is a critical growth factor in early human T-cell development. Blood 1996;88:4239–45.
81. Alpdogan O, Muriglan SJ, Eng JM, Willis LM, Greenberg AS, Kappel BJ, et al. IL-7 enhances peripheral T cell reconstitution after allogeneic hematopoietic stem cell transplantation. J Clin Invest. 2003;112:1095–107.
82. Boerman OC, Gregorio TA, Grzegorzewski KJ, Faltynek CR, Kenny JJ, Wiltrout RH, et al. Recombinant human IL-7 administration in mice affects colony-forming units-spleen and lymphoid precursor cell localization and accelerates engraftment of bone marrow transplants. J Leukoc Biol. 1995;58:151–8.
83. Bolotin E, Smogorzewska M, Smith S, Widmer M, Weinberg K. Enhancement of thymopoiesis after bone marrow transplant by in vivo interleukin-7. Blood 1996;88:1887–94.
84. Mackall CL, Fry TJ, Bare C, Morgan P, Galbraith A, Gress RE. IL-7 increases both thymic-dependent and thymic-independent T-cell regeneration after bone marrow transplantation. Blood 2001;97:1491–7.
85. Storek J, Gillespy T, 3rd, Lu H, Joseph A, Dawson MA, Gough M, et al. Interleukin-7 improves CD4 T-cell reconstitution after autologous CD34 cell transplantation in monkeys. Blood 2003;101:4209–18.
86. Fry TJ, Moniuszko M, Creekmore S, Donohue SJ, Douek DC, Giardina S, et al. IL-7 therapy dramatically alters peripheral T-cell homeostasis in normal and SIV-infected nonhuman primates. Blood 2003;101:2294–9.
87. Sinha ML, Fry TJ, Fowler DH, Miller G, Mackall CL. Interleukin 7 worsens graft-versus-host disease. Blood 2002;100:2642–9.
88. Blazar BR, McKenna HJ, Panoskaltsis-Mortari A, Taylor PA. Flt3 ligand (FL) treatment of murine donors does not modify graft-versus-host disease (GVHD) but FL

treatment of recipients post-bone marrow transplantation accelerates GVHD lethality. Biol Blood Marrow Transplant. 2001;7:197–207.

89. Alpdogan O, Schmaltz C, Muriglan SJ, Kappel BJ, Perales MA, Rotolo JA, et al. Administration of interleukin-7 after allogeneic bone marrow transplantation improves immune reconstitution without aggravating graft-versus-host disease. Blood 2001;98:2256–65.
90. Alpdogan O, Eng JM, Muriglan SJ, Willis LM, Hubbard VM, Tjoe KH, et al. Interleukin-15 enhances immune reconstitution after allogeneic bone marrow transplantation. Blood 2005;105:865–73.
91. Katsanis E, Xu Z, Panoskaltsis-Mortari A, Weisdorf DJ, Widmer MB, Blazar BR. IL-15 administration following syngeneic bone marrow transplantation prolongs survival of lymphoma bearing mice. Transplantation 1996;62:872–5.
92. Chen X, Barfield R, Benaim E, Leung W, Knowles J, Lawrence D, et al. Prediction of T-cell reconstitution by assessment of T-cell receptor excision circle before allogeneic hematopoietic stem cell transplantation in pediatric patients. Blood 2005;105:886–93.
93. Tomita Y, Khan A, Sykes M. Role of intrathymic clonal deletion and peripheral anergy in transplantation tolerance induced by bone marrow transplantation in mice conditioned with a nonmyeloablative regimen. J Immunol. 1994;153:1087–98.
94. Hollander GA, Wang B, Nichogiannopoulou A, Platenburg PP, van Ewijk W, Burakoff SJ, et al. Developmental control point in induction of thymic cortex regulated by a subpopulation of prothymocytes. Nature 1995;373:350–3.
95. Lind EF, Prockop SE, Porritt HE, Petrie HT. Mapping precursor movement through the postnatal thymus reveals specific microenvironments supporting defined stages of early lymphoid development. J Exp Med. 2001;194:127–34.
96. Weinberg K, Blazar BR, Wagner JE, Agura E, Hill BJ, Smogorzewska M, et al. Factors affecting thymic function after allogeneic hematopoietic stem cell transplantation. Blood 2001;97:1458–66.
97. Rubin JS, Osada H, Finch PW, Taylor WG, Rudikoff S, Aaronson SA. Purification and characterization of a newly identified growth factor specific for epithelial cells. Proc Natl Acad Sci USA. 1989;86:802–6.
98. Min D, Taylor PA, Panoskaltsis-Mortari A, Chung B, Danilenko DM, Farrell C, et al. Protection from thymic epithelial cell injury by keratinocyte growth factor: a new approach to improve thymic and peripheral T-cell reconstitution after bone marrow transplantation. Blood 2002;99:4592–600.
99. Rossi S, Blazar BR, Farrell CL, Danilenko DM, Lacey DL, Weinberg KI, et al. Keratinocyte growth factor preserves normal thymopoiesis and thymic microenvironment during experimental graft-versus-host disease. Blood 2002;100:682–91.
100. Alpdogan O, Hubbard VM, Smith OM, Patel N, Lu S, Goldberg GL, et al. Keratinocyte growth factor (KGF) is required for postnatal thymic regeneration. Blood 2006;107:2453–60.
101. Rossi SW, Jeker LT, Ueno T, Kuse S, Keller MP, Zuklys S, et al. Keratinocyte growth factor (KGF) enhances postnatal T-cell development via enhancements in proliferation and function of thymic epithelial cells. Blood 2007;109:3803–11.
102. Min D, Panoskaltsis-Mortari A, Kuro OM, Hollander GA, Blazar BR, Weinberg KI. Sustained thymopoiesis and improvement in functional immunity induced by exogenous KGF administration in murine models of aging. Blood 2007;109:2529–37.
103. Gattinoni L, Finkelstein SE, Klebanoff CA, Antony PA, Palmer DC, Spiess PJ, et al. Removal of homeostatic cytokine sinks by lymphodepletion enhances the efficacy of adoptively transferred tumor-specific CD8+ T cells. J Exp Med. 2005;202:907–12.
104. Klebanoff CA, Khong HT, Antony PA, Palmer DC, Restifo NP. Sinks, suppressors and antigen presenters: how lymphodepletion enhances T cell-mediated tumor immunotherapy. Trends Immunol. 2005;26:111–7.

105. Wrzesinski C, Paulos CM, Gattinoni L, Palmer DC, Kaiser A, Yu Z, et al. Hematopoietic stem cells promote the expansion and function of adoptively transferred antitumor CD8 T cells. J Clin Invest. 2007;117:492–501.
106. Heslop HE, Ng CY, Li C, Smith CA, Loftin SK, Krance RA, et al. Long-term restoration of immunity against Epstein-Barr virus infection by adoptive transfer of gene-modified virus-specific T lymphocytes. Nat Med. 1996;2:551–5.
107. Peggs KS, Verfuerth S, Pizzey A, Khan N, Guiver M, Moss PA, et al. Adoptive cellular therapy for early cytomegalovirus infection after allogeneic stem-cell transplantation with virus-specific T-cell lines. Lancet 2003;362:1375–7.
108. Feuchtinger T, Matthes-Martin S, Richard C, Lion T, Fuhrer M, Hamprecht K, et al. Safe adoptive transfer of virus-specific T-cell immunity for the treatment of systemic adenovirus infection after allogeneic stem cell transplantation. Br J Haematol. 2006;134:64–76.
109. Leen AM, Myers GD, Sili U, Huls MH, Weiss H, Leung KS, et al. Monoculture-derived T lymphocytes specific for multiple viruses expand and produce clinically relevant effects in immunocompromised individuals. Nat Med. 2006;12:1160–6.
110. Rauser G, Einsele H, Sinzger C, Wernet D, Kuntz G, Assenmacher M, et al. Rapid generation of combined CMV-specific CD4+ and CD8+ T-cell lines for adoptive transfer into recipients of allogeneic stem cell transplants. Blood 2004;103:3565–72.
111. Szmania S, Galloway A, Bruorton M, Musk P, Aubert G, Arthur A, et al. Isolation and expansion of cytomegalovirus-specific cytotoxic T lymphocytes to clinical scale from a single blood draw using dendritic cells and HLA-tetramers. Blood 2001;98:505–12.
112. Cobbold M, Khan N, Pourgheysari B, Tauro S, McDonald D, Osman H, et al. Adoptive transfer of cytomegalovirus-specific CTL to stem cell transplant patients after selection by HLA-peptide tetramers. J Exp Med. 2005;202:379–86.
113. Park KD, Marti L, Kurtzberg J, Szabolcs P. In vitro priming and expansion of cytomegalovirus-specific Th1 and Tc1 T cells from naive cord blood lymphocytes. Blood 2006;108:1770–3.
114. Rosenberg SA, Sportes C, Ahmadzadeh M, Fry TJ, Ngo LT, Schwarz SL, et al. IL-7 administration to humans leads to expansion of CD8+ and CD4+ cells but a relative decrease of CD4+ T-regulatory cells. J Immunother (1997). 2006;29:313–9.
115. Dudley ME, Wunderlich JR, Robbins PF, Yang JC, Hwu P, Schwartzentruber DJ, et al. Cancer regression and autoimmunity in patients after clonal repopulation with antitumor lymphocytes. Science 2002;298:850–4.
116. Becker C, Pohla H, Frankenberger B, Schuler T, Assenmacher M, Schendel DJ, et al. Adoptive tumor therapy with T lymphocytes enriched through an IFN-gamma capture assay. Nat Med. 2001;7:1159–62.
117. Morgan RA, Dudley ME, Wunderlich JR, Hughes MS, Yang JC, Sherry RM, et al. Cancer regression in patients after transfer of genetically engineered lymphocytes. Science 2006;314:126–9.
118. Stanislawski T, Voss RH, Lotz C, Sadovnikova E, Willemsen RA, Kuball J, et al. Circumventing tolerance to a human MDM2-derived tumor antigen by TCR gene transfer. Nat Immunol. 2001;2:962–70.
119. Bozza S, Perruccio K, Montagnoli C, Gaziano R, Bellocchio S, Burchielli E, et al. A dendritic cell vaccine against invasive aspergillosis in allogeneic hematopoietic transplantation. Blood 2003;102:3807–14.
120. Rapoport AP, Stadtmauer EA, Aqui N, Badros A, Cotte J, Chrisley L, et al. Restoration of immunity in lymphopenic individuals with cancer by vaccination and adoptive T-cell transfer. Nat Med. 2005;11:1230–7.
121. Prlic M, Blazar BR, Khoruts A, Zell T, Jameson SC. Homeostatic expansion occurs independently of costimulatory signals. J Immunol. 2001;167:5664–8.
122. Amrolia PJ, Muccioli-Casadei G, Huls H, Adams S, Durett A, Gee A, et al. Adoptive immunotherapy with allodepleted donor T-cells improves immune reconstitution after haploidentical stem cell transplantation. Blood 2006;108:1797–808.

123. Andre-Schmutz I, Le Deist F, Hacein-Bey-Abina S, Vitetta E, Schindler J, Chedeville G, et al. Immune reconstitution without graft-versus-host disease after haemopoietic stem-cell transplantation: a phase 1/2 study. Lancet 2002;360:130–7.
124. Solomon SR, Mielke S, Savani BN, Montero A, Wisch L, Childs R, et al. Selective depletion of alloreactive donor lymphocytes: a novel method to reduce the severity of graft-versus-host disease in older patients undergoing matched sibling donor stem cell transplantation. Blood 2005;106:1123–9.
125. Amrolia PJ, Muccioli-Casadei G, Yvon E, Huls H, Sili U, Wieder ED, et al. Selective depletion of donor alloreactive T cells without loss of antiviral or antileukemic responses. Blood 2003;102:2292–9.
126. Martins SL, St John LS, Champlin RE, Wieder ED, McMannis J, Molldrem JJ, et al. Functional assessment and specific depletion of alloreactive human T cells using flow cytometry. Blood 2004;104:3429–36.
127. Michalek J, Collins RH, Durrani HP, Vaclavkova P, Ruff LE, Douek DC, et al. Definitive separation of graft-versus-leukemia- and graft-versus-host-specific CD4+ T cells by virtue of their receptor beta loci sequences. Proc Natl Acad Sci USA. 2003;100:1180–4.
128. Mielke S, Rezvani K, Savani BN, Nunes R, Yong AS, Schindler J, et al. Reconstitution of FOXP3+ regulatory T cells (Tregs) after CD25-depleted allotransplantation in elderly patients and association with acute graft-versus-host disease. Blood 2007 Sep 1;110(5):1689–97.

Chapter 7
Functionally Defined T Cell Subsets in Transplantation Biology and Therapy: Regulatory T Cells and Th2 Cells

Daniel Fowler, Petra Hoffmann, and Matthias Edinger

7.1 Regulatory T Cells

7.1.1 Biology of CD4$^+$CD25$^+$ Regulatory T Cells (Treg Cells)

Peripheral tolerance mechanisms include deletion by activation induced cell death, anergy and dominant suppression. Although the important contribution of suppression for the maintenance of peripheral T-cell tolerance was repeatedly proven in experimental systems, it was discredited for many years as no defined suppressor cell population could be identified. In 1995, Sakaguchi and coworkers rejuvenated interest in T-cell-mediated immunosuppression when they showed that thymectomy in neonatal mice caused autoimmunity that could be prevented by adoptive transfer of CD25-coexpressing CD4$^+$ T cells isolated from adult animals [1]. These findings advanced the field in several aspects: (1) For the first time, phenotypic markers (CD4$^+$CD25$^+$) identified a cell population endowed with potent suppressive activity; (2) the suppressive cell population seemed to be thymus-derived; (3) its export from the thymus seemed to be delayed for up to 8 days after birth compared to conventional T cells; (4) the suppressive function of this cell population is nonredundant, as no other tolerance mechanism compensated for their absence in the periphery; and (5) once exported, the suppressor population seemed to be long-lived, as thymectomy after day 8 no longer induced autoimmunity.

In subsequent years, other investigators confirmed Sakaguchi's main findings and the respective cell population was named "natural regulatory T cells" [2]. "Natural" indicates that these cells develop in the thymus as a separate lineage, which distinguishes them from "induced" or "adaptive" suppressor cells generated in the periphery from conventional T cells (Tconv) under physiological or experimental conditions, e.g., in the presence of IL-10 or TGF-β [3]. The term

D. Fowler (✉)
Experimental Transplantation and Immunology Branch, Center for Cancer Research, National Cancer Institute, Bethesda, MD, USA
e-mail: fowlerda@mail.nih.gov

M.R. Bishop (ed.), *Hematopoietic Stem Cell Transplantation*, Cancer Treatment and Research 144, DOI 10.1007/978-0-387-78580-6_7,

"regulatory" was introduced to segregate the cells from the discredited suppressor T cell field, although $CD4^+CD25^+$ Treg cells do not "regulate" in a sense that they boost weak and inhibit overwhelming immune responses, but they solely dampen or block immune reactions and are thus bona fide suppressor cells. Final proof for the relevance of Treg cells in self-tolerance came with the discovery that they constitutively express the forkhead family transcription factor Foxp3 (forkhead box protein 3) [4]. Foxp3 is encoded on the X chromosome and loss of function mutations found in "scurfy" (*sf*) mice cause a lymphoproliferative disorder and rapidly lethal autoimmunity in male animals [5]. Similar Foxp3 mutations in humans cause the immunodysregulation, polyendocrinopathy and enteropathy, X-linked syndrome (IPEX) [6]. In both mouse and man, Foxp3 mutants lack a functional Treg cell compartment. The crucial contribution of Foxp3 for Treg cell generation and function has been confirmed experimentally in genetically modified mouse strains. Foxp3 reporter mice revealed the almost exclusive expression of Foxp3 in $CD4^+CD25^+$ T cells [7], whereas Foxp3-deficient animals lack $CD4^+CD25^+$ Treg cells and develop lethal autoimmunity similar to *sf* mice [4]. Likewise, experimental shut-down of Foxp3 expression in adult conditional knock-out animals induces autoimmunity [8], demonstrating that continuous Foxp3 expression [9] at sufficiently high levels [10] is required for Treg cell-mediated suppression. Thus, Foxp3 is a lineage specification factor for Treg cells and required for their thymic development and peripheral function. The yet unidentified suppressive mechanism of Treg cells seems to be conserved across species and is pivotal for immune homeostasis and the maintenance of peripheral self-tolerance.

Natural $CD4^+CD25^+$ Treg cells represent only 5–10% of the peripheral $CD4^+$ T cell pool. Despite intensive investigations, no exclusive surface marker has been identified to date and thus Treg cell isolation still relies on the use of surrogate markers such as CD25 (IL-2R α-chain). In normal mice, almost all $CD4^+CD25^+$ T cells represent Treg cells (as verified by Foxp3 expression) and in peripheral blood of healthy human individuals Treg cells reside predominantly within the $CD4^+CD25^{high}$ subpopulation [11]. However, CD25 is also expressed on activated conventional T cells (Tconv; up to 50% of human peripheral blood $CD4^+$ T cells express intermediate levels of CD25), which limits the use of CD25 alone as a Treg cell marker. Similar limitations exist for other markers preferentially or constitutively expressed by Treg cells, including glucocorticoid-induced TNF receptor (GITR), cytotoxic T lymphocyte-associated antigen 4 (CTLA-4), and certain chemokine (CCR4, CCR6, CCR7) or homing receptors (CD103, CD62L) [12]. Recently, the groups of Fazekas de St. Groth and Bluestone demonstrated that the combination of CD25 and CD127 (IL-7R α-chain) permits the discrimination of Treg cells from activated Tconv cells: Whereas activated—and thus $CD25^+$-Tconv cells—express high CD127 levels, $CD25^+$ Treg cells express only low or no CD127 [13, 14] (see Fig. 7.1).

An alternative Treg cell isolation strategy is based on the fact that activated Tconv cells no longer display a naïve phenotype after their encounter with antigen. Although early studies concluded that Treg cells continuously respond

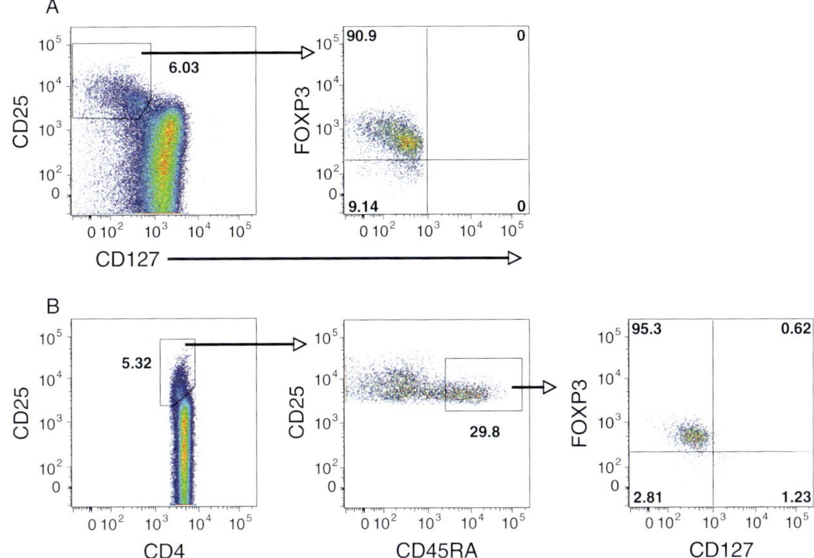

Fig. 7.1 Human Treg cell isolation strategies. Human peripheral blood mononuclear cells (PBMC) were isolated by FICOLL gradient centrifugation, stained for CD4, CD25, CD45RA and CD127 on the cell surface, fixed/permeabilized and intracellularly stained for FoxP3 (clone PCH101). (**a**) Gating strategy for isolation of $CD4^+CD25^+CD127^-$ T cells and FOXP3 expression of gated target cells. (**b**) Gating strategy for isolation of $CD4^+CD25^{high}CD45RA^+$ T cells and FoxP3 expression of gated target cells. Left plots in A and B are gated on $CD4^+$ cells among PBMC

to self-antigens and therefore exclusively belong to the memory T cell pool, later reports illustrated that the T cell receptor (TCR) repertoire of Treg cells is diverse and largely overlapping with that of Tconv cells [15, 16]. Importantly, the Treg population in adult human peripheral blood also contains recent thymic emigrants that display a naïve phenotype characterized by low CD45RO expression and high expression of CD45RA, CCR7, and CD62L [17]. By isolating $CD4^+$ T cells that coexpress CD25 and CD45RA, we found that this naïve subset yields a pure Treg cell product that maintains a stable phenotype and suppressive function even after repetitive stimulation and extensive proliferation in vitro [18] (and Fig. 7.1). Thus, human Treg cells can be isolated to high purity despite the lack of exclusive Treg cell surface markers.

Originally, murine and human Treg cells were described as being anergic due to their hypoproliferative response in vitro as compared to Tconv cells [19]. For their survival in vitro and in vivo, Treg cells depend on exogenous IL-2 because they inadequately remodel their chromatin in the IL-2 promoter region upon stimulation and therefore do not produce IL-2 themselves [20]. Upon IL-2- or TCR-mediated stimulation in vitro, Treg cells hardly proliferate as signaling pathways supporting cell proliferation are blocked, while the survival-promoting JAK/STAT5 pathway is intact [21, 22]. As a result, Treg cells are virtually absent in the periphery of IL-2- and IL-2R-deficient mice even though IL-2 is not absolutely required for their development in the thymus [23]. In contrast, natural Treg cells proliferate vigorously in vivo upon interaction with their cognate antigen and in parts even under steady state conditions [24, 25]. Meanwhile, several research groups, including our own, showed that Treg cells also proliferate in vitro provided strong costimulation via CD28 and high concentrations of IL-2 compliment TCR stimulation [26–28].

Once activated through their TCR, Treg cells acquire suppressive activity and inhibit the proliferation and cytokine production of cocultured CD4^{+} and CD8^{+} Tconv cells [29]. Other targets of Treg cell-mediated suppression include B cells [30] and natural killer (NK) cells [31] as well as monocytes and dendritic cells (DC) [32]. The mode of suppression by Treg cells has not yet been identified unequivocally on a molecular level, but in vitro it seems to be cell contact dependent and cytokine independent [33]. Potential mechanisms that have been proposed include membrane-bound TGF-β [34], CTLA-4 [35], transfer of cAMP from Treg to Tconv cells via gap junctions [36], generation of adenosine by CD39 and CD73 expressed on the Treg cell surface [37], contact dependent induction of ICER/CREM in target T cells [38], competitive IL-2 consumption [39], induction of cytokine deprivation-mediated apoptosis [40], and even cytolysis via granzyme B and perforin [41]. Considering the diversity of the proposed cellular and molecular mechanisms, it seems likely that Treg cells suppress by different pathways depending on the target cell and the respective microenvironment. Treg cell-mediated suppression in vivo has been shown to occur in lymphoid as well as in non-lymphoid tissues [42]. In lymph nodes, Treg cells suppress the activation, proliferation and export of Tconv cells and thereby inhibit the initiation of an immune response [43]. Apart from direct Treg–Tconv cell interactions, indirect Treg cell effects contribute to suppression at those sites, such as the modulation of DC function [44, 45]. At extralymphatic sites of inflammation, suppression seems to depend predominantly on the secretion of suppressive cytokines, e.g., IL-10 and TGF-β, which inhibit effector cell function, block the recruitment of additional effector cells, or even convert Tconv cells into suppressor cells [46–49].

7.1.2 Peripheral Induction of Treg and Th17 Cells

In addition to “natural” CD4^{+}CD25^{+}Foxp3^{+} Treg cells that develop in the thymus, T cells with suppressive capacity can also be generated by peripheral induction. Stimulation of CD4^{+}CD25^{-} Tconv cells in vitro or in vivo in the presence of IL-10 induces their differentiation to so-called Tr1 cells. In contrast to natural CD4^{+}CD25^{+} Treg cells, Tr1 cells do not express Foxp3 and mediate their effects via secretion of immunosuppressive cytokines, mainly IL-10; they have been reviewed in detail elsewhere [50]. In addition, the groups of Wahl and Ziegler in 2003 both described the conversion of naïve CD4^{+} Tconv cells to Foxp3-expressing cells with suppressive activity if stimulated in vitro in the presence of TGF-β [3, 51]. Since then a number of reports confirmed the generation of "induced" or "converted" Treg cells in vitro (especially with cells of human origin), but also in vivo under defined experimental conditions in mice. However, there is still considerable debate about the stability of such an induced regulatory phenotype [52, 53], the suppressive activity of those cells [54, 55], and most importantly, the relevance and frequency of this developmental pathway in vivo [56]. Yet, recent work from the groups of Powrie and Belkaid convincingly showed that in the gastrointestinal tract and its associated lymphoid tissue, extrathymic Treg cell development is a frequent process that depends on the presence of TGF-β and the vitamin A metabolite retinoic acid (RA) and is supported by a subpopulation of mucosal DC that expresses high levels of CD103 [57, 58]. Likewise, Benson et al. demonstrated that the addition of RA to T cell cultures stabilized the TGF-β induced Treg phenotype and made the cells refractory to reversion in vivo [59]. These findings suggest that TGF-β is necessary but not sufficient for a stable Tconv to Treg cell conversion and that additional factors such as the presence of specialized DC populations or the particular microenvironment also influence the final developmental fate of Tconv cells.

The finding that addition of IL-6 to T cell conversion cultures completely abrogates Treg induction but supports the differentiation of T cells towards a Th17 phenotype further supports these conclusions [60–64]. Th17 cells produce two of the six members of the IL-17 cytokine family (IL-17A and IL-17F) [65] and in analogy to T-bet for Th1, GATA-3 for Th2 and Foxp3 for Treg cells, their development depends on the presence of a master transcription factor, ROR-γt [66] (Fig. 7.2). Whereas IL-1 and TNF further support Th17 cell development but do not induce them on their own [62], the combination of

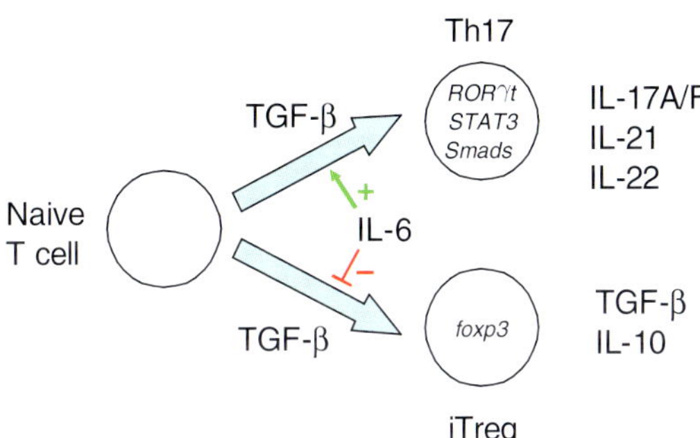

Fig. 7.2 Differential development of Treg cells and Th17 cells. TGF-β is present during the differentiation of naïve T cells to both the Th17 pathway and the inducible Treg cell pathway (iTreg cells). The presence or absence of IL-6 appears to represent the key factor in the differentiation of Th17 and Treg cells, respectively. iTreg cells express the master transcription factor Foxp3, whereas Th17 cells express the ROR-γt transcription factor. Th17 cells are also characterized by their dependence upon the STAT3 and SMAD signalling pathways and their relatively unique secretion of IL-17A/F, IL-21 and IL-22; in contrast, iTreg cells can be further characterized by their preferential secretion of TGF-β and IL-10

TGF-β and IL-21 suffices for this task, as shown in IL-6$^{-/-}$ mice [67]. In contrast IL-23, which was originally also regarded a Th17 differentiation cytokine, is now known to be required mainly for Th17 cell survival and function, but not for their *de novo* induction from naïve T cells [68]. Physiologically, Th17 cells protect from Gram-negative bacteria and fungi, but they also contribute to autoimmune diseases under pathological conditions [65]. Th17 cells have potent proinflammatory activity and activate and recruit other effector cells, especially neutrophils and Th1 cells, by inducing an array of cytokines and chemokines, such as IL-6, IL8, G-CSF, GM-CSF, CXCL1 and CXCL10 in various target cell populations, including endothelial and epithelial cells, neutrophils, macrophages and DC [65, 68].

In summary, TGF-β seems pivotal for the induction of presumably opposing cell types such as Treg and Th17 cells and it is intriguing to speculate that a pro-inflammatory immune response simultaneously triggers its own termination under physiological conditions. The contribution of induced Treg and Th17 cells to the pathophysiology of graft-versus-host disease (GvHD) has not yet been fully examined in appropriate animal models.

7.1.3 Evaluation of Natural Treg Cells in Experimental Models of Bone Marrow Transplantation

CD4^{+}CD25^{+} Treg cells do not mediate pro-inflammatory effects but actively suppress the proliferation of CD4^{+} and CD8^{+} Tconv cells in mixed lymphocyte reactions. These functional characteristics prompted several groups to explore their suppressive activity in murine models of allogeneic hematopoietic stem cell transplantation (HSCT). When cotransplanted with T-cell depleted bone marrow, donor-type Treg cells did not induce GvHD even when transplanted in large numbers and across complete MHC barriers. Yet, their cotransplantation in high ratios (1:1 or 1:2) with either CD4^{+} or CD4^{+} and CD8^{+} Tconv cells protected mice from lethal GvHD that was otherwise observed in Tconv cell recipients [43, 69, 70]. Both freshly isolated polyclonal Treg cells as well as pre-activated and in vitro expanded donor Treg cells protected from GvHD, while Treg cell depletion from a conventional stem cell graft aggravated GvHD [70–73]. Inhibition of GvHD by Treg cells was observed after minor mismatched, selectively MHC class II mismatched, and even after completely MHC mismatched transplantation. Furthermore, Treg cells prevented GvHD induction in CD4- and CD8-dependent disease models and clinical effects ranged from reduced body weight loss and prolonged mean survival time to full protection from GvHD lethality. Only donor, but not host Treg cells were protective [69] and Treg cell-derived IL-10 partially contributed to this effect, as Treg cells from IL-10-deficient donor mice showed diminished capacity to inhibit GvHD lethality [69]. The target cell populations for this IL-10 effect are thus far unknown, but the modulation of antigen presenting cell function probably plays a role, as previously also shown for models of autoimmunity [74]. As Treg cells are only suppressive after their own activation, Nguyen and coworkers hypothesized that the protective effect might be enhanced if Treg cells were pre-stimulated in vivo before their encounter with GvHD-inducing Tconv cells. When Treg cells were infused 48 h prior to Tconv cells, full protection from GvHD was in fact achieved even at physiological ratios of Treg cells to Tconv cells (1:10) [75]. Thus, the composition of a stem cell graft as well as the temporal activation of suppressor and effector T cell populations seems to determine the outcome after allogeneic HSCT. Importantly, the suppressive activity of cotransplanted Treg cells did not impair but rather facilitated stem cell engraftment in models of allograft rejection [76, 77]. Furthermore, addition of Treg cells to the bone marrow graft did not impair but rather fostered immune reconstitution after transplantation [78, 79]. Improved immune reconstitution in Treg cell recipients was probably a consequence of diminished lymphoid tissue destruction in GvHD-free animals. The relevant site for suppression of Tconv cells by Treg cells in the induction phase of GvHD seemed to be lymphoid organs, as only Treg cells with lymph node homing capacity efficiently protected from GvHD. This was shown in experiments where Treg cells were separated with respect to their CD62L expression that, in combination with other homing receptors, ensures their efficient entry into secondary lymphoid organs. Although the suppressive activity in vitro did not differ between CD62L^{-} and CD62L^{+} Treg cells, the latter showed enhanced lymph node migration and superior protection in GvHD models [80, 81]. Thus, cotransplanted Treg cells seem to become primed and activated at the same sites as GvHD-inducing Tconv cells and probably respond to the same residual host antigen-presenting cells (APC) [82]. In later stages, Treg cells leave these lymphoid priming sites and home to GvHD target tissues where they contribute to long lasting protection [83]. The similar migration pattern of donor Treg and Tconv cells has recently been confirmed in elegant in vivo imaging studies [75].

When the protective effect of donor Treg cells in GvHD was first examined, it was shown that the rapid proliferative response of alloreactive Tconv cells was inhibited, thereby impairing the massive donor T cell infiltration of the gut that is a hallmark of GvHD induction and mainly responsible for GvHD lethality in these models. Of note, donor Tconv cells re-isolated from transplant recipients that did or did not receive additional Treg cells expressed similar patterns of activation markers, secreted the same pro-inflammatory cytokines, and responded similarly to alloantigens after in vitro re-stimulation [43]. Thus, Treg cells protect from GvHD primarily by confining the clonal size of the alloaggressive T cell pool rather than by deletional mechanisms or the induction of anergy in Tconv cells. Whether alloreactive Tconv cells, restricted in their clonal expansion by cotransplanted Treg cells, were still able to mediate graft-versus-leukemia/lymphoma effects (GvL) was examined in several tumor models. Not unexpectedly, low numbers of cotransplanted Tconv cells were unable to eradicate residual disease. However, Treg cell therapy permitted the administration of sufficiently high Tconv cell numbers for the eradication of residual leukemia even in the absence of GvHD [43, 73]. Thus, Treg cell transplantation does not induce complete immune paralysis. Rather, Treg cells restrict the alloresponse to its most sensitive target, namely residual host hematopoiesis, while inhibiting excessive Tconv cell proliferation, GvHD target organ infiltration and destruction.

Most of the studies cited above explored the adoptive transfer of donor Treg cells for GvHD prophylaxis, but not their therapeutic application. Yet, Jones et al. observed protection from GvHD even after delayed transfer of Treg cells in a slowly progressive GvHD model [73]. Although not yet confirmed by other groups, these observations suggest that Treg cells not only prevent alloaggression after HSCT, but might even ameliorate ongoing GvHD, as previously also shown for the treatment of autoimmunity [84].

Important findings regarding the immune modulating influence of Treg cells reconstituting from the transplanted bone marrow came from the groups of Johnson and Truitt. Initially, these investigators described an increased host tolerance towards donor T cell infusions after hematopoietic reconstitution (3–4 weeks after HSCT) as compared to T cell administration on the day of HSCT [85]. In follow up studies, they discovered that the reduced susceptibility for the induction of GvHD was not only the result of diminished tissue inflammation late after conditioning, but in large parts mediated by bone marrow-derived $CD4^+CD25^+$ Treg cells [86, 87]. Thus, the successful thymic maturation of Treg cells seems to contribute to long-term tolerance not only in ontogeny (as seen in scurfy mice), but also after allogeneic HSCT.

7.1.4 Evaluation of Treg Cells in Human Hematopoietic Stem Cell Transplantation

Encouraged by the findings in murine HSCT models, several groups examined the influence of Treg cells on the outcome of hematopoietic stem cell transplants in humans. For this purpose, absolute numbers and relative proportions of Treg cells in stem cell grafts and/or the quantitative reconstitution of the Treg cell compartment after transplantation have been correlated with the incidence and severity of acute and chronic GvHD. Initially, Stanzani et al. described that high numbers of $CD25^+$ T cells in the graft actually increased the risk for GvHD [88]. However, these initial studies were hampered by technical problems caused by the use of previously frozen stem cell samples and the lack of antibodies for the determination of Foxp3. Indeed, subsequent studies by several other groups found an inverse correlation between the number of transplanted Treg cells and incidence of acute GvHD [89–91]. Interestingly, two clinical trials exploring CD25-targeted antibodies for the elimination of allo-activated T cells were halted due to an unexpected high incidence of GvHD in a prophylaxis study [92] and adverse outcome after the combined administration with steroids as first line treatment for acute GvHD [93]. In these reports, the authors speculated that the unintended depletion of Treg cells might have contributed to the unexpected outcome. Of course, none of these correlative studies ultimately proves that Treg cells ameliorate acute GvHD in human HSCT, but they do support the hypothesis that cotransplanted Treg cells may contribute to mutual tolerance induction.

Studies that examined the reconstitution of the Treg cell compartment after SCT came to controversial conclusions. Miura et al. found decreased Foxp3 message by quantitative PCR in peripheral blood of acute and chronic GvHD patients as compared to transplant recipients without GvHD. Furthermore, diminished Foxp3 expression correlated with reduced T cell receptor excision circles (TREC), indicating that impaired thymic function was associated with a lack of Treg cell generation [94]. This observation is consistent with the notion that GvHD-induced thymic damage might further perpetuate GvHD by inhibiting recovery of the Treg cell compartment. While several other groups also observed an inverse correlation of Treg cell numbers in host peripheral blood and the incidence of acute GvHD [95, 96], others did not find such an association [97, 98]. Yet, an imbalance between Treg and effector T cells in patients with GvHD has been described by some investigators [97], and Rieger et al. found a deficiency of Treg cells in the gut of affected GvHD patients, but not in patients with other types of colitis [99]. Association of Treg cell numbers with chronic GvHD has been highly variable, with different studies describing increased Treg cell numbers [100], decreased Treg cell numbers [101], or no apparent association of Treg cell numbers [102] with chronic GvHD. Although these studies are not directly comparable due to different patient selection criteria and experimental methods, they illustrate that larger monitoring trials using standardized techniques and identification criteria are required to elucidate the influence of Treg cell reconstitution on acute and chronic GvHD and vice versa.

In our (biased) view, the data from mouse models and published clinical trials suggest that the contribution of natural Treg cells to the modulation of an alloresponse after allogeneic HSCT has to be evaluated separately for transferred versus regenerating Treg cells. Adoptively transferred Treg cells (and thus maturated in the healthy donor) do not induce GvHD (as proven in mouse models), but presumably recognize the same or a similar repertoire of host antigens as GvHD-inducing Tconv cells. Since Treg cells are only suppressive after their own activation, a high precursor frequency of alloreactive Treg cells seems favorable for the suppression of GvHD. These assumptions predict that donor Treg cells will be most efficient in transplant settings where they are most desperately needed, that is, after HLA-mismatched or haplo-identical HSCT. As most clinical studies concluded that HSC grafts containing high Treg cell numbers are protective against GvHD, it seems reasonable to further explore this strategy by transplanting Treg cell-enriched grafts either without pharmacological immunosuppression or under the cover of tolerance permissive drugs such as sirolimus.

The role of regenerating Treg cells after allogeneic HSCT seems more complex. Evidently, the severe autoimmune syndrome seen in *scurfy* mice and IPEX patients reveals the pivotal role of Treg cells for the development and maintenance of self-tolerance in ontogeny, and there is no reason to believe that their regeneration is dispensable for lymphoid reconstitution and tolerance induction after HSCT. In mouse models, Treg cells regenerated from transplanted bone marrow and matured in the host thymus ameliorated alloresponses after delayed DLI [86, 87]. However, one limitation of such models is the absence of prior acute GvHD, which is known to affect the thymus [103]. Thus, Treg cell-mediated suppression in GvHD patients could be disturbed due to impaired Treg regeneration after thymic damage caused either by the conditioning regimen or by GvHD. Alternatively, thymic damage might perpetuate immune dysfunction (manifesting itself as chronic GvHD) due to altered positive and negative selection of both Tconv and Treg cells. In such a case, Treg cells might not necessarily be protective in chronic GvHD, but may even contribute to disease manifestation through the dysregulated secretion of cytokines such as TGF-β or IL-10. If true, this might partially explain the controversial results obtained in chronic GvHD patients, as functional characteristics of Treg cells, dictated by their skewed TCR repertoire, might be more relevant than their mere numbers in peripheral blood or GvHD target organs. Furthermore, it should be kept in mind that chronic GvHD is not a single disease but has a plethora of manifestations that might be differentially affected by Treg cells. These issues remain to be examined in appropriate animal models.

7.1.5 Strategies and Challenges in Regulatory T Cell Research and Therapy

Since human Treg cells show similar phenotypic, functional and molecular characteristics as murine Treg cells, their adoptive transfer seems a promising strategy for the prevention of GvHD after allogeneic HSCT. In fact, first clinical trials are currently performed at our institution in Regensburg, Germany, and at other institutions (University of Minnesota, Department of Pediatrics, B. Blazar, personal communication) and in preparation at other sites (Stanford School of Medicine, Division of BMT, R.S. Negrin, personal communication). In our clinical trial unmanipulated donor Treg cells isolated by magnetic bead selection are administered in a setting of pre-emptive donor lymphocyte infusions. Blazar and colleagues study in vitro expanded third party cord blood Treg cells at the time of HSCT with concomitant pharmacologic immunosuppression. Negrin and colleagues plan to use highly FACS-purified Treg cells in haploidentical donor/recipient pairs. All these phase I clinical trials focus on safety and feasibility issues and will not instantly reveal an efficacy of Treg cell transfers for the prevention of GvHD. The different approaches, however, illustrate some of the challenges associated with the translation of those concepts into clinical trials. Technical issues primarily relate to the isolation and expansion of Treg cells. With GMP-compatible bead separation technologies, Treg cells can be enriched to more than 50% purity. This seems sufficient for their prophylactic use because it results in the administration of Treg cells and Tconv cells at a 1:1 ratio [28] (PH & GE, unpublished results). However, 50% purity is insufficient for potential therapeutic applications in GvHD patients or for the in vitro expansion of Treg cells, as contaminating Tconv cells might outgrow Treg cells after combined stimulation with anti-CD3 and anti-CD28 antibodies and high-dose IL-2. Godfrey and coworkers attempt to circumvent this problem by using cord blood cells that presumably contain less activated Tconv cells within the $CD25^+$ T cell fraction [104]. Other investigators proposed to expand Treg cells in the presence of rapamycin, which has been shown to preferentially kill Tconv cells but spare Treg cells [105]. Alternative FACS-based isolation strategies such as the exclusion of $CD25^+CD127^+$ T cells or sorting for $CD45RA^+$ $CD4^+CD25^{high}$ T cells significantly improve Treg cell purity, but are in part limited by costs, as only few facilities are in possession of GMP-compatible FACS-sorting equipment. Broader accessibility to such sorting technologies can only be expected if pioneering trials undoubtedly prove a benefit and industrial partners are willing to invest in this approach. The generation of sufficient Treg cell numbers for clinical trials seems currently feasible, as GMP-compatible expansion protocols have been developed [27, 106]. For this purpose, we deliberately promote the use of polyclonal Treg cell products in allogeneic HSCT trials even though others favor the use of alloantigen-specific Treg cells [78, 107, 108]. In mouse models, in vivo selection of alloreactive donor Treg cells from a polyclonal Treg cell pool was sufficient for prevention of GvHD. In contrast, we would expect that donor Treg cells primed in vitro with host peripheral blood mononuclear cells recognize predominantly hematopoietic alloantigens, but not necessarily non-hematopoietic antigens that induce GvHD in target tissues but are not permanently presented by recipient blood cells. Thus, alloantigen-primed Treg cells might potently suppress the desired graft-versus-hematopoiesis effect but lose TCR-specificities required for tissue-specific GvHD inhibition; by comparison, polyclonally expanded Treg cells should maintain all specificities. Yet, it remains to be seen whether polyclonal cell products contain a sufficient frequency of alloreactive Treg cells for GvHD inhibition, as most transplants in humans are performed between HLA-identical donor/recipient pairs where the frequency of responding Treg cells is expected to be lower than in the MHC-disparate mouse models used for proof of concept studies. The administration of Treg cell products early after transplantation might be advantageous in this setting, as lymphopenia of the conditioned recipients might boost the in vivo expansion of reactive Treg clones [109]. The peculiar ability of Treg cells to maintain expression of lymph node homing receptors such as CD62L and CCR7 in culture suggests that their initial migration to and survival in lymphoid organs might not be affected by their prior in vitro expansion [28, 106].

More challenging than technical aspects concerning Treg cell isolation and expansion is the identification of clinical situations that permit a stepwise examination of the safety and efficacy of Treg cell therapies. Thus far, many of the drugs used for conditioning and immunosuppression of transplant recipients interfere with Treg cell function and survival. Because peripheral tolerance is not only a passive process but an active accomplishment of the immune system, protocols that do not interfere but favour Treg cell function would be preferable. The observation that mTOR inhibitors affect Treg cells less than calcineurin inhibitors is encouraging in this respect, as it suggests that tolerance-promoting regimens could be developed. The ongoing efforts to identify the differing signalling pathways in Treg and Tconv cells might ultimately lead to the development of reagents that more specifically target either alloaggressive or suppressive T cell populations. Such strategies could complement or even replace adoptive Treg cell therapies for the prevention of GvHD after allogeneic HSCT.

7.2 Th2 Cells

7.2.1 *Th1/Th2 Cell Biology*

In 1986, Mosmann discovered dichotomous murine $CD4^+$ T cell clones that were antigen specific yet differentially secreted either IL-2 or IL-4 [110]. Evaluation of Th2 cell biology was facilitated by discovery of the key cytokines promoting their development, IL-2 and IL-4 [111]; NK cells may link innate immunity to adaptive T cell immunity via type I NK cell secretion of IL-4 that subsequently promotes Th2 cell development [112]. Th2 cell polarization typically occurs in the context of clonal expansion via antigen-presenting-cell (APC) interaction; APC costimulation through CD28 can certainly promote Th2 polarization through induction of the Th2-specific transcription factor GATA-3 [113], although Th1 responses are also typically promoted [114]. In addition to IL-4 exposure in the antigenic microenvironment, it has been found that a "DC2" subset of dendritic cells exist that promote Th2 responses through a poorly understood, non-IL-4 mechanism [115]; it is possible that DC relatively deficient in IL-12 secretion constitute a functional DC2 cell that promotes Th2 polarity through a "default" mechanism [116]. Th2 cell differentiation consists of an initial "central memory" stage (T_{CM} cells [117]) characterized by a favorable pattern of lymph node homing receptors, including L-selection (CD62L) and the chemokine receptor CCR7, and limited effector function characterized low level secretion of the primordial Th2 cytokine, IL-4. With further Th2 effector differentiation towards an effector memory (T_{EM}) phenotype, downstream type II cytokines including IL-5, IL-10, and IL-13 are coordinately upregulated [118]. The paradigm of cytokine-secreting subsets extends as well to $CD8^+$ T cells, which can exist as T cytotoxic type I cells (Tc1 cells) that secrete the type I cytokines IL-2 and IFN-γ and mediate target cell lysis primarily through fas ligand or Tc2 cells that secrete type II cytokines and lyse targets primarily via a perforin-dependent mechanism [119, 120].

By comparison, Th1 cell differentiation occurs in an antigenic microenvironment rich in IL-12, which is either provided by a DC1-type dendritic cell or through IL-12 secreting NK type I cells [121]. Undifferentiated T cells express the IL-12 receptor, which when triggered by IL-12, activates the STAT-1 signaling pathway that dictates expression of the Th1 hallmark transcription factor, T-bet [122]. It should be noted that Th1 and Th2 cells differ not only with respect to cytokine secretion and cytolytic effector mechanism, but also in terms of chemokine receptor expression [123]; indeed, microarray experiments have identified extensive differential gene expression in Th1 vs. Th2 cells [124].

Importantly, early in the period of Th1/Th2 research, it was found that these subsets were cross-regulatory in murine models of infectious disease [125], thereby providing a rationale for adoptive T cell therapy attempts using cytokine polarized T cells. Of equal importance to translational research efforts was the early description that human T cells also could exist in Th1 vs. Th2 polarized states [126]. Cytokine polarization in humans may manifest differently or be less robust relative to murine systems; for example, early studies identified the existence of human Th1-type cells that also secreted high levels of the Th2 cytokine IL-10 [127]. Nonetheless, the basic tenets of Th2 cell biology hold true for human $CD4^+$ T cell development, with IL-4 priming and GATA-3 transcription factor expression dictating the coordinate secretion of multiple Th2 cytokines [128]. Fig. 7.3 summarizes the basic aspects of Th1 vs. Th2 differentiation.

7.2.2 Th1/Th2 Balance in Transplantation Biology

7.2.2.1 Th2 Cells for GvHD Prevention

In murine models, the biology of acute GvHD has in general been characterized as primarily a Th1-type process. That is, $CD4^+$ T cell production of IL-2 [129] and expression of CD40 ligand [130] play a key role in GvHD natural history; importantly, CD40 ligand primes APC for IL-12 production, which then propagates Th1-driven acute GvHD [131]. Th1 cells also preferentially lyse targets via fas ligand, which contributes to skin, gut, and liver GvHD [132, 133]. $CD8^+$ T cells, which differentiate along a Tc1 pathway during acute GvHD, operate through fas ligand cytolysis and high level IFN-γ secretion, which primes monocytes and macrophages for pro-inflammatory cytokine secretion [134] that is a hallmark of the more distal, "cytokine storm" phase of acute GvHD [135]. It should be noted that several results caution against strict interpretation of acute GvHD as a Th1-driven process: Specifically, it has been shown that (1) STAT-4 deficient T cells that are restricted in Th1 differentiation maintain some GvHD potential [136]; (2) specific deletion of IL-2 or IL-4 secreting

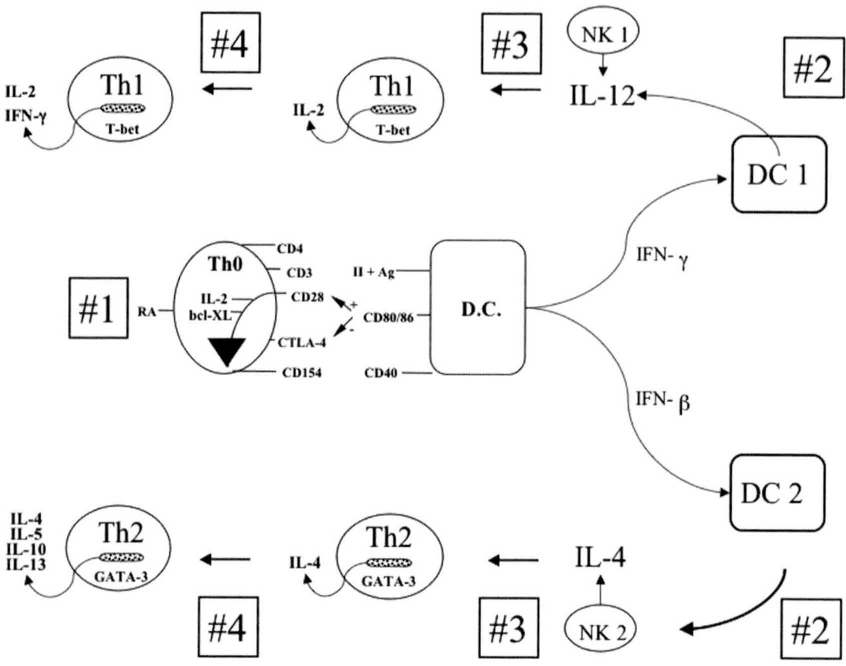

Fig. 7.3 Complexity of Th1 vs. Th2 polarization in vivo. (Point #1) Naïve CD4+ T cells (Th0) interact with dendritic cells (D.C.) and receive positive signals via CD28 and down-regulatory signals via CTLA-4; the D.C. receives positive signals via T cell expression of CD40 ligand (CD154). D.C. maturation in environments rich in IFN-γ vs. IFN-β promotes either a DC1 or DC2 dendritic cell phenotype that promote Th1 or Th2 differentiation, respectively. (Point #2) DC1 cell or type I NK cell secretion of IL-12 is required for Th1 polarization; in contrast, DC2 cells (through an as yet to be described, non-IL-4 mechanism) or type II NK cell secretion of IL-4 is required for Th2 polarization. (Point #3) IL-12 dictates Th1 cell acquisition of the T-bet transcription factor, whereas IL-4 dictates Th2 cell GATA-3 transcription factor expression. Early in polarization, Th1 or Th2 cells express a T central memory phenotype characterized in part by a limited repertoire of effector cytokine secretion. (Point #4) With continued T cell expansion and differentiation, Th1 or Th2 cells express a T effector memory phenotype typified by a high level secretion of diverse Th1 or Th2 cytokines

donor T cells can reduce GvHD [137]; and (3) IFN-γ or IL-4 deficient donor T cells can reduce or increase GvHD, respectively [138]. In contrast to these results using cytokine- or signaling-molecule deficient donor T cells, adoptive transfer experiments using wild-type, polarized donor T cells have found that Th1 and Tc1 cells mediate increased GvHD relative to Th2 and Tc2 cells and determined that Th2-type cells can actively down-regulate GvHD inducing donor T cell inocula [139–142].

In summary, these data provide a rationale for using the adoptive transfer of Th2 polarized donor T cells as a novel strategy to prevent GvHD. One additional important consideration is the potential influence of such an approach on chronic GvHD; this is a relatively complex issue because of the inter-relationship between acute and chronic GvHD and the less understood biology of chronic GvHD. In light of the known association of chronic GvHD to B cell-driven autoimmunity [131], it is possible that Th2 strategies may exacerbate chronic GvHD. On the other hand, if a Th2 strategy were to prevent acute GvHD damage to the thymus, it is possible that an absence of forbidden clones and improved immune reconstitution may limit chronic GvHD [143].

7.2.2.2 Th2 Cells to Balance GvHD and GvT Effects

In the setting of transplantation for therapy of malignant disease, it is essential to also determine the effect of any given anti-GvHD strategy on graft-versus-tumor (GvT) effects. Using the adoptive transfer of ex vivo generated, cytokine polarized murine T cells, we found that dissection of GvT effects from GvHD is problematic using Th1 vs. Th2 cells. That is, in a murine model of leukemia, we found that the anti-GvHD effect of Th2 and Tc2 cells was associated with significant blunting of the post-transplant anti-tumor effect [141, 144]; in contrast, Th1 and Tc1 cells mediated potent anti-tumor effects at the expense of lethal GvHD. Similarly, in a murine model of metastatic breast carcinoma, we determined that Th1/Tc1 cells mediated potent GvT effects and lethal GvHD; by comparison, Th2/Tc2 cells mediated greatly reduced GvHD but also limited GvT effects. Such difficult dissection of GvHD and GvT effects points towards their shared biology [145]. Additional lines of investigation have demonstrated the importance of Th1-type effector molecules such as IFN-γ and fas ligand in anti-tumor responses that occur after allogeneic [146] or syngeneic transplantation [147].

In light of this biology, we have developed murine models of allograft engineering that seek to provide a post-transplant balance of both Th1- and Th2-type effector mechanisms such that some component of GvT effects can occur through a Th1 mechanism with concomitant GvHD regulation via a Th2 mechanism. Because unmanipulated donor T cells primarily differentiate along a Th1 pathway in vivo, such a balance may be induced through the augmentation of a T cell replete allograft with donor Th2 cells. We have also evaluated whether it is possible to further dissect GvT effects from GvHD by a sequential Th1 → Th2 strategy that first incorporates unmanipulated donor T cell infusion with subsequent administration of Th2 polarized donor T cells. Along these lines, using ex vivo generated donor Th2 cells expanded in high-dose rapamycin, we have recently found that Th2 cell allograft augmentation or the strategy of delayed Th2 cell infusion can yield a GvT effect with concomitant or sequential regulation of GvHD [148].

Two important principles derived from these experiments are of relevance to current translational research efforts using adoptive T cell transfer. First, with respect to Th2 cell expansion methods, we observed an inverse correlation between the magnitude of Th2 cell cytokine production from the T cell product just prior to infusion (Fig. 7.4a) and the resultant post-transplant capacity to promote Th2 cytokines (Fig. 7.4b). Of note, in other studies, we have

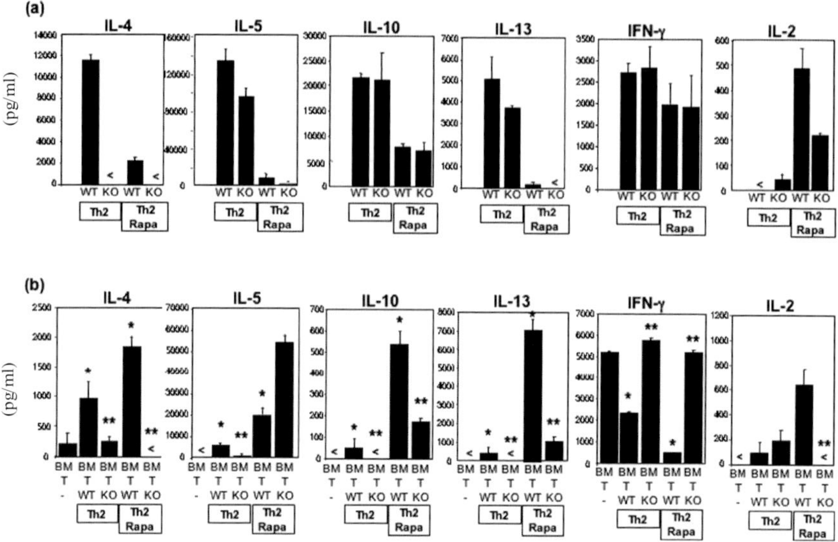

Fig. 7.4 Inverse correlation between Th2 cell product cytokine production and in vivo cytokine production. Murine Th2 cells were generated without ex vivo rapamycin ("Th2") or with ex vivo rapamycin ("Th2 Rapa"). CD4 cells were obtained from wild-type donors ("WT") or IL-4 knock-out donors ("KO"). Fig. 7.2a shows cytokine production from four different Th2 cell products prior to in vivo administration, including the Th1 cytokines IL-2 and IFN-γ and the Th2 cytokines IL-4, IL-5, IL-10, and IL-13. The rapamycin-generated Th2 cell product actually had reduced magnitude of Th2 cell cytokine secretion relative to control Th2 cells. Fig. 7.2b shows in vivo cytokine production in murine recipients of semi-allogeneic bone marrow ("BM"), and unmanipulated T cells ("T") either alone or with one of four generated Th2 cell products. Adoptive transfer of rapamycin-generated Th2 cells induced a more potent shift towards the Th2 cytokines post-transplant; this in vivo effect was dependent upon Th2 cell IL-4 secretion (Data from Foley et al. [148])

characterized rapamycin-generated Th2 cells as possessing a T_{CM} effector phenotype, including increased CD62 ligand expression [149], which is associated with increased efficacy of adoptive T cell therapy [150], including Treg cell prevention of GvHD [80, 81]. Second, the capacity of the Th2 cell product to polarize towards Th2 cytokines post-transplant, and also to prevent GvHD, was IL-4 dependent. This result indicates that IL-4 secretion capacity, perhaps in the relative absence of a more diverse pattern of Th2 cytokine expression, may represent the most important bio-marker for Th2 cell therapy products. Such IL-4 dependency, in addition to our additional finding that rapamycin-generated Th2 cells have nominal Foxp3 transcription factor expression, also argues against a significant contribution from a Treg cell mechanism that may be induced in some models by ex vivo rapamycin [151]. In fact, we have found no evidence that rapamycin specifically induces the generation of Treg cells, as we have been able to generate Th1, Th2, Tc1, and Tc2 cells in high dose rapamycin that each mediates increased in vivo effects [149].

7.2.2.3 Th2 Cells to Promote Engraftment with Reduced GvHD

Although clinical graft rejection is relatively uncommon, the host-versus-graft reactivity (HVGR) that forms the biologic basis of rejection represents a major barrier to the broader and safer clinical application of allogeneic HSCT, particularly in settings such as the aging cancer population, the use of reduced-intensity conditioning regimens, and transplantation across increased donor/host genetic disparity [152]. In practice, such HVG reactivity is mitigated by the inclusion of unmanipulated donor T cells in the allograft and by utilization of intensive preparative regimens that initiate GvHD and contribute to transplant-related morbidity and mortality. As such, investigators have attempted to define donor T cell subsets that abrogate HVGR with reduced GvHD; such investigations have focused primarily on donor CD8$^+$ T cells, including

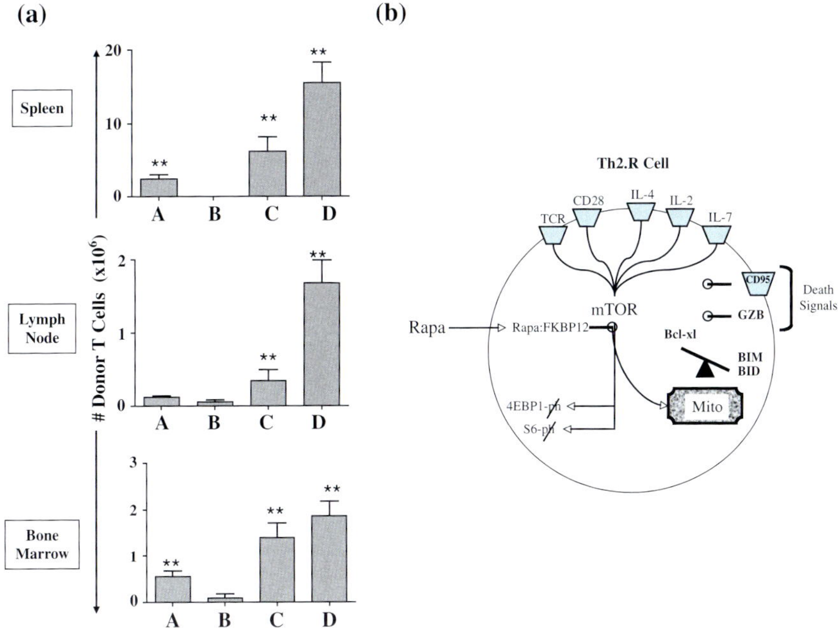

Fig. 7.5 Th2 cells for prevention of fully MHC-dependent graft rejection with reduced GvHD. Results from a B6-into-BALB/c graft rejection model are shown (*left panels*); cohort A is an engraftment control cohort, whereas cohorts B, C, and D received post-irradiation host T cells to initiate graft rejection. Cohorts A, B, C, and D receiving hematopoietic stem cell transplantation with: A (no further donor inocula); B (+ "control" donor Th2/Tc2 cells); C (+ donor Th2/Tc2.R cells) and D (+ donor CD4$^+$ Th2.R cells). At day 14 (a time point where rejection controls had died), only the rapamycin-generated T cells were present in significant numbers in the spleen, lymph node, and bone marrow; recipients of control Th2/Tc2 cells rejected the graft, whereas recipients of Th2/Tc2.R or Th2.R cells achieved alloengraftment without lethal GvHD. As modeled in the right frame, Th2.R cells had inhibition of targets down-stream to mTOR (4EBP-1 and S6), were resistant to fas- and granzyme-based apoptotic stimuli, and expressed an anti-apoptotic pattern of bcl-2 family genes

non-alloreactive or Tc2-type cells [153–155]. More recently, the role of functional subsets of donor $CD4^+$ T cells in rejection abrogation has emerged in studies involving Treg cells [76, 80] or most recently from our laboratory, rapamycin-expanded Th2 cells [156]. Several important points can be derived from this latter work, which are illustrated below in Fig. 7.5. First, in this model of fully MHC-disparate graft rejection, the capacity of the ex vivo generated donor T cells to prevent graft rejection was associated with the donor T cell capacity to persist in vivo: polarized T cells generated ex vivo in rapamycin, in particular, the $CD4^+$ Th2 cell subset, had a marked degree of expansion and persistence in vivo and were highly efficacious in the prevention of rejection [156]. Second, as modeled in Fig. 7.5 (right panel), we found that Th2 cells generated in rapamycin were resistant to subsequent rapamycin exposure and also manifested a multi-faceted resistance to apoptosis that was associated with marked alteration of the bcl-2 family gene expression, including up-regulation of anti-apoptotic bcl-xl and down-regulation of pro-apoptotic BIM and BID. In sum, these data indicate that Th2 cells demonstrate great potential for the promotion of engraftment with reduced GvHD, and indicate that Th2 adoptive cell therapy efforts should focus on the manufacture of T cell products with an enhanced capacity to persist in vivo, such as T cells exposed to high-dose rapamycin.

7.2.2.4 Recent Advances in Th2 Cell Therapy

In 1999, we initiated the first clinical trial of allogeneic Th2 cell therapy at the Experimental Transplantation and Immunology Branch, Center for Cancer Research, National Institutes of Health. The results from this trial have recently been published [157]. This protocol represented a clinical translation of our murine experiments using the technique of Th2 cell allograft augmentation: That is, subjects received both the full complement of donor T cells contained within the G-CSF mobilized, HLA-matched sibling, hematopoietic stem cell product and the ex vivo generated donor Th2 cells. Transplantation was performed after host immune ablation with fludarabine-containing outpatient induction and inpatient preparative chemotherapy. In this first-generation clinical trial, Th2 cells were manufactured by the following method: (a) $CD4^+$ cells were isolated by steady-state lymphopheresis and subsequent elutriation and negative selection; (b) $CD4^+$ cells were costimulated both at day 0 of culture and also for a second time at approximately day 12 of culture; and (c) T cells were expanded in the presence of IL-4 and IL-2 (no rapamycin). The resultant T cell product was partially shifted towards a Th2 phenotype relative to culture input donor $CD4^+$ T cells; however, such polarization was relatively incomplete relative to the extreme polarity that can be achieved in murine models. Donor Th2 cells were transfused in a phase I dose escalation manner at 5, 25, or 125×10^6 Th2 cells per kg recipient body weight with $n = 3$, $n = 19$, and $n = 6$ subjects in each cohort, respectively; there were no apparent clinical toxicities attributable to the Th2 cell infusion. Post-transplant immune monitoring determined that Th2 cell recipients expressed a mixed pattern of both Th1 and Th2 cytokine production post-transplant. However, relative to a protocol control cohort that did not receive Th2 cells, monocyte inflammatory cytokines IL-1-α and TNF-α were not reduced in Th2 cell recipients; in addition, acute GvHD was not significantly reduced in Th2 cell recipients. In sum, these results demonstrated the feasibility, safety, and apparent biologic activity of Th2 cell allograft augmentation, yet also identified the need for further improvements in this strategy if the goal of improving transplant outcomes might be realized.

In parallel with this first-generation clinical trial implementation, we determined that murine Th2 cells generated in high-dose rapamycin were more effective than control Th2 cells relative to in vivo cytokine-polarization capacity and with respect to prevention of acute GvHD [148]. In light of these murine results, we developed a clinical-scale manufacturing method for the generation of human Th2 cells in rapamycin (see Fig. 7.6). This method has several potential advantages relative to our initial method. First, Th2 cells are generated after a single-round of costimulation, which greatly increases the feasibility of the culture method; after only 12 days in culture, contamination with the Th1-type cytokine IFN-γ is relatively nominal. In addition, because of the

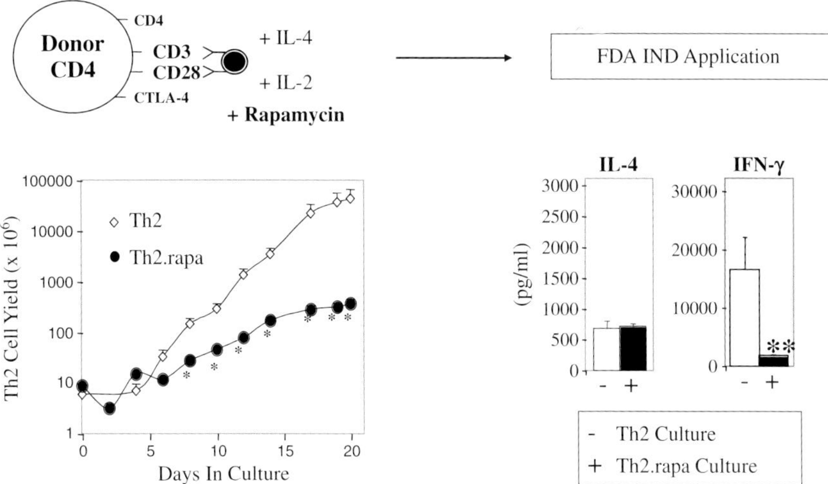

Fig. 7.6 Ex vivo generation of donor Th2 cells in high-dose rapamycin. [*Top panel*] In the current clinical trial evaluating Th2 cell allograft augmentation, Th2 cells are generated by: (**a**) $CD4^+$ T cell positive selection by Miltenyi® device; (**b**) costimulation by tosyl-activated magnetic beads conjugated with anti-CD3 and anti-CD28 antibodies; and (**c**) expansion in the presence of IL-4, IL-2, and rapamycin (1 μM). The T cell manufacturing method and clinical protocol are submitted to an Investigational New Drug (IND) application file with the U.S. Food and Drug Administration (FDA). [*Lower left panel*] Expansion of Th2 cells in rapamycin yields one- to two-log reduced yield relative to Th2 cells not expanded in rapamycin; however, CD4 isolation from a 5–10 l steady state apheresis product is typically sufficient to allow Th2 cell therapy at a dose of 2.5×10^7 Th2 cells per kg recipient body weight. [*Lower right panel*] At the end of culture, rapamycin-generated donor Th2 cells have reduced cytokine secretion relative to control Th2 cells, particularly with respect to the Th1-type cytokine IFN-γ

reduced time in culture, the Th2 cells express a more "central memory" differentiation status including up-regulation of molecules such as CD62L and CCR7. The method has the potential disadvantage of greatly reduced T cell expansion in rapamycin; however, $CD4^+$ cell harvest from a 5–10 l apheresis product typically will allow Th2 cell therapy at the intermediate dose established in our initial Th2 cell clinical trial, 2.5×10^7 Th2 cells/kg. This second generation Th2 cell clinical trial, in addition to evaluating a new method of Th2 cell manufacture, is also evaluating a new post-transplant GvHD chemoprophylaxis regimen consisting of cyclosporine plus a short-course of sirolimus (through day 14 post-transplant). This regimen was chosen because our murine experiments determined that Th2 cells generated in rapamycin were relatively resistant to inhibition by post-transplant rapamycin therapy.

Because rapamycin has been associated with the preferential expansion of Treg cells [151], one important issue is to evaluate the potential contribution of Treg cells to any observed effect of Th2 cells generated in rapamycin. On this point, we have evaluated Th2 cells generated with or without rapamycin for their expression of the Foxp3 transcription factor. As Fig. 7.7 shows, we have found a nominal level of expression of this Treg cell marker in both populations, with only a modest increase in Th2 cell Foxp3 expression with high-dose rapamycin exposure.

Because both Th2 cells and Treg cells represent candidate populations capable of improving the therapeutic index of allogeneic T cell therapy, understanding the mechanism(s) of action of each population and determining the potential interaction of these two cell populations is an important research goal. Toward this end, we have initiated murine experiments in the setting of Th2 cell therapy of established GvHD (see Fig. 7.8). In the murine system, the rapamycin-generated

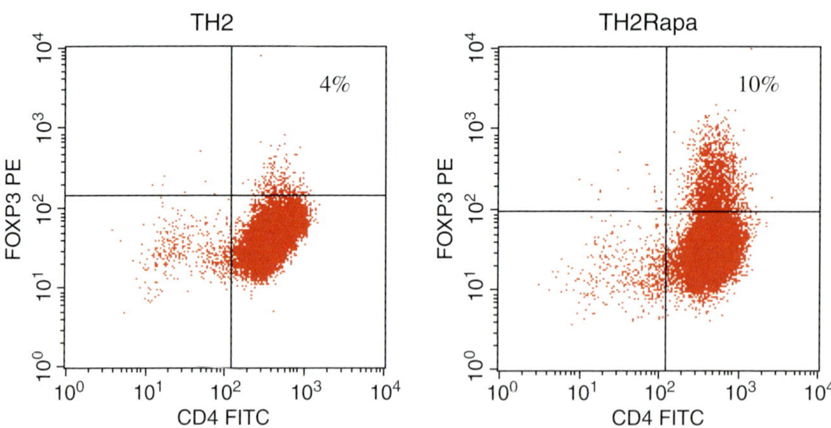

Fig. 7.7 Th2 cells have nominal expression of the Treg cell transcription factor, Foxp3. Donor Th2 cells were generated by costimulation in the presence of IL-4 and IL-2 either with rapamycin (1 μM) or without rapamycin. At day 12 of culture, cells were evaluated by flow cytometry for surface CD4 expression and intra-cellular expression of Foxp3

	Transplant Components				Post-BMT Cytokine Production			
	Host	Donor						
Cohort #	Tumor	BM	T Cells	Th2 Cells	IL-2	IFN-γ	IL-4	IL-10
1	-	+	-	-	2 ± 0.4	2 ± 0.4	4 ± 1	2 ± 1
2	+	+	-	-	1 ± .1	1 ± .1	9 ± 0.4	3 ± 0.5
3	+	+	+	-	11 ± 4	388 ± 55	67 ± 10	26 ± 7
4	+	+	+	Th2.R	12 ± 4	83 ± 5**	497 ± 47**	160 ± 33**
5	+	+	+	Th2.R (10% Treg)	7 ± 2	230 ± 40	100 ± 15	27 ± 8

Fig. 7.8 Exploring the inter-relationship between Th2 cell and Treg cell therapy of GHVD. A murine model of established GvHD was utilized (B6 donor-into-lethally irradiated BALB/c hosts). Cohorts 1 to 5 received donor bone marrow either alone or in combination with GvHD-inducing donor splenic T cells; at day 14 post-transplant, at a time of severe acute GvHD, cohorts 4 and 5 received additional donor Th2 cells generated ex vivo in rapamycin (Th2.R cells). Cohort 4 received 10×10^6 Th2 cells, whereas cohort 5 received 9×10^6 Th2 cells and 1×10^6 donor splenic Treg cells (non-expanded Treg cells). At day 19 post-transplant (5 days after Th2 cell infusion), splenic T cells were harvested (n = 5 per cohort) and a 24-h-supernatant was generated by T cell activation with host dendritic cells. As this figure shows, GvHD controls (cohort #3) had primarily T cell IFN-γ secretion; day 14 Th2 cell therapy (cohort #4) greatly reduced post-transplant IFN- γ, and greatly increased production of the Th2 cytokines IL-4 and IL-10. Remarkably, addition of only 10% natural Treg cells greatly reduced the capacity of Th2 cells to polarize the post-transplant cytokine phenotype. (Data presented by Foley et al. [159])

Th2 cell product is nominally "contaminated" by Treg cells (typically $< 1\%$ of the population expresses Foxp3). Therefore, we determined the effect of adding Treg cells to the Th2 cell product, with a Treg to Th2 cell ratio of 1:10. Remarkably, addition of this relatively low-level of natural Treg cells nearly completely abrogated the capacity of Th2 cells to yield a post-transplant Th2 cytokine phenotype, and also abrogated the ability of Th2 cells to improve survival in this model of established GvHD. This result suggests that Treg cell contamination does not contribute greatly to the Th2 cell effect, and that depletion of Treg cells from Th2 cell products may represent a strategy for further improving the potency of Th2 cell therapy; importantly, it has been previously observed that Treg cells can potently suppress Th2 responses [158].

7.3 Strategies and Challenges in Th2 Cell Research and Therapy

7.3.1 Biology

Over 20 years ago, Dr. William Paul described a soluble T cell factor (IL-4) that promoted B cell antibody responses and subsequently became known as the primordial Th2 cytokine that, along with IL-2, primed for the full spectrum of

Th2 cytokine secretion, including IL-5, IL-10, and IL-13. Remarkably, these observations regarding the central role of IL-4 still represent the most important tenet of Th2 cell biology. Of course, a great deal of information has been garnered since these origins of the field. One of the more important advances relates to the association of the GATA-3 transcription factor with the Th2 cell program, in contradistinction to t-bet for Th1 cells, Foxp3 for Treg cells, and ROR-γ for the newly described Th17 cells. Interestingly, it has recently been shown that T cell notch signaling can promote GATA-3 expression in an IL-4 independent manner, thereby providing a potential pathway for an initial burst of IL-4 production that subsequently sustains the Th2 pathway [160]. Ongoing research in CD4 cell fate decisions based on differential transcription factor expression will certainly help elucidate the role of CD4 cell subsets in transplant biology.

A second important issue with instant clinical implication relates to the in vivo immune modulation effects of rapamycin (sirolimus) in terms of the balance of Th1, Th2, and Treg cells. It has long been known that Th1/Tc1 cells are preferentially inhibited during rapamycin post-transplant therapy, thereby leading to a Th2 bias [161]. On this point, we have recently found that even Th1/Tc1 cells rendered resistant to rapamycin in vitro are highly susceptible to rapamycin in vivo; this observation is consistent with the possibility that rapamycin inhibition of Th1/Tc1 cells may be indirect through modulation of APC, such as reduction in IL-12 production [162]. Of note, rapamycin, but not cyclosporine, is permissive for Treg cell inhibition of experimental GvHD [163]. Finally, a third area of recent research relates to the biology of adoptive T cell therapy, with the realization that there exists an inverse correlation between the magnitude T cell product effector function relative to subsequent in vivo efficacy because T central memory effectors appear to represent an advantageous subset relative to T effector memory cells [80, 81, 149, 150].

7.3.2 *Therapeutic Issues*

The current climate seems promising for investigators to bring Th2 or Treg cell therapies to clinical fruition: There exists a detailed understanding of the biology of Th1, Th2, and Treg cells; feasible methods have been developed to activate and expand T cells ex vivo; and there is an improved understanding of the T cell differentiation characteristics that translate into improved in vivo efficacy after adoptive transfer. Having said this, numerous challenges still await this burgeoning field of research. First, from a practical standpoint, it is imperative that a full repertoire of reagents such as monoclonal antibodies for cell selection, and cytokines and costimulatory molecules for cell activation and propagation be available in clinically relevant grade and scale. Second, further knowledge from murine pre-clinical models will provide rationales for clinical trial design. Specifically, such studies should further delineate optimal combinations of pharmacologic immune modulation agents with T cell products; hopefully, advances in cell therapy will facilitate reduced reliance upon conventional immune suppressive therapies. It will be crucial to further identify the differential mechanism(s) of candidate populations such as Treg cells and Th2 cells, with an eye towards evaluating whether such subsets may operate in a synergistic or antagonistic manner. Advances in the understanding and modeling of acute vs. chronic GvHD will be essential to improve the odds that a particular T cell therapy may prove efficacious for a given GvHD biology.

7.3.3 Feasibility Issues

Adoptive T cell therapy using functionally defined T cell subsets must be both efficacious and feasible. The efficacy issue in the allogeneic HSCT context has been outlined: Such a T cell therapy must associate with a favorable balance of GvT effect to GvHD or pro-engraftment effect to GvHD. Feasibility has already been demonstrated in numerous pilot clinical trials of adoptive T cell therapy. It is estimated that the cost of a patient-specific T cell collection, isolation, and expansion is in the range of $10,000 (U.S.); if the product is truly efficacious, it is quite likely that such an expenditure would be cost effective relative to pharmacologic or other biologic interventions. Ongoing research should seek to limit the donor-to-donor variability that can exist with donor-specific therapies; it seems that the use of robust T cell expansion methods such as antibody-based costimulation in preference to antigen-presenting-cell methods represents one significant step in this direction. Alternatively, novel transplantation strategies may be developed that utilize "off-the-shelf" T cell therapies using universal donors.

References

1. Sakaguchi S. Sakaguchi N. Asano M. Itoh M. Toda M. Immunologic self-tolerance maintained by activated T cells expressing IL-2 receptor alpha-chains (CD25). Breakdown of a single mechanism of self-tolerance causes various autoimmune diseases. J Immunol. 1995;155:1151–64.
2. Bluestone JA. Abbas AK. Natural versus adaptive regulatory T cells. Nat Rev Immunol. 2003;3:253–7.
3. Chen W. Jin W. Hardegen N, et al. Conversion of peripheral CD4 + CD25– naive T cells to CD4 + CD25 + regulatory T cells by TGF-beta induction of transcription factor Foxp3. J Exp Med. 2003;198:1875–86.
4. Fontenot JD. Gavin MA. Rudensky AY. Foxp3 programs the development and function of CD4 + CD25 + regulatory T cells. Nat Immunol. 2003;4:330–6.
5. Brunkow ME. Jeffery EW. Hjerrild KA, et al. Disruption of a new forkhead/winged-helix protein, scurfin, results in the fatal lymphoproliferative disorder of the scurfy mouse. Nat Genet. 2001;27:68–73.

6. Bennett CL. Christie J. Ramsdell F, et al. The immune dysregulation, polyendocrinopathy, enteropathy, X-linked syndrome (IPEX) is caused by mutations of FOXP3. Nat Genet. 2001;27:20–1.
7. Fontenot JD. Rasmussen JP. Williams LM. Dooley JL. Farr AG. Rudensky AY. Regulatory T cell lineage specification by the forkhead transcription factor foxp3. Immunity 2005;22:329–41.
8. Lahl K. Loddenkemper C. Drouin C, et al. Selective depletion of Foxp3+ regulatory T cells induces a scurfy-like disease. J Exp Med. 2007;204:57–63.
9. Williams LM. Rudensky AY. Maintenance of the Foxp3-dependent developmental program in mature regulatory T cells requires continued expression of Foxp3. Nat Immunol. 2007;8:277–84.
10. Wan YY. Flavell RA. Regulatory T-cell functions are subverted and converted owing to attenuated Foxp3 expression. Nature 2007;445:766–70.
11. Baecher-Allan C. Brown JA. Freeman GJ. Hafler DA. CD4+CD25 high regulatory cells in human peripheral blood. J Immunol. 2001;167:1245–53.
12. Wing K. Suri-Payer E. Rudin A. CD4+CD25+ -regulatory T cells from mouse to man. Scand J Immunol. 2005;62:1–15.
13. Liu W. Putnam AL. Xu-Yu Z, et al. CD127 expression inversely correlates with FoxP3 and suppressive function of human CD4+ T reg cells. J Exp Med. 2006;203:1701–11.
14. Seddiki N. Santner-Nanan B. Martinson J, et al. Expression of interleukin (IL)-2 and IL-7 receptors discriminates between human regulatory and activated T cells. J Exp Med. 2006;203:1693–1700.
15. Pacholczyk R. Kern J. Singh N. Iwashima M. Kraj P. Ignatowicz L. Nonself-antigens are the cognate specificities of Foxp3+ regulatory T cells. Immunity 2007;27:493–504.
16. Wong J. Obst R. Correia-Neves M. Losyev G. Mathis D. Benoist C. Adaptation of TCR repertoires to self-peptides in regulatory and nonregulatory CD4+ T cells. J Immunol. 2007;178:7032–41.
17. Valmori D. Merlo A. Souleimanian NE. Hesdorffer CS. Ayyoub M. A peripheral circulating compartment of natural naive CD4 Tregs. J Clin Invest. 2005;115:1953–62.
18. Hoffmann P. Eder R. Boeld TJ, et al. Only the CD45RA+ subpopulation of CD4+CD25high T cells gives rise to homogeneous regulatory T-cell lines upon in vitro expansion. Blood 2006;108:4260–7.
19. Thornton AM. Shevach EM. Suppressor effector function of CD4+CD25+ immunoregulatory T cells is antigen nonspecific. J Immunol. 2000;164:183–90.
20. Su L. Creusot RJ. Gallo EM, et al. Murine CD4+CD25+ regulatory T cells fail to undergo chromatin remodeling across the proximal promoter region of the IL-2 gene. J Immunol. 2004;173:4994–5001.
21. Bensinger SJ. Walsh PT. Zhang J, et al. Distinct IL-2 receptor signaling pattern in CD4+CD25+ regulatory T cells. J Immunol. 2004;172:5287–96.
22. Hickman SP. Yang J. Thomas RM. Wells AD. Turka LA. Defective activation of protein kinase C and Ras-ERK pathways limits IL-2 production and proliferation by CD4+CD25+ regulatory T cells. J Immunol. 2006;177:2186–94.
23. Fontenot JD. Rasmussen JP. Gavin MA. Rudensky AY. A function for interleukin 2 in Foxp3-expressing regulatory T cells. Nat Immunol. 2005;6:1142–51.
24. Klein L. Khazaie K, von Boehmer H. In vivo dynamics of antigen-specific regulatory T cells not predicted from behavior in vitro. Proc Natl Acad Sci USA. 2003;100:8886 91.
25. Fisson S. Darrasse-Jeze G. Litvinova E, et al. Continuous activation of autoreactive CD4+CD25+ regulatory T cells in the steady state. J Exp Med. 2003;198:737–46.
26. Earle KE. Tang Q. Zhou X, et al. In vitro expanded human CD4+CD25+ regulatory T cells suppress effector T cell proliferation. Clin Immunol. 2005;115:3–9.
27. Hoffmann P. Eder R. Kunz-Schughart LA. Andreesen R. Edinger M. Large-scale in vitro expansion of polyclonal human CD4(+)CD25high regulatory T cells. Blood 2004;104:895–903.

28. Hoffmann P. Boeld TJ. Eder R, et al. Isolation of CD4(+)CD25(+) Regulatory T Cells for Clinical Trials. Biol Blood Marrow Transplant. 2006;12:267–74.
29. Thornton AM. Shevach EM. CD4+CD25+ immunoregulatory T cells suppress polyclonal T cell activation in vitro by inhibiting interleukin 2 production. J Exp Med. 1998;188:287–96.
30. Zhao DM. Thornton AM. DiPaolo RJ. Shevach EM. Activated CD4+CD25+ T cells selectively kill B lymphocytes. Blood 2006;107:3925–32.
31. Romagnani C. Della Chiesa M. Kohler S, et al. Activation of human NK cells by plasmacytoid dendritic cells and its modulation by CD4+ T helper cells and CD4+CD25hi T regulatory cells. Eur J Immunol. 2005;35:2452–8.
32. Misra N. Bayry J. Lacroix-Desmazes S. Kazatchkine MD. Kaveri SV. Cutting edge: human CD4+CD25+ T cells restrain the maturation and antigen-presenting function of dendritic cells. J Immunol. 2004;172:4676–80.
33. von Boehmer H. Mechanisms of suppression by suppressor T cells. Nat Immunol. 2005;6:338–44.
34. Nakamura K. Kitani A. Fuss I, et al. TGF-beta 1 plays an important role in the mechanism of CD4+CD25+ regulatory T cell activity in both humans and mice. J Immunol. 2004;172:834–42.
35. Birebent B. Lorho R. Lechartier H, et al. Suppressive properties of human CD4+CD25+ regulatory T cells are dependent on CTLA-4 expression. Eur J Immunol. 2004;34:3485–96.
36. Bopp T. Becker C. Klein M, et al. Cyclic adenosine monophosphate is a key component of regulatory T cell-mediated suppression. J Exp Med. 2007;204:1303–10.
37. Deaglio S. Dwyer KM. Gao W, et al. Adenosine generation catalyzed by CD39 and CD73 expressed on regulatory T cells mediates immune suppression. J Exp Med. 2007;204:1257–65.
38. Bodor J. Fehervari Z. Diamond B. Sakaguchi S. ICER/CREM-mediated transcriptional attenuation of IL-2 and its role in suppression by regulatory T cells. Eur J Immunol. 2007;37:884–95.
39. de la Rosa M. Rutz S. Dorninger H. Scheffold A. Interleukin-2 is essential for CD4+CD25+ regulatory T cell function. Eur J Immunol. 2004;34:2480–8.
40. Pandiyan P. Zheng L. Ishihara S. Reed J. Lenardo MJ. CD4(+)CD25(+)Foxp3(+) regulatory T cells induce cytokine deprivation-mediated apoptosis of effector CD4(+) T cells. Nat Immunol. 2007;8:1353–62.
41. Cao X. Cai SF. Fehniger TA, et al. Granzyme B and perforin are important for regulatory T cell-mediated suppression of tumor clearance. Immunity 2007;27:635–46.
42. Rudensky AY. Campbell DJ. In vivo sites and cellular mechanisms of T reg cell-mediated suppression. J Exp Med. 2006;203:489–92.
43. Edinger M. Hoffmann P. Ermann J, et al. CD4(+)CD25(+) regulatory T cells preserve graft-versus-tumor activity while inhibiting graft-versus-host disease after bone marrow transplantation. Nat Med. 2003;9:1144–50.
44. Tang Q. Adams JY. Tooley AJ, et al. Visualizing regulatory T cell control of autoimmune responses in nonobese diabetic mice. Nat Immunol. 2006;7:83–92.
45. Tadokoro CE. Shakhar G. Shen S, et al. Regulatory T cells inhibit stable contacts between CD4+ T cells and dendritic cells in vivo. J Exp Med. 2006;203:505–11.
46. Chen ML. Pittet MJ. Gorelik L, et al. Regulatory T cells suppress tumor-specific CD8 T cell cytotoxicity through TGF-beta signals in vivo. Proc Natl Acad Sci USA. 2005;102:419–24.
47. Chen Z. Herman AE. Matos M. Mathis D. Benoist C. Where CD4+CD25+ T reg cells impinge on autoimmune diabetes. J Exp Med. 2005;202:1387–97.
48. Siegmund K. Feuerer M. Siewert C, et al. Migration matters: regulatory T-cell compartmentalization determines suppressive activity in vivo. Blood 2005;106:3097–104.

49. Waldmann H. Adams E. Fairchild P. Cobbold S. Infectious tolerance and the long-term acceptance of transplanted tissue. Immunol Rev. 2006;212:301–13.
50. Roncarolo MG. Gregori S. Battaglia M. Bacchetta R. Fleischhauer K. Levings MK. Interleukin-10-secreting type 1 regulatory T cells in rodents and humans. Immunol Rev. 2006;212:28–50.
51. Walker MR. Kasprowicz DJ. Gersuk VH, et al. Induction of FoxP3 and acquisition of T regulatory activity by stimulated human CD4+CD25– T cells. J Clin Invest. 2003;112:1437–43.
52. Kretschmer K. Apostolou I. Hawiger D. Khazaie K. Nussenzweig MC, von Boehmer H. Inducing and expanding regulatory T cell populations by foreign antigen. Nat Immunol. 2005;6:1219–27.
53. Floess S. Freyer J. Siewert C, et al. Epigenetic control of the foxp3 locus in regulatory T cells. PLoS Biol. 2007;5:e38.
54. Fantini MC. Becker C. Monteleone G. Pallone F. Galle PR. Neurath MF. Cutting edge: TGF-beta induces a regulatory phenotype in CD4+CD25– T cells through Foxp3 induction and down-regulation of Smad7. J Immunol. 2004;172:5149–53.
55. Tran DQ. Ramsey H. Shevach EM. Induction of FOXP3 expression in naive human CD4+FOXP3 T cells by T-cell receptor stimulation is transforming growth factor-beta dependent but does not confer a regulatory phenotype. Blood 2007;110:2983–90.
56. Pillai V. Karandikar NJ. Human regulatory T cells: a unique, stable thymic subset or a reversible peripheral state of differentiation? Immunol Lett. 2007;114:9–15.
57. Sun CM. Hall JA. Blank RB, et al. Small intestine lamina propria dendritic cells promote de novo generation of Foxp3 T reg cells via retinoic acid. J Exp Med. 2007;204:1775–85.
58. Coombes JL. Siddiqui KR. Arancibia-Carcamo CV, et al. A functionally specialized population of mucosal CD103+ DCs induces Foxp3+ regulatory T cells via a TGF-beta and retinoic acid-dependent mechanism. J Exp Med. 2007;204:1757–64.
59. Benson MJ. Pino-Lagos K. Rosemblatt M. Noelle RJ. All-trans retinoic acid mediates enhanced T reg cell growth, differentiation, and gut homing in the face of high levels of co-stimulation. J Exp Med. 2007;204:1765–74.
60. Weaver CT. Harrington LE. Mangan PR. Gavrieli M. Murphy KM. Th17: an effector CD4 T cell lineage with regulatory T cell ties. Immunity 2006;24:677–88.
61. Cua DJ. Sherlock J. Chen Y, et al. Interleukin-23 rather than interleukin-12 is the critical cytokine for autoimmune inflammation of the brain. Nature 2003;421:744–8.
62. Veldhoen M. Hocking RJ. Atkins CJ. Locksley RM. Stockinger B. TGFbeta in the context of an inflammatory cytokine milieu supports de novo differentiation of IL-17-producing T cells. Immunity 2006;24:179–89.
63. Mangan PR. Harrington LE. O'Quinn DB, et al. Transforming growth factor-beta induces development of the T(H)17 lineage. Nature 2006;441:231–4.
64. Bettelli E. Carrier Y. Gao W, et al. Reciprocal developmental pathways for the generation of pathogenic effector TH17 and regulatory T cells. Nature 2006;441:235–8.
65. Stockinger B. Veldhoen M. Differentiation and function of Th17 T cells. Curr Opin Immunol. 2007;19:281–6.
66. Ivanov, II. McKenzie BS. Zhou L, et al. The orphan nuclear receptor RORgammat directs the differentiation program of proinflammatory IL-17+ T helper cells. Cell 2006;126:1121–33.
67. Korn T. Bettelli E. Gao W, et al. IL-21 initiates an alternative pathway to induce proinflammatory T(H)17 cells. Nature 2007;448:484–7.
68. Bettelli E. Korn T. Kuchroo VK. Th17: the third member of the effector T cell trilogy. Curr Opin Immunol. 2007;19:652–7.
69. Hoffmann P. Ermann J. Edinger M. Fathman CG. Strober S. Donor-type CD4(+)CD25(+) regulatory T cells suppress lethal acute graft-versus-host disease after allogeneic bone marrow transplantation. J Exp Med. 2002;196:389–99.

70. Cohen JL. Trenado A. Vasey D. Klatzmann D. Salomon BL. CD4(+)CD25(+) immunoregulatory T cells: new therapeutics for graft-versus-host disease. J Exp Med. 2002;196:401–6.
71. Taylor PA. Friedman TM. Korngold R. Noelle RJ. Blazar BR. Tolerance induction of alloreactive T cells via ex vivo blockade of the CD40:CD40L costimulatory pathway results in the generation of a potent immune regulatory cell. Blood 2002;99:4601–9.
72. Taylor PA. Lees CJ. Blazar BR. The infusion of ex vivo activated and expanded CD4(+)CD25(+) immune regulatory cells inhibits graft-versus-host disease lethality. Blood 2002;99:3493–9.
73. Jones SC. Murphy GF. Korngold R. Post-hematopoietic cell transplantation control of graft-versus-host disease by donor CD4(+)25(+) T cells to allow an effective graft-versus-leukemia response. Biol Blood Marrow Transplant. 2003;9:243–56.
74. Moore KW, de Waal Malefyt R. Coffman RL. O'Garra A. Interleukin-10 and the interleukin-10 receptor. Annu Rev Immunol. 2001;19:683–765.
75. Nguyen VH. Zeiser R. Dasilva DL, et al. In vivo dynamics of regulatory T-cell trafficking and survival predict effective strategies to control graft-versus-host disease following allogeneic transplantation. Blood 2007;109:2649–56.
76. Hanash AM. Levy RB. Donor CD4+CD25+ T cells promote engraftment and tolerance following MHC-mismatched hematopoietic cell transplantation. Blood 2005;105: 1828–36.
77. Steiner D. Brunicki N. Bachar-Lustig E. Taylor PA. Blazar BR. Reisner Y. Overcoming T cell-mediated rejection of bone marrow allografts by T-regulatory cells: synergism with veto cells and rapamycin. Exp Hematol. 2006;34:802–8.
78. Trenado A. Charlotte F. Fisson S, et al. Recipient-type specific CD4+CD25+ regulatory T cells favor immune reconstitution and control graft-versus-host disease while maintaining graft-versus-leukemia. J Clin Invest. 2003;112:1688–96.
79. Nguyen VH. Shashidhar S. Chang DS, et al. The impact of regulatory T cells on T-cell immunity following hematopoietic cell transplantation. Blood 2008;111:945–53.
80. Taylor PA. Panoskaltsis-Mortari A. Swedin JM, et al. L-Selectin(hi) but not the L-selectin(lo) CD4+25+ T-regulatory cells are potent inhibitors of GVHD and BM graft rejection. Blood 2004;104:3804–12.
81. Ermann J. Hoffmann P. Edinger M, et al. Only the CD62L+ subpopulation of CD4+CD25+ regulatory T cells protects from lethal acute GVHD. Blood 2005;105: 2220–6.
82. Shlomchik WD. Couzens MS. Tang CB, et al. Prevention of graft versus host disease by inactivation of host antigen-presenting cells. Science 1999;285:412–5.
83. Wysocki CA. Jiang Q. Panoskaltsis-Mortari A, et al. Critical role for CCR5 in the function of donor CD4+CD25+ regulatory T cells during acute graft-versus-host disease. Blood 2005;106:3300–7.
84. Mottet C. Uhlig HH. Powrie F. Cutting edge: cure of colitis by CD4+CD25+ regulatory T cells. J Immunol. 2003;170:3939–43.
85. Johnson BD. Truitt RL. Delayed infusion of immunocompetent donor cells after bone marrow transplantation breaks graft-host tolerance allows for persistent antileukemic reactivity without severe graft-versus-host disease. Blood 1995;85:3302–12.
86. Johnson BD. Becker EE. LaBelle JL. Truitt RL. Role of immunoregulatory donor T cells in suppression of graft-versus-host disease following donor leukocyte infusion therapy. J Immunol. 1999;163:6479–87.
87. Johnson BD. Konkol MC. Truitt RL. CD25+ immunoregulatory T-cells of donor origin suppress alloreactivity after BMT. Biol Blood Marrow Transplant. 2002;8: 525–35.
88. Stanzani M. Martins SL. Saliba RM, et al. CD25 expression on donor CD4+ or CD8+ T cells is associated with an increased risk for graft-versus-host disease after HLA-identical stem cell transplantation in humans. Blood 2004;103:1140–6.

89. Rezvani K. Mielke S. Ahmadzadeh M, et al. High donor FOXP3-positive regulatory T-cell (Treg) content is associated with a low risk of GVHD following HLA-matched allogeneic SCT. Blood 2006;108:1291–7.
90. Pabst C. Schirutschke H. Ehninger G. Bornhauser M. Platzbecker U. The graft content of donor T cells expressing gamma delta TCR+ and CD4+foxp3+ predicts the risk of acute graft versus host disease after transplantation of allogeneic peripheral blood stem cells from unrelated donors. Clin Cancer Res. 2007;13:2916–22.
91. Wolf D. Wolf AM. Fong D, et al. Regulatory T-cells in the graft and the risk of acute graft-versus-host disease after allogeneic stem cell transplantation. Transplantation 2007;83:1107–13.
92. Martin PJ. Pei J. Gooley T, et al. Evaluation of a CD25-specific immunotoxin for prevention of graft-versus-host disease after unrelated marrow transplantation. Biol Blood Marrow Transplant. 2004;10:552–60.
93. Lee SJ. Zahrieh D. Agura E, et al. Effect of up-front daclizumab when combined with steroids for the treatment of acute graft-versus-host disease: results of a randomized trial. Blood 2004;104:1559–64.
94. Miura Y. Thoburn CJ. Bright EC, et al. Association of Foxp3 regulatory gene expression with graft-versus-host disease. Blood 2004;104:2187–93.
95. Schneider M. Munder M. Karakhanova S. Ho AD. Goerner M. The initial phase of graft-versus-host disease is associated with a decrease of CD4+CD25+ regulatory T cells in the peripheral blood of patients after allogeneic stem cell transplantation. Clin Lab Haematol. 2006;28:382–90.
96. Mielke S. Rezvani K. Savani BN, et al. Reconstitution of FOXP3+ regulatory T cells (Tregs) after CD25-depleted allotransplantation in elderly patients and association with acute graft-versus-host disease. Blood 2007;110:1689–97.
97. Sanchez J. Casano J. Alvarez MA, et al. Kinetic of regulatory CD25high and activated CD134+ (OX40) T lymphocytes during acute and chronic graft-versus-host disease after allogeneic bone marrow transplantation. Br J Haematol. 2004;126:697–703.
98. Arimoto K. Kadowaki N. Ishikawa T. Ichinohe T. Uchiyama T. FOXP3 expression in peripheral blood rapidly recovers and lacks correlation with the occurrence of graft-versus-host disease after allogeneic stem cell transplantation. Int J Hematol. 2007;85:154–62.
99. Rieger K. Loddenkemper C. Maul J, et al. Mucosal FOXP3+ regulatory T cells are numerically deficient in acute and chronic GvHD. Blood 2006;107:1717–23.
100. Clark FJ. Gregg R. Piper K, et al. Chronic graft-versus-host disease is associated with increased numbers of peripheral blood CD4+CD25high regulatory T cells. Blood 2004;103:2410–6.
101. Zorn E. Kim HT. Lee SJ, et al. Reduced frequency of FOXP3+ CD4+CD25+ regulatory T cells in patients with chronic graft-versus-host disease. Blood 2005;106:2903–11.
102. Meignin V. Peffault de Latour R. Zuber J, et al. Numbers of Foxp3-expressing CD4+CD25high T cells do not correlate with the establishment of long-term tolerance after allogeneic stem cell transplantation. Exp Hematol. 2005;33:894–900.
103. Hauri-Hohl MM. Keller MP. Gill J, et al. Donor T-cell alloreactivity against host thymic epithelium limits T-cell development after bone marrow transplantation. Blood 2007;109:4080–8.
104. Godfrey WR. Spoden DJ. Ge YG, et al. Cord blood CD4(+)CD25(+)-derived T regulatory cell lines express FoxP3 protein and manifest potent suppressor function. Blood 2005;105:750–8.
105. Battaglia M. Stabilini A. Migliavacca B. Horejs-Hoeck J. Kaupper T. Roncarolo MG. Rapamycin promotes expansion of functional CD4+CD25+FOXP3+ regulatory T cells of both healthy subjects and type 1 diabetic patients. J Immunol. 2006;177:8338–47.

106. Godfrey WR. Ge YG. Spoden DJ, et al. In vitro-expanded human CD4(+)CD25(+) T-regulatory cells can markedly inhibit allogeneic dendritic cell-stimulated MLR cultures. Blood 2004;104:453–61.
107. Jiang S. Tsang J. Game DS. Stevenson S. Lombardi G. Lechler RI. Generation and expansion of human CD4+ CD25+ regulatory T cells with indirect allospecificity: potential reagents to promote donor-specific transplantation tolerance. Transplantation 2006;82:1738–43.
108. Roncarolo MG. Battaglia M. Regulatory T-cell immunotherapy for tolerance to self antigens and alloantigens in humans. Nat Rev Immunol. 2007;7:585–98.
109. Zhang H. Chua KS. Guimond M, et al. Lymphopenia and interleukin-2 therapy alter homeostasis of CD4+CD25+ regulatory T cells. Nat Med. 2005;11:1238–43.
110. Mosmann TR. Cherwinski H. Bond MW. Giedlin MA. Coffman RL. Two types of murine helper T cell clone. I. Definition according to profiles of lymphokine activities and secreted proteins. J Immunol. 1986;136:2348–57.
111. Le Gros G. Ben-Sasson SZ. Seder R. Finkelman FD. Paul WE. Generation of interleukin 4 (IL-4)-producing cells in vivo and in vitro: IL-2 and IL-4 are required for in vitro generation of IL-4-producing cells. J Exp Med. 1990;172:921–9.
112. Yoshimoto T. Bendelac A. Watson C. Hu-Li J. Paul WE. Role of NK1.1+ T cells in a TH2 response and in immunoglobulin E production. Science 1995;270:1845–7.
113. Rodriguez-Palmero M. Hara T. Thumbs A. Hunig T. Triggering of T cell proliferation through CD28 induces GATA-3 and promotes T helper type 2 differentiation in vitro and in vivo. Eur J Immunol. 1999;29:3914–24.
114. Brown DR. Green JM. Moskowitz NH. Davis M. Thompson CB. Reiner SL. Limited role of CD28-mediated signals in T helper subset differentiation. J Exp Med. 1996;184:803–10.
115. Rissoan MC. Soumelis V. Kadowaki N, et al. Reciprocal control of T helper cell and dendritic cell differentiation. Science 1999;283:1183–6.
116. Kalinski P. Hilkens CM. Snijders A. Snijdewint FG. Kapsenberg ML. IL-12-deficient dendritic cells, generated in the presence of prostaglandin E2, promote type 2 cytokine production in maturing human naive T helper cells. J Immunol. 1997;159:28–35.
117. Sallusto F. Lenig D. Forster R. Lipp M. Lanzavecchia A. Two subsets of memory T lymphocytes with distinct homing potentials and effector functions. Nature 1999;401:708–12.
118. Kelly BL. Locksley RM. Coordinate regulation of the IL-4, IL-13, and IL-5 cytokine cluster in Th2 clones revealed by allelic expression patterns. J Immunol. 2000;165:2982–6.
119. Croft M. Carter L. Swain SL. Dutton RW. Generation of polarized antigen-specific CD8 effector populations: reciprocal action of interleukin (IL)-4 and IL-12 in promoting type 2 versus type 1 cytokine profiles. J Exp Med. 1994;180:1715–28.
120. Carter LL. Dutton RW. Relative perforin- and Fas-mediated lysis in T1 and T2 CD8 effector populations. J Immunol. 1995;155:1028–31.
121. Peritt D. Robertson S. Gri G. Showe L. Aste-Amezaga M. Trinchieri G. Differentiation of human NK cells into NK1 and NK2 subsets. J Immunol. 1998;161:5821–4.
122. Afkarian M. Sedy JR. Yang J, et al. T-bet is a STAT1-induced regulator of IL-12R expression in naive CD4+ T cells. [comment]. Nat Immunol. 2002;3:549–57.
123. Sallusto F. Lenig D. Mackay CR. Lanzavecchia A. Flexible programs of chemokine receptor expression on human polarized T helper 1 and 2 lymphocytes. J Exp Med. 1998;187:875–83.
124. Chtanova T. Kemp RA. Sutherland AP. Ronchese F. Mackay CR. Gene microarrays reveal extensive differential gene expression in both CD4(+) and CD8(+) type 1 and type 2 T cells. J Immunol. 2001;167:3057–63.

125. Sher A. Gazzinelli RT. Oswald IP, et al. Role of T-cell derived cytokines in the down-regulation of immune responses in parasitic and retroviral infection. Immunol Rev. 1992;127:183–204.
126. Salgame P. Abrams JS. Clayberger C, et al. Differing lymphokine profiles of functional subsets of human CD4 and CD8 T cell clones. Science 1991;254:279–82.
127. Windhagen A. Anderson DE. Carrizosa A. Williams RE. Hafler DA. IL-12 induces human T cells secreting IL-10 with IFN-gamma. J Immunol. 1996;157:1127–31.
128. Cousins DJ. Lee TH. Staynov DZ. Cytokine coexpression during human Th1/Th2 cell differentiation: direct evidence for coordinated expression of Th2 cytokines. J Immunol. 2002;169:2498–506.
129. Via CS. Finkelman FD. Critical role of interleukin-2 in the development of acute graft-versus-host disease. Int Immunol. 1993;5:565–72.
130. Blazar BR. Taylor PA. Panoskaltsis-Mortari A, et al. Blockade of CD40 ligand-CD40 interaction impairs CD4+ T cell-mediated alloreactivity by inhibiting mature donor T cell expansion and function after bone marrow transplantation. J Immunol. 1997;158:29–39.
131. Via CS. Rus V. Gately MK. Finkelman FD. IL-12 stimulates the development of acute graft-versus-host disease in mice that normally would develop chronic, autoimmune graft-versus-host disease. J Immunol. 1994;153:4040–7.
132. Baker MB. Altman NH. Podack ER. Levy RB. The role of cell-mediated cytotoxicity in acute GVHD after MHC-matched allogeneic bone marrow transplantation in mice. J Exp Med. 1996;183:2645–56.
133. Kataoka Y. Iwasaki T. Kuroiwa T, et al. The role of donor T cells for target organ injuries in acute and chronic graft-versus-host disease. Immunology 2001;103:310–8.
134. Nestel FP. Price KS. Seemayer TA. Lapp WS. Macrophage priming and lipopolysaccharide-triggered release of tumor necrosis factor alpha during graft-versus-host disease. J Exp Med. 1992;175:405–13.
135. Abhyankar S. Gilliland DG. Ferrara JL. Interleukin-1 is a critical effector molecule during cytokine dysregulation in graft versus host disease to minor histocompatibility antigens. Transplantation 1993;56:1518–23.
136. Nikolic B. Lee S. Bronson RT. Grusby MJ. Sykes M. Th1 and Th2 mediate acute graft-versus-host disease, each with distinct end-organ targets. J Clin Invest. 2000;105:1289–98.
137. Liu J. Anderson BE. Robert ME, et al. Selective T-cell subset ablation demonstrates a role for T1 and T2 cells in ongoing acute graft-versus-host disease: a model system for the reversal of disease. Blood 2001;98:3367–75.
138. Murphy WJ. Welniak LA. Taub DD, et al. Differential effects of the absence of interferon-gamma and IL-4 in acute graft-versus-host disease after allogeneic bone marrow transplantation in mice. J Clin Invest. 1998;102:1742–8.
139. Fowler DH. Kurasawa K. Husebekk A. Cohen PA. Gress RE. Cells of Th2 cytokine phenotype prevent LPS-induced lethality during murine graft-versus-host reaction. Regulation of cytokines and CD8+ lymphoid engraftment. J Immunol. 1994;152:1004–13.
140. Krenger W. Snyder KM. Byon JC. Falzarano G. Ferrara JL. Polarized type 2 alloreactive CD4+ and CD8+ donor T cells fail to induce experimental acute graft-versus-host disease. J Immunol. 1995;155:585–93.
141. Fowler DH. Breglio J. Nagel G. Eckhaus MA. Gress RE. Allospecific CD8+ Tc1 and Tc2 populations in graft-versus-leukemia effect and graft-versus-host disease. J Immunol. 1996;157:4811–21.
142. Jung U. Foley JE. Erdmann AA. Eckhaus MA. Fowler DH. CD3/CD28-costimulated T1 and T2 subsets: differential in vivo allosensitization generates distinct GVT and GVHD effects. Blood 2003;102:3439–46.

143. van den Brink MR. Moore E. Ferrara JL. Burakoff SJ. Graft-versus-host-disease-associated thymic damage results in the appearance of T cell clones with anti-host reactivity. Transplantation 2000;69:446–9.
144. Fowler DH. Breglio J. Nagel G. Hirose C. Gress RE. Allospecific CD4 +, Th1/Th2 and CD8 +, Tc1/Tc2 populations in murine GVL: type I cells generate GVL and type II cells abrogate GVL. Biol Blood Marrow Transplant. 1996;2:118–25.
145. Fowler DH. Shared biology of GVHD and GVT effects: potential methods of separation. Crit Rev Oncol Hematol. 2006;57:225–44.
146. Ramirez-Montagut T. Chow A. Kochman AA, et al. IFN-gamma and Fas ligand are required for graft-versus-tumor activity against renal cell carcinoma in the absence of lethal graft-versus-host disease. J Immunol. 2007;179:1669–80.
147. Dobrzanski MJ. Reome JB. Dutton RW. Therapeutic effects of tumor-reactive type 1 and type 2 CD8 + T cell subpopulations in established pulmonary metastases. J Immunol. 1999;162:6671–80.
148. Foley JE. Jung U. Miera A, et al. Ex vivo rapamycin generates donor Th2 cells that potently inhibit graft-versus-host disease and graft-versus-tumor effects via an IL-4-dependent mechanism. J Immunol. 2005;175:5732–43.
149. Jung U. Foley JE. Erdmann AA, et al. Ex vivo rapamycin generates Th1/Tc1 or Th2/Tc2 Effector T cells with enhanced in vivo function and differential sensitivity to post-transplant rapamycin therapy. Biol Blood Marrow Transplant. 2006;12:905–18.
150. Klebanoff CA. Gattinoni L. Torabi-Parizi P, et al. Central memory self/tumor-reactive CD8 + T cells confer superior antitumor immunity compared with effector memory T cells. Proc Natl Acad Sci USA. 2005;102:9571–6.
151. Battaglia M. Stabilini A. Roncarolo MG. Rapamycin selectively expands CD4 + CD25 + FoxP3 + regulatory T cells. Blood 2005;105:4743–8.
152. Teshima T, Matsuo K, Matsue K, et al. Impact of human leucocyte antigen mismatch on graft-versus-host disease and graft failure after reduced intensity conditioning allogeneic haematopoietic stem cell transplantation from related donors. Br J Haematol. 2005;130:575–87.
153. Martin PJ, Akatsuka Y, Hahne M, Sale G. Involvement of donor T-cell cytotoxic effector mechanisms in preventing allogeneic marrow graft rejection. Blood 1998;92:2177–81.
154. Fowler DH, Whitfield B, Livingston M, Chrobak P, Gress RE. Non-host-reactive donor CD8 + T cells of Tc2 phenotype potently inhibit marrow graft rejection. Blood 1998;91:4045–50.
155. Bachar-Lustig E, Reich-Zeliger S, Reisner Y. Anti-third-party veto CTLs overcome rejection of hematopoietic allografts: synergism with rapamycin and BM cell dose. Blood 2003;102:1943–50.
156. Mariotti J, Foley J, Jung U, et al. Ex vivo rapamycin generates apoptosis-resistant donor th2 cells that persist in vivo and prevent hemopoietic stem cell graft rejection. J Immunol. 2008;180:89–105.
157. Fowler DH, Odom J, Steinberg SM, et al. Phase I clinical trial of costimulated, IL-4 polarized donor CD4 + T cells as augmentation of allogeneic hematopoietic cell transplantation. Biol Blood Marrow Transplant. 2006;12:1150–60.
158. Beiting DP, Gagliardo LF, Hesse M, Bliss SK, Meskill D, Appleton JA. Coordinated control of immunity to muscle stage Trichinella spiralis by IL-10, regulatory T cells, and TGF-beta. J Immunol. 2007;178:1039–47.
159. Foley JE, Mariotti J, Amarnath S, Han S, Eckhaus M, Fowler DH. TH2.rapa cell treatment of established murine acute GvHD is abrogated by IL-2 therapy and T regulatory cells. Blood (ASH Annual Meeting Abstracts), 2007;110:2169.
160. Amsen D, Antov A, Jankovic D, et al. Direct regulation of Gata3 expression determines the T helper differentiation potential of Notch. Immunity 2007;27:89–99.

161. Blazar BR, Taylor PA, Panoskaltsis-Mortari A, Vallera DA. Rapamycin inhibits the generation of graft-versus-host disease- and graft-versus-leukemia-causing T cells by interfering with the production of Th1 or Th1 cytotoxic cytokines. J Immunol. 1998;160:5355–65.
162. Hackstein H, Taner T, Zahorchak AF, et al. Rapamycin inhibits IL-4-induced dendritic cell maturation in vitro and dendritic cell mobilization and function in vivo. Blood 2003;101:4457–63.
163. Zeiser R, Nguyen VH, Beilhack A, et al. Inhibition of CD4+CD25+ regulatory T-cell function by calcineurin-dependent interleukin-2 production. Blood 2006;108:390–9.

Chapter 8
Understanding and Enhancing the Graft-Versus-Leukemia Effect After Hematopoietic Stem Cell Transplantation

Jeffrey Molldrem and Stanley Riddell

8.1 Introduction

The graft-versus-leukemia (GvL) effect of allogeneic hematopoietic stem cell transplantation (HSCT) was first identified by studies in mice showing that transplanted leukemia could be cured by a lethal dose of total body irradiation (TBI) and the infusion of allogeneic bone marrow to restore hematopoiesis. Mice given TBI treatment but infused with syngeneic marrow almost always succumbed to recurrent leukemia [1]. Initial efforts to use allogeneic HSCT to treat human leukemia also gave intensive conditioning to kill malignant cells and prevent rejection of the stem cell graft, but leukemia relapse has remained a major cause of failure, particularly for patients transplanted for advanced disease [2, 3]. It soon became apparent that the development of acute and/or chronic GvHD was associated with a lower probability of leukemia relapse [4, 5], confirming the prediction of murine studies that immunologic non-identity between the donor and recipient would provide a GvL effect. The development of registries enabled analysis of outcomes for large cohorts of HSCT recipients with chronic myeloid leukemia (CML), acute myeloid leukemia (AML), and acute lymphoblastic leukemia (ALL). These studies concluded the GvL effect was associated with acute and/or chronic GvHD and that the risk of leukemia relapse was higher for patients that received allogeneic T cell depleted (TCD) or syngeneic HSCT than for patients that received unmodified allogeneic HSCT [6–9]. A reduction in relapse in CML and AML patients that did not develop GvHD was also observed, suggesting it might be possible to enhance the GvL effect without GvHD [9]. While this goal has yet to be realized in clinical HSCT, it has been possible to exploit the GvL effect, and laboratory studies have begun to elucidate mechanisms and identify targets that may augment GvL activity.

J. Molldrem (✉)
Professor of Medicine, Section Chief, Transplant Immunology, M.D. Anderson Cancer Center, Houston, TX, USA
e-mail: jmolldre@mdanderson.org

M.R. Bishop (ed.), *Hematopoietic Stem Cell Transplantation*, Cancer Treatment and Research 144, DOI 10.1007/978-0-387-78580-6_8,

8.2 Donor Lymphocyte Infusions to Promote a GvL Effect

A role for donor class I MHC-restricted $CD8^+$ and class II MHC-restricted $CD4^+$ T cells in allogeneic GvHD and GvL responses was demonstrated in animal models and inferred from human studies in which T cells were depleted from the graft to prevent GvHD [10]. TCD was effective for GvHD prevention, but the risk of relapse was higher compared with non-T cell depleted transplant, particularly for leukemias that were most susceptible to the GvL effect [9, 11]. These findings led to efforts to augment the GvL effect in patients with advanced leukemia by giving only a short course of post transplant immunosuppression, or administering a donor lymphocyte infusion (DLI) early after HSCT. Unfortunately, these approaches resulted in a high incidence of grade II–IV GvHD and an increase in non-relapse mortality [12].

Although DLI given early after HSCT caused severe GvHD, pioneering studies by Kolb demonstrated that administering DLI later after HSCT could induce durable remission in patients with relapsed CML with manageable GvHD in most patients [13]. Subsequent studies in canine and murine allogeneic HSCT models confirmed that the DLI given late after HSCT caused less GvHD [14, 15]. DLI is now a standard approach to treat relapse after allogeneic HSCT, and several multicenter surveys have confirmed its efficacy for a variety of hematologic malignancies [16–21]. DLI results in a durable compete remission in 75–80% of patients with relapse of chronic phase CML, and in 12–30% of patients with advanced phase CML [16–20]. The response rate is 25–40% for patients with relapse of AML or myelodysplastic syndrome, with the highest response rates observed when DLI is given after cytoreductive chemotherapy [22]. B-cell lymphoma, chronic lymphocytic leukemia (CLL), and Hodgkin disease are susceptible to the GvL effect, and patients with relapse of these malignancies can also respond to DLI. The most disappointing results are in the treatment of relapsed ALL where the 3-year-disease free survival is less than 15%, even if DLI is given after chemotherapy, providing further evidence that ALL is particularly resistant to eradication by immune mechanisms [16].

8.2.1 Strategies for Reducing GvHD After DLI

The major complications of DLI are myelosuppression and GvHD. Myelosuppression is usually transient if there is persistent donor hematopoiesis prior to therapy, and can be managed with transfusion support and hematopoietic growth factors [23]. The infusion of additional donor hematopoietic stem cells with DLI did not reduce the frequency of myelosuppression [24]. Grade II–IV GvHD occurs in approximately 60% of patients treated with DLI, and contributes significantly to morbidity and mortality [17–22]. In patients with relapse of chronic phase CML where disease progression is slow and tumor burden can be monitored, the infusion of escalating doses of DLI and then allowing 8–12 weeks to assess disease response before infusing a higher cell dose, has reduced the mortality related to GvHD [25]. This strategy is difficult to use in blast phase CML or acute leukemia because of the rapid tempo of disease progression.

The introduction of a conditional suicide gene into donor T cells has been employed to abrogate GvHD after DLI. Conceptually, this strategy could allow for the ablation of T cells that cause GvHD and retain the GvL effect if the tumor was completely eradicated at the time the suicide gene was activated. The herpes virus thymidine kinase gene (TK) confers sensitivity to ganciclovir and was the first suicide gene used for this purpose. A phase I study in which DLI modified to express TK was given to treat post transplant relapse or EBV lymphoproliferative disease showed that ganciclovir was effective in reversing GvHD [26]. The efficacy of TK gene therapy for reversing GvHD has been confirmed in phase II studies [27]. A major limitation of the viral TK is that it is immunogenic in humans, and immune competent patients develop a TK-specific cytotoxic T cell response that prematurely eliminates TK-modified cells and interferes with the GvL effect [28, 29].

Alternative suicide genes that encode modified human proteins such as inducible Fas or caspase 9 that naturally signal programmed cell death have been developed. The Fas or caspase 9 proteins are inactive until induced to dimerize using a nontoxic synthetic drug [30, 31]. The Fas construct (termed LV'VFas) was designed to contain a truncated cell surface human nerve growth factor receptor (LNGFR) to facilitate selection of transduced cells, two copies of FKBP modified at a single amino acid to provide a pocket for high affinity binding of the dimerizer drug, and the intracellular domain of Fas. T cells modified with either LV'VFas or with a caspase 9 vector undergo apoptosis after exposure to the dimerizer drug in vitro and LV'VFas modified cells were eliminated without toxicity in non-human primates [30]. Because the protein components of these constructs are human, only fusion sites and the point mutation in FKBP could potentially be immunogenic. The further evaluation of suicide genes for controlling severe GvHD after HSCT is in progress in haploidentical HSCT recipients [32].

8.3 Effector Mechanisms and Molecular Targets of the GvL Effect

The GvL effect can provide potent antitumor activity as demonstrated by the success of DLI and reduced intensity conditioning (Chap. 9), but HSCT recipients continue to have an unacceptably high rate of relapse, and current approaches to HSCT remain incapable of enhancing the GvL effect and segregating it from GvHD. A focus of laboratory research has been to elucidate the mechanisms involved in the GvL effect and identify targets that might be used to augment antileukemic activity without GvHD. A variety of immune cells have been implicated in the GvL effect including NK and NKT cells [33–36],

T cells that recognize recipient minor histocompatibility (H) antigens [37, 38], and T cells that recognize nonpolymorphic leukemia associated antigens (LAA) [39, 40].

8.3.1 NK and NKT Cells

NK cells are large granular lymphocytes that make up 3–15% of peripheral blood lymphocytes, 5% of splenocytes, and approximately 25% of liver lymphocytes [41]. NK cells express IgG Fc-receptor IIIA (CD16) and the neural cell adhesion molecule (NCAM, CD56), but lack CD3 [42]. A distinguishing feature of NK cells is the ability to lyse target cells without prior sensitization, and to recognize cells that lack HLA or are HLA-mismatched [43]. The spontaneous cytotoxicity of NK cells is critical for their role in the innate immune response to pathogens. In contrast, T-cells must be exposed to antigens to be activated, and expand and differentiate over a period of days [44]. The function of NK cells is determined by the integration of signals from both inhibitory and activating receptors including killer immunoglobulin receptors (KIRs) [45], which are members of the immunoglobulin superfamily and bind to HLA-A, B, or C molecules; natural killer group 2 NKG2/CD94 receptors that bind the non-classical HLA-E, F, or G molecules [46–48]; and several activating receptors for which ligands are still being elucidated [49].

A role for NK cells in a GvL effect in the absence of GvHD has been established in the setting of haploidentical HSCT. The lack of appropriate class I HLA molecules in the recipient to engage KIR receptors on donor NK cells proved to be a highly independent predictor of survival in AML [36]. A similar effect was not observed in ALL suggesting that ALL cells must lack a necessary activating ligand or adhesion molecule. The adoptive transfer of NK cells to enhance antitumor effects has also been evaluated after haploidentical HSCT. Transferred NK cells were able to expand in vivo when subcutaneous IL-2 was administered and 5 of 19 poor-prognosis AML patients treated with haploidentical HSCT, IL-2 and NK cell infusion achieved a complete remission [50]. Transferring autologous NK cells has not shown significant antitumor activity [51], but the rapid recovery of NK cells after T cell depleted HLA matched HSCT correlated with improved outcome in AML, suggesting a potential role for NK infusions in this setting [52].

NKT cells are a unique subset of $CD3^+$ T cells that express the Vα24 T cell receptor (TCR) and recognize glycolipid antigens presented by CD1d, a non-classical MHC molecule. CD1d is expressed on hematopoietic cells, including circulating T and B cells, and professional APC [53–55], and is highly expressed on myeloid and lymphoid leukemia cells [56, 57]. NKT cells can be activated by stimulation with the glycolipid antigen α-galactosylceramide (α-GalCer), which binds CD1d [58] and treatment with α-GalCer pulsed DC has shown anti-tumor activity against a spectrum of solid tumors in murine models and humans [59, 60]. Imatinib-treated CML patients in complete cytogenetic response were shown to have NKT cells capable of producing IFN-γ, in contrast to patients in partial remission [61]. These data, in addition to prior reports demonstrating CD1d expression by AML cells [57] provide a rationale for pursuing α-GalCer pulsed DC for therapy of AML, including in the HSCT setting.

8.3.2 T Cells Specific for Minor Histocompatibility Antigens

In the setting of allogeneic HLA matched HSCT, endogenous proteins in recipient cells that differ from those of the donor can provide distinct HLA binding peptides that serve as minor H antigens recognized by donor T cells, and have been presumed to be primarily responsible for the GvL effect. Minor H antigens may be ubiquitously expressed on cells and tissues, including those involved in GvHD. However, some minor H antigens are preferentially or selectively expressed by hematopoietic cells and have limited or absent expression in tissues that are targets of GvHD. In murine models of HSCT, the adoptive transfer of donor T cells specific for a single minor H antigen that is abundantly expressed on hematopoietic cells eradicated leukemia without causing GvHD [62]. This data has raised speculation that the tissue expression of minor H antigens will enable the selection of targets for T cell therapy to provide a GvL effect without GvHD.

Several characteristics of minor H antigens make them attractive targets for immunotherapy to enhance the GvL effect. Because minor H antigens are foreign to the donor, they elicit high avidity $CD8^+$ and $CD4^+$ T-cells and can recognize tumor cells that might have reduced levels of MHC. Human leukemic stem cells (LSC), which are resistant to chemotherapy due to enhanced drug efflux mechanisms, express minor H antigens and can be lysed in vitro and eradicated in NOD/SCID mice by $CD8^+$ T cells that recognize a single minor H antigen [63]. Leukemic cells express multiple minor H antigens, including those that may be derived from proteins that are essential for cell function, which should reduce the probability that leukemic cells could escape elimination by loss of a single antigen or MHC allele. Finally, unlike targeting nonpolymorphic LAA where toxicity to normal tissues is a potential concern, targeting hematopoietic restricted minor H antigens should not cause toxicity since the goal of allogeneic HSCT is to replace recipient hematopoiesis with that of the donor.

Several groups have derived minor H antigen-specific T cells from post transplant blood of HSCT recipients, determined the recognition of cells from various tissues, and identified the genes encoding minor H antigens using a variety of methods [37, 64–69]. Most minor H antigens result from nonsynonymous single nucleotide polymorphisms (SNPs) in the coding sequence of donor and recipient genes that alter the HLA binding or TCR contact of HLA bound peptides [64–67, 70–74]. There are approximately 7 million SNPs with an allele frequency of >5% in the human genome, including approximately 50,000 SNPs that lead to amino acid changes in proteins [75]. Thus, it is likely only a small fraction of the minor H antigens involved in immune interactions after allogeneic HSCT in humans have so far been discovered.

8.3.2.1 HY Encoded Minor H Antigens

HSCT from a female donor into a male recipient is a special situation where minor H antigens may be derived from genes encoded by the Y chromosome that are polymorphic with their X-homologues. Such H-Y antigens were among the first minor H antigens to be identified in mouse and man, and exert a surprisingly strong effect in human HSCT [76–78]. Compared with HSCT between other donor/recipient gender combinations, HSCT from a female donor into a male recipient is associated with increased GvHD and a reduced risk of leukemic relapse even after controlling for GvHD [78]. In humans, there are at least 15 Y chromosome genes that could encode minor H antigens and epitopes recognized by T cells isolated from transplant recipients have already been identified in six of these genes including *RPS4Y1*, *USP9Y*, *DDX3Y*, *UTY*, *TMSB4Y*, and *SMCY* [67, 73, 74, 76, 79–81]. The molecular identification of individual epitopes has facilitated studies to examine the contribution of HY-specific T cells to GvL and GvHD. $CD8^+$ T cells specific for an HLA A2-restricted epitope derived from the ubiquitously expressed SMCY protein cause histologic changes of GvHD in a skin explant model, and expansion of these T cells in vivo correlated with the onset of GvHD [77, 82]. $CD8^+$ T cells specific for an epitope presented by HLA B8 and derived from UTY were isolated from a male recipient who did not develop GvHD after HSCT, and recognize male hematopoietic cells including LSC but not nonhematopoietic cells [63]. UTY transcripts are not entirely restricted to hematopoietic cells, but the absence of GvHD suggests the level of gene expression in nonhematopoietic tissues may be below the threshold necessary for T cell recognition of this antigen, or that the frequency of UTY-specific T cells in this patient remained below the threshold required to cause GvHD.

8.3.2.2 Autosomal Encoded Minor H Antigens

Autosomal genes that are selectively or preferentially expressed on hematopoietic cells and encode minor H antigens recognized by T cells have also been discovered and could participate in GvL reactions in all donor recipient gender combinations [64–66, 70, 71, 83]. There is persuasive evidence that several of these hematopoietic lineage-restricted minor H antigens can be effective targets for a GvL response. T cells specific for *SP110* eliminate LSC in NOD/SCID mice, and the expansion of *HA-1*, *HA-2*, and *P2X5*-specific T-cells has been observed in the blood of patients that achieved a complete remission after DLI [63, 71, 84].

Despite the attributes of minor H antigens, several issues have impeded efforts to target these antigens to enhance the GvL effect. It is essential the recipient express the correct HLA molecule and be disparate for minor H antigen expression with the donor, and the proportion of individuals that meet these criteria is relatively small for the minor H antigens that are defined currently [85]. The identification of additional hematopoietic lineage restricted minor H antigens and determining how best to enhance T cell responses to minor H antigens remain areas where additional investigation is necessary. Most minor H antigen discovery has focused on $CD8^+$ T cells but $CD4^+$ T cells are likely to play a key role either as direct effector cells in the GvL response, or to support the function and persistence of $CD8^+$ T cells, and efforts to define class II MHC-restricted minor H antigens are in progress.

8.3.3 T Cells Specific for Nonpolymorphic Leukemia Associated Antigens

Nonpolymorphic proteins that are highly expressed in leukemic cells have been shown to provide peptides that can be presented by class I and class II MHC molecules to $CD8^+$ and $CD4^+$ T cells. There is increasing evidence that some of these proteins can be immunogenic and that specific T cell responses can be elicited by vaccination and have antileukemic activity, providing a potential path for enhancing the GvL effect in HSCT recipients without GvHD.

8.3.4 BCR-ABL

A widely studied leukemic antigen is the BCR-ABL protein in CML. The fusion region encoded by the b3a2 or b2a2 translocation is unique in leukemia cells containing the Philadelphia chromosome t(9;22)(q34;q11), and expression of BCR-ABL is essential and sufficient for the development of CML. Peptides derived from the fusion region were shown to bind to HLA molecules, including HLA-A2, A3, A11, and B8, and to elicit T cells in-vitro that recognize peptide-pulsed target cells [86–90]. BCR-ABL-specific T cells were detected in the blood of CML patients and in some healthy donors by tetramer staining [91–94]. The presence of these tetramer positive cells was associated with a lower tumor burden, suggesting that BCR-ABL-specific T cells may participate in disease control. Immunity to b3a2 fusion peptides was elicited in 16 CML patients treated with imatinib or interferon-alpha after vaccination in incomplete Freund's adjuvant. Cytogenetic responses, including two patients with complete cytogenetic responses were observed in patients with demonstrable immunity [95]. The use of additional treatments confounded analysis of a correlation between the induced T-cell responses and the antitumor effect, but ongoing trials should answer this important question.

8.3.5 WT-1

The Wilms tumor gene (WT-1) encodes a zinc finger transcription factor involved in apoptosis, cell proliferation, and organ development [96]. WT-1 is overexpressed in many tumors including lymphoid and myeloid leukemias, and is linked to leukemogenesis [97]. A number of putative HLA-binding peptides have been documented within the WT-1 protein, some of which elicit a peptide specific CTL response [98]. T cells engineered to express a WT-1 specific TCR have antileukemic activity in vitro, and in NOD/SCID mice inoculated with human leukemia [99, 100]. Recent work has also suggested that the emergence of WT-1-specific T cells after HLA identical sibling HSCT for ALL correlates with a GvL effect [40]. It remains to be determined if the responses that are detected are responsible for the GvL effect or result from epitope spreading as a consequence of destruction of leukemic cells by other mechanisms.

Efforts to elicit WT-1 specific T cells by vaccination in non-transplant patients with advanced disease are providing increasing support for a direct role of WT-1-specific T cells. WT-1-specific T cells were elicited in AML and MDS patients following vaccination with an HLA A24-restricted WT-1 peptide, and antitumor effects were correlated with the induction of these CTL [101]. A CR was achieved in a single patient with relapsed AML who received multiple vaccinations with an HLA A2-restricted WT-1 peptide plus the T helper protein keyhole limpet hemocyanin (KLH) and GM-CSF [102]. More recently, the results of a phase II trial of 16 HLA-A2-positive patients with AML and one patient with MDS who received multiple vaccinations of WT-1 peptide with KLH and GM-CSF were reported. Twelve patients had elevated blast counts at study entry and five patients were in CR with a high relapse risk. In patients with elevated blast counts, six demonstrated evidence of anti-leukemia activity; one patient achieved CR for 12 months. Furthermore, tetramer and intracellular cytokine staining demonstrated WT-1-specific T cell responses in peripheral blood and bone marrow [103].

8.3.6 PR1

PR1 is an HLA-A201 restricted nonomer peptide (VLQELNVTV) that is derived from the differentiation stage-specific neutral serine proteases proteinase 3 (P3) and neutrophil elastase (NE), which share 54% amino acid sequence homology and are normally stored in primary azurophil granules of myeloid progenitor cells [39]. The pre-pro-forms of both proteins contain a leader peptide which traffics them to the endoplasmic reticulum (ER) for processing [104, 105]. P3 and NE are aberrantly expressed in myeloid leukemia (2- to 5-fold higher versus normal cells) and rheumatologic disorders such as Wegener's granulomatosis and small vessel vasculitis [106–109]. The leukemogenic and immunogenic properties of these proteins makes them ideal targets for the development of anti-leukemia immunotherapy. Indeed, there is now substantial evidence that T cell immunity to PR-1 has antileukemic activity. PR1-specific CTL that recognize and kill PR1 expressing HLA-A2 CML cells were detected in 11 of 12 CML patients that responded to IFN-α2b therapy but were absent in all seven non-responders [39, 110]. Similarly, PR1 specific CTL were detected in six of eight patients with CML that responded to allogeneic HSCT, but were absent in allogeneic HSCT patients who failed to respond.

Direct evidence for a role for PR-1 specific T cell immunity also comes from vaccine trials. A Phase I/II vaccine study in patients with refractory or relapsed myeloid leukemia combined PR1 peptide and GM-CSF in 15 CML and AML patients with progressive disease. PR1-specific CTL, measured using PR1/HLA-A2 tetramers, were detected in eight patients, five of whom obtained a clinical response [111]. In a follow-up to this initial trial, a total of 66 patients (AML, CML, and MDS) were treated with the PR1 peptide vaccine and immune responses were noted in 58%, which correlated with clinical responses including complete molecular remissions of t(15;17) AML, inv(16) AML, and t(9;22) CML assessed by RT-PCR that persisted for up to 7 years [112]. The effectiveness of peptide vaccination for inducing T-cell immunity and clinical responses has been confirmed in a separate trial in which combined vaccination with WT-1 and PR1 resulted in immune responses in eight of eight patients with myeloid malignancies and a reduction of WT-1 RNA in some patients as a marker of minimal residual disease [113].

8.3.7 RHAMM/CD168

The receptor for hyaluronic acid (HA) mediated motility (RHAMM/CD168) has also been used as a target for vaccine therapy for AML. RHAMM is a glycophosphatidylinositol (GPI)-anchored receptor that is involved in cell motility [114]. In addition, it is oncogenic when overexpressed, is critical for *ras*-mediated transformation [115], and has been reported in blasts of more than 80% of patients with AML, MDS, and multiple myeloma (MM) [116]. In a phase I/II vaccine study, clinical and immunological responses were noted following administration of RHAMM R3 peptide emulsified with incomplete Freund's adjuvant and GM-CSF to patients with AML, MDS, and MM over-expressing RHAMM/CD168 [116].

8.4 Strategies for Augmenting GvL Responses Without GvHD

Progress in discovering polymorphic minor H antigens that are restricted to hematopoietic lineage cells and nonpolymorphic LAA are providing new opportunities to enhance the GvL effect after HSCT to reduce relapse. However, allogeneic HSCT using peripheral blood stem cells (PBSC) that contain

T cells represents a challenging setting in which to execute specific immunotherapy due to the confounding effects of immunosuppressive drugs that must be administered to prevent or treat GvHD. Dissociating the GvL effect from GvHD will only be accomplished if HSCT regimens are first developed that reduce GvHD. Complete T cell depletion of the graft eliminates GvHD and the need for immunosuppression [11, 117, 118], and would provide a superior platform for adoptive T cell immunotherapy compared with unmodified PBSC grafts. The initial problems of graft rejection and relapse with TCD have been overcome by modifying the conditioning regimen [118], but poor reconstitution of T cell immunity to pathogens and opportunistic infections are likely to remain critical issues for patients that receive T cell depleted grafts [119].

8.4.1 Depletion of Alloreactive T Cells from Hematopoietic Stem Cell Grafts

A conceptually attractive approach to reduce GvHD without compromising immune reconstitution is the selective removal of alloreactive T cells. This would provide an environment in which T cells specific for LAA or hematopoietic restricted minor H antigens could then be introduced or elicited to promote a selective GvL effect.

8.4.1.1 Immunotoxins and Monoclonal Antibodies

One approach to specifically remove alloreactive donor T cells involves coculturing donor T cells with irradiated recipient mononuclear cells in vitro to induce activation markers such as CD25, CD69, and CD137 that can be used for depletion of the alloreactive subset using immunomagnetic beads or an immunotoxin [120–122]. This approach may be best suited to HLA mismatched HSCT where the frequency of alloreactive T cells in highest. The elimination of $CD25^+$ cells with an immunotoxin has been used in a clinical trial of HLA mismatched HSCT in children. GvHD was lower than expected in this study and there was evidence of T cell immune reconstitution to viruses [120]. The majority of patients in this trial with a malignancy relapsed, illustrating the need to incorporate tumor-reactive T cells to augment the GvL effect.

8.4.1.2 Depletion of Naïve T cells

The identification of functional subsets of T lineage cells including regulatory cells (T_{REG}), antigen inexperienced naïve T cells (T_N), and antigen experienced memory T cells, which can be divided into central memory (T_{CM}) and effector memory (T_{EM}) subsets, has provided opportunities for manipulation of allogeneic grafts that might reduce GvHD after HLA matched HSCT. Depletion of donor T_N cells abrogated GvHD in a MHC-matched, minor H antigen-mismatched mouse model and allowed the efficient transfer of T cell memory to a model antigen [123]. This result was confirmed in additional murine minor H antigen-mismatched models of GvHD, and in rats [124–126]. Although the intent was to deplete T_N, the depletion procedure targeted CD62L and also eliminated the T_{CM} subset of T_M. The potential for T_{CM} from unprimed donors to induce GvHD in these models remains to be clearly established, but the available data suggests that T_N cause significantly greater GvHD than T_{CM} [127].

Human T_N and T_M can also be distinguished based on phenotype [128–130], and inferential data suggests the frequency of minor H antigen specific T cells in donors who have not been primed to these antigens by pregnancy or blood transfusion is different between these subsets. Sequencing of TCR genes from purified human T_N and T_M to estimate the diversity of $\alpha\beta$ TCRs showed the T_N repertoire contains $>2.5 \times 10^7$ different TCR combinations or >99% of overall TCR diversity, while the T_M subset contains only 1×10^5 to 2×10^5 TCR combinations and <1% of diversity [131]. A major component of the $CD4^+$ and $CD8^+$ T_M repertoire is specific for persistent viruses such as CMV, EBV, HSV, and VZV [132–136]. There are reports that virus-specific T-cells cross react with allogeneic HLA molecules, but cross reactivity with minor H antigens has not been reported [137, 138]. Allogeneic HSCT grafts engineered to lack T_N but containing virus-specific T_M will soon be evaluated for their ability to engraft and provide immune reconstitution to pathogens in HLA matched transplant recipients. This approach may reduce GvHD and provide a setting in which targeted therapy with T cells specific for LAA or minor H antigens can be applied in the absence of GvHD or immunosuppression.

8.4.2 Vaccination to Augment a GvL Effect

The discovery of antigens on leukemic cells has provided a foundation for immunotherapy trials using component antigens for vaccination to elicit leukemia-reactive T cells. Efforts to exploit vaccination with LAA such as PR-1 and WT-1 to treat leukemia are well underway. The results of phase I and II trials have shown little toxicity and promising antitumor activity with these vaccines. Because most patients with AML relapse despite achieving CR, efforts to employ vaccination for AML have been extended to patients in CR and if effective, might reduce the need for allogeneic HSCT. For those patients that undergo allogeneic HSCT, these antigens may be ideal targets for inducing a GvL effect without GvHD.

Barriers to successful vaccination remain, particularly if they are to be employed after allogeneic HSCT. It is unclear whether component vaccines, dendritic cell-based vaccines, or alternative strategies might be most effective, and analysis of the quality and function of T cell responses that are elicited have been limited. Dose, scheduling, and adjuvants have not yet been rigorously addressed, and strategies such as vaccinating before and after lymphodepletion chemotherapy might improve results [139]. From the perspective of allogeneic HSCT, it is unclear whether the current vaccines would be immunogenic if given early after transplant when immunosuppressive drugs must be administered to prevent GvHD. The consequences of removing alloreactive T cells to reduce GvHD and the need for immunosuppression may also compromise the T cell repertoire and the ability to respond to vaccination. Eventually, vaccination of healthy donors with LAA or minor H antigens could be used to boost T-cell immunity in the donor prior to allogeneic HSCT. Toxicity would not be expected from minor H antigens since these are foreign and priming to minor H antigens as a consequence of pregnancy or blood transfusion has not been associated with toxicity. PR-1 and other leukemia-specific antigens are self-proteins, but no autoimmunity has been reported so far after PR1 or WT1 vaccination.

8.4.3 Adoptive T Cell Therapy Targeting Leukemia Associated Antigens

The adoptive transfer of donor virus-specific T cells is effective for preventing CMV and EBV disease after allogeneic HSCT without causing GvHD [140–142]. Thus, a direct approach for enhancing the GvL effect would be to adoptively transfer donor T cells that are specific for LAA or minor H antigens expressed by leukemic cells. The clinical application of T cell therapy targeting minor H antigens has been impeded by the lack of a sufficient number of antigens that are selectively expressed on hematopoietic lineage cells. This is less of an issue for non-polymorphic LAA such as proteinase-3 and WT-1, although the identification of epitopes presented by additional HLA alleles will be important to broaden the potential utility of these antigens. An area of progress has been the development of methods to selectively isolate antigen-specific T cells for therapy. Stimulation of T cells with autologous or artificial APC pulsed with antigenic peptides or transfected with genes that encode the target antigen has been used to enrich polyclonal T cells for a desired specificity. Peptide-MHC tetramers, bispecific antibodies, and antibodies that bind to T cell molecules that are upregulated after antigen stimulation have been used to select T cells of a defined specificity [143–145]. Culture techniques for expanding these cells have been developed and pilot clinical trials of T cell therapy to promote GvL effects have been initiated at several centers.

Even if T cells that recognize leukemia can be reliably isolated and expanded, sustained antitumor efficacy will depend on the ability of the transferred T cells to persist in vivo long enough to eradicate all of the malignant cells. Unfortunately, the persistence of cultured effector T cells (T_E) in trials of adoptive therapy for human cancer is often short [146]. T cell persistence can be improved by depletion of host lymphocytes before cell transfer to eliminate regulatory cells and competition for cytokines, and by the administration of IL-2 after cell transfer [147, 148], but these interventions have not resulted in persistence of transferred T cells in all patients, and lack of persistence has predicted lack of efficacy. A recent study in nonhuman primates found that antigen-specific $CD8^+$ T_E derived from the T_{EM} subset of memory T cells survived in the blood for only a short duration after adoptive transfer and failed to home to lymph nodes. By contrast, T_E derived from T_{CM} persisted long-term after adoptive transfer, migrated to memory T cell niches, and reacquired phenotypic properties of T_M [149]. These results suggest that intrinsic qualities of the T cells that enable their persistence in vivo must be considered when selecting cells for immunotherapy. The potential for T_E derived from T_N cells to persist in vivo has not been determined in humans, but studies in murine models suggest that T_N differentiated toward a memory phenotype by culture in IL-15 or IL-21 are more effective in tumor therapy than T cells cultured in IL-2 [150, 151].

8.4.4 Adoptive T Cell Therapy Using Gene-Modified T Cells

For leukemias that express TAA or minor H antigens that are shared among many patients, the requirement to isolate T cells from each donor could be overcome if T cells were engineered to have the desired antigen specificity. This can be accomplished by transferring the TCR α and β genes that confer antigen recognition into donor T lymphocytes. TCR gene transfer has been successful for engineering T cells to be specific for melanoma, viruses, minor H antigens, and oncoproteins [152, 153], although sustained expression of the transferred TCR chains is not always achieved with currently available vectors. The introduced TCRs can also cross-pair with the endogenous TCR chains resulting in formation of hybrid receptors with a potentially deleterious specificity. This problem may be resolved using murine rather than human constant regions in the introduced TCR chains, or by incorporating cysteine residues in the human constant regions of both the α and β chains to allow disulphide bonds to form and preferentially pair the introduced TCRs [154, 155].

T cells can also be genetically modified to confer tumor recognition through the introduction of a chimeric antigen receptor (CAR) specific for a tumor cell surface molecule, which overcomes the requirement for MHC restriction. Typically, CARs contain an extracellular domain comprised of a single chain antibody (scFv) that incorporates the heavy and light variable chains of a monoclonal antibody specific for a tumor cell molecule fused to an intracellular signaling domain such as the ζ chain of the TCR to trigger T cell activation [156, 157]. This strategy seems ideal for targeting B cell malignancies since CD20 has been validated as a target in follicular, diffuse large cell, and mantle cell lymphoma, and monoclonal antibodies specific for CD19 could be used to engineer T cells to target B-cell ALL. Preclinical studies in murine models have demonstrated that T cells modified to express CARs can efficiently eliminate tumors in vivo and phase I clinical trials of adoptively transferred CAR-modified T cells are in progress in patients with lymphoma and leukemia.

The use of genes encoding CARs to target T cells to tumors resolves the need to isolate or engineer MHC-restricted T cells and may be useful to enhance the GvL effect after allogeneic HSCT, particularly for ALL, which is especially resistant to the GvL effect that develops naturally after HSCT. One strategy would be to introduce the CARs into donor T cells of a known antigen-specificity such as EBV or CMV, to avoid a risk of GvHD and take advantage of additional signaling that could be provided through the endogenous TCR [158]. T cell activation normally involves signaling through both TCR and costimulatory molecules, and CARs that only encode the CD3-ζ signaling domain would fail to provide a costimulatory signal. CARs that encode domains to provide costimulatory signals have been developed and have superior antitumor activity in animal models [158]. CAR antibody domains may need to be humanized to reduce immunogenicity, since many CARs are derived from murine antibodies. Finally, several of the molecules that are being targeted by CARs including CD19 and CD20 are expressed by normal cells in addition to tumor cells, and the adoptive transfer of CAR-modified T cells may cause a prolonged B-cell deficiency. This might eventually be overcome using inducible suicide genes.

8.5 Conclusion

The existence of the GvL effect is one of the most compelling demonstrations that the human immune system is capable of eradicating malignancy and has already fostered new approaches to allogeneic HSCT that exploit the GvL effect rather than cytotoxic chemoradiotherapy to promote antitumor effects. These efforts have substantiated the importance of the GvL effect for curing patients after allogeneic HSCT but have not enabled the separation of the GvL effect from GvHD or completely solved the problem of recurrent disease. The identification of antigens expressed on leukemic cells but not tissues involved in GvHD, combined with advances in vaccination, genetic modification of T cells, and adoptive T cell transfer have set the stage for the development of targeted therapy to promote a selective GvL effect. These efforts are not only relevant for improving the outcome of patients undergoing allogeneic HSCT, but should provide insights for therapy of leukemia in the non-transplant setting.

References

1. Barnes DW, Corp MJ, Loutit JF, Neal FE. Treatment of murine leukemia with X-rays and homologous bone marrow. Br Med J. 1956;2:626–27.
2. Thomas E, Storb R, Clift RA, et al. Bone-marrow transplantation (first of two parts). N Engl J Med. 1975;292:832–43.

3. Thomas ED, Storb R, Clift RA, et al. Bone-marrow transplantation (second of two parts). N Engl J Med. 1975;292:895–902.
4. Weiden PL, Flournoy N, Thomas ED, et al. Antileukemic effect of graft-versus-host disease in human recipients of allogeneic-marrow grafts. N Engl J Med. 1979;300:1068–73.
5. Weiden PL, Sullivan KM, Flournoy N, et al. Antileukemic effect of chronic graft-versus-host disease: contribution to improved survival after allogeneic marrow transplantation. N Engl J Med. 1981;304:1529–33.
6. Butterini A, Bortin MM, Gale RP. Graft-versus-leukemia following bone marrow transplantation. Bone Marrow Transplantation. 1987;2:233–42.
7. Fefer A, Sullivan KM, Weiden P, et al. Graft versus leukemia effect in man: the relapse rate of acute leukemia is lower after allogeneic than after syngeneic marrow transplantation. Prog Clin Biol Res. 1987;244:401–8.
8. Gale RP, Horowitz MM. Graft-versus-leukemia in bone marrow transplantation. The Advisory Committee of the International Bone Marrow Transplant Registry. Bone Marrow Transplant. 1990;6 Suppl 1:94–7.
9. Horowitz MM, Gale RP, Sondel PM, et al. Graft-versus-leukemia reactions after bone marrow transplantation. Blood 1990;75:555–62.
10. Korngold R, Leighton C, Manser T. Graft-versus-myeloid leukemia responses following syngeneic and allogeneic bone marrow transplantation. Transplantation 1994;58(3): 278–87.
11. Marmont AM, Horowitz MM, Gale RP, et al. T-cell depletion of HLA-identical transplants in leukemia. Blood 1991;78(8):2120–30.
12. Sullivan KM, Storb R, Buckner CD, et al. Graft-versus-host disease as adoptive immunotherapy in patients with advanced hematologic neoplasms. N Engl J Med. 1989;320(13):828–34.
13. Kolb HJ, Mittermuller J, Clemm C, et al. Donor leukocyte transfusions for treatment of recurrent chronic myelogenous leukemia in marrow transplant patients. Blood 1990;76(12):2462–5.
14. Johnson BD, Drobyski WR, Truitt RL. Delayed infusion of normal donor cells after MHC-matched bone marrow transplantation provides an antileukemia reaction without graft-versus-host disease. Bone Marrow Transplant. 1993;11(4):329–36.
15. Kolb HJ, Gunther W, Schumm M, Holler E, Wilmanns W, Thierfelder S. Adoptive immunotherapy in canine chimeras. Transplantation 1997;63(3):430–6.
16. Collins RH Jr, Goldstein S, Giralt S, et al. Donor leukocyte infusions in acute lymphocytic leukemia. Bone Marrow Transplant. 2000;26:511–6.
17. Collins RH Jr, Shpilberg O, Drobyski WR, et al. Donor leukocyte infusions in 140 patients with relapsed malignancy after allogeneic bone marrow transplantation. J Clin Oncol. 1997;15:433–44.
18. Kolb HJ, Schattenberg A, Goldman JM, et al. Graft-versus-leukemia effect of donor lymphocyte transfusions in marrow grafted patients. Blood 1995;86:2041–50.
19. Peggs KS, Mackinnon S. Cellular therapy: donor lymphocyte infusion. Curr Opin Hematol. 2001;8:349–54.
20. Porter DL, Collins RH Jr, Shpilberg O, et al. Long-term follow-up of patients who achieved complete remission after donor leukocyte infusions. Biol Blood Marrow Transplant. 1999;5:253–61.
21. Lokhorst HM, Schattenberg A, Cornelissen JJ, et al. Donor lymphocyte infusions for relapsed multiple myeloma after allogeneic stem-cell transplantation: predictive factors for response and long-term outcome. J Clin Oncol. 2000;18:3031–7.
22. Levine JE, Braun T, Penza SL, et al. Prospective trial of chemotherapy and donor leukocyte infusions for relapse of advanced myeloid malignancies after allogeneic stem-cell transplantation. J Clin Oncol. 2002;20:405–12.
23. Keil F, Haas OA, Fritsch G, et al. Donor leukocyte infusion for leukemic relapse after allogeneic marrow transplantation: lack of residual donor hematopoiesis predicts aplasia. Blood 1997;89:3113–7.

24. Flowers ME, Leisenring W, Beach K, et al. Granulocyte colony-stimulating factor given to donors before apheresis does not prevent aplasia in patients treated with donor leukocyte infusion for recurrent chronic myeloid leukemia after bone marrow transplantation. Biol Blood Marrow Transplant. 2000;6:321–6.
25. Mackinnon S, Papadopoulos EB, Carabasi MH, et al. Adoptive immunotherapy evaluating escalating doses of donor leukocytes for relapse of chronic myeloid leukemia after bone marrow transplantation: separation of graft-versus-leukemia responses from graft-versus-host disease. Blood 1995;86:1261–8.
26. Bonini C, Ferrari G, Verzeletti S, et al. HSV-TK gene transfer into donor lymphocytes for control of allogeneic graft-versus-leukemia. Science 1997;276:1719–24.
27. Bonini C, Bondanza A, Perna SK, et al. The suicide gene therapy challenge: how to improve a successful gene therapy approach. Mol Ther. 2007;15:1248–52.
28. Berger C, Flowers ME, Warren EH, Riddell SR. Analysis of transgene-specific immune responses that limit the in vivo persistence of adoptively transferred HSV-TK-modified donor T cells after allogeneic hematopoietic cell transplantation. Blood 2006;107: 2294–302.
29. Riddell SR, Elliott M, Lewinsohn DA, et al. T-cell mediated rejection of gene-modified HIV-specific cytotoxic T lymphocytes in HIV-infected patients. Nat Med. 1996;2:216–23.
30. Berger C, Blau CA, Huang ML, et al. Pharmacologically regulated Fas-mediated death of adoptively transferred T cells in a nonhuman primate model. Blood 2004;103:1261–9.
31. Straathof KC, Pule MA, Yotnda P, et al. An inducible caspase 9 safety switch for T-cell therapy. Blood 2005;105:4247–54.
32. Tey SK, Dotti G, Rooney CM, Heslop HE, Brenner MK. Inducible caspase 9 suicide gene to improve the safety of allodepleted T cells after haploidentical stem cell transplantation. Biol Blood Marrow Transplant. 2007;13:913–24.
33. Hsu KC, Gooley T, Malkki M, et al. KIR ligands and prediction of relapse after unrelated donor hematopoietic cell transplantation for hematologic malignancy. Biol Blood Marrow Transplant. 2006;12:828–36.
34. Hsu KC, Keever-Taylor CA, Wilton A, et al. Improved outcome in HLA-identical sibling hematopoietic stem-cell transplantation for acute myelogenous leukemia predicted by KIR and HLA genotypes. Blood 2005;105:4878–84.
35. Miller JS, Cooley S, Parham P, et al. Missing KIR ligands are associated with less relapse and increased graft-versus-host disease (GVHD) following unrelated donor allogeneic HCT. Blood 2007;109:5058–61.
36. Ruggeri L, Capanni M, Urbani E, et al. Effectiveness of donor natural killer cell alloreactivity in mismatched hematopoietic transplants. Science 2002;295:2097–100.
37. Bleakley M, Riddell SR. Molecules and mechanisms of the graft-versus-leukaemia effect. Nat Rev Cancer. 2004;4:371–80.
38. Falkenburg JH, van de Corput L, Marijt EW, Willemze R. Minor histocompatibility antigens in human stem cell transplantation. Exp Hematol. 2003;31:743–51.
39. Molldrem JJ, Lee PP, Wang C, et al. Evidence that specific T lymphocytes may participate in the elimination of chronic myelogenous leukemia. Nat Med. 2000;6:1018–23.
40. Rezvani K, Yong AS, Savani BN, et al. Graft-versus-leukemia effects associated with detectable Wilms tumor-1 specific T lymphocytes after allogeneic stem-cell transplantation for acute lymphoblastic leukemia. Blood 2007;110:1924–32.
41. Timonen T, Ortaldo JR, Herberman RB. Characteristics of human large granular lymphocytes and relationship to natural killer and K cells. J Exp Med. 1981;153:569–82.
42. Miller JS. The biology of natural killer cells in cancer, infection, and pregnancy. Exp Hematol. 2001;29:1157–68.
43. Robertson MJ, Ritz J. Biology and clinical relevance of human natural killer cells. Blood 1990;76:2421–38.
44. Herberman RB, Ortaldo JR. Natural killer cells: their roles in defenses against disease. Science 1981;214:24–30.

45. Uhrberg M, Valiante NM, Shum BP, et al. Human diversity in killer cell inhibitory receptor genes. Immunity 1997;7:753–63.
46. Lazetic S, Chang C, Houchins JP, Lanier LL, Phillips JH. Human natural killer cell receptors involved in MHC class I recognition are disulfide-linked heterodimers of CD94 and NKG2 subunits. J Immunol. 1996;157:4741–5.
47. Braud VM, Allan DS, O'Callaghan CA, et al. HLA-E binds to natural killer cell receptors CD94/NKG2A, B and C. Nature 1998;391:795–9.
48. Borrego F, Masilamani M, Marusina AI, Tang X, Coligan JE. The CD94/NKG2 family of receptors: from molecules and cells to clinical relevance. Immunol Res. 2006;35:263–78.
49. Kirwan SE, Burshtyn DN. Regulation of natural killer cell activity. Curr Opin Immunol. 2007;19:46–54.
50. Miller JS, Soignier Y, Panoskaltsis-Mortari A, et al. Successful adoptive transfer and in vivo expansion of human haploidentical NK cells in patients with cancer. Blood 2005;105:3051–7.
51. Miller JS, Tessmer-Tuck J, Pierson BA, et al. Low dose subcutaneous interleukin-2 after autologous transplantation generates sustained in vivo natural killer cell activity. Biol Blood Marrow Transplant. 1997;3:34–44.
52. Savani BN, Mielke S, Adams S, et al. Rapid natural killer cell recovery determines outcome after T-cell-depleted HLA-identical stem cell transplantation in patients with myeloid leukemias but not with acute lymphoblastic leukemia. Leukemia 2007;21: 2145–52.
53. Exley M, Garcia J, Wilson SB, et al. CD1d structure and regulation on human thymocytes, peripheral blood T cells, B cells and monocytes. Immunology 2000;100:37–47.
54. Pulendran B, Lingappa J, Kennedy MK, et al. Developmental pathways of dendritic cells in vivo: distinct function, phenotype, and localization of dendritic cell subsets in FLT3 ligand-treated mice. J Immunol. 1997;159:2222–31.
55. Spada FM, Borriello F, Sugita M, Watts GF, Koezuka Y, Porcelli SA. Low expression level but potent antigen presenting function of CD1d on monocyte lineage cells. Eur J Immunol. 2000;30:3468–77.
56. Fais F, Tenca C, Cimino G, et al. CD1d expression on B-precursor acute lymphoblastic leukemia subsets with poor prognosis. Leukemia 2005;19:551–6.
57. Metelitsa LS, Weinberg KI, Emanuel PD, Seeger RC. Expression of CD1d by myelomonocytic leukemias provides a target for cytotoxic NKT cells. Leukemia 2003;17:1068–77.
58. Hayakawa Y, Godfrey DI, Smyth MJ. Alpha-galactosylceramide: potential immunomodulatory activity and future application. Curr Med Chem. 2004;11:241–52.
59. Giaccone G, Punt CJ, Ando Y, et al. A phase I study of the natural killer T-cell ligand alpha-galactosylceramide (KRN7000) in patients with solid tumors. Clin Cancer Res. 2002;8:3702–9.
60. Toura I, Kawano T, Akutsu Y, Nakayama T, Ochiai T, Taniguchi M. Cutting edge: inhibition of experimental tumor metastasis by dendritic cells pulsed with alpha-galactosylceramide. J Immunol. 1999;163:2387–91.
61. Shimizu K, Hidaka M, Kadowaki N, et al. Evaluation of the function of human invariant NKT cells from cancer patients using alpha-galactosylceramide-loaded murine dendritic cells. J Immunol. 2006;177:3484–92.
62. Fontaine P, Roy-Proulx G, Knafo L, Baron C, Roy DC, Perreault C. Adoptive transfer of minor histocompatibility antigen-specific T lymphocytes eradicates leukemia cells without causing graft-versus-host disease. Nat Med. 2001;7:789–94.
63. Bonnet D, Warren EH, Greenberg PD, Dick JE, Riddell SR. CD8(+) minor histocompatibility antigen-specific cytotoxic T lymphocyte clones eliminate human acute myeloid leukemia stem cells. Proc Natl Acad Sci USA. 1999;96:8639–44.
64. Akatsuka Y, Nishida T, Kondo E, et al. Identification of a polymorphic gene, BCL2A1, encoding two novel hematopoietic lineage-specific minor histocompatibility antigens. J Exp Med. 2003;197:1489–500.

65. den Haan JM, Meadows LM, Wang W, et al. The minor histocompatibility antigen HA-1: a diallelic gene with a single amino acid polymorphism. Science 1998;279:1054–7.
66. Dolstra H, Fredrix H, Maas F, et al. A human minor histocompatibility antigen specific for B cell acute lymphoblastic leukemia. J Exp Med. 1999;189:301–8.
67. Meadows L, Wang W, den Haan JM, et al. The HLA-A*0201-restricted H-Y antigen contains a posttranslationally modified cysteine that significantly affects T cell recognition. Immunity 1997;6:273–81.
68. Murata M, Warren EH, Riddell SR. A human minor histocompatibility antigen resulting from differential expression due to a gene deletion. J Exp Med. 2003; 197:1279–89.
69. Kawase T, Nannya Y, Torikai H, et al. Identification of human minor histocompatibility antigens based on genetic association with highly parallel genotyping of pooled DNA. Blood 2008;111:3286–94.
70. Brickner AG, Evans AM, Mito JK, et al. The PANE1 gene encodes a novel human minor histocompatibility antigen that is selectively expressed in B-lymphoid cells and B-CLL. Blood 2006;107:3779–86.
71. de Rijke B, van Horssen-Zoetbrood A, Beekman JM, et al. A frameshift polymorphism in P2X5 elicits an allogeneic cytotoxic T lymphocyte response associated with remission of chronic myeloid leukemia. J Clin Invest. 2005;115:3506–16.
72. Pierce RA, Field ED, Mutis T, et al. The HA-2 minor histocompatibility antigen is derived from a diallelic gene encoding a novel human class I myosin protein. J Immunol. 2001;167:3223–30.
73. Torikai H, Akatsuka Y, Miyazaki M, et al. A novel HLA-A*3303-restricted minor histocompatibility antigen encoded by an unconventional open reading frame of human TMSB4Y gene. J Immunol. 2004;173:7046–54.
74. Warren EH, Gavin MA, Simpson E, et al. The human UTY gene encodes a novel HLA-B8-restricted H-Y antigen. J Immunol. 2000;164:2807–14.
75. Carlson CS, Eberle MA, Rieder MJ, Smith JD, Kruglyak L, Nickerson DA. Additional SNPs and linkage-disequilibrium analyses are necessary for whole-genome association studies in humans. Nat Genet. 2003;33:518–21.
76. Wang W, Meadows LR, den Haan JM, et al. Human H-Y: a male-specific histocompatibility antigen derived from the SMCY protein. Science 1995;269:1588–90.
77. Mutis T, Gillespie G, Schrama E, Falkenburg JH, Moss P, Goulmy E. Tetrameric HLA class I-minor histocompatibility antigen peptide complexes demonstrate minor histocompatibility antigen-specific cytotoxic T lymphocytes in patients with graft-versus-host disease. Nat Med. 1999;5:839–42.
78. Randolph SS, Gooley TA, Warren EH, Appelbaum FR, Riddell SR. Female donors contribute to a selective graft-versus-leukemia effect in male recipients of HLA-matched, related hematopoietic stem cell transplants. Blood 2004;103:347–52.
79. Ivanov R, Aarts T, Hol S, et al. Identification of a 40S ribosomal protein S4-derived H-Y epitope able to elicit a lymphoblast-specific cytotoxic T lymphocyte response. Clin Cancer Res. 2005;11:1694–703.
80. Pierce RA, Field ED, den Haan JM, et al. Cutting edge: the HLA-A*0101-restricted HY minor histocompatibility antigen originates from DFFRY and contains a cysteinylated cysteine residue as identified by a novel mass spectrometric technique. J Immunol. 1999;163:6360–4.
81. Rosinski KV, Fujii N, Mito JK, et al. DDX3Y encodes a class I MHC-restricted H-Y antigen that is expressed in leukemic stem cells. Blood 2008;111:4817–26.
82. Dickinson AM, Wang XN, Sviland L, et al. In situ dissection of the graft-versus-host activities of cytotoxic T cells specific for minor histocompatibility antigens. Nat Med. 2002;8:410–4.
83. Warren EH, Vigneron NJ, Gavin MA, et al. An antigen produced by splicing of non-contiguous peptides in the reverse order. Science 2006;313:1444–7.

84. Marijt WA, Heemskerk MH, Kloosterboer FM, et al. Hematopoiesis-restricted minor histocompatibility antigens HA-1- or HA-2-specific T cells can induce complete remissions of relapsed leukemia. Proc Natl Acad Sci USA. 2003;100:2742–7.
85. Spierings E, Hendriks M, Absi L, et al. Phenotype frequencies of autosomal minor histocompatibility antigens display significant differences among populations. PLoS Genet. 2007;3:e103.
86. Bocchia M, Wentworth PA, Southwood S, et al. Specific binding of leukemia oncogene fusion protein peptides to HLA class I molecules. Blood 1995;85:2680–4.
87. Bocchia M, Korontsvit T, Xu Q, et al. Specific human cellular immunity to bcr-abl oncogene-derived peptides. Blood 1996;87:3587–92.
88. Buzyn A, Ostankovitch M, Zerbib A, et al. Peptides derived from the whole sequence of BCR-ABL bind to several class I molecules allowing specific induction of human cytotoxic T lymphocytes. Eur J Immunol. 1997;27:2066–72.
89. Yotnda P, Firat H, Garcia-Pons F, et al. Cytotoxic T cell response against the chimeric p210 BCR-ABL protein in patients with chronic myelogenous leukemia. J Clin Invest. 1998;101:2290–6.
90. Osman Y, Takahashi M, Zheng Z, et al. Generation of bcr-abl specific cytotoxic T-lymphocytes by using dendritic cells pulsed with bcr-abl (b3a2) peptide: its applicability for donor leukocyte transfusions in marrow grafted CML patients. Leukemia 1999;13:166–74.
91. Clark RE, Dodi IA, Hill SC, et al. Direct evidence that leukemic cells present HLA-associated immunogenic peptides derived from the BCR-ABL b3a2 fusion protein. Blood 2001;98:2887–93.
92. Butt NM, Wang L, Abu-Eisha HM, Christmas SE, Clark RE. BCR-ABL-specific T cells can be detected in healthy donors and in chronic myeloid leukemia patients following allogeneic stem cell transplantation. Blood 2004;103:3245.
93. Westermann J, Schlimper C, Richter G, Mohm J, Dorken B, Pezzutto A. T cell recognition of bcr/abl in healthy donors and in patients with chronic myeloid leukaemia. Br J Haematol. 2004;125:213–6.
94. Butt NM, Rojas JM, Wang L, Christmas SE, Abu-Eisha HM, Clark RE. Circulating bcr-abl-specific CD8+ T cells in chronic myeloid leukemia patients and healthy subjects. Haematologica 2005;90:1315–23.
95. Bocchia M, Gentili S, Abruzzese E, et al. Effect of a p210 multipeptide vaccine associated with imatinib or interferon in patients with chronic myeloid leukaemia and persistent residual disease: a multicentre observational trial. Lancet 2005;365:657–62.
96. Hewitt SM, Hamada S, McDonnell TJ, Rauscher FJ 3rd, Saunders GF. Regulation of the proto-oncogenes bcl-2 and c-myc by the Wilms' tumor suppressor gene WT1. Cancer Res. 1995;55:5386–9.
97. Tsuboi A, Oka Y, Ogawa H, et al. Constitutive expression of the Wilms' tumor gene WT1 inhibits the differentiation of myeloid progenitor cells but promotes their proliferation in response to granulocyte-colony stimulating factor (G-CSF). Leuk Res. 1999;23:499–505.
98. Bellantuono I, Gao L, Parry S, et al. Two distinct HLA-A0201-presented epitopes of the Wilms tumor antigen 1 can function as targets for leukemia-reactive CTL. Blood 2002;100:3835–7.
99. Xue SA, Gao L, Hart D, et al. Elimination of human leukemia cells in NOD/SCID mice by WT1-TCR gene-transduced human T cells. Blood 2005;106:3062–7.
100. Tsuji T, Yasukawa M, Matsuzaki J, et al. Generation of tumor-specific, HLA class I-restricted human Th1 and Tc1 cells by cell engineering with tumor peptide-specific T-cell receptor genes. Blood 2005;106:470–6.
101. Oka Y, Tsuboi A, Taguchi T, et al. Induction of WT1 (Wilms' tumor gene)-specific cytotoxic T lymphocytes by WT1 peptide vaccine and the resultant cancer regression. Proc Natl Acad Sci USA. 2004;101:13885–90.

102. Mailander V, Scheibenbogen C, Thiel E, Letsch A, Blau IW, Keilholz U. Complete remission in a patient with recurrent acute myeloid leukemia induced by vaccination with WT1 peptide in the absence of hematological or renal toxicity. Leukemia 2004;18:165–6.
103. Keilholz U, Letsch A, Asemissen A, et al. Clinical and immune responses of WT-1 peptide vaccination in patients with acute myeloid leukemia. American Society of Clinical Oncology Annual Meeting Proceedings. J Clin Oncol. 2006;24:2511a.
104. Rao NV, Rao GV, Marshall BC, Hoidal JR. Biosynthesis and processing of proteinase 3 in U937 cells. Processing pathways are distinct from those of cathepsin G. J Biol Chem. 1996;271:2972–8.
105. Lindmark A, Gullberg U, Olsson I. Processing and intracellular transport of cathepsin G and neutrophil elastase in the leukemic myeloid cell line U-937-modulation by brefeldin A, ammonium chloride, and monensin. J Leukoc Biol. 1994;55:50–7.
106. Franssen CF, Stegeman CA, Kallenberg CG, et al. Antiproteinase 3- and antimyeloperoxidase-associated vasculitis. Kidney Int. 2000;57:2195–206.
107. Borregaard N, Cowland JB. Granules of the human neutrophilic polymorphonuclear leukocyte. Blood 1997;89:3503–21.
108. Brouwer E, Stegeman CA, Huitema MG, Limburg PC, Kallenberg CG. T cell reactivity to proteinase 3 and myeloperoxidase in patients with Wegener's granulomatosis (WG). Clin Exp Immunol. 1994;98:448–53.
109. Dengler R, Munstermann U, al-Batran S, et al. Immunocytochemical and flow cytometric detection of proteinase 3 (myeloblastin) in normal and leukaemic myeloid cells. Br J Haematol. 1995;89:250–7.
110. Molldrem JJ Lee PP, Wang C, Champlin RE, Davis MM. A PR1-human leukocyte antigen-A2 tetramer can be used to isolate low-frequency cytotoxic T lymphocytes from healthy donors that selectively lyse chronic myelogenous leukemia. Cancer Res. 1999;59:2675–81.
111. Heslop HE, Stevenson FK, Molldrem JJ. Immunotherapy of hematologic malignancy. Hematology Am Soc Hematol Educ Program. 2003;331–49.
112. Qazilbash MH, Wieder E, Rios R, Lu S, Kant S, Giralt S, Estey E, Thall P, de Lima M, Couriel D, Champlin RE, Komanduri K, Molldrem JJ. Vaccination with the PR1 leukemia-associated antigen can induce complete remission in patients with myeloid leukemia. Blood 2004;104:259a.
113. Rezvani K, Yong AS, Mielke S, et al. Leukemia-associated antigen-specific T-cell responses following combined PR1 and WT1 peptide vaccination in patients with myeloid malignancies. Blood 2008;111:236–42.
114. Entwistle J, Zhang S, Yang B, et al. Characterization of the murine gene encoding the hyaluronan receptor RHAMM. Gene 1995;163:233–8.
115. Hall CL, Yang B, Yang X, et al. Overexpression of the hyaluronan receptor RHAMM is transforming and is also required for H-ras transformation. Cell 1995;8:19–26.
116. Greiner J, Li L, Ringhoffer M, et al. Identification and characterization of epitopes of the receptor for hyaluronic acid-mediated motility (RHAMM/CD168) recognized by CD8+ T cells of HLA-A2-positive patients with acute myeloid leukemia. Blood 2005;106:938–45.
117. Ho VT, Soiffer RJ. The history and future of T-cell depletion as graft-versus-host disease prophylaxis for allogeneic hematopoietic stem cell transplantation. Blood 2001;98:3192–204.
118. Jakubowski AA, Small TN, Young JW, et al. T cell depleted stem-cell transplantation for adults with hematologic malignancies: sustained engraftment of HLA-matched related donor grafts without the use of antithymocyte globulin. Blood 2007;110:4552–9.
119. Almyroudis NG, Jakubowski A, Jaffe D, et al. Predictors for persistent cytomegalovirus reactivation after T-cell-depleted allogeneic hematopoietic stem cell transplantation. Transpl Infect Dis. 2007;9:286–94.

120. Andre-Schmutz I, Le Deist F, Hacein-Bey-Abina S, et al. Immune reconstitution without graft-versus-host disease after haemopoietic stem-cell transplantation: a phase 1/2 study. Lancet 2002;360:130–7.
121. Hartwig UF, Nonn M, Khan S, Meyer RG, Huber C, Herr W. Depletion of alloreactive T cells via CD69: implications on antiviral, antileukemic and immunoregulatory T lymphocytes. Bone Marrow Transplant. 2006;37:297–305.
122. Wehler TC, Nonn M, Brandt B, et al. Targeting the activation-induced antigen CD137 can selectively deplete alloreactive T cells from antileukemic and antitumor donor T-cell lines. Blood 2007;109:365–73.
123. Anderson BE, McNiff J, Yan J, et al. Memory CD4+ T cells do not induce graft-versus-host disease. J Clin Invest. 2003;112:101–8.
124. Chen BJ, Cui X, Sempowski GD, Liu C, Chao NJ. Transfer of allogeneic CD62L- memory T cells without graft-versus-host disease. Blood 2004;103:1534–41.
125. Xystrakis E, Bernard I, Dejean AS, Alsaati T, Druet P, Saoudi A. Alloreactive CD4 T lymphocytes responsible for acute and chronic graft-versus-host disease are contained within the CD45RChigh but not the CD45RClow subset. Eur J Immunol. 2004;34:408–17.
126. Zheng H, Matte-Martone C, Li H, et al. Effector memory CD4+ T cells mediate graft-versus-leukemia without inducing graft-versus-host disease. Blood 2008;111:2476–84.
127. Shlomchik WD. Graft-versus-host disease. Nat Rev Immunol. 2007;7:340–52.
128. Sallusto F, Geginat J, Lanzavecchia A. Central memory and effector memory T cell subsets: function, generation, and maintenance. Annu Rev Immunol. 2004;22:745–63.
129. Sallusto F, Langenkamp A, Geginat J, Lanzavecchia A. Functional subsets of memory T cells identified by CCR7 expression. Curr Top Microbiol Immunol. 2000;251:167–71.
130. Willinger T, Freeman T, Hasegawa H, McMichael AJ, Callan MF. Molecular signatures distinguish human central memory from effector memory CD8 T cell subsets. J Immunol. 2005;175:5895–903.
131. Arstila TP, Casrouge A, Baron V, Even J, Kanellopoulos J, Kourilsky P. A direct estimate of the human alphabeta T cell receptor diversity. Science 1999;286:958–61.
132. Bitmansour AD, Waldrop SL, Pitcher CJ, et al. Clonotypic structure of the human CD4+ memory T cell response to cytomegalovirus. J Immunol. 2001;167:1151–63.
133. Koelle DM, Liu Z, McClurkan CL, et al. Immunodominance among herpes simplex virus-specific CD8 T cells expressing a tissue-specific homing receptor. Proc Natl Acad Sci USA. 2003;100:12899–904.
134. Manley TJ, Luy L, Jones T, Boeckh M, Mutimer H, Riddell SR. Immune evasion proteins of human cytomegalovirus do not prevent a diverse CD8+ cytotoxic T-cell response in natural infection. Blood 2004;104:1075–82.
135. Frey CR, Sharp MA, Min AS, Schmid DS, Loparev V, Arvin AM. Identification of CD8+ T cell epitopes in the immediate early 62 protein (IE62) of varicella-zoster virus, and evaluation of frequency of CD8+ T cell response to IE62, by use of IE62 peptides after varicella vaccination. J Infect Dis. 2003;188:40–52.
136. Hislop AD, Gudgeon NH, Callan MF, et al. EBV-specific CD8+ T cell memory: relationships between epitope specificity, cell phenotype, and immediate effector function. J Immunol. 2001;167:2019–29.
137. Burrows SR, Silins SL, Khanna R, et al. Cross-reactive memory T cells for Epstein-Barr virus augment the alloresponse to common human leukocyte antigens: degenerate recognition of major histocompatibility complex-bound peptide by T cells and its role in alloreactivity. Eur J Immunol. 1997;27:1726–36.
138. Elkington R, Khanna R. Cross-recognition of human alloantigen by cytomegalovirus glycoprotein-specific CD4+ cytotoxic T lymphocytes: implications for graft-versus-host disease. Blood 2005;105:1362–4.
139. Rapoport AP, Stadtmauer EA, Aqui N, et al. Restoration of immunity in lymphopenic individuals with cancer by vaccination and adoptive T-cell transfer. Nat Med. 2005;11:1230–7.

140. Leen AM, Myers GD, Sili U, et al. Monoculture-derived T lymphocytes specific for multiple viruses expand and produce clinically relevant effects in immunocompromised individuals. Nat Med. 2006;12:1160–6.
141. Rooney CM, Smith CA, Ng CY, et al. Infusion of cytotoxic T cells for the prevention and treatment of Epstein-Barr virus-induced lymphoma in allogeneic transplant recipients. Blood 1998;92:1549–55.
142. Walter EA, Greenberg PD, Gilbert MJ, et al. Reconstitution of cellular immunity against cytomegalovirus in recipients of allogeneic bone marrow by transfer of T-cell clones from the donor. N Engl J Med. 1995;333:1038–44.
143. Dunbar PR, Ogg GS, Chen J, Rust N, van der Bruggen P, Cerundolo V. Direct isolation, phenotyping and cloning of low-frequency antigen-specific cytotoxic T lymphocytes from peripheral blood. Curr Biol. 1998;8:413–6.
144. Ho WY, Nguyen HN, Wolfl M, Kuball J, Greenberg PD. In vitro methods for generating CD8+ T-cell clones for immunotherapy from the naive repertoire. J Immunol Methods. 2006;310:40–52.
145. Wolfl M, Kuball J, Ho WY, et al. Activation-induced expression of CD137 permits detection, isolation, and expansion of the full repertoire of CD8+ T cells responding to antigen without requiring knowledge of epitope specificities. Blood 2007;110:201–10.
146. Yee C, Thompson JA, Byrd D, et al. Adoptive T cell therapy using antigen-specific CD8+ T cell clones for the treatment of patients with metastatic melanoma: in vivo persistence, migration, and antitumor effect of transferred T cells. Proc Natl Acad Sci USA. 2002;99:16168–73.
147. Dudley ME, Wunderlich JR, Robbins PF, et al. Cancer regression and autoimmunity in patients after clonal repopulation with antitumor lymphocytes. Science 2002;298:850–4.
148. Gattinoni L, Powell DJ Jr, Rosenberg SA, Restifo NP. Adoptive immunotherapy for cancer: building on success. Nat Rev Immunol. 2006;6:383–93.
149. Berger C, Jensen MC, Lansdorp PM, Gough M, Elliott C, Riddell SR. Adoptive transfer of effector CD8+ T cells derived from central memory cells establishes persistent T cell memory in primates. J Clin Invest. 2008;118:294–305.
150. Hinrichs CS, Spolski R, Paulos CM, et al. IL-2 and IL-21 confer opposing differentiation programs to CD8+ T cells for adoptive immunotherapy. Blood 2008;111:5326–33.
151. Klebanoff CA, Gattinoni L, Torabi-Parizi P, et al. Central memory self/tumor-reactive CD8+ T cells confer superior antitumor immunity compared with effector memory T cells. Proc Natl Acad Sci USA. 2005;102:9571–6.
152. Clay TM, Custer MC, Sachs J, Hwu P, Rosenberg SA, Nishimura MI. Efficient transfer of a tumor antigen-reactive TCR to human peripheral blood lymphocytes confers antitumor reactivity. J Immunol. 1999;163:507–13.
153. Stanislawski T, Voss RH, Lotz C, et al. Circumventing tolerance to a human MDM2-derived tumor antigen by TCR gene transfer. Nat Immunol. 2001;2:962–70.
154. Cohen CJ, Zhao Y, Zheng Z, Rosenberg SA, Morgan RA. Enhanced antitumor activity of murine-human hybrid T-cell receptor (TCR) in human lymphocytes is associated with improved pairing and TCR/CD3 stability. Cancer Res. 2006;66:8878–86.
155. Kuball J, Dossett ML, Wolfl M, et al. Facilitating matched pairing and expression of TCR chains introduced into human T cells. Blood 2007;109:2331–8.
156. Eshhar Z, Waks T, Gross G, Schindler DG. Specific activation and targeting of cytotoxic lymphocytes through chimeric single chains consisting of antibody-binding domains and the gamma or zeta subunits of the immunoglobulin and T-cell receptors. Proc Natl Acad Sci USA. 1993;90:720–4.
157. Sadelain M, Riviere I, Brentjens R. Targeting tumours with genetically enhanced T lymphocytes. Nat Rev Cancer. 2003;3:35–45.
158. Stephan MT, Ponomarev V, Brentjens RJ, et al. T cell-encoded CD80 and 4-1BBL induce auto- and transcostimulation, resulting in potent tumor rejection. Nat Med. 2007;13:1440–9.

Chapter 9
Reduced-Intensity and Nonmyeloablative Conditioning Regimens

Francine Foss and Koen van Besien

9.1 Alternative Conditioning Regimens for Allogeneic Hematopoietic Stem Cell Transplantation

Preparative regimens for allogeneic hematopoietic stem cell transplantation (HSCT) must address two immunologic barriers to establish successful hematopoietic engraftment: the host-versus-graft effect (HvG) and the graft-versus-host (GvH) effect. High-dose chemotherapy combined with sublethal doses of radiation therapy has been used to immune suppress the host sufficiently to prevent rejection of donor cells. Although effective in most patients, the original myeloablative regimens based on high dose TBI or busulfan are toxic to non-hematopoietic tissues and are associated with high transplant-associated morbidity and mortality, limiting the potential of this curative treatment to younger patients without underlying end organ dysfunction. Further, conventional ablative regimens require long-term immunosuppression to control GvHD, with resulting immune compromise and toxicity related to these agents.

With the recognition that the graft-versus-tumor (GvT) effect is responsible for many of the observed cures following allogeneic transplantation, less intensive and nonmyeloablative preparative regimens have been developed that rely on the graft-versus-disease effect while lessening the myeloablative effect of the transplant. Compared to conventional marrow toxic conditioning regimens in which host hematopoiesis is, in principle fully ablated, “mini-transplant,” or nonmyeloablative regimens utilize immunosuppressive strategies, including low-dose total body irradiation (TBI) and T-cell depleting agents to allow engraftment of allogeneic stem cells, in many instances establishing mixed donor/host lymphohematopoietic chimerism. The goals in the development of these strategies have been 2-fold: to facilitate engraftment of allogeneic stem cells with minimal end organ toxicity, and to modulate graft-versus-host alloreactivity in the direction of GvT while minimizing GvHD.

F. Foss (✉)
Medical Oncology and Bone Marrow Transplantation, Yale University School of Medicine, New Haven, CT 06520, USA
e-mail: Francine.foss@yale.edu

M.R. Bishop (ed.), *Hematopoietic Stem Cell Transplantation*,
Cancer Treatment and Research 144, DOI 10.1007/978-0-387-78580-6_9,

Alternative conditioning regimens have been characterized as "reduced-intensity" or "nonmyeloablative" based on their immunosuppressive and myelosuppressive properties. Nonmyeloablative conditioning, as defined by Storb et al., is characterized by persistence of host hematopoiesis and the presence of early mixed chimerism (coexistence of host and donor hematopoiesis) [1]. The goals of nonmyeloablative regimens are to establish donor hematopoiesis without introducing potentially toxic doses of radiation or chemotherapy and thus, nonmyeloablative strategies do not produce major anti-tumor effects. These regimens rely on immunosuppression to minimize host-versus-graft effects and facilitate donor engraftment. In the absence of immunosuppression or donor cell infusion, host hematopoiesis is restored. Reduced-intensity regimens, on the other hand, contain immunosuppressive agents to create marrow space for donor cells as well as lower doses of radiation or cytotoxic chemotherapeutic agents that have anti-tumor effects. Engraftment is facilitated due to the lymphohematopoietic depletion resulting from radiation and cytotoxic agents.

9.1.1 Nonmyeloablative Conditioning Regimens

The basis for the development of nonmyeloablative regimens was the demonstration in preclinical studies that donor engraftment and sustained mixed chimerism can be established in mice following low dose TBI (300 cGy) or cyclophosphamide (200 mg/kg), monoclonal anti-T-cell antibody therapy, thymic irradiation, and cyclosporine [2]. Canine studies have demonstrated that mixed lymphohematopoietic chimerism could be established using as little as 200 cGy of TBI followed by post-transplant immunosuppression with mycophenolate mofetil and cyclosporine A [3–8]. In these studies, it was demonstrated that a dose of 9.0 Gy was necessary to reliably permit engraftment of donor cells, whereas at 4.5 Gy, only 41% of the animals had sustained engraftment. But with the addition of immunosuppression (cyclosporine A), full engraftment was sustained in all of the animals. Further studies demonstrated that mixed chimerism could be sustained with as little as 2 Gy of radiation along with both cyclosporine A and mycophenolate mofetil (MMF) [9].

Based on the preclinical data indicating that stable mixed chimerism could be established with nonmyeloablative doses of TBI along with immunosuppression, a number of nonmyeloablative conditioning regimens have been developed, primarily for patients who were ineligible for more aggressive regimens due to age, extensive prior therapies, including prior autologous or allogeneic stem cell transplantation, or comorbid medical conditions. The initial Seattle trials used 2 Gy of TBI followed by MMF at 15 mg/kg b.i.d. for 28 days and cyclosporine at full dose until day + 35 or + 56 post-transplant [10]. While the majority of patients sustained full donor granulocyte chimerism (defined as >95% donor cells), they were mixed chimeric in the lymphocyte compartment up to day + 180. Unfortunately, 9 of 44 patients undergoing this regimen eventually experienced graft failure.

In the next trials, low dose fludarabine, a potent immunosuppressant, and extended administration of MMF was introduced in the conditioning regimen to further immunosuppress the patient and thereby decrease the frequency of graft rejection. In the setting of HLA-identical donors, sustained engraftment occurred in 97% of patients conditioned with fludarabine 30 mg/m^2 daily for 3 days, followed by 2 Gy TBI (Fig. 9.1a). In addition to fludarabine,

(a)

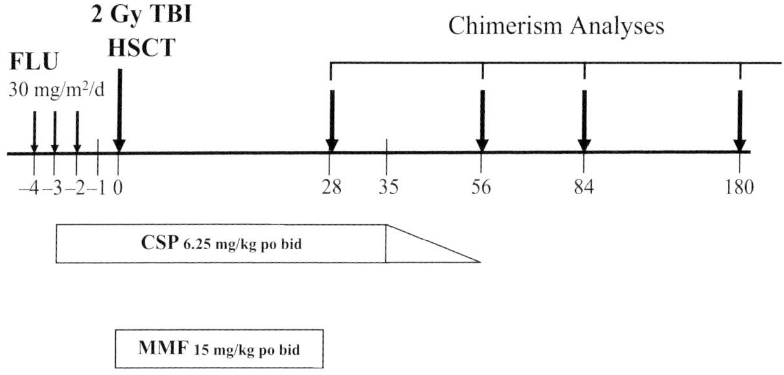

Fig. 9.1 Commonly used reduced-intensity and non myeloablative conditioning regimens: (**a**) Schema of non myeloablative conditioning regimen developed at Fred Hutchinson Cancer Center. Patients receive 2 Gy TBI, often combined with fludarabine. GHVD prophylaxis consists of a combination of cyclosporine A and mycophenolate mofetil, both of which are tapered by day 100. *Flu* fludarabine, *TBI* total body irradiation, *CSA* cyclosporine A, *MMF* mycophenolate mofetil. (**b**) Schema of reduced intensity conditioning regimen developed by Giralt et al. Patients receive fludarabine combined with high dose melphalan. GvHD prophylaxis consists of tacrolimus and methotrexate 5 mg/m^2 on days 1, 3 and 6. ATG is given to recipients of unrelated donor transplantation. (**c**) Schema of reduced intensity conditioning regimen developed by Mackinnon et al. The conditioning regimen is virtually identical to that studied at MD Anderson. GvHD prophylaxis consists of pre-transplant alemtuzumab and post transplant tacrolimus. Methotrexate is not used. (**d**) Schema of reduced intensity conditioning regimen developed by Slavin et al. Patients receive fludarabine combined with intermediate dose busulfan 2 mg/kg/day for four consecutive days. GvHD prophylaxis consists of cyclosporine and methotrexate 5 mg/m^2 on days 1, 3 and 6. ATG is given to recipients of unrelated donor transplantation. (**e**) Schema of reduced intensity conditioning regimen developed by Miller et al. This is an intermediate intensity conditioning regimen. Pentostatin, a nucleoside analog is combined with intermediate dose TBI. The conditioning regimen is preceded by 2 days of extracorporeal photopheresis (ECP) (see text). GvHD prophylaxis consists of cyclosporine and methotrexate

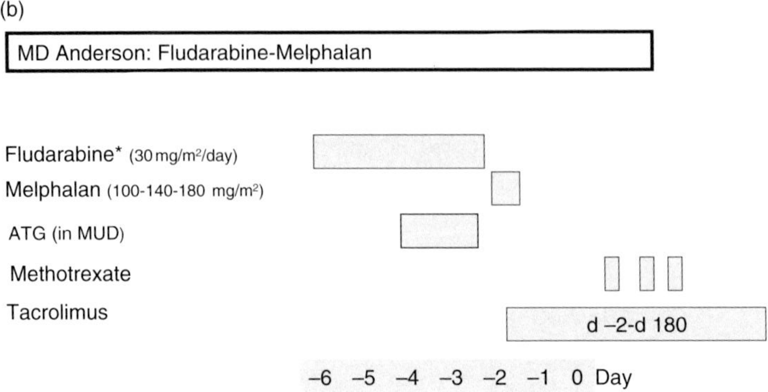

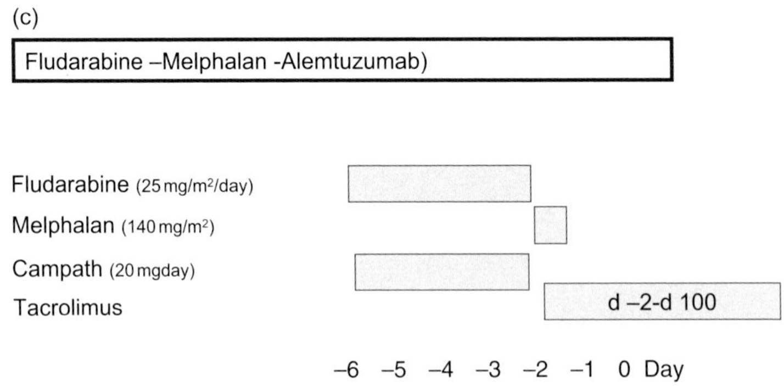

Fig. 9.1 (continued)

HLA-matched unrelated donor recipients received MMF up to day + 40 with a taper to day 96, along with a longer administration of cyclosporine to day + 100 with taper through day + 180. Durable engraftment occurred in 85% of patients who received peripheral blood stem cells and 56% of those who

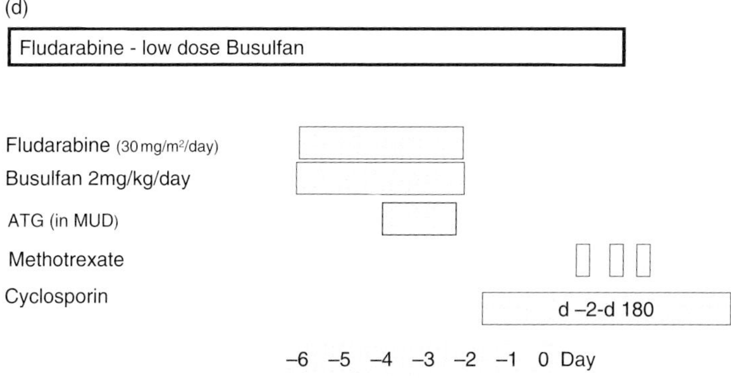

Slavin et al, Blood, 91, 756, 1998

(e)

ECP Based Conditioning

Preparative Regimen	
Day −7, −6	Extracorporeal photopheresis
Day −5, −4	Pentostatin 4mg/m²/day × 2 days by continuous infusion
Day −3, −2	TBI 200 cGy ×3 (600 cGy total)
Day −1	Rest
Day 0	Hematopoietic Stem Cell Infusion

Miller et al, BMT 33. 881, 2004

Fig. 9.1 (continued)

received bone marrow grafts. Further studies of MMF pharmacokinetics revealed that the $t^{1/2}$ was 3 h, and increasing administration to 15 mg/kg TID enhanced durable engraftment to 95%.

Baron et al. reported outcomes of 157 patients who underwent TBI (2 Gy) based nonmyeloablative regimen with MMF and cyclosporine A as GvHD prophylaxis [11]. The predominant predictors of graft rejection were donor T-cell and NK cell chimerism less than 50% at day + 14. High levels of donor natural killer (NK) cell chimerism early after transplant predicted for improved GvT effect and progression-free survival. High T-cell chimerism on day + 14 was associated with an increased probability of grade II–IV acute GvHD. The incidence and severity of acute and chronic GvHD in nonmyeloablative transplants was compared to standard ablative regimens by Mielcarek et al., who evaluated age matched recipients of related and unrelated grafts and demonstrated that the cumulative incidence of grades II–IV acute GvHD was significantly lower (64% vs. 85%, $P = 0.001$) favoring the nonmyeloablative group, whereas the incidence of chronic GvHD was similar (73% vs. 71%, $P = 0.96$) [12]. Transplant-related mortality and 1-year survival were better in the nonmyeloablative group (24% vs. 35%, $P = 0.27$; 68% vs. 50%, $P = 0.04$). With respect to transplant related toxicities, transfusion requirements and end organ damage to liver, kidney, and lung were significantly less in the nonmyeloablative group, despite the fact that the patients were older, had more advanced disease and more comorbidities [2, 3, 13, 14].

A recent retrospective study has compared outcomes for nonmyeloablative transplants based on donor status with related ($n = 221$) and unrelated ($n = 184$) donors [4]. After adjusting for comorbidity index, relapse risk, age, stem cell source, and cytomegalovirus (CMV) status in multivariate analysis, there was no statistically significant difference in nonrelapse mortality (hazard ratio [HR] = 0.98; 95% confidence interval [CI] = 0.6–1.6; $P = 0.94$), relapse (HR = 1.04; 95% CI = 0.7–1.5; $P = 0.82$), or overall mortality (HR = 0.99; 95% CI = 0.7–1.4; $P = 0.94$). Overall rates of severe acute GvHD and extensive chronic GvHD also were not significantly different between the two groups.

9.1.2 Reduced-Intensity Regimens

While nonmyeloablative regimens were designed to primarily induce immunosuppression sufficient to permit engraftment of donor cells, reduced-intensity conditioning regimens utilize drugs active against the underlying disease. Many of these regimens have combined purine analogs to induce immunosuppression along with other cytotoxic agents or low doses of TBI. These regimens can be categorized based on their degree of intensity, with those which contain busulfan at doses up to 10 mg/kg, melphalan at doses up to 180 mg/kg, or TBI at doses up to 8 Gy as the most intensive, and those containing cyclophosphamide, thymic irradiation, and antibodies as the least intensive. The use of fludarabine as an immunosuppressive agent in these regimens has been well characterized and a threshold dose of 125–150 mg/m^2 has been established to establish donor engraftment.

In one of the first of these trials, Khouri et al. reported results in 15 lymphoma and chronic lymphocytic leukemia patients treated with fludarabine 30 mg/m^2 for 3 days and either cyclophosphamide 300 mg/m^2/day for 3 days, or cisplatin 25 mg/m^2/day for 4 days and cytosine arabinoside 500 mg/m^2/day for 2 days[5]. Eleven of 15 patients had at least 50% donor engraftment, four had no engraftment, and five developed acute GvHD. Eight had a complete response. Giralt et al. treated 15 patients with leukemia or myelodysplastic syndrome with either fludarabine 30 mg/m^2/day for 4 days and idarubicin 12 mg/m^2/day for 3 days or high-dose melphalan 140 mg/m^2/day, or 2-CDA 12 mg/m^2/day for 5 days and cytosine arabinoside 1000 mg/m^2/day for 5 days [6] (Fig. 9.1b). Thirteen patients demonstrated engraftment, seven had 90% donor hematopoiesis by day + 30, and three had acute GvHD. Childs et al. treated 15 patients including three with renal cell carcinoma and four with melanoma with a regimen of cyclophosphamide 60 mg/kg/day for 4 days and fludarabine 25 mg/kg/day for 5 days in the setting of HLA-matched or single mismatched donor peripheral blood stem cells and reported stable engraftment in 14 of 15 patients and acute GvHD in all seven patients who had established 100% donor T-cell chimerism by day + 30 [15]. Busulfan was introduced by Slavin et al. who treated 22 patients with busulfan 8 mg/kg and fludarabine 180 mg/m^2, along with anti-thymocyte globulin (ATG) and granulocyte-colony-stimulating factor (G-CSF)-mobilized peripheral stem cells. Donor engraftment occurred in all patients, and acute GvHD was observed in 12 of 26 [7] (Fig. 9.1d).

The most commonly used reduced-intensity regimens are fludarabine plus melphalan and fludarabine plus busulfan, both of which have similar immunosuppressive intensity. Selection of one regimen over the other may be dictated to some degree by disease type. In a historical comparison of outcomes with these two regimens in 151 patients treated at a single institution, fludarabine/melphalan was associated with more grade III/IV organ toxicity ($P = 0.005$) and grade II–IV acute GvHD ($P = 0.01$) compared to fludarabine/busulfan, but was also more cytoreductive against underlying hematologic malignancies. Patients receiving fludarabine/melphalan experienced more significant myelosuppression, while several who received busulfan did not experience significant pancytopenia. Melphalan has been shown to have broad stem cell toxicity to both primitive and committed stem cells, whereas busulfan spares committed stem cells. In multivariate analysis, fludarabine plus melphalan was associated with a higher incidence of transplant-related mortality but a reduced incidence of disease relapse.

Another approach in reduced-intensity transplantation is to establish stable mixed chimerism using low dose cyclophosphamide, thymic irradiation, and ATG. This platform is based on the establishment of graft tolerance, with later use of donor lymphocyte infusions (DLI) to augment GvT effects. Using this strategy, Sykes et al. reported establishment of stable mixed chimerism in 20 of 23 HLA-matched and 7 of 10 mismatched recipients [8]. Many of the patients were converted to full donor chimerism by DLI without significant GvHD and had complete remission of their disease, suggesting that significant GVL effect could be achieved without significant GvHD. Daly et al. reported similar results in 13 patients with a regimen of cyclophosphamide 150–200 mg/kg, ATG, and thymic irradiation along with a short course of cyclosporine for GvHD prophylaxis [9]. Seven patients with no acute GvHD had DLI beginning 5–6 weeks after transplant to convert mixed to full donor chimerism and augment GVL. In this study, seven patients had a complete disease response with a median disease-free survival probability at 2 years of 37.5%, but disappointingly, grade II–IV acute GvHD occurred in most of the patients related to DLI.

9.1.3 Reducing GvHD in Reduced-Intensity Regimens

Despite the reduction in transplant related mortality from regimen-related toxicity with reduced-intensity transplants, acute and chronic GvHD remain a major problem. The incidence of grade II–IV acute GvHD with fludarbine based regimens has ranged from 30–50% and chronic GvHD from 40–60% (Table 9.1). The onset of GvHD after 100 days has been a characteristic of many

Table 9.1 Incidence of GvHD with reduced-intensity regimens

References	Regimen	Acute GvHD (%) grade II–IV	Chronic GvHD (%)
[10, 90, 99, 108, 125, 126]	TBI 2 Gy, Flu 90 mg/m^2	19–63	40–63
[127]	TBI 8 Gy, Flu 120 mg/m^2 ± ATG	17	46
[76]	TBI 5.5 Gy, Cy 120 mg/m^2	45	59
[60]	TBI 8 Gy, Cy 120 mg/m^2	48	64
[88, 92, 98]	Flu 90 mg/m^2, Cy 2000–2250 mg/m^2	5–12	36–64
[15, 58]	Flu 125 mg/m^2, Cy 120 mg/kg	50–55	26–53
[70, 128]	Flu 100–150 mg/m^2, Mel 100–140 mg/m^2	20–40	26–33
[20, 21, 93]	Flu 150 mg/m^2, Mel 140 mg/m^2, Campath	15–41	7–33
[71, 72]	Flu 120–180 mg/m^2, Bu 8 mg/kg po, 6.4 mg/kg IV	37–48	48
[79, 129]	Flu 150 mg/m^2, Bu 8 mg/kg	27	62
[56, 129]	Flu 150 mg/m^2, Bu 8 mg/kg, Campath	27	62
[130]	Cy 150–200 mg/kg, ATG, thymic radiation	29	NA
[49]	ECP/Pentostatin, 6 Gy	9	43

Flu fludarabine, *Cy* cyclophosphamide, *Bu* busulfan, *TBI* total body irradiation, *ATG* anti-thymocyte globulin, *ECP* extracorporeal photopheresis reduced-intensity regimens. Patients may manifest features of both acute and chronic GvHD. A number of strategies have been employed to reduce the incidence of acute GvHD. The in vitro depletion of T cells occurs with the addition of ATG to the conditioning regimen. The impact of ATG in this setting has been mostly in patients with unrelated donor transplants. A recent review of 83 patients, who received peripheral blood stem cells from HLA-identical siblings after conditioning with either busulfan (8 mg/kg) and fludarabine (150 mg/m^2) ($n = 45$) or busulfan (8 mg/kg) fludarabine (180 mg/m^2) and ATG (40 mg/kg) ($n = 38$) reported no difference in incidence of acute GvHD or chronic GvHD in the ATG patients, and no overall survival difference [16]. In studies with unrelated donors, however, the addition of ATG has reduced the incidence of graft failure and acute GvHD [17].

Alemtuzumab (anti-CD52 antibody, CAMPATH-1H) has also been extensively studied as a T-cell depleting agent. The CD52 antigen is expressed on all T and B cells, and the majority of monocytes, macrophages, eosinophils, NK cells, and dendritic cells. Alemtuzumab is capable of inducing antibody-dependent cell-mediated cytotoxicity, thus eliminating both T cells and CD52-expressing dendritic cells in vitro and in vivo. When alemtuzumab was added to a fludarabine plus melphalan regimen (alemtuzumab 20 mg on days −8 to −4, fludarabine 30 mg/m^2 days −7 to −3, melphalan 140 mg/m^2 day −2, the incidence of acute and chronic GvHD decreased significantly [18–20] (Fig. 9.1c). Of the 34 patients who were evaluated for chimerism at 1 month, 29 (85%) had achieved full donor chimerism; at 5 months, five of these patients had converted to mixed chimerism. A review of 88 lymphoma patients treated with this regimen reported graft failure in only three and grades II–IV acute GvHD in 15% [21]. A high frequency of mixed hematopoietic chimerism (19 of 69 evaluable patients) was noted 1–3 months post-transplant due to the in vivo T-cell depleting effects of alemtuzumab on the stem cell graft; conversion to full donor chimerism was achieved with DLI in 8 of 15 patients. Similarly, the effects of T-cell depletion on the GvT effect required DLI for persistent disease in a number of patients. In other studies alemtuzumab has been used “in the bag” to purge stem cell products and thus reduce the incidence of acute GvHD after ablative conditioning regimens [22–24].

While alemtuzumab containing regimens have been well-tolerated and associated with a low incidence of life-threatening acute GvHD and a low incidence of chronic GvHD, the incidence of serious infections has been high related to immunosuppression. In one study, CMV reactivation was observed in 63% of at-risk patients [21]. Pre-emptive monitoring and treatment of CMV has now become a standard for patients receiving alemtuzumab [25]. Other infectious complications seen with these regimens included invasive aspergillosis, toxoplasmosis, and disseminated adenovirus [26, 27]. On the other hand, the low incidence of extensive chronic GvHD with these regimens mitigates the risk for late infections, and the overall risk for treatment related mortality may be reduced [28].

9.1.4 Dendritic Cells and Reduced-Intensity Regimens

The importance of host dendritic cells (DC) in establishment of GvHD was defined by Shlomchik et al. in a murine HLA-matched allogeneic transplant model, in which it was demonstrated that $CD8^+$ T-cell mediated GvHD and GvT required donor T-cell recognition of host antigens in the context of host antigen-presenting cells, suggesting that acute GvHD may be driven by persistence of functional host antigen presenting cells after allogeneic stem cell infusion [29]. These results suggested that incidence and severity of GvHD may be influenced by the quality of host/donor DC chimerism achieved after engraftment. In this model, host DC capable of presenting minor histocompatibility antigens to infused donor T cells would initiate T-cell activation and a Th-1 cytokine cascade implicated in the pathogenesis of acute GvHD.

While conventional immunosuppressive regimens containing cyclosporine, tacrolimus, and sirolimus may effectively reduce the activation of donor T cells, they have little effect on residual host antigen-presenting cells. The clinical effectiveness of the addition of alemtuzumab in reducing the incidence of acute GvHD may be due, in part, to its direct effects on DC populations [30–42]. Other monoclonal antibodies are being developed to target and eradicate DC [30].

Another novel strategy to modify host DC populations involves the use of extracorporeal photopheresis (ECP), a therapy that involves the ex vivo exposure of leukapheresed peripheral blood mononuclear cells to 8-methoxypsoralen, a DNA-damaging agent, in the presence of ultraviolet light in a plastic chamber. ECP has been demonstrated to be an effective therapy for acute and chronic GvHD by a mechanism which involved the induction of tolerogenic dendritic cells [43–48]. ECP induces induction of apoptosis in T cells, which are ingested by monocytoid DC and induce the expression of tolerizing cytokines, such as IL-10 [43, 45]. Functional studies have shown decresased capacity of these ECP treated DC to induce T-cell proliferation [43].

A Phase I/II study using a reduced-intensity conditioning regimen was conducted to explore the role of ECP as a strategy to modulate host DC prior to the infusion of allogeneic stem cells. The regimen consisted of 2 days of ECP followed by infusional pentostatin at a dose of 8 mg/m^2 over 48 h and 6 Gy of TBI [49] (Fig. 9.1e). Of 92 patients enrolled, 22 had a prior transplant and 53 had refractory disease at the time of transplant. Engraftment was seen in all but one patient; four patients with active, refractory acute myelogenous leukemia (AML) at the time of transplant had progressive disease before engraftment. The median time to engraftment of leukocytes and platelets was 14 and 17 days, respectively. The regimen was well-tolerated even in this high risk group of patients. The most significant outcome of this trial was the low incidence of acute and chronic GvHD with a 13% incidence of grade III–IV acute GvHD and a 12% incidence of extensive chronic GvHD. A randomized trial of this regimen with and without ECP is underway to explore whether the reduced incidence of GvHD was associated with the use of ECP.

9.2 Outcomes of Reduced-Intensity Conditioning and Nonmyeloablative Transplantation in Specific Diseases

The reduced-intensity and nonmyeloablative regimens have been widely adopted because of their relative lack of early toxicity and the reliable engraftment observed with a variety of donor types. In certain instances and institutions, they have replaced myeloablative conditioning [50, 51]. Yet, despite prolonged and intensive investigation, the definitive role of nonmyeloablative transplantation has not been established in any particular disease. Randomized studies comparing with conventional conditioning regimens are non-existent. Encouraging phase II data are not routinely confirmed in multi-institutional or registry analysis, and some analyses suggest worse outcomes for subsets of patients.

These conflicting results are explained to a large extent by differences in patient selection, the profusion of conditioning regimens, and the important role of other treatment components such as donor type, and GvHD prophylaxis for the outcome of transplantation. Despite these limitations, there continues to be major interest in the further development of reduced-intensity conditioning.

9.2.1 Chronic Myelogenous Leukemia and Other Myeloproliferative Disorders

Allogeneic transplantation was until recently the standard of care for patients with chronic myelogenous leukemia (CML). Myeloablative transplantation with related or unrelated donors resulted in very high cure rates for young patients [52]. In the middle-aged and older, cure rates of 50–60% were routinely reported, but treatment-related mortality was considerable [53]. Given the susceptibility of CML to GvT effects, the exploration of nonmyeloablative conditioning represented an attractive option. Kebriaei et al. recently reported long-term outcomes in 64 patients treated at the M.D. Anderson Cancer Center with nonmyeloablative conditioning [54]. Only 20% of patients were in first chronic phase, the rest were in second chronic phase, accelerated phase, or blast crisis. Among chronic-phase patients, progression-free survival at 2 and 5 years was 47% and 31%, respectively, compared with 15% and 11%, respectively, for patients with accelerated- or blast-phase disease ($P = 0.03$). Several years earlier, the Seattle group had reported on a similar group of 24 older patients with CML who received conditioning with low-dose TBI or fludarabine and TBI [55]. Four of the 8 receiving low-dose TBI alone experienced graft rejection, which might indicate that low-dose TBI is not sufficiently immunosuppressive for allogeneic HSCT in patients with previously untreated CML. After the addition of fludarabine to the conditioning regimen, no further instances of graft rejection were observed. With a median follow up of 36 months, 13 of 24 patients remained alive and in complete remission. A study by Or and colleagues in Jerusalem found excellent results in younger patients using a low dose busulfan conditioning regimen [56].

By contrast Das and colleagues in India reported very poor results with only 6 of 17 patients surviving [57]. Sloand et al. also reported high rates of recurrence after reduced-intensity conditioning in patients in first or second chronic phase CML [58]. Such contradictory results are best brought in perspective by a registry analysis on 186 patients reported by the European Group for Blood and Marrow Transplantaiton. They found a cumulative treatment-related mortality of 21%, despite limited early treatment-related mortality. Progression-free survival at 3 years was 37% and was worse in patients with advanced disease [59]. Weisser et al. reported encouraging results with a reduced-intensity regimen consisting of TBI (8 Gy), fludarabine, and cyclophosphamide (80 mg/kg) combined with ATG. They treated 35 elderly CML and reported a low rate of recurrence and 68% survival at 2.5 years [60].

The tyrosine kinase inhibitors have revolutionized management of CML and currently the majority of CML patients referred for transplant are either refractory or intolerant to imatinib. Cohort analysis indicates that prior exposure to imatinib by itself does not affect tolerance to transplant conditioning, engraftment and complication rates [61]. However, those referred after failing imatinib may be predisposed to higher complication and failure rates. Data with nonmyeloablative transplant in this setting are virtually absent, but it is to be expected that recurrence rates will be high. Consideration should be given to maintaining such patients on imatinib post-transplant [62, 63].

Among the other myeloproliferative disorders, myelofibrosis has been the topic of considerable interest. After an initial report of successful allogeneic transplantation in a group of four patients [64], results have been updated in a survey by Rondelli et al. [65]. They identified 21 patients—most with advanced disease. Eigtheen patients had durable engraftment and prolonged responses. This compared favorably to the high treatment-related mortality observed in advanced myelofibrosis with myeloablative conditioning [66].

9.2.2 *Acute Leukemias and Myelodysplastic Syndromes*

Nonmyeloablative allogeneic HSCT has been widely utilized in the management of acute leukemia, in particular AML. The Seattle consortium using mostly fludarabine and low-dose TBI recently reported long term outcomes in patients with myeloid malignancies [67]. Long-term survival rates were in the 30% range and ranged from approximately 20% for those with myelodysplastic syndromes (MDS) and therapy-related AML (t-AML) to approximately 40% for those with myeloproliferative disorders. Of interest, graft rejection occurred in 23 (16%) of the patients regardless of donor type. Occurrence of chronic GvHD was associated with a reduced risk of recurrence, but not with improved survival. Similar results were reported by Koh et al. using the Seattle fludarabine-TBI regimen [68]. In their series, GvHD accounted for most of the treatment-related mortality (TRM) and could be reduced by intensifying GvHD prophylaxis.

The M.D. Anderson Cancer Center group investigated the use of allogeneic HSCT following a reduced-intensity regimen of fludarabine plus melphalan regimen, as well as a less-intensive regimen of fludarabine, idarubicin, and cytosine arabinoside, for high-risk AML and MDS. The fludarabine-melphalan regimen resulted in approximately 60% disease-free survival at 2 years for patients transplanted in complete remission [69]. For those patients transplanted with active disease, disease-free survival was much lower. The less-intensive regimen of fludarabine-idarubicin-cytosine arabinoside was associated with an increased rate of recurrence, underscoring the importance of chemotherapy intensity to overall outcome [70]. Kroger et al. used a reduced-intensity regimen consisting of busulfan (8 mg/kg) and fludarabine in the treatment of MDS or t-AML and reported an estimated 38% 3-year disease-free survival [71]. But Shimoni et al., reported that a reduced dose busulfan conditioning regimen was less effective than myeloablative doses of busulfan for transplant of patients with active AML [72]. Campath based T-cell depletion has been studied in AML and MDS by our group as well as by the UK consortium [73, 74]. While relapse rate is increased, GvHD related complications and transplant related mortality are lower and overall results are comparable to those obtained with fludarabine-melphalan conditioning [28]. Other regimens have been investigated as well. For example Maruyama et al. reported a large retrospective analysis of patients, mostly with acute leukemias and MDS, who were not in remission at the time of transplant. The conditioning regimen consisted of fludarabine or cladribine combined with low-dose busulfan and sometimes with low dose TBI. They found no striking differences in toxicity or overall efficacy of these reduced-intensity regimens compared with conventional conditioning [75]. Girgis et al. and Hallemeier et al. developed a conditioning regimen of low-dose cyclophosphamide and TBI, with excellent long-term outcomes in patients with good-risk disease [76, 77]. A recurrent observation in each of these studies is the high rate of recurrence in patients with advanced disease, an issue that is being addressed by more intensive pre-transplant induction or by post-transplant maintenance therapy. The use of pre-transplant induction was studied as part of a multicenter trial from Germany and Austria in which patients with refractory AML underwent allogeneic HSCT with a reduced-intensity conditioning regimen 4 days after cytarabine and amsacrine induction [78]. Those without GvHD received prophylactic DLIs as of day 120. One hundred and three patients were studied; two-thirds had unrelated donors. One-year survival in this group of patients was an encouraging 54%. Similar, but more preliminary, data were reported by Blaise and colleagues in Marseille [79]. Others have evaluated the use of post-transplant prophylactic DLI or other forms of adoptive immunotherapy [78, 80], vaccinations [81], or more recently, maintenance chemotherapeutic treatment [82]. Intensification of the conditioning regimen is achieved by the addition of agents such as gemtuzumab ozogamycin that are highly leukemia specific [83], or the incorporation of new chemotherapeutic agents such as treosulfan [84].

9.2.3 Lymphoma and Chronic Lymphocytic Leukemia

Myeloablative transplantation can be curative for chronic lymphocytic leukemia (CLL) and low-grade non-Hodgkin's lymphoma (NHL), but very high rates of TRM were reported in early series [85–87]. Both the M.D. Anderson and the Seattle groups report encouraging outcomes with nonmyeloablative transplantation in low-grade NHL and CLL [5, 88–92]. In a multi-institutional trial from the United Kingdom UK group, the use of an alemtuzumab (Campath)-based conditioning regimen resulted in slightly higher rates of disease recurrence, but overall similar outcomes in patients with follicular NHL [21]. In patients with CLL, a surprisingly high incidence of opportunistic infections was encountered after Campath-based conditioning, perhaps because of excessive immunosuppression [93].

The encouraging phase II and single institution results contrast with an analysis by the International Bone Marrow Transplant Registry (IBMTR) that found no advantage for nonmyeloablative transplantation [51]. Performance status and disease status, not the type of conditioning regimen, were predictors for outcome. There was even a trend for higher recurrence rates after nonmyeloablative or reduced-intensity conditioning. No effect of GvHD on relapse rates could be detected in this or in earlier IBMTR analyses. The Seattle group also compared the outcomes after allogeneic HSCT with nonmyeloablative or myeloablative conditioning regimens in lymphoid malignancies [94]. Patients with comorbidities, two-thirds of their entire patient group, benefited from reduced-intensity conditioning because of decreased treatment related mortality. The results of nonmyeloablative and myeloablative conditioning were similar in the one-third of patients without comorbidities. The Seattle study suggested that GvT effects rather than conditioning intensity was the major determinant for outcome of allogeneic HSCT in lymphoma. Neither of these studies can be considered definitive because they are based on retrospective comparisons between groups with major imbalances in patient and disease characteristics. In both studies, patients undergoing nonmyeloablative transplantation tended to be older but also were more often transplanted in remission. Adjustment for such covariates can only partially address these issues, and it cannot at all account for the omission of important covariates such as comorbidities in the IBMTR study and performance score in the Seattle study.

Nonmyeloablative allogeneic HSCT has also been studied in other subtypes of lymphoma including mantle cell lymphoma, transformed lymphoma, diffuse large B-cell lymphoma, and peripheral T-cell lymphoma. The results are widely variable, but there is a consensus that transplantation of patients with aggressive NHL and active disease does not result in high cure rates [21, 95–99].

In Hodgkin's lymphoma, the historical results with myeloablative allogeneic HSCT are dismal, perhaps because it has mainly been utilized in patients with very advanced disease including those who relapse after autologous transplantation [100]. Single institution studies or consortium studies show excellent results with nonmyeloablative conditioning for recurrent Hodgkin's lymphoma [101, 102]. Nonmyeloablative allogeneic HSCT may be particularly useful in those who have failed autologous transplantation. Although only a minority of patients is cured, the survival after allogeneic transplantation is clearly superior to that obtained with further conventional chemotherapy [103]. An analysis from the European Group for Blood and Marrow Transplantation (EBMT) registry confirmed the advantage of nonmyeloablative over myeloablative sibling transplantation in Hodgkin's lymphoma [104]. This was not confirmed in an IBMTR analysis of unrelated donor transplantation [105].

9.2.4 Multiple Myeloma

Despite its curative potential, myeloablative allogeneic transplantation has never found wide application in multiple myeloma because of the serious toxicity and excessive treatment-related mortality in this frail patient population [106]. Nonmyeloablative transplantation has therefore rapidly found widespread interest. Reduced intensity comes, however, with increased recurrence [107]. An EBMT analysis of 320 patients confirmed the low TRM rate, but also a much higher recurrence rate than after myeloablative conditioning and overall no benefit [50]. There is, however, an increasing interest in the use of sequential autologous followed by nonmyeloablative transplant consolidation [108, 109]. It is hoped that the separation of the toxicity of high dose conditioning from the immunosuppression associated with nonmyeloablative transplantation will result in less overall toxicity. A randomized study from Italy showed a benefit of sequential autologous followed by allogeneic transplantation over double autologous transplantation in patients with myeloma in first response [110]. A similar study restricted to patients with high-risk disease failed to show a benefit for allogeneic transplantation [111]. Several randomized studies are currently ongoing to address this issue.

9.2.5 Benign Hematologic Disorders

Nonmyeloablative allogeneic HSCT holds particular appeal for patients with so-called benign hematological disorders, where the conditioning regimen is required only to assure engraftment and not to assure disease control. Allogeneic HSCT can be curative for sickle cell disease and thalassemia, but it is only rarely performed in patients with advanced disease because of excessive toxicity. Using a fludarabine-melphalan conditioning regimen, we reported engraftment in two patients with advanced sickle cell disease [112]. Unfortunately both died of complications related to GvHD. More recently using a Campath-based GvHD prophylaxis durable engraftment after reduced-intensity conditioning was reported in two patients, including one who was in renal failure and on dialysis

[113]. But graft failure has also been frequently observed after nonmyeloablative transplantation for sickle cell disease, and the lack of related or matched unrelated donors in many patients with sickle cell disease poses considerable challenges for implementing this strategy [114]. Nonmyeloablative allogeneic HSCT has also been tested in thalassemia, particularly in those with advanced disease who are poor candidates for conventional myeloablative conditioning, but it has been associated with an excessive incidence of graft rejection [115].

9.3 Predicting Toxicity

Originally developed as a method to extend allogeneic HSCT to the frail and elderly, nonmyeloablative and reduced-intensity conditioning regimens have only partially fulfilled that promise. The contradictory results of various studies in nonmyeloablative transplantation stem in large part from differences in patient selection. Initial studies often selected patients on the basis of age alone, and age has even constituted the basis for randomization between myeloablative and reduced-intensity conditioning [116]. But age is a poor predictor of transplant tolerance [117]. In an effort to better define the risk for transplant-related morbidity and mortality, tools for measuring comorbidities developed in geriatric medicine have been utilized and adapted for transplant [118]. Sorror et al. developed the transplant specific comorbidity index, which was shown to be an independent predictor of transplant outcome across studies and institutions [119]. Artz et al. found that combining a measure of comorbidity (the Kaplan Feinstein index) with the commonly used WHO performance status adds additional power to predict treatment related mortality, an observation that was recently confirmed by the Seattle group who also found a correlation with survival [120, 121]. Measurement of comorbidity scores and performance scores lack accuracy and reproducibility. There is an interest in creating simpler and more reliable measures of fitness. Investigators from the Dana-Farber Cancer Institue reported that serum ferritin, an acute phase reactant, but also a measure of iron overload, predicts for transplant-related toxicity [122]. Our group at the University of Chicago, as well as the M.D. Anderson group, has presented preliminary evidence on the correlation between C-reactive protein levels and toxicity [123, 124]. The further refinement of prognostic tools and scores is essential for improvement in treatment strategies in allogeneic transplantation.

References

1. Storb RF, Champlin R, Riddell SR, et al. Non-myeloablative transplants for malignant disease. Hematology Am Soc Hematol Educ Program. 2001:375–91.
2. Diaconescu R, Flowers CR, Storer B, et al. Morbidity and mortality with nonmyeloablative compared with myeloablative conditioning before hematopoietic cell transplantation from HLA-matched related donors. Blood 2004;104:1550–8.

3. Chien JW, Maris MB, Sandmaier BM, et al. Comparison of lung function after myeloablative and 2 Gy of total body irradiation-based regimens for hematopoietic stem cell transplantation. Biol Blood Marrow Transplant. 2005;11:288–96.
4. Mielcarek M, Storer BE, Sandmaier BM, et al. Comparable outcomes after nonmyeloablative hematopoietic cell transplantation with unrelated and related donors. Biol Blood Marrow Transplant. 2007;13:1499–507.
5. Khouri I, Keating M, Korbling M, et al. Transplant-lite: induction of graft-versus-malignancy using fludarabine-based nonablative chemotherapy and allogeneic blood progenitor-cell transplantation as treatment for lymphoid malignancies. J Clin Oncol. 1998;16:2817–24.
6. Giralt S, Estey E, Albitar M, et al. Engraftment of allogeneic hematopoietic progenitor cells with purine analog-containing chemotherapy: harnessing graft-versus-leukemia without myeloablative therapy. Blood 1997;89:4531–6.
7. Slavin S, Nagler A, Naparstek E, et al. Nonmyeloablative stem cell transplantation and cell therapy as an alternative to conventional bone marrow transplantation with lethal cytoreduction for the treatment of malignant and nonmalignant hematologic diseases. Blood 1998;91:756–63.
8. Sykes M, Preffer F, McAfee S, et al. Mixed lymphohaematopoietic chimerism and graft-versus-lymphoma effects after non-myeloablative therapy and HLA-mismatched bone marrow transplantation. Lancet 1999;353:1755–9.
9. Daly A, McAfee S, Dey B, et al. Nonmyeloablative bone marrow transplantation: infectious complications in 65 recipients of HLA-identical and mismatched transplants. Biol Blood Marrow Transplant. 2003;9:373–82.
10. McSweeney PA, Niederwieser D, Shizuru JA, et al. Hematopoietic cell transplantation in older patients with hematologic malignancies: replacing high-dose cytotoxic therapy with graft-versus-tumor effects. Blood 2001;97:3390–400.
11. Baron F, Baker JE, Storb R, et al. Kinetics of engraftment in patients with hematologic malignancies given allogeneic hematopoietic cell transplantation after nonmyeloablative conditioning. Blood 2004;104:2254–62.
12. Mielcarek M, Martin PJ, Leisenring W, et al. Graft-versus-host disease after nonmyeloablative versus conventional hematopoietic stem cell transplantation. Blood 2003;102:756–62.
13. Hogan WJ, Maris M, Storer B, et al. Hepatic injury after nonmyeloablative conditioning followed by allogeneic hematopoietic cell transplantation: a study of 193 patients. Blood 2004;103:78–84.
14. Sorror ML, Maris MB, Storer B, et al. Comparing morbidity and mortality of HLA-matched unrelated donor hematopoietic cell transplantation after nonmyeloablative and myeloablative conditioning: influence of pretransplantation comorbidities. Blood 2004;104:961–8.
15. Childs R, Chernoff A, Contentin N, et al. Regression of metastatic renal-cell carcinoma after nonmyeloablative allogeneic peripheral-blood stem-cell transplantation. N Engl J Med. 2000;343:750–8.
16. Schetelig J, Bornhauser M, Kiehl M, et al. Reduced-intensity conditioning with busulfan and fludarabine with or without antithymocyte globulin in HLA-identical sibling transplantation—a retrospective analysis. Bone Marrow Transplant. 2004;33:483–90.
17. Bertz H, Potthoff K, Finke J. Allogeneic stem-cell transplantation from related and unrelated donors in older patients with myeloid leukemia. J Clin Oncol. 2003;21:1480–4.
18. Kottaridis PD, Milligan DW, Chopra R, et al. In vivo CAMPATH-1H prevents GvHD following nonmyeloablative stem-cell transplantation. Cytotherapy 2001;3:197–201.
19. Chakraverty R, Peggs K, Chopra R, et al. Limiting transplantation-related mortality following unrelated donor stem cell transplantation by using a nonmyeloablative conditioning regimen. Blood 2002;99:1071–8.

20. van Besien K, Artz A, Smith S, et al. Fludarabine, melphalan, and alemtuzumab conditioning in adults with standard-risk advanced acute myeloid leukemia and myelodysplastic syndrome. J Clin Oncol. 2005;23:5728–38.
21. Morris E, Thomson K, Craddock C, et al. Outcome following Alemtuzumab (CAMPATH-1H)-containing reduced intensity allogeneic transplant regimen for relapsed and refractory non-Hodgkin's lymphoma (NHL). Blood 2004;104:3865–71.
22. Novitzky N, Thomas V, du TC. Prevention of graft vs. host disease with alemtuzumab "in the bag" decreases early toxicity of stem cell transplantation and in multiple myeloma is associated with improved long-term outcome. Cytotherapy 2008;10:45–53.
23. Novitzky N, Thomas V. Allogeneic stem cell transplantation with T cell-depleted grafts for lymphoproliferative malignancies. Biol Blood Marrow Transplant. 2007;13:107–15.
24. Hale G, Jacobs P, Wood L, et al. CD52 antibodies for prevention of graft-versus-host disease and graft rejection following transplantation of allogeneic peripheral blood stem cells. Bone Marrow Transplant. 2000;26:69–76.
25. Kline J, Pollyea DA, Stock W, et al. Pre-transplant ganciclovir and post transplant high-dose valacyclovir reduce CMV infections after alemtuzumab-based conditioning. Bone Marrow Transplant. 2006;37:307–10.
26. Chakrabarti S, Mackinnon S, Chopra R, et al. High incidence of cytomegalovirus infection after nonmyeloablative stem cell transplantation: potential role of Campath-1H in delaying immune reconstitution. Blood 2002;99:4357–63.
27. Avivi I, Chakrabarti S, Milligan DW, et al. Incidence and outcome of adenovirus disease in transplant recipients after reduced-intensity conditioning with alemtuzumab. Biol Blood Marrow Transplant. 2004;10:186–94.
28. van Besien K, de Lima M, Artz A, et al. Alemtuzumab reduces chronic graft versus host disease (cGVHD) and treatment related mortality (TRM) after reduced intensity conditioning for AML and MDS. Blood (ASH Annual Meeting Abstracts). 2007;110:1076.
29. Shlomchik WD, Couzens MS, Tang CB, et al. Prevention of graft versus host disease by inactivation of host antigen-presenting cells. Science 1999;285:412–5.
30. Zhang PL, Malek SK, Prichard JW, et al. Monocyte-mediated acute renal rejection after combined treatment with preoperative Campath-1H (alemtuzumab) and postoperative immunosuppression. Ann Clin Lab Sci. 2004;34:209–13.
31. Trzonkowski P, Zilvetti M, Friend P, Wood KJ. Recipient memory-like lymphocytes remain unresponsive to graft antigens after CAMPATH-1H induction with reduced maintenance immunosuppression. Transplantation 2006;82:1342–51.
32. Simpson D. T-cell depleting antibodies: new hope for induction of allograft tolerance in bone marrow transplantation? BioDrugs 2003;17:147–54.
33. Ratzinger G, Reagan JL, Heller G, Busam KJ, Young JW. Differential CD52 expression by distinct myeloid dendritic cell subsets: implications for alemtuzumab activity at the level of antigen presentation in allogeneic graft-host interactions in transplantation. Blood 2003;101:1422–9.
34. Orsini E, Pasquale A, Maggio R, et al. Phenotypic and functional characterization of monocyte-derived dendritic cells in chronic lymphocytic leukaemia patients: influence of neoplastic CD19 cells in vivo and in vitro. Br J Haematol. 2004;125:720–8.
35. Morse MA, Mosca PJ, Clay TM, Lyerly HK. Dendritic cell maturation in active immunotherapy strategies. Expert Opin Biol Ther. 2002;2:35–43.
36. Kirsch BM, Haidinger M, Zeyda M, et al. Alemtuzumab (Campath-1H) induction therapy and dendritic cells: impact on peripheral dendritic cell repertoire in renal allograft recipients. Transpl Immunol. 2006;16:254–7.
37. Jordan MB, McClain KL, Yan X, Hicks J, Jaffe R. Anti-CD52 antibody, alemtuzumab, binds to Langerhans cells in Langerhans cell histiocytosis. Pediatr Blood Cancer. 2005;44:251–4.

38. Collin MP, Munster D, Clark G, et al. In vitro depletion of tissue-derived dendritic cells by CMRF-44 antibody and alemtuzumab: implications for the control of graft-versus-host disease. Transplantation 2005;79:722–5.
39. Buggins AG, Mufti GJ, Salisbury J, et al. Peripheral blood but not tissue dendritic cells express CD52 and are depleted by treatment with alemtuzumab. Blood 2002;100:1715–20.
40. Bayes M, Rabasseda X, Prous JR. Gateways to clinical trials. Methods Find Exp Clin Pharmacol. 2004;26:473–503.
41. Auffermann-Gretzinger S, Eger L, Schetelig J, et al. Alemtuzumab depletes dendritic cells more effectively in blood than in skin: a pilot study in patients with chronic lymphocytic leukemia. Transplantation 2007;83:1268–72.
42. Auffermann-Gretzinger S, Eger L, Bornhauser M, et al. Fast appearance of donor dendritic cells in human skin: dynamics of skin and blood dendritic cells after allogeneic hematopoietic cell transplantation. Transplantation 2006;81:866–73.
43. Gorgun G, Miller KB, Foss FM. Immunologic mechanisms of extracorporeal photochemotherapy in chronic graft-versus-host disease. Blood 2002;100:941–7.
44. Spisek R, Gasova Z, Bartunkova J. Maturation state of dendritic cells during the extracorporeal photopheresis and its relevance for the treatment of chronic graft-versus-host disease. Transfusion 2006;46:55–65.
45. Lamioni A, Parisi F, Isacchi G, et al. The immunological effects of extracorporeal photopheresis unraveled: induction of tolerogenic dendritic cells in vitro and regulatory T cells in vivo. Transplantation 2005;79:846–50.
46. Foss FM, Gorgun G, Miller KB. Extracorporeal photopheresis in chronic graft-versus-host disease. Bone Marrow Transplant. 2002;29:719–25.
47. Fimiani M, Di RM, Rubegni P. Mechanism of action of extracorporeal photochemotherapy in chronic graft-versus-host disease. Br J Dermatol. 2004;150:1055–60.
48. Di Renzo M, Sbano P, De Aloe G, et al. Extracorporeal photopheresis affects co-stimulatory molecule expression and interleukin-10 production by dendritic cells in graft-versus-host disease patients. Clin Exp Immunol. 2008;151:407–13.
49. Miller KB, Roberts TF, Chan G, et al. A novel reduced intensity regimen for allogeneic hematopoietic stem cell transplantation associated with a reduced incidence of graft-versus-host disease. Bone Marrow Transplant. 2004;33:881–9.
50. Crawley C, Iacobelli S, Bjorkstrand B, et al. Reduced-intensity conditioning for myeloma: lower nonrelapse mortality but higher relapse rates compared with myeloablative conditioning. Blood 2007;109:3588–94.
51. Hari P, Carreras J, Zhang MJ, et al. Allogeneic transplants in follicular lymphoma: higher risk of disease progression after reduced-intensity compared to myeloablative conditioning. Biol Blood Marrow Transplant. 2008;14:236–45.
52. Hansen JA, Gooley TA, Martin PJ, et al. Bone marrow transplants from unrelated donors for patients with chronic myeloid leukemia. N Engl J Med. 1998;338:962–8.
53. Giralt SA, Kantarjian HM, Talpaz M, et al. Effect of prior interferon alfa therapy on the outcome of allogeneic bone marrow transplantation for chronic myelogenous leukemia. J Clin Oncol. 1993;11:1055–61.
54. Kebriaei P, Detry MA, Giralt S, et al. Long-term follow-up of allogeneic hematopoietic stem-cell transplantation with reduced-intensity conditioning for patients with chronic myeloid leukemia. Blood 2007;110:3456–62.
55. Kerbauy FR, Storb R, Hegenbart U, et al. Hematopoietic cell transplantation from HLA-identical sibling donors after low-dose radiation-based conditioning for treatment of CML. Leukemia 2005;19:990–7.
56. Or R, Shapira MY, Resnick I, et al. Nonmyeloablative allogeneic stem cell transplantation for the treatment of chronic myeloid leukemia in first chronic phase. Blood 2003;101:441–5.

57. Das M, Saikia TK, Advani SH, Parikh PM, Tawde S. Use of a reduced-intensity conditioning regimen for allogeneic transplantation in patients with chronic myeloid leukemia. Bone Marrow Transplant. 2003;32:125–9.
58. Sloand E, Childs RW, Solomon S, et al. The graft-versus-leukemia effect of nonmyeloablative stem cell allografts may not be sufficient to cure chronic myelogenous leukemia. Bone Marrow Transplant. 2003;32:897–901.
59. Crawley C, Szydlo R, Lalancette M, et al. Outcomes of reduced-intensity transplantation for chronic myeloid leukemia: an analysis of prognostic factors from the Chronic Leukemia Working Party of the EBMT. Blood 2005;106:2969–76.
60. Weisser M, Schleuning M, Ledderose G, et al. Reduced-intensity conditioning using TBI (8 Gy), fludarabine, cyclophosphamide and ATG in elderly CML patients provides excellent results especially when performed in the early course of the disease. Bone Marrow Transplant. 2004;34:1083–8.
61. Oehler VG, Gooley T, Snyder DS, et al. The effects of imatinib mesylate treatment before allogeneic transplantation for chronic myeloid leukemia. Blood 2007;109:1782–9.
62. Anderlini P, Sheth S, Hicks K, et al. Re: imatinib mesylate administration in the first 100 days after stem cell transplantation. Biol Blood Marrow Transplant. 2004;10:883–4.
63. Olavarria E, Siddique S, Griffiths MJ, et al. Posttransplantation imatinib as a strategy to postpone the requirement for immunotherapy in patients undergoing reduced-intensity allografts for chronic myeloid leukemia. Blood 2007;110:4614–7.
64. Devine SM, Hoffman R, Verma A, et al. Allogeneic blood cell transplantation following reduced-intensity conditioning is effective therapy for older patients with myelofibrosis with myeloid metaplasia. Blood 2002;99:2255–8.
65. Rondelli D, Barosi G, Bacigalupo A, et al. Allogeneic hematopoietic stem-cell transplantation with reduced-intensity conditioning in intermediate- or high-risk patients with myelofibrosis with myeloid metaplasia. Blood 2005;105:4115–9.
66. Deeg HJ, Gooley TA, Flowers ME, et al. Allogeneic hematopoietic stem cell transplantation for myelofibrosis. Blood 2003;102:3912–8.
67. Laport GG, Sandmaier BM, Storer BE, et al. Reduced-intensity conditioning followed by allogeneic hematopoietic cell transplantation for adult patients with myelodysplastic syndrome and myeloproliferative disorders. Biol Blood Marrow Transplant. 2008;14:246–55.
68. Koh LP, Chen CS, Tai BC, et al. Impact of postgrafting immunosuppressive regimens on nonrelapse mortality and survival after nonmyeloablative allogeneic hematopoietic stem cell transplant using the fludarabine and low-dose total-body irradiation 200-cGy. Biol Blood Marrow Transplant. 2007;13:790–805.
69. Oran B, Giralt S, Saliba R, et al. Allogeneic hematopoietic stem cell transplantation for the treatment of high-risk acute myelogenous leukemia and myelodysplastic syndrome using reduced-intensity conditioning with fludarabine and melphalan. Biol Blood Marrow Transplant. 2007;13:454–62.
70. de Lima M, Anagnostopoulos A, Munsell M, et al. Non-Ablative versus reduced intensity conditioning regimens in the treatment of acute myeloid leukemia and high-risk myelodysplastic syndrome. Dose is relevant for long-term disease control after allogeneic hematopoietic stem cell transplantation. Blood 2004;104:865–72.
71. Kroger N, Bornhauser M, Ehninger G, et al. Allogeneic stem cell transplantation after a fludarabine/busulfan-based reduced-intensity conditioning in patients with myelodysplastic syndrome or secondary acute myeloid leukemia. Ann Hematol. 2003;82:336–42.
72. Shimoni A, Hardan I, Shem-Tov N, et al. Allogeneic hematopoietic stem-cell transplantation in AML and MDS using myeloablative versus reduced-intensity conditioning: the role of dose intensity. Leukemia 2006;20:322–8.
73. van Besien K, Artz A, Smith S, et al. Fludarabine, melphalan, and alemtuzumab conditioning in adults with standard-risk advanced acute myeloid leukemia and myelodysplastic syndrome. J Clin Oncol. 2005;23:5728–38.

74. Tauro S, Craddock C, Peggs K, et al. Allogeneic stem-cell transplantation using a reduced-intensity conditioning regimen has the capacity to produce durable remissions and long-term disease-free survival in patients with high-risk acute myeloid leukemia and myelodysplasia. J Clin Oncol. 2005;23:9387–93.
75. Maruyama D, Fukuda T, Kato R, et al. Comparable antileukemia/lymphoma effects in nonremission patients undergoing allogeneic hematopoietic cell transplantation with a conventional cytoreductive or reduced-intensity regimen. Biol Blood Marrow Transplant. 2007;13:932–41.
76. Girgis M, Hallemeier C, Blum W, et al. Chimerism and clinical outcomes of 110 recipients of unrelated donor bone marrow transplants who underwent conditioning with low-dose, single-exposure total body irradiation and cyclophosphamide. Blood 2005;105:3035–41.
77. Hallemeier C, Girgis M, Blum W, et al. Outcomes of adults with acute myelogenous leukemia in remission given 550 cGy of single-exposure total body irradiation, cyclophosphamide, and unrelated donor bone marrow transplants. Biol Blood Marrow Transplant. 2004;10:310–9.
78. Schmid C, Schleuning M, Schwerdtfeger R, et al. Long term survival in refractory acute myeloid leukemia after sequential treatment with chemotherapy and reduced intensity conditioning for allogeneic stem cell transplantation. Blood 2006;108:1092–9.
79. Blaise DP, Michel Boiron J, Faucher C, et al. Reduced intensity conditioning prior to allogeneic stem cell transplantation for patients with acute myeloblastic leukemia as a first-line treatment. Cancer 2005;104:1931–8.
80. Mutis T, Goulmy E. Hematopoietic system-specific antigens as targets for cellular immunotherapy of hematological malignancies. Semin Hematol. 2002;39:23–31.
81. Molldrem JJ. Vaccination for leukemia. Biol Blood Marrow Transplant. 2006;12:13–8.
82. de Lima M, Padua L, Giralt S, et al. A dose and schedule finding study of maintenance therapy with low-dose 5-azacitidine (AZA) after allogeneic hematopoietic stem cell transplantation (HSCT) for high-risk AML or MDS. Blood (ASH Annual Meeting Abstracts). 2007;110:3012.
83. de Lima M, Champlin RE, Thall PF, et al. Phase I/II study of gemtuzumab ozogamicin added to fludarabine, melphalan and allogeneic hematopoietic stem cell transplantation for high-risk CD33 positive myeloid leukemias and myelodysplastic syndrome. Leukemia 2008;22:258–64.
84. Casper J, Knauf W, Kiefer T, et al. Treosulfan and fludarabine: a new toxicity-reduced conditioning regimen for allogeneic hematopoietic stem cell transplantation. Blood 2004;103:725–31.
85. van Besien KW, Khouri IF, Giralt SA, et al. Allogeneic bone marrow transplantation for refractory and recurrent low grade lymphoma—the case for aggressive management. J Clin Oncol. 1995;13:1096–102.
86. van Besien K, Keralavarma B, Devine S, Stock W. Allogeneic and autologous transplantation for chronic lymphocytic leukemia. Leukemia 2001;15:1317–25.
87. van Besien K, Loberiza FR, Bajorunaite R, et al. Comparison of autologous and allogeneic hematopoietic stem cell transplantation for follicular lymphoma. Blood 2003;102:3521–9.
88. Khouri IF, Lee MS, Saliba RM, et al. Nonablative allogeneic stem cell transplantation for chronic lymphocytic leukemia: impact of rituximab on immunomodulation and survival. Exp Hematol. 2004;32:28–35.
89. Khouri IF, Saliba RM, Admirand J, et al. Graft-versus-leukaemia effect after non-myeloablative haematopoietic transplantation can overcome the unfavourable expression of ZAP-70 in refractory chronic lymphocytic leukaemia. Br J Haematol. 2007;137:355–63.
90. Sorror ML, Maris MB, Sandmaier BM, et al. Hematopoietic cell transplantation after nonmyeloablative conditioning for advanced chronic lymphocytic leukemia. J Clin Oncol. 2005;23:3819–29.

91. Rezvani AR, Storer B, Maris M, et al. Nonmyeloablative allogeneic hematopoietic cell transplantation in relapsed, refractory, and transformed indolent non-Hodgkin's lymphoma. J Clin Oncol. 2008;26:211–7.
92. Khouri IF, Saliba RM, Giralt SA, et al. Nonablative allogeneic hematopoietic transplantation as adoptive immunotherapy for indolent lymphoma: low incidence of toxicity, acute graft-versus-host disease, and treatment-related mortality. Blood 2001;98:3595–9.
93. Delgado J, Thomson K, Russell N, et al. Results of alemtuzumab-based reduced-intensity allogeneic transplantation for chronic lymphocytic leukemia: a British Society of Blood and Marrow Transplantation Study. Blood 2006;107:1724–30.
94. Sorror ML, Storer BE, Maloney DG, et al. Outcomes after allogeneic hematopoietic cell transplantation with nonmyeloablative or myeloablative conditioning regimens for treatment of lymphoma and chronic lymphocytic leukemia. Blood 2008;111:446–52.
95. Kahl C, Storer BE, Sandmaier BM, et al. Relapse risk in patients with malignant diseases given allogeneic hematopoietic cell transplantation after nonmyeloablative conditioning. Blood 2007;110:2744–8.
96. Faulkner RD, Craddock C, Byrne JL, et al. BEAM-alemtuzumab reduced-intensity allogeneic stem cell transplantation for lymphoproliferative diseases: GVHD, toxicity, and survival in 65 patients. Blood 2004;103:428–34.
97. Robinson SP, Goldstone AH, Mackinnon S, et al. Chemoresistant or aggressive lymphoma predicts for a poor outcome following reduced-intensity allogeneic progenitor cell transplantation: an analysis from the Lymphoma Working Party of the European Group for Blood and Bone Marrow Transplantation. Blood 2002;100:4310–6.
98. Khouri IF, Lee MS, Saliba RM, et al. Nonablative allogeneic stem-cell transplantation for advanced/recurrent mantle-cell lymphoma. J Clin Oncol. 2003;21:4407–12.
99. Maris MB, Sandmaier BM, Storer BE, et al. Allogeneic hematopoietic cell transplantation after fludarabine and 2 Gy total body irradiation for relapsed and refractory mantle cell lymphoma. Blood 2004;104:3535–42.
100. Gajewski JL, Phillips GL, Sobocinski KA, et al. Bone marrow transplants from HLA-identical siblings in advanced Hodgkin's disease. J Clin Oncol. 1996;14:572–8.
101. Anderlini P, Saliba R, Acholonu S, et al. Reduced-intensity allogeneic stem cell transplantation in relapsed and refractory Hodgkin's disease: low transplant-related mortality and impact of intensity of conditioning regimen. Bone Marrow Transplant. 2005;35:943–51.
102. Peggs KS, Hunter A, Chopra R, et al. Clinical evidence of a graft-versus-Hodgkin's-lymphoma effect after reduced-intensity allogeneic transplantation. Lancet 2005;365:1934–41.
103. Thomson KJ, Peggs KS, Smith P, et al. Superiority of reduced-intensity allogeneic transplantation over conventional treatment for relapse of Hodgkin's lymphoma following autologous stem cell transplantation. Bone Marrow Transplant. 2008 May; 41(9):765–70. Epub 2008 Jan 14.
104. Sureda A, Robinson S, Canals C, et al. Reduced-intensity conditioning compared with conventional allogeneic stem-cell transplantation in relapsed or refractory Hodgkin's lymphoma: an analysis from the Lymphoma Working Party of the European Group for Blood and Marrow Transplantation. J Clin Oncol. 2008;26:455–62.
105. Devetten MP, Hari P, Carerras J, et al. Unrelated donor nonmyeloablative/reduced intensity (NST/RIC) hematopoietic stem cell transplantation (HCT) for patients with relapsed and refractory Hodgkin's lymphoma (HL). Blood (ASH Annual Meeting Abstracts). 2006;108:601.
106. Pant S, Copelan EA. Hematopoietic stem cell transplantation in multiple myeloma. Biol Blood Marrow Transplant. 2007;13:877–85.

107. Bensinger WI. The current status of reduced-intensity allogeneic hematopoietic stem cell transplantation for multiple myeloma. Leukemia 2006;20:1683–9.
108. Maloney DG, Molina AJ, Sahebi F, et al. Allografting with nonmyeloablative conditioning following cytoreductive autografts for the treatment of patients with multiple myeloma. Blood 2003;102:3447–54.
109. Kroger N, Schwerdtfeger R, Kiehl M, et al. Autologous stem cell transplantation followed by a dose-reduced allograft induces high complete remission rate in multiple myeloma. Blood 2002;100:755–60.
110. Bruno B, Rotta M, Patriarca F, et al. A comparison of allografting with autografting for newly diagnosed myeloma. N Engl J Med. 2007;356:1110–20.
111. Garban F, Attal M, Michallet M, et al. Prospective comparison of autologous stem cell transplantation followed by dose-reduced allograft (IFM99-03 trial) with tandem autologous stem cell transplantation (IFM99-04 trial) in high-risk de novo multiple myeloma. Blood 2006;107:3474–80.
112. van Besien K, Bartholomew A, Stock W, et al. Fludarabine-based conditioning for allogeneic transplantation in adults with sickle cell disease. Bone Marrow Transplant. 2000;26:445–9.
113. Horwitz ME, Spasojevic I, Morris A, et al. Fludarabine-based nonmyeloablative stem cell transplantation for sickle cell disease with and without renal failure: clinical outcome and pharmacokinetics. Biol Blood Marrow Transplant. 2007;13:1422–6.
114. Walters MC, Patience M, Leisenring W, et al. Barriers to bone marrow transplantation for sickle cell anemia. Biol Blood Marrow Transplant. 1996;2:100–4.
115. Lucarelli G, Gaziev J. Advances in the allogeneic transplantation for thalassemia. Blood Rev. 2008;22:53–63.
116. Martino R, Valcarcel D, Brunet S, Sureda A, Sierra J. Comparable non-relapse mortality and survival after HLA-identical sibling blood stem cell transplantation with reduced or conventional-intensity preparative regimens for high-risk myelodysplasia or acute myeloid leukemia in first remission. Bone Marrow Transplant. 2008;41:33–8.
117. van Besien K, Artz A, Stock W. Unrelated donor transplantation over the age of 55. Are we merely getting (b)older? Leukemia. 2005;19:31–3.
118. Sorror ML, Maris MB, Storb R, et al. Hematopoietic cell transplantation (HCT)-specific comorbidity index: a new tool for risk assessment before allogeneic HCT. Blood 2005;106:2912–9.
119. Sorror ML, Giralt S, Sandmaier BM, et al. Hematopoietic cell transplantation specific comorbidity index as an outcome predictor for patients with acute myeloid leukemia in first remission: combined FHCRC and MDACC experiences. Blood 2007;110:4606–13.
120. Sorror M, Storer B, Sandmaier BM, et al. Hematopoietic cell transplantation-comorbidity index and Karnofsky performance status are independent predictors of morbidity and mortality after allogeneic nonmyeloablative hematopoietic cell transplantation. Cancer 2008 May 1;112(9):1992–2001.
121. Artz A, Pollyea D, Kocherginsky M, et al. Performance status and comorbidity predict transplant related mortality after allogeneic hematopoietic cell transplantation. Biol Blood Marrow Transplant. 2006 Sep;12(9):954–64.
122. Armand P, Kim HT, Cutler CS, et al. Prognostic impact of elevated pretransplantation serum ferritin in patients undergoing myeloablative stem cell transplantation. Blood 2007;109:4586–8.
123. Dinner SN, Artz A, Kocherginsky M, et al. Biomarkers to predict outcome after allogeneic hematopoietic cell transplant (HCT). Blood (ASH Annual Meeting Abstracts). 2007;110:1100.
124. Giralt S, Saliba RM, Mendoza F, et al. Pre transplant values of C reactive protein (CRP) and brain natriuretic peptide (BNP) as predictors of transplant outcomes in patients

with acute myelogenous leukemia or myelodysplastic syndromes (AML/MDS) undergoing allogeneic stem cell transplantation (AlloSCT). Blood (ASH Annual Meeting Abstracts). 2007;110:1984.
125. Sandmaier BM, Mackinnon S, Childs RW. Reduced intensity conditioning for allogeneic hematopoietic cell transplantation: current perspectives. Biol Blood Marrow Transplant. 2007;13:87–97.
126. Nieto Y, Patton N, Hawkins T, et al. Tacrolimus and mycophenolate mofetil after nonmyeloablative matched-sibling donor allogeneic stem-cell transplantations conditioned with fludarabine and low-dose total body irradiation. Biol Blood Marrow Transplant. 2006;12:217–25.
127. Stelljes M, Bornhauser M, Kroger M, et al. Conditioning with 8-Gy total body irradiation and fludarabine for allogeneic hematopoietic stem cell transplantation in acute myeloid leukemia. Blood 2005;106:3314–21.
128. Dasgupta RK, Rule S, Johnson P, et al. Fludarabine phosphate and melphalan: a reduced intensity conditioning regimen suitable for allogeneic transplantation that maintains the graft versus malignancy effect. Bone Marrow Transplant. 2006;37:455–61.
129. Shaw BE, Russell NH, Devereux S, et al. The impact of donor factors on primary non-engraftment in recipients of reduced intensity conditioned transplants from unrelated donors. Haematologica 2005;90:1562–9.
130. Spitzer TR, McAfee S, Sackstein R, et al. Intentional induction of mixed chimerism and achievement of antitumor responses after nonmyeloablative conditioning therapy and HLA-matched donor bone marrow transplantation for refractory hematologic malignancies. Biol Blood Marrow Transplant. 2000;6:309–20.

Chapter 10
Umbilical Cord Blood Transplantation

John E. Wagner, Claudio Brunstein, William Tse, and Mary Laughlin

10.1 Introduction

Use of umbilical cord blood (UCB) as a clinical source of hematopoietic stem cells (HSC) was first considered in the late 1960s. In the first known published report of its use, Ende et al. [1] infused freshly procured UCB samples from eight donors to a 16-year-old male with acute lymphocytic leukemia. While long-term hematopoietic reconstitution was not demonstrated, Ende et al. documented transient alteration in red cell antigens in the peripheral blood, suggesting a transient mixed chimerism from at least one UCB unit. Studies subsequently performed by Koike et al. [2] and Vidal et al. [3] in the late 1970s and early 1980s, however, provided for the first real evidence that UCB may contain sufficient numbers of hematopoietic progenitor cells for transplantation. However, it was not until experiments performed by Broxmeyer et al. [4] that ultimately led to the first UCB transplantation, which took place on October 6, 1988 at the Hôpital St. Louis in Paris for a child with Fanconi anemia [5]. Over the succeeding two decades, UCB was found to have several unique biological properties that established it as a major source of HSC for pediatric and adult transplantation [4, 6]. We summarize the current state of knowledge that supports its routine use, provide a rationale for an UCB selection algorithm, and suggest a list of research priorities for optimizing survival in recipients of UCB HSCs.

10.2 Attributes of UCB as a Graft Source for Transplantation

Broxmeyer et al. postulated that the number of hematopoietic progenitors in UCB had a greater capacity for expansion than those in bone marrow (BM), suggesting that UCB might be a suitable HSC source [4, 6]. Cardoso et al. also

J.E. Wagner (✉)
University of Minnesota, Minneapolis, MN, USA
e-mail: wagne002@maroon.tc.umn.edu

M.R. Bishop (ed.), *Hematopoietic Stem Cell Transplantation*,
Cancer Treatment and Research 144, DOI 10.1007/978-0-387-78580-6_10,

showed that the total CFU-GM production of UCB $CD34^+$ $CD38^-$ cells was 7.6-fold greater than that in a corresponding population in adult BM [7]. Consistent with these in vitro findings, UCB was also found to have a higher engrafting capability in a murine model than adult BM cells [8]. Through limiting dilution analysis, the frequency of SRC in UCB appeared to be 1 in 9.3×10^5 cells as compared to 1 in 3×10^6 in adult BM, and 1 in 6×10^6 in mobilized adult peripheral blood; overall UCB appeared to have about three to six times higher SRC content than adult BM and mobilized peripheral blood, respectively. On the basis of these and other observations, UCB was noted to contain higher concentrations of primitive hematopoietic progenitors with greater proliferative capacity as compared to adult HSC. These unique biological features suggested that UCB could be a useful clinical source of hematopoietic stem and progenitor cells for both children and adults.

Allogeneic BM transplantation (BMT) is associated with a high risk of acute and chronic graft-versus-host disease (GvHD), particularly in recipients who receive unmanipulated HLA-mismatched BM. Stringent HLA matching between donor-recipient significantly limits the wide use of BM from unrelated donors. While preclinical data strongly suggest that UCB may be a reliable source of HSC for hematopoietic reconstitution in myeloablated recipients, clinical investigators have argued that alloreactivity would be less pronounced due to the unique qualities of the neonatal immune system [9]. As UCB recipients in initial studies have been noted to tolerate one to two HLA antigens mismatched grafts UCB has emerge as an attractive alternative source of HSC for patients without HLA matched sibling donors.

Rainaut et al. and Hannet et al. found that, as compared to adult peripheral blood, UCB had a significantly lower percentage of $CD8^+$ T cells, and UCB lymphocytes had phenotypic characteristics of T cell "immaturity" [10, 11]. Hannet et al. observed co-expression of CD45RA on the majority of $CD4^+$ UCB lymphocytes (91% as compared to 40% of adult $CD4^+$ lymphocytes), fewer $CD3^+$ T cells with IL-2 receptors (8% vs. 18%), and fewer $CD3^+$ T cells with the activation markers (2% vs. 10%). Clement et al. demonstrated that $CD4^+CD45RA^+$ UCB T cells had no detectable helper function and their dominant immunoregulatory activity was suppression [12]. These observations suggested the "naïve" features of T-cells in UCB grafts might contribute to immune tolerance and have better transplant outcomes despite donor-recipient HLA disparity.

Later, Godfrey et al. [13] demonstrated a high frequency of regulatory T cells in UCB. These cells, characterized by the co-expression of CD4, CD25 and FoxP3, had been shown to be critically important in self-tolerance and the prevention of autoimmunity [14–18]. Several investigators showed that regulatory T cells markedly impaired the activation and expansion of alloreactive $CD4^+$ and $CD8^+$ T cells and GvHD decreased lethality in animal models [14–17].

Today, it is known that a single UCB unit usually contains a sufficient number of HSC for reliable engraftment in children but often insufficient for adults due to recipient's body size. The exact cell dose threshold is arguably at least 2.5×10^7 nucleated cells/kg recipient weight in order to attain a >90% likelihood of donor engraftment. It is also known that full HLA match is not required. While the maximally allowable HLA mismatch is not known, UCB units with one to two out of six mismatched antigens for HLA-A, -B and -DRB1 are acceptable.

10.3 Sibling Donor UCB Transplantation: Outcomes in Children

The first registry data reported the UCB transplantation outcomes from HLA matched and mismatched sibling donors in 1995 [19] and was updated in 1998 [20]. Seventy-four patients were transplanted with sibling UCB with the median age of 4.9 years (range 0.5–16.3). Among them, 56 patients received HLA zero to one antigen mismatched grafts and 18 received HLA two to three antigen mismatched grafts. For recipients of HLA zero to one antigen mismatched sibling UCB grafts, the probability of neutrophil recovery (defined as an absolute neutrophil count of $\geq 5 \times 10^8$/L) was 91% (±2) at 60 days after transplantation at a median of 22 days (range, 9–46). Despite overall high engraftment rates, there was a trend toward a greater risk of graft failure in recipients with nonmalignant hematologic disorders including marrow failure syndromes, hemoglobinopathies, or inherited metabolic disorders.

Gluckman et al. subsequently reported transplant outcomes in 74 recipients of related UCB [21]. The median age of the population was 5 years (range 0.2–20) with 46 patients having malignancies, 17 with BM failure syndromes, eight with hemoglobinopathy, and seven with inborn errors of metabolism. Sixty of the 74 patients received HLA-identical grafts. In contrast to the prior report [20], the probability of neutrophil engraftment was only 79%. Myeloid recovery and engraftment was favorably influenced by younger recipient age ($p = 0.02$), lower recipient body weight ($p = 0.02$), and HLA-identity ($p = 0.04$) with a trend toward better outcome in those with a higher nucleated cell dose ($p = 0.06$). This was the first report that suggested a possible relationship between nucleated cell dose of the UCB graft and myeloid engraftment. This finding suggested that a UCB graft with lower nucleated cell dose might have a higher risk of graft failure or markedly delayed myeloid recovery.

Importantly, in each of these initial reports, the incidence and severity of acute and chronic GvHD were surprisingly lower than expected among UCB recipients who received zero to one HLA mismatched sibling grafts. In the report by Wagner et al. [19], the probability of grade II–IV and grade III–IV GvHD was only 3% (±2) and 2% (±2), respectively. Limited chronic GvHD was only reported in three patients and no extensive chronic GvHD was observed. In the report by Gluckman et al. [21], the probability of grade II–IV

GvHD was 9% in recipients of HLA-matched UCB, with chronic GvHD observed only in eight of 56 patients who survived beyond day + 100 after transplantation.

Wagner et al. [20] reported a survival of 61% (±12) in recipients of zero to one HLA-antigen mismatched UCB grafts at a median follow-up of 2 years and similarly, Gluckman et al. [21] reported a survival of 63% at 1 year. Factors that favorably influenced survival were younger age ($p < 0.001$), lower recipient body weight ($p < 0.001$), HLA-identity ($p < 0.006$), and negativity of recipient pretransplant cytomegalovirus (CMV) serology ($p = 0.002$). While lower body weight was associated with improved outcome, cell dose was not identified as a key factor in these two studies, perhaps due to the limited number of patients and narrow range in the cell doses infused.

In the absence of a prospective randomized trial, a retrospective analysis of registry data was performed in order to assess the relative risks of delayed myeloid recovery or graft failure, GvHD, and mortality between UCB and adult donor HSC sources. In a joint study of the International Bone Marrow Transplant Registry and Eurocord, Rocha et al. compared the clinical outcomes in 113 HLA matched UCB recipients with 2052 HLA matched BM recipients [22]. It was the first report that documented a delayed myeloid recovery in UCB recipients (incidence 89% at a median of 26 days as compared to 98% at a median of 18 days, $p < 0.001$). Perhaps most importantly, it was also the first time showing that UCB recipients had lower incidence and severity of GvHD. Risk of grade II–IV acute GvHD was 14% in UCB recipients compared to 24% in BM recipients ($p = 0.02$). Survival rates after UCB and BM transplantation were similar at 3 years (64% vs. 66%, $p = 0.93$). Because of lower incidence of GvHD, concern was raised whether the UCB recipients might be at higher risk of disease relapse. In this analysis, however, relapse as a cause of death was no different in recipients of UCB compared to recipients of BM, suggesting that graft-versus-leukemia (GvL) was intact.

10.4 Unrelated Donor UCB Transplantation: Outcomes in Children

As a result of the early successes with sibling donor UCB transplantation, cord blood banking programs were rapidly initiated and expanded throughout U.S. and Europe. These efforts ultimately led to the first two reports on use of unrelated UCB transplantation in children in 1996 [23, 24]. These two studies clearly demonstrated that hematopoietic recovery and sustained engraftment could be achieved at least in children and possibly in smaller adults. Furthermore, incidence and severity of acute GvHD were surprisingly lower than expected, particularly given the fact that vast majority of patients received one to two HLA mismatched UCB units. Gluckman et al. subsequently reported the outcomes in 65 patients (median age = 9 years) transplanted with unrelated UCB [21]. Similar to the observations in the sibling UCB recipients, the probability of myeloid recovery was 87%. Notably, the UCB recipients who received median cell dose more than 3.7×10^7 NC/kg were more likely to have faster myeloid engraftment (25 days vs. 35 days) and higher probability of myeloid recovery (94% vs. 76%), clearly confirming the importance of UCB nucleated cell dose.

Rubinstein et al., next published a landmark study on unrelated UCB transplantation [25]. In this study patients either had a hematological malignancy ($n = 581$, 67%), genetic disease ($n = 209$, 24%), or acquired BM failure ($n = 79$, 9%) in the majority of pediatric patients (79%). In this report, the overall probability of myeloid recovery was 93%. This report again showed the importance of UCB cell dose on engraftment, risk of adverse events and survival. While a stepwise increase in graft nucleated cell dose was associated with a progressively shortened time to myeloid recovery, the incidence of myeloid recovery didn't significantly change once the nucleated cell dose exceeded 2.5×10^7/kg. In addition, HLA match level (HLA 0 vs. ≥ 1 mismatch) was also associated with myeloid engraftment. The median time to myeloid recovery in recipients of a 6/6 HLA matched UCB unit was 23 days as compared to 28 days in those transplanted with HLA mismatched units ($p = 0.0027$). However, engraftment was similar in recipients of 1 vs. 2 vs. 3 antigen mismatched UCB grafts.

Risk of acute GvHD varied between reports. In the study reported by Gluckman et al. and others, although a smaller series failed to detect any difference in risk of GvHD in recipients of HLA 1 vs. 2 antigens mismatched UCB grafts, Rubinstein et al. [25] found that risk of grade III–IV GvHD increased with increasing of mismatch level, i.e., 8% in 6/6 HLA-matched UCB, 19% in 5/6 HLA-matched UCB, and 28% in 4/6 HLA-matched UCB ($p = 0.006$). Even today, there are still conflicting results on the impact of HLA mismatch related to GvHD. Nonetheless, it is general consensus that the risk of GvHD is considerably lower than anticipated at the level of HLA mismatch in most UCB recipients compared with recipients of unrelated adult donor grafts.

In terms of survival, Gluckman et al. reported survival of 34% at 1 year and it was adversely affected by recipients with older age, female sex, and advanced stage of disease [26]. Notably, neither degree of HLA-mismatching nor cell dose was shown to influence survival. Rubinstein et al. reported 3-year survival of 48% in patients with genetic disease and 27% in patients with hematological malignancy. Risk factors for adverse transplant-related events were UCB graft low cell dose and HLA-mismatch [27]. This was the first time that survival of the UCB recipients was noted to be influenced by cell dose and HLA disparity. The literature on the use of unrelated donor UCB transplantation in children is summarized in Table 10.1.

Table 10.1 Unrelated UCB transplantation for children

	n	Age in years; median (range)	Cell dose $\times 10^7$/kg (range)	Median time to neutrophil recovery in days	Neutrophil engraftment (%)	Platelet engraftment (%)	Acute GVHD II–IV (%)	Acute GVHD III–IV (%)	GVHD chronic (%)	TRM (%)	Survival (%)
Wagner et al. [24] (Minnesota and Orange County)	18	2.6; (0.1–21.3)	4.1 (1.4–40.0)	24	100	77	50	11	NA	39	65% at 6 months
Kurtzberg et al. [23] (Duke)	25	7; (0.8–24)	3.0 (0.7–11)	22	92	NA	43	10	10	44 at 6 months	64% at 100 days
Gluckman et al. [21] (Registry)	65	9; (0.3–45)	3.7 (0.7–30)	30	87	39 at 60 days	40	NA	0	NA	29% at 1 year
Rubinstein et al. [27] (Registry)	864	NA; (79% <18)	NA	NA	93	NA	48	24	31	NA	27% at 3 year (leukemia), 48% at 3 year (genetic disease), 29% at 3 year (BM failure)
Wagner et al. [28] (Minnesota)	102	7; (0.2–57)	3.1 (0.7–58)	23	88	65 at 180 days	39	11	10	30 at 1 year	58% at 1 year, 70% at 1 year if dose > 1.7 $\times 10^5$ CD34$^+$/kg, 60% at 2 year (nonmalignant disease), 38% at 2 year (malignant disease)
Gluckman et al. [26] (Registry)	550	9.4; (4.5–21.1)	3.11 (1.9–5.2)	NA	76	43 at 60 days	36	20	26	34	34% at 3 years
Kurtzberg et al. [29] (COBLT)	191	7.7; (0.9–17.9)	5.1 (1.5–23.7)	27	80	50% at 180 days	42	21	20	17% at 100 days	50% at 2 year, influenced by CMV serostatus, ABO match, gender, and TNC.

GVHD graft-versus-host disease, *TRM* treatment-related mortality, *NA* not available, *BM* bone marrow, *TNC* total nucleated cell dose

10.5 Unrelated Donor UCB Transplantation: Outcomes in Adults

After the initial successes in children, UCB transplantation was extensively investigated in adults for whom a volunteer unrelated adult BM donor was not available. The first series of reports of unrelated UCB transplantation experience in adults were published together with pediatric population in 1996 [23, 24, 30]. In 2000 and 2001, the first three series specifically focused on the outcomes of UCB transplantation in adults were reported [31–33]. Laughlin et al. [31] reported the results in 68 adults (median age 31, range 17–58) with high-risk hematologic diseases who received 3–6/6 HLA matched UCB grafts. The probability of myeloid recovery was 90% at a median of 27 days. However, it is important to note that the Kaplan-Meyer estimate was as high as those reported in children, in part due to the high incidence of early death during the first 28 days, and these patients were censored in the analysis. In addition, the report does not indicate the number of potential adult recipients excluded on the basis of cell dose. Moreover, the incidence of grades II–IV and III–IV acute GvHD was higher than those previously reported in children (60% and 16%, respectively). Similar to observations in children, the incidence of severe acute GvHD was also not associated with UCB graft HLA disparity. The incidence of chronic GvHD was 33% for those survivors beyond day 100. Event free survival was only 26%, reflective in part of patient selection to include those with advanced disease and extensive pretreatment. Importantly, higher survival was observed in recipients who received cell doses $\geq 1.2 \times 10^5$/CD34/kg. Similarly, Rocha et al. [32] reported results in 108 adults (median age 26, range 15–53), with hematological malignancies who underwent UCB transplantation. The median time to myeloid recovery was 32 days. Grades II–IV acute GvHD was observed in 41% and chronic GvHD in 26% of the patients. Overall, 1-year survival was 27%.

Since the first successful UCB transplant in an adult with chronic myelogenous leukemia and emerging acute myeloid leukemia in 1996, and further publications focused on adults transplanted with UCB [34], to date nearly 3000 UCB transplants have been performed in adults >18 years of age. For patients with acute leukemia, the EFS has ranged from 15% to 50% [31, 33, 35–40] with some small series reporting up to 70% [41, 42]. Younger patients [33, 38] receiving higher UCB cell doses (nucleated cells, CD34, CFU-GM) with pretransplant CMV serum negativity [37] and pretransplant complete remission status [35, 41] generally have better outcomes. Over the past 5 years, there has been a growing interest in using UCB as an HSC source for adults. Despite the UCB cell dose barrier limiting its wide use in adult patients, UCB has received increasing attention in adult transplantation since UCB is readily available for transplantation without requirement for prolonged unrelated adult donor searching; this being beneficial for those patients requiring urgent treatment. The literature on the use of unrelated donor UCB transplantation in adults is summarized in Table 10.2.

Table 10.2 Unrelated UCB transplantation in adults

Reference	N	Median age (years)	Nucleated cell dose ($\times 10^7$/kg)	Median time to ANC $\geq$ 500/μL (days)	Median time to platelet recovery (20 or 50 $\times 10^9$/L)	Grades II–IV acute GVHD (%)	Extensive chronic GVHD (%)	DFS relapse	TRM (%)	EFS/OS	Comment
Rocha et al. [32]	108	26	1.7 (0.2–6.0)	32	129 (20)	41	26	NA	24	1-year OS 27%	None
Sanz et al. [33]	22	29	1.7 (1.0–5.0)	22	69 (20)	73	45	1-year DFS 53%	43 at 100 days	NA	Patients younger than 30 years have better DFS Alive at 1 year without disease: AML 3/3, MDS 1/1, CML 5/12
Laughlin et al. [31]	68	31	1.6 (0.6–4.0)	27	99 (50)	60	33	22 months DFS 26%	50 at 100 days	OS 28% 22 months[c]	Higher CD34$^+$ cell dose improves EFS
Ooi et al. [39]	7	38	2.2 (2.1–4.0)	24	49(50)	2/7	1/6	Relapse 2/7	NA	OS 5/7 12 months[c]	None
Long et al. [38]	57	31	1.5 (0.5–2.8)	28	84 (20)	30	32	3-year EFS 15%	50% at 100 days	3-year OS 19%	Patients younger than 31 years have better EFS
Ooi et al. [43]	18	43	2.5[b] (1.2–5.5)	23	49 (50)	65	NA	2-year LFS 77%	NA	14/18 pts	De novo acute myeloid leukemia
Iori et al. [37]	42	12	3.2 (1.3–10.9)	29	63 (20)	21	20	4-year LFS 47%, 4-year relapse 28%	28 at 4 years	4-year EFS 46%, 4-year OS 45%	Relapse for AML:1/13 Higher CFU-GM and negative CMV sorology associated with improved OS
Kai et al.[a] [44]	11	33	3.9[b] (2.8–4.8)	21	53 (50)	44	Zero	NA	NA	NA	Abstract
Barker et al.[a] [41]	23	24	3.5 (1.1–6.3)	23	71%(50) at 6 months	65	23	1-year DFS 57%	22	NA	1-year DFS for patients in remission 72% and in relapse 25%

Table 10.2 (continued)

Reference	N	Median age (years)	Nucleated cell dose ($\times 10^7$/kg)	Median time to ANC $\geq$ 500/μL (days)	Median time to platelet recovery (20 or 50×10^9/L)	Grades II–IV acute GVHD (%)	Extensive chronic GVHD (%)	DFS relapse	TRM (%)	EFS/OS	Comment
Cornetta et al. [36]	34	34	2.3[b] (1.4–5.5)	31	117 (20)	34	21	1-year relapse 46%	NA	1-year OS 17%	COBLT
Ooi et al. [45]	22	40	2.4[b] (1.8–4.1)	21	49 (50)	33	42	4-year DFS 76% relapse 4/22	NA	NA	Myelodysplastic syndrome
Konuma et al. [42]	11	51	2.5[b] (2.1–3.5)	19.5	42 (50)	4/10	2/8	2-year DFS 73% relapse 3/11	0	OS 8/11 24 months[c]	Patients 50–55 years old undergoing myeloablative conditioning 2-year DFS for AML 34%, MDS 25%, CML 19%, and sAL 22%
Arcese et al. [35]	171	29	2.1 (0.8–7.3)	28	84 (20)	25	36	2-year DFS 27%, 2-year relapse 22%	51% at 2 years	2-year OS 33%	2-year relapse for CML 5.5% and MDS 31% Advanced disease and non-CML higher relapse risk Advanced disease, pt female gender and major ABO incompatibility poorer DFS

HSC hematopoietic stem cell, *DFS* disease-free survival, *LFS* leukemia-free survival, *EFS* event-free survival, *OS* overall survival, *URD* unrelated, *UCB* umbilical cord blood, *CML* chronic myelogenous leukemia, *UCBT* umbilical cord blood transplantation, *AML* acute myeloid leukemia, *MDS* myelodysplastic syndrome, *NA* not available, *sAML* secondary acute myeloid leukemia

[a]Double UCB unit graft

[b]Cryopreserved cell dose

[c]Median follow-up

10.5.1 UCB: A New "Standard of Care" for Children and Adults

Until 2000, BM from HLA matched related and unrelated donors were considered to be the "gold standard" and the first choice of HSC source for hematologic malignancies and metabolic disorders. UCB has emerged as an alternative HSC source over the past decade. The increasing use of UCB is mainly attributed to the following: (1) evidence of favorable results in children, (2) growing availability of UCB units with larger cell doses, (3) emerging acceptance of "double" UCB platform (i.e., use of two UCB units from two partially HLA matched donors in rapid series), (4) rapid donor identification and cell acquisition, and (5) better tolerance of HLA disparity. Due to the fact that for the majority of ethnic minority patients in the USA today identification of HLA matched donors either within the family or in adult marrow donor registries is difficult, there is a continued need to investigate UCB as alternative stem cell sources for these patients.

Based on the data available today, we describe the views of two transplant teams experienced in both marrow and UCB transplantation, with focus on (1) the place of UCB as a source of HSC for specific circumstances, (2) approach to selecting the best UCB unit(s) for potential patients, and (3) research priorities in the field of UCB transplantation.

10.5.2 For Pediatric Patients with Acute Leukemia, What is the Best HSC Source?

Minnesota Position: A 4–6/6 HLA matched UCB is the first choice even if an 8/8 allele HLA matched BM donor is available. When the transplant is urgent or a 6/6 HLA matched UCB unit is available, UCB has the advantage.

Several studies have been reported comparing outcomes in pediatric recipients of UCB and unrelated BM. One of the first reports was a matched-pair analysis (matching: age, diagnosis and disease stage) at the University of Minnesota, comparing the outcomes principally in pediatric patients transplanted either with zero to three HLA-A, -B, -DRB1 mismatched UCB or HLA-A, -B, -DRB1-matched BM [46]. While myeloid recovery was significantly slower after UCB transplantation, incidence of engraftment by day 45 was similar. Likewise, incidences of acute and chronic GvHD were similar. Overall, the probability of survival after UCB transplantation was 53% vs. 41% in BM recipients ($p = 0.40$). This study suggested that despite increased HLA disparity in recipients of UCB, survival rates were similar to recipients of HLA-matched unrelated donor BM.

More recently a collaboration of the New York Blood Center and the Center for International Blood and Marrow Transplant Research (CIBMTR) compared the outcomes of children receiving HLA-matched and mismatched UCB ($n = 503$) or 8/8 allele HLA matched unrelated donor BM ($n = 116$) [47]. All patients had acute leukemia and were younger than 16 years undergoing myeloablative transplantation. In comparison with allele-matched BM transplants, 5-year leukemia-free survival (LFS) was similar to that after transplants with UCB mismatched at one to two loci with potentially superior results in recipients of HLA matched UCB. For recipients of 8/8 allele HLA matched marrow, 6/6 antigen HLA matched UCB, 5/6 antigen HLA matched UCB (cell dose $> 3.0 \times 10^7$ NC/kg) and 4/6 antigen HLA matched UCB (any cell dose), the adjusted LFS rates were 38%, 60%, 45%, and 33%.

In summary, these data establish the role of UCB in transplant medicine and support its use as front line therapy for pediatric patients with malignancy (especially when transplant is urgent) even when marrow donors are potentially available. This position is further supported by a recent report by the Institute of Medicine of the U.S. National Academy of Sciences, which demonstrates that UCB use matches that of BM as a source of HSCs for unrelated donor transplantation in children [48].

Case Western Position: An 8/8 or 10/10 matched BM is still the first choice. However, if there is 6/6 HLA matched UCB unit with cell count $> 3.0 \times 10^7$/kg available, it may be the preferable choice. When the transplant is urgent and a 4–6/6 HLA matched UCB unit is available, UCB has the advantage.

With the concern of low cell dose, its effect on prolonged neutrophil recovery, and treatment-related mortality (TRM), the Case group still chooses 8/8 or 10/10 matched BM as the first choice at the present time. However, emerging data from the CIBMTR suggest an advantage of using 6/6 matched UCB [47], especially when BM is not immediately available. In 35 pediatric leukemia patients who received 6/6 matched UCB, the risk of transplanted-related mortality was very low compared to recipients who received 8/8 matched BM [47]. Despite having increased TRM in 4–5/6 mismatched UCB recipients of any cell dose, treatment failure in these patients was mostly due to low cell dose. However, mismatched UCB seemed to provide lower risk of relapse. The CIBMTR data provided encouraging results that one to two mismatched single units of UCB have comparable 5-year LFS [47]. With increasing data on the use of two UCB units double UCB transplantation may be an alternative strategy to overcome the limitations of cell dose.

For patients with high risk features and for whom transplants are urgently needed, such as those with acute leukemia beyond CR1, 4–6/6 HLA matched UCB has clear advantages over HLA-matched BM from unrelated adult donors. When multiple UCB units are available, priority is given to those units with allele level matching at HLA-DRB1 (New York Blood Center, MD, C. Stevens, personal communication).

In summary, retrospective data from large data registries support the use of HLA matched and mismatched UCB as an alternative HSC source for pediatric leukemia patients. Recently published CIBMTR data also provided evidence for the use of HLA 6/6 matched UCB over HLA-matched BM when available.

10.5.3 For Pediatric Patients with Nonmalignant Disease, What is the Best HSC Source?

Minnesota Position: An 8/8 allele HLA matched BM is the optimal graft in most circumstances. If transplant is urgent or a 6/6 HLA matched UCB unit what is adequate cell dose is available, UCB has the advantage.

In recent years, there have been more reports on the use of UCB for the treatment of nonmalignant diseases. Based on the types of diseases (e.g., metabolic diseases, hemoglobinopathies, and immune deficiencies), most such transplants are performed in children. Reports of UCB transplantation for the treatment of children in patients with sickle cell disease and β-thalassemia have shown high rates of engraftment and encouraging survival [49–53]. More recently, Walters et al. [54] have shown that engraftment and survival rates are similar in those transplanted with UCB and BM from HLA matched donors. In addition, unrelated donor UCB has been shown to be useful in the treatment of patients with specific inborn errors of metabolism. As hematopoietic elements circulate throughout the body, including the central nervous system, partial or complete chimerism is often associated with stabilization (and in some cases improvement) in the central and peripheral manifestations of these disorders. In the COBLT study that included patients with lysosomal and peroxisomal storage diseases, the 1-year survival was 72% [55]. However, results vary with stage of disease and age of the recipient [56, 57].

Certainly, larger numbers of patients and longer follow-up are needed to understand the true benefit of UCB in the setting of nonmalignant disease. Furthermore, comparative studies are required to determine how the outcomes of UCB transplant compare to BM. Whether UCB offers advantages over BM remains to be proven. However, it is unequivocally clear that UCB is (1) associated with less GvHD, which has no beneficial effect in this setting (in contrast to the setting of malignant disease); and (2) more rapidly available (which is particularly critical for rapidly progressive neurological diseases). However, if graft rejection occurs after UCB transplantation, the donor is not available for reharvesting or donor lymphocyte collection. Overall, the available clinical data support the use of UCB as a source of HSC for the transplantation of children with nonmalignant diseases—perhaps as a secondary choice if an 8/8 allele HLA-matched donor is unavailable.

Case Western Position: A 6/6 matched UCB with cell dose $>3.0 \times 10^7$/kg is the preferred first choice even when a 6/6 or 8/8 matched BM/PBSC unit is available. When the transplant is urgent or a $\geq$4/6 HLA matched UCB unit is available, UCB has the advantage.

The experience of using UCB as an HSC source for pediatric nonhematologic diseases is less comprehensive as compared to that for pediatric leukemia. Two recent reports by the Duke Pediatric Program support the use of UCB for infants with inherited metabolic disorders. First, Infantile Krabbe's disease produces progressive neurologic deterioration and death in early childhood.

Eleven asymptomatic newborns (age range, 12–44 days) and 14 symptomatic infants (age range, 142–352 days) with infantile Krabbe's disease underwent transplantation of UCB from unrelated donors after myeloablative chemotherapy. The rates of engraftment and survival were 100% and 100%, respectively, among the asymptomatic newborns (median follow-up, 3.0 years) and 100% and 43%, respectively, among the symptomatic infants (median follow-up, 3.4 years). Infants who underwent transplantation before the development of symptoms showed progressive central myelination and continued gains in developmental skills, and most had age-appropriate cognitive function and receptive language skills, but a few had mild-to-moderate delays in expressive language and mild-to-severe delays in gross motor function. Children who underwent transplantation after the onset of symptoms had minimal neurologic improvement [56].

Hurler syndrome (the most severe form of mucopolysaccharidosis type I) causes progressive deterioration of the central nervous system and death in childhood. Twenty consecutive children with Hurler syndrome received busulfan, cyclophosphamide, and antithymocyte globulin before receiving UCB transplants from unrelated donors. UCB donors had normal alpha-L-iduronidase activity (mean number of cells = 10.53×10^7/kg of body weight) and were discordant for up to three of six HLA markers. Neutrophil engraftment occurred at a median of 24 days after transplantation. Five patients had grade II or grade III acute GvHD; none had extensive chronic GvHD. Seventeen of the 20 children were alive at a median of 905 days after transplantation, with complete donor chimerism and normal peripheral-blood alpha-L-iduronidase activity noted (event-free survival rate = 85%). Transplantation improved neurocognitive performance and decreased somatic features of Hurler's syndrome [57]. Taken together, transplantation of UCB from unrelated donors in inherited metabolic disorders favorably alters the natural history of the disease.

10.5.4 For Adult Patients with Acute Leukemia, What is the Best HSC Source?

Minnesota Position: A 4–6/6 HLA matched UCB and graft cell dose exceeding 3×10^7 nucleated cells/kg should be considered at least as a reasonable alternative if an 8/8 allele HLA matched BM is not available or if transplant is urgent. However, practice at Minnesota is to use 1–2 units of partially HLA matched UCB in preference to 8/8 matched marrow.

Studies comparing outcomes in adult recipients of UCB have demonstrated similar or inferior results in recipients of HLA matched BM. Rocha et al. reported a matched-pair analysis comparing outcomes in adult recipients of UCB ($n = 81$) and BM ($n = 162$) with acute leukemia [58]. They reported that myeloid recovery, as in children, was significantly delayed (median 28 days vs. 19 days), and acute GvHD was less (31% vs. 41%, $p = 0.05$). Incidences of chronic GvHD, TRM and relapse were comparable between groups as was disease-free survival (26% in recipients of UCB and 33% in recipients of BM, $p = 0.28$). In contrast, Laughlin et al. [59] found that recipients of UCB had inferior leukemia free-survival as compared to recipients of HLA matched BM, while Takahashi et al. [60] found that recipients of UCB had superior survival. In a meta-analysis performed by Hwang et al. [61], the authors suggested that the differences between these three studies in terms of survival could not be entirely explained by differences in recipient HLA match, body weight, and cell doses. The reasons for the different outcomes between studies remain to be determined.

In summary, these reports support the use of UCB in adults at least for those who cannot identify a suitably HLA matched unrelated volunteer donor in the time interval mandated by the individual patient's disease status. Because of the unavailability of randomized, controlled trials comparing UCB and BM or peripheral blood from unrelated donors, we must rely on retrospective analyses. It is unlikely that a randomized trial will be performed until most adults can find a "suitable" UCB graft. While cord blood banks are now focused on the storage of larger units, still only 30% of adults are able to identify an appropriately HLA matched single unit of sufficient cell dose. New strategies are being developed that may reduce or eliminate the cell dose limitation (see Research Priorities, below).

Case Western Position: An 8/8 or 10/10 matched BM remains the first choice. However, if there is 6/6 HLA matched UCB unit with cell count $> 2.5 \times 10^7$/kg available, it may be an equally preferable choice because of its desirable early post-transplant survival. When the transplant is urgent or a 4–6/6 HLA matched UCB unit is available, UCB has the advantage.

However, local studies support the use of partially HLA matched single unit UCB if the cell dose is $>3 \times 10^7$/kg. Otherwise, the use of two partially HLA matched units that together provide a cell dose $>3.0 \times 10^7$/kg with results similar to those observed with sibling donors discuss further in section 10.6.

Laughlin and Rocha reported the UCB transplant experiences in adult hematologic malignancies from North America and Europe and further confirmed that UCB is a valuable alternative source of HSC for adult patients when HLA matched HSC is not readily available [59, 58, 62]. However, the incidence of chronic GvHD was higher among recipients of mismatched UCB in the North American study, which might partly explain the inferior outcomes in recipients of mismatched UCB compared with recipients of matched HSC. With increasing experience of using UCB and improving peritransplantation supportive care for adult leukemia patients, it is important to examine the clinical outcome in adult leukemia patients who receive HLA matched UCB containing higher cell doses.

10.5.5 For Adult Patients with Nonmalignant Disease, What is the Best HSC Source?

Minnesota Position: Use of UCB should be considered only in the absence of an 8/8 allele HLA matched BM.

At this time, there are too few reports available to make an informed statement regarding the use of UCB. At a minimum, only 4–6/6 HLA matched units with cell doses greater than 2.5×10^7 nucleated cells/kg should be routinely offered to adult patients with nonmalignant diseases if an 8/8 HLA matched marrow donor is not available.

Case Western Position: When a 6/6 matched UCB unit or 4–5/6 mismatched UCB unit with cell dose $> 2.5 \times 10^7$cells/kg is available, UCB as an alternative HSC source should be considered for adult patients with nonmalignant disease. However, using 8/8 or 10/10 HLA matched BM remains the first choice.

Allogeneic HSCT for nonmalignant diseases is less frequently used compared to adults. However, there is no need for a graft-versus-tumor effect. Therefore, UCB grafts are especially attractive because of lower incidence of severe GvHD even in recipients receiving mismatched UCB units. However, there is scarce clinical data in this area, and multi-institutional clinical trials to address this area are warranted.

10.6 Identification of the Optimal UCB Graft

As of 2008, it remains unclear as to what "makes" the best UCB unit for a specific patient. However, it is clear that there are at least three factors, namely, donor–recipient HLA match, graft cell dose, and recipient diagnosis disease status, all of which play important roles in survival outcome. The debate today relates to the relative weight assignment for each of the two graft factors.

Minnesota Position: For patients with malignant disease, UCB grafts most often are composed of 2 units from partially HLA matched donors because of possible augmentation in GvL effect. For patients with nonmalignant disease, UCB grafts are most often are composed of a single unit with high cell dose, if available. Because of increased risk of grade II acute GvHD in recipients of two units, which is not advantageous in patients with nonmalignant disease.

At the University of Minnesota, the initial search is limited to all UCB units with at least a 4–6/6 HLA match (with antigen level typing at HLA-A and -B, and allele level typing at HLA-DRB1 with no recognition of HLA-C, -DQ or -DP at the time of donor selection) and cell dose greater than 1.5×10^7 nucleated cells/kg actual recipient body weight. If a unit exists that has a cell dose greater than 3.0×10^7 nucleated cells/kg and 6/6 HLA match, dose greater than 4.0×10^7 nucleated cells/kg and 5/6 HLA match or dose greater than 5.0×10^7 nucleated cells/kg and 4/6 HLA match, a single unit may be selected with highest priority given to the best matched unit. While the optimal cell dose for each degree of HLA match or mismatch is unknown, the principal is clear that higher cell doses minimize the adverse effect of HLA mismatch.

In patients with malignant disease, GvL appears to be enhanced in recipients of two units. For this reason, it could be argued that such patients should be offered two units even if a single unit exists with the cell doses described above.

In patients with nonmalignant disease, better HLA match as well as higher cell dose unit are associated with less transplant related mortality. As risk of GvHD is higher in recipients of two units, it could be argued that such patients should preferentially be offered a large single unit if it is available.

The complexity of choosing two UCB units is problematic because there is no way to predict which unit will predominate. It is clear that in >95% of recipients of two UCB units, only one unit will contribute to hematopoiesis by day 100 regardless of type of preparative therapy (myeloablative versus non myeloablative therapy). Despite unproven assumptions, the following is the current method for selecting the two UCB units.

Step (1) Unit 1 is the "best" single unit that is available—having the best HLA match followed by the best cell dose

Step (2) Unit 2 is the second "best" unit that is available that not only has the best HLA match and best cell dose for the recipient but one that is also partially HLA matched with unit 1.

The best unit is defined in order of priority (1–15 below, see Table 10.3)

It is important to point out that unit 2 is often not the next best unit because of the intra-unit HLA matching requirement. In addition, there are other factors that may influence the final selection of units 1 and 2; these include (a) attributes of the cord blood bank (i.e., some cord blood banks do not meet all the criteria of the Minnesota Program; some banks have a track record of slow response time and poor service), (b) lack of infectious disease serology, (c) lack of attached segments for quality control testing (i.e., proof of unit identity and HLA type), (d) high cost (i.e., poor exchange rates, payment requirement prior to unit confirmation), (e) high numbers of nucleated red cells, (f) positive cultures. Selection of the two units, however, has become easier with the advent of the National Marrow Donor Program cord blood search tools.

Case Western Position:

Recent data in UCB allogeneic transplantation in adult hematologic malignancy patients supports a strong rationale for use of two UCB grafts, HLA matched at four of six loci or better to the patient, in the circumstance where a single UCB unit of sufficient cell dose exceeding 2.5×10^7/kg is not available.

Therefore, current institutional protocols at Case Western stipulate that final selection of the optimal UCB graft is based on consideration of the nucleated cell content of the unit and type and degree of HLA disparity. With

Table 10.3 UCB Graft Selection Prioritization

	Cell dose levels						
HLA match	1.5–2.0	2.1–2.5	2.6–3.0	3.1–3.5	3.6–4.0	4.1–4.5	4.6–5.0
HLA 6/6	3	2	1				
HLA 5/6	8	7	6	5	4		
HLA 4/6	15	14	13	12	11	10	9

The best unit is defined in order of priority (1–15)

low resolution typing, six loci are considered while in high resolution typing, 12 loci are considered. When more than one similarly matching unit is available, cell dose $\geq 2.5 \times 10^7$ cells/kg and genetic identity at the DR > B > A loci are preferred. For those patients lacking an identified single UCB graft containing a minimum nucleated cell dose exceeding 2.5×10^7/kg actual patient body weight, two UCB units are selected using the following criteria:

- Each unit must be at least a 4/6 HLA-A/B/DRB1 match to the recipient. A 6/6 matched unit is selected before a 5/6, which will be selected before a 4/6 antigen matched unit.
- The two units selected must be at least a 4/6 match with each other.
- Each unit must have a combined cryopreserved dose of at least 1.5×10^7 TNC/kg. based on actual body weight for calculating the graft cell dose.

The doses of graft-nucleated cells and $CD34^+$ hematopoietic progenitor cells are predictors of allogeneic engraftment and survival in UCB recipients. In a recent single institution prospective phase II trial published by the Case Western group, flow cytometric analyses of $CD34^+$ progenitor and lymphocyte populations in unmodified single units of HLA-disparate UCB grafts that were infused into 31 consecutive adults (median age = 41 years; range, 20–64) receiving myeloablative conditioning were compared with transplant outcomes including engraftment, GvHD, and survival. Median infused UCB graft-nucleated cells and $CD34^+$ cell dose was 2.2×10^7/kg and 1.2×10^5/kg, respectively. Days to absolute neutrophil count equal to or greater than 0.5×10^9/L in recipients reached full donor chimerism averaged 27 day (range 12–41). Univariate analyses demonstrated that UCB graft-infused cell doses of $CD34^+$ ($p = 0.015$), $CD3^+$ ($p = 0.024$), and $CD34^+HLADR^+CD38^+$ progenitors ($p = 0.043$) correlated with neutrophil engraftment. This analysis did not demonstrate a correlation between $CD34^+$ ($p = 0.11$), $CD3^+$ ($p = 0.28$), or $CD34^+HLADR^+CD38^+$ ($p = 0.108$) cell dose and event-free survival (EFS). High-resolution matching for HLA-class II (DRB1) resulted in improved EFS ($p = 0.02$) and decreased risk for acute GvHD ($p = 0.004$). Early mortality (prior to post-transplant day + 28) occurred in three patients, while 26 patients achieved myeloid engraftment. These results suggest that UCB graft matching at DRB1 is an important risk factor for acute GvHD and survival, while higher UCB graft cell doses of $CD34^+$, committed $CD34^+$ progenitors, and $CD3^+$ T cells favorably influence UCB allogeneic engraftment [63].

10.7 Research Priorities

10.7.1 Augmentation of Cell Dose

Clearly, cell dose is the most critical factor that prevents increasing utilization of UCB. Low cell dose UCB magnifies the deleterious effect of HLA mismatch and is responsible for delayed hematopoietic recovery, poor engraftment, high TRM, and poor survival. Therefore, novel strategies are urgently needed to augment the “effective” cell dose of the UCB graft. There are several possible approaches that can be considered, the most obvious being ex vivo expansion culture, strategies to reduce nonspecific losses of UCB HSC and enhance homing to the marrow microenvironment, and co-infusion of a “carrier” population to provide a more rapid early wave of hematopoietic recovery. In addition, novel strategies are needed for reducing TRM and speeding immune recovery, which is particularly important for adults.

Among many strategies currently being explored to enhance engraftment, utilization of two partially HLA matched UCB units as a graft source needs to be considered a high priority [64–66]. In the myeloablative and nonmyeloablative setting, the use of the “double UCB platform” has met with considerable success. Results thus far in more than 350 double UCB transplants have demonstrated a high probability of hematopoietic recovery, low TRM, and low risk of relapse. Due to the absence of life-threatening toxicity, this approach has substantially increased the availability of UCB transplantation to most adults, with 93% having successful searches at the U of M. Still, there is room for improvement. Based on the Minnesota experience in nearly 100 patients transplanted after myeloablation, the median time to myeloid recovery is 21 days with sustained engraftment observed in 87% of recipients. While markedly improved from historical experiences in adults, more rapid recovery and 100% engraftment are goals yet to be achieved. At this time, a phase II trial of “double UCB transplantation” in adults is in the final stages of development, and a prospective, randomized phase III clinical trial in children has 1-year leukemia free survival as the primary end point, comparing single versus double UCB transplantation as part of the NIH-sponsored Blood and Marrow Transplant Clinical Trials Network (BMT-CTN). The goal is to establish greater experience with the double UCB platform and prove its safety and efficacy, respectively.

10.7.2 Reduction in Risk of TRM

At the University of Minnesota, more than 170 UCB transplants have been performed after a non myeloablative conditioning, primarily in older adults. Analysis of the outcomes in the first 110 patients [64] receiving fludarabine 40 mg/m^2/day for 5 days, cyclophosphamide 50 mg/kg/day for 1 day and low-dose TBI (200 cGy) in a single fraction without shielding has demonstrated myeloid recovery in 92% at a median of 12 days (range: 0–32). Incidences at day 100 of grades II–IV and grades III–IV acute GvHD were 59% (95%CI: 49–69%) and 22% (95%CI: 14–30%), respectively. Incidence of TRM, however, was 19% (95%CI: 12–26%) at day 180. The only risk factor for TRM in Cox regression analysis was the presence of pretransplant comorbidities. For this heterogeneous group of older adults or patients with comorbidities or extensive prior therapy, the probability of survival was 45% and progressive free survival was 38% (95% CI: 28–48%). In multivariate analysis, presence of comorbidities adversely influenced PFS, and use of two UCB units was associated with a trend toward improved PFS ($p = 0.06$).

Based on the report by Rocha et al. [67], the combination of cyclophosphamide, fludarabine, and TBI (200 cGy) may be the most effective to date in terms of engraftment and survival after UCB transplantation for adults with lymphoid malignancy. While this approach has markedly extended the age limit and donor availability for many patients potentially cured by hematopoietic stem cell transplantation clearly additional strategies are needed to reduce TRM for those with comorbidities.

10.7.3 Reduction in the Interval of Immunodeficiency

The transplant program at Case Western has conducted a retrospective study of rates and kinetics of bacterial, fungal, and viral infections in 51 adult patients with hematologic disorders treated concurrently and consecutively at this institution with myeloablation and transplantation with either unrelated HLA partially matched UCB (28 patients) or HLA-matched adult URD grafts (23 patients) [68]. These transplant recipients were evaluated for life-threatening infections, hematologic reconstitution, GvHD, relapse, and event-free (EFS) survival. UCB recipients received grafts containing a lower nucleated cell dose (mean $2.1 \times 10^7/\text{kg} \pm 0.93$) compared with recipients of HSC from unrelated adult donors ($78.6 \times 10^7/\text{kg} \pm 73.8$), and the median duration of neutropenia after transplantation was longer (29 days vs. 14 days) in the UCB group ($p = 0.0001$). Probability of neutrophil engraftment by day 42 was 0.86 (95% CI: 0.71, 1.0) in UCB recipients versus 0.96 (95% CI: 0.87, 1.0) in adult URD recipients surviving >28 days. Overall infection rates and rates of bacterial infections, especially gram-positive organisms after transplant, were higher in UCB recipients, particularly at early time points (prior to day + 50). Bacterial infection rate prior to day + 50 in UCB recipients was 3.1 compared with 1.25 in URD recipients ($p = 0.003$). Graft failure occurred in five UCB recipients and two URD recipients and was noted to be associated with the occurrence of bacteremia during neutropenia ($p = 0.04$) [68]. Taken together, UCB transplantation in adults is marked by delayed neutrophil recovery compared to adult URD grafting, and is associated with higher rates of bacteremia at early time points after transplantation.

It is clear that delayed engraftment associated infection is a major cause of morbidity and mortality after UCB transplantation. Whether the risks of infection are greater with UCB, additional studies are needed with systematic collection of all infectious disease complications with subsequent correlations with assays of immune reconstitution and identification of pre and post-transplant risk factors. Regardless of stem cell source, new strategies are needed to speed immune recovery.

10.8 Conclusion

Since the first UCB transplant nearly two decades ago, multiple investigators have since proven the place of UCB as a clinically useful source of HSC. While it turned out that a single unmanipulated UCB unit was not sufficient for the majority of adults, new strategies are underway that will not only improve the efficacy of UCB transplantation in general but will also increase the engraftment potential of a single or double UCB graft. Clearly, UCB has increased the option of HSCT. The next step is to reduce the associated risks and costs.

References

1. Ende M, Ende N. Hematopoietic transplantation by means of fetal (cord) blood. Va Med J. 1972;99:276–80.
2. Koike K. Cryopreservation of pluripotent and committed hemopoietic progenitor cells from human bone marrow and cord blood. Acta Paediatr Jpn. 1983;25:275.
3. Vidal JB. Nature and characterization of granulocyte-macrophage precursors in cord blood. Universtiy of Valencia School of Medicine (Doctoral Dissertation); 1985.
4. Broxmeyer HE, et al. Human umbilical cord blood as a potential source of transplantable hematopoietic stem/progenitor cells. Proc Natl Acad Sci USA. 1989;86:3828–32.
5. Broxmeyer HE, et al. Growth characteristics and expansion of human umbilical cord blood and estimation of its potential for transplantation in adults. Proc Natl Acad Sci USA. 1992;89:4109–13.
6. Gluckman E, et al. Hematopoietic reconstitution in a patient with Fanconi's anemia by means of umbilical-cord blood from an HLA-identical sibling. N Engl J Med. 1989;321:1174–8.
7. Cardoso AA, et al. Release from quiescence of CD34+ CD38– human umbilical cord blood cells reveals their potentiality to engraft adults. Proc Natl Acad Sci USA. 1993;90:8707–11.
8. Yahata T, et al. A highly sensitive strategy for SCID-repopulating cell assay by direct injection of primitive human hematopoietic cells into NOD/SCID mice bone marrow. Blood 2003;101:2905–13.
9. Broxmeyer HE. Introduction: The past, present, and future of cord blood transplantation. In: Broxmeyer HE, editor. Cellular characteristics of cord blood and cord blood transplantation. Bethesda, MA: AABB Press; 1998. p. 1–9.
10. Hannet I, et al. Developmental and maturational changes in human blood lymphocyte subpopulations. Immunol Today. 1992;13:215, 218.
11. Rainaut M, et al. Characterization of mononuclear cell subpopulations in normal fetal peripheral blood. Hum Immunol. 1987;18:331–7.
12. Clement LT, Vink PE, Bradley GE. Novel immunoregulatory functions of phenotypically distinct subpopulations of CD4+ cells in the human neonate. J Immunol. 1990;145:102–8.
13. Godfrey WR, et al. Cord blood CD4(+)CD25(+)-derived T regulatory cell lines express FoxP3 protein and manifest potent suppressor function. Blood 2005;105:750–8.
14. Cohen JL, et al. CD4(+)CD25(+) immunoregulatory T cells: new therapeutics for graft-versus-host disease. J Exp Med. 2002;196:401–6.

15. Hoffmann P, et al. Donor-type CD4(+)CD25(+) regulatory T cells suppress lethal acute graft-versus-host disease after allogeneic bone marrow transplantation. J Exp Med. 2002;196:389–99.
16. Taylor PA, Lees CJ, Blazar BR. The infusion of ex vivo activated and expanded CD4(+)CD25(+) immune regulatory cells inhibits graft-versus-host disease lethality. Blood 2002;99:3493–9.
17. Taylor PA, et al. L-Selectin(hi) but not the L-selectin(lo) CD4+25+ T-regulatory cells are potent inhibitors of GvHD and BM graft rejection. Blood 2004;104:3804–12.
18. Trenado A, et al. Recipient-type specific CD4+CD25+ regulatory T cells favor immune reconstitution and control graft-versus-host disease while maintaining graft-versus-leukemia. J Clin Invest. 2003;112:1688–96.
19. Wagner JE, et al. Allogeneic sibling umbilical-cord-blood transplantation in children with malignant and non-malignant disease. Lancet 1995;346:214–9.
20. Wagner JE, Kurtzberg J. Allogeneic umbilical cord blood transplantation. In: Broxmeyer HE, editor. Cellular characteristics of cord blood and cord blood transplantation. Bethesda, MA: AABB Press; 1998. p. 113–46.
21. Gluckman E, et al. Outcome of cord-blood transplantation from related and unrelated donors. Eurocord Transplant Group and the European Blood and Marrow Transplantation Group. N Engl J Med. 1997;337:373–81.
22. Rocha V, et al. Graft-versus-host disease in children who have received a cord-blood or bone marrow transplant from an HLA-identical sibling. Eurocord and International Bone Marrow Transplant Registry Working Committee on Alternative Donor and Stem Cell Sources. N Engl J Med. 2000;342:1846–54.
23. Kurtzberg J, et al. Placental blood as a source of hematopoietic stem cells for transplantation into unrelated recipients. N Engl J Med. 1996;335:157–66.
24. Wagner JE, et al. Successful transplantation of HLA-matched and HLA-mismatched umbilical cord blood from unrelated donors: analysis of engraftment and acute graft-versus-host disease. Blood 1996;88:795–802.
25. Rubinstein P, et al. Outcomes among 562 recipients of placental-blood transplants from unrelated donors. N Engl J Med. 1998;339:1565–77.
26. Gluckman E, et al. Factors associated with outcomes of unrelated cord blood transplant: guidelines for donor choice. Exp Hematol. 2004;32:397–407.
27. Rubinstein P, Stevens CE. Placental blood for bone marrow replacement: the New York Blood Center's program and clinical results. Baillieres Best Pract Res Clin Haematol. 2000;13:565–84.
28. Wagner JE, et al. Transplantation of unrelated donor umbilical cord blood in 102 patients with malignant and nonmalignant diseases: influence of CD34 cell dose and HLA disparity on treatment-related mortality and survival. Blood 2002;100:1611–8.
29. Martin PL, Carter SL, Kernan NA, Sahdev I, Wall D, Pietryga D, Wagner JE, Kurtzberg J. Results of the cord blood transplantation study (COBLT): outcomes of unrelated donor umbilical cord blood transplantation in pediatric patients with lysosomal and peroxisomal storage diseases. Biol Blood Marrow Transplant. 2006 Feb;12(2):184–94.
30. Laporte JP, et al. Cord-blood transplantation from an unrelated donor in an adult with chronic myelogenous leukemia. N Engl J Med. 1996;335:167–70.
31. Laughlin MJ, et al. Hematopoietic engraftment and survival in adult recipients of umbilical-cord blood from unrelated donors. N Engl J Med. 2001;344:1815–22.
32. Rocha V, et al. Prognostic factors of outcome after unrelated cord blood transplant (UCBT) in adults with hematologic malignancies. Blood 2000;96:587a.
33. Sanz GF, et al. Standardized, unrelated donor cord blood transplantation in adults with hematologic malignancies. Blood 2001;98:2332–8.
34. Laporte JP, et al. Unrelated mismatched cord blood transplantation in patients with hematological malignancies: a single institution experience. Bone Marrow Transplant. 1998;22 Suppl 1:S76–7.

35. Arcese W, et al. Unrelated cord blood transplants in adults with hematologic malignancies. Haematologica 2006;91:223–30.
36. Cornetta K, et al. Umbilical cord blood transplantation in adults: results of the prospective cord blood transplantation (COBLT). Biol Blood Marrow Transplant. 2005;11:149–60.
37. Iori AP, et al. Pre-transplant prognostic factors for patients with high-risk leukemia undergoing an unrelated cord blood transplantation. Bone Marrow Transplant. 2004;33:1097–105.
38. Long GD, et al. Unrelated umbilical cord blood transplantation in adult patients. Biol Blood Marrow Transplant. 2003;9:772–80.
39. Ooi J, et al. Unrelated cord blood transplantation for adult patients with myelodysplastic syndrome-related secondary acute myeloid leukaemia. Br J Haematol. 2001;114:834–6.
40. Tomonari A, et al. Cord blood transplantation for acute myelogenous leukemia using a conditioning regimen consisting of granulocyte colony-stimulating factor-combined high-dose cytarabine, fludarabine, and total body irradiation. Eur J Haematol. 2006;77:46–50.
41. Barker JN, et al. Transplantation of 2 partially HLA-matched umbilical cord blood units to enhance engraftment in adults with hematologic malignancy. Blood 2005;105:1343–7.
42. Konuma T, et al. Unrelated cord blood transplantation after myeloablative conditioning in patients with acute leukemia aged between 50 and 55 years. Bone Marrow Transplant. 2006;37:803–4.
43. Ooi J, et al. Unrelated cord blood transplantation for adult patients with de novo acute myeloid leukemia. Blood 2004;103:489–91.
44. Kai S, et al. Double-unit cord blood transplantation in Japan. Blood 2004;104:5166a.
45. Ooi J. The efficacy of unrelated cord blood transplantation for adult myelodysplastic syndrome. Leuk Lymphoma. 2006;47:599–602.
46. Barker JN, et al. Survival after transplantation of unrelated donor umbilical cord blood is comparable to that of human leukocyte antigen-matched unrelated donor bone marrow: results of a matched-pair analysis. Blood 2001;97:2957–61.
47. Eapen M, et al. Outcomes of transplantation of unrelated donor umbilical cord blood and bone marrow in children with acute leukaemia: a comparison study. Lancet 2007;369:1947–54.
48. Meyer EA, et al. Cord blood: establishing a national cord blood stem cell bank program. Washington: The National Academy Press; 2005.
49. Adamkiewicz TV, et al. Unrelated cord blood transplantation in children with sickle cell disease: US centers experience. Blood 2005;106:2044.
50. Fang J, et al. Umbilical cord blood transplantation in Chinese children with beta-thalassemia. J Pediatr Hematol Oncol. 2004;26:185–9.
51. Jaing TH, et al. Rapid and complete donor chimerism after unrelated mismatched cord blood transplantation in 5 children with beta-thalassemia major. Biol Blood Marrow Transplant. 2005;11:349–53.
52. Locatelli F, et al. Related umbilical cord blood transplantation in patients with thalassemia and sickle cell disease. Blood 2003;101:2137–43.
53. Miniero R, et al. Cord blood transplantation (CBT) in hemoglobinopathies. Eurocord. Bone Marrow Transplant. 1998;22 Suppl 1:S78–9.
54. Walters MC, et al. Sibling donor cord blood transplantation for thalassemia major: experience of the sibling donor cord blood program. Ann N Y Acad Sci. 2005;1054:206–13.
55. Martin PL, et al. Results of the cord blood transplantation study (COBLT): outcomes of unrelated donor umbilical cord blood transplantation in pediatric patients with lysosomal and peroxisomal storage diseases. Biol Blood Marrow Transplant. 2006;12:184–94.
56. Escolar ML, et al. Transplantation of umbilical-cord blood in babies with infantile Krabbe's disease. N Engl J Med. 2005;352:2069–81.

57. Staba SL, et al. Cord-blood transplants from unrelated donors in patients with Hurler's syndrome. N Engl J Med. 2004;350:1960–9.
58. Rocha V, et al. Results of unrelated cord blood versus unrelated bone marrow transplant in adults with acute leukemia. A matched pair analysis. Blood 2002;100:42a.
59. Laughlin MJ, et al. Outcomes after transplantation of cord blood or bone marrow from unrelated donors in adults with leukemia. N Engl J Med. 2004;351:2265–75.
60. Takahashi S, et al. Single-institute comparative analysis of unrelated bone marrow transplantation and cord blood transplantation for adult patients with hematologic malignancies. Blood 2004;104:3813–20.
61. Hwang WY, et al. A meta-analysis of unrelated donor umbilical cord blood transplantation versus unrelated donor bone marrow transplantation in adult and pediatric patients. Biol Blood Marrow Transplant. 2007;13:444–53.
62. Rocha V, et al. Transplants of umbilical-cord blood or bone marrow from unrelated donors in adults with acute leukemia. N Engl J Med. 2004;351:2276–85.
63. van Heeckeren WJ, et al. Influence of human leucocyte antigen disparity and graft lymphocytes on allogeneic engraftment and survival after umbilical cord blood transplant in adults. Br J Haematol. 2007;139:464–74.
64. Brunstein CG, et al. Umbilical cord blood transplantation after nonmyeloablative conditioning: impact on transplant outcomes in 110 adults with hematological disease. Blood 2007;110(8):3064–70.
65. Brunstein CG, Wagner JE. Cord blood transplantation for adults. Vox Sang. 2006;91:195–205.
66. Majhail NS, Brunstein CG, Wagner JE. Double umbilical cord blood transplantation. Curr Opin Immunol. 2006;18:571–5.
67. Rocha V, et al. Reduced intensity conditioning regimen in single unrelated cord blood transplantation in adults with hematological malignant disorders. An Eurocord-Netcord and SFGM-TC survey. Blood 2006;108:897a.
68. Hamza NS, et al. Kinetics of myeloid and lymphocyte recovery and infectious complications after unrelated umbilical cord blood versus HLA-matched unrelated donor allogeneic transplantation in adults. Br J Haematol. 2004;124:488–98.

Chapter 11
Biology and Management of Acute Graft-Versus-Host Disease

Robert Korngold and Joseph H. Antin

11.1 Introduction

Extensive investigations over the last 25 years of the basic biology of acute graft-versus-host disease (GvHD) in murine models of allogeneic blood and marrow transplantation (BMT), particularly in major histocompatibility complex (MHC)-matched, minor histocompatibility antigen (miHA) different strain combinations, has brought us to an understanding of much of the etiology and pathogenesis of this disease. The relative contributions of mature donor $CD4^+$ and $CD8^+$ T cells in causing the development of GvHD across different histocompatibility barriers has been clarified and the involvement of host conditioning factors and the requirements for inflammatory cytokines at early stages after transplant are now appreciated. We also now have a reasonable understanding of what miHA are and how T cells recognize them, although which particular minor H antigens elicit severe GvHD responses in mice is still far from clear. Overall, the elucidation of the complex aspects of GvHD immunobiology has led to many novel approaches to intervene in the process and to attempt to block GvHD development. For clinical application, the primary goal is to obtain GvHD minimization without compromising the subsequent ability of donor T cells to mount responses against opportunistic infections or to mediate a graft-versus-tumor (GvT) effect. Since there may be both overlapping and specific populations of T cells that can be involved in all of these responses, achieving this goal, which would clearly improve patient outcomes, has proven difficult.

11.2 T-Cell Responses in GvHD

T cells can be divided into two major subsets that have different phenotypes and functions. Those cells expressing the CD4 coreceptor are capable of recognizing small peptide antigens derived from the cellular environment and presented in

J.H. Antin (✉)
Dana-Farber Cancer Institute, 44 Binney St, Boston, MA 02115, USA
e-mail: jantin@partners.org

M.R. Bishop (ed.), *Hematopoietic Stem Cell Transplantation*,
Cancer Treatment and Research 144, DOI 10.1007/978-0-387-78580-6_11,

the context of MHC class II molecules on antigen presenting cells (APC). Once stimulated, $CD4^+$ T cells can respond by rapid proliferation and production of cytokines, such as interleukin-2 (IL-2), that can provide the milieu for responses of other antigen-specific $CD4^+$ T cells, as well as several other immune cells. A large proportion of $CD4^+$ T cells contributes to inflammatory responses, whereas, others are regulatory in nature or help to generate B-cell production of certain classes of antibodies. In contrast, $CD8^+$ T cells recognize small peptide antigens derived from degradation of proteins within cells and presented in the context of MHC class I molecules. $CD8^+$ T cells often have cytotoxic functionality, although they too are a source of inflammatory cytokines, such as interferon-gamma (IFNγ). Often, $CD8^+$ T cells require the presence of IL-2 from reacting $CD4^+$ T cells in order for them to proliferate and to develop their effector functions. However, in some circumstances, $CD8^+$ T cells can develop a response independent of $CD4^+$ cells, producing enough of their own IL-2 [1]. In addition, $CD8^+$ T cells can mediate direct cytotoxic effects against target cells expressing specific antigen by induction of apoptosis, primarily via the perforin/granzyme pathway, but also through tumor necrosis factor (TNF) and TNF-like family members (TRAIL), or by Fas ligand (FasL)/fas interactions [2]. It should be noted that some $CD4^+$ T cells also have these cytotoxic capabilities [3] and together with $CD8^+$ T cells account for much of the immunopathological tissue injury in the target organs of GvHD [4].

11.2.1 GvHD to miHA

In experimental GvHD models and in the clinical situation, it was observed early on that transfer of bone marrow populations containing T cells into MHC different irradiated recipients was regularly associated with severe GvHD and usually fatality [5, 6]. By the late 1970s, similar severe results were also recognized in BMT across multiple miHA barriers in mice [7, 8], and the extent of GvHD was directly proportional to the number of T cells present in the donor inoculum [7]. On the other hand, the depletion of mature T cells from donor marrow inoculum resulted in survival of the irradiated recipients, firmly establishing the etiology of GvHD in miHA mismatches [7] MiHA were also recognized as a major cause of GvHD in the clinical setting [9, 10].

MiHA are derived from the degradation of normal cellular proteins. Depending upon their specific residue sequence, those small peptides that are cytosolic and are processed through proteosomes find their way to be presented on MHC class I molecules on the cell surface, whereas those peptides derived from the extracellular environment and processed by lysosomal enzymatic activity become presented on MHC class II molecules [11]. In MHC-matched individuals, miHA are these presented peptides that may be derived from genes active in the recipient but not the donor, or from mostly single nucleotide polymorhisms (SNPs) that can be recognized by donor T cells. In mice, there can be a wide range of the number of miHA that can be present between two MHC-matched strains. This is also true in humans, with for example, H-Y, originating from the SMCY gene of the Y chromosome, serving as a miHA that is recognized by female donor cells [12], and HA-1, which is an example of a miHA derived from an SNP, present in recipients [13].

Translation of the findings in murine models that T cells were responsible for miHA-directed GvHD and similar observations of this association in the clinical setting led to a number of T cell depletion trials, which did succeed in reducing GvHD development, but did not effectively change patient survival outcomes because of increased risks of leukemic relapse and infections [14]. As it turns out, immune reconstitution in BMT patients is slow to recover [15] and without any donor T cells provided in the inocula, there is very little to counter opportunistic infections and the regrowth of residual malignant cells.

11.2.2 T Cell Subsets in GvHD

The role of T-cell subsets in the pathogenesis of GvHD directed to multiple miHA has been established for a number of murine allogeneic model systems. In most situations, $CD8^+$ T cells, alone, can mediate a varying degree of severe GvHD, as exemplified in the $H2^k$-compatible B10.BR → CBA model [16]. In some cases, $CD8^+$ T cells can only mediate GvHD in the presence of $CD4^+$ T cells; e.g., in the C57BL/6 → BALB.B model [17]. Transplantation of only $CD4^+$ T cells often fails to cause severe GvHD, although these donor cells may proliferate to some extent in vivo in response to specific host miHA [16]. In contrast, in some strain combinations (B10.D2 → DBA/2 or C57BL/6 → BALB.B), $CD4^+$ T cells can directly mediate severe GvHD-related immunopathology, particularly in gastrointestinal tissue, and can be lethal [18, 19]. The nature of these particular vehement responses and what drives them is currently under study.

The primary target tissues for effector T cells mediating GvHD histopathology are the lymphoid organs, the skin, gastrointestinal tract, and the liver. Initial responses of T cells upon transplantation against APC presenting foreign miHA occur in the peripheral lymphoid system. For $CD4^+$ responding cells, APC are likely host-derived in the early phases after BMT, but may later switch over to donor APC, since they are both MHC-compatible and can process and present extracellular antigens derived from the host [20, 21]. As might be expected, $CD8^+$ T cell responses require stimulation by host-derived APC. As both subsets of T cells become activated in the periphery and turn into effector cells, they home to target tissues in whose vascular endothelial cells have been pre-activated by inflammatory cytokines and chemokines released from local dendritic and other myeloid and stromal cells in response to the recipient conditioning regimen (irradiation or myeloablative chemotherapy). These mediators upregulate appropriate adhesion molecules on the endothelium that attracts activated T cells and allows them to infiltrate into the tissues [22]. Interestingly, at this stage, the effector cells need to be reactivated by recognition of the specific miHA on APC or target epithelial cells, and then they can perform their cytotoxic or inflammatory functions. However, it is clear for both $CD4^+$ and $CD8^+$ effector cells, that target tissue injury only occurs if the nonhematopoietic derived parenchymal tissue express the relevant miHA [23, 24].

11.2.3 Regulatory T Cells

Regulatory T cells (Treg) with a $CD4^+CD25^+$ phenotype and expressing the FoxP3 transcription factor are known to be involved in self-tolerance and the avoidance of autoimmunity [25, 26]. Treg are also thought to be capable of controlling alloreactive responses [27]. In BMT models, Treg were found to regenerate quickly post-transplant and were believed to be responsible for tempering the induction of GvHD by delayed donor lymphocyte infusions 1–2 months later [28]. Several groups have also demonstrated their capacity to inhibit the development of GvHD in MHC and miHA-disparate combinations when given at time of transplant [29–31]. In addition, the infusion of Treg cells after a 10-day delay into myeloid leukemia-challenged, BMT-recipient mice ameliorated the development of acute GvHD in a miHA model and allowed for retention of a significant GvT effect [32]. This observation may have potential application in the clinical situation.

11.3 Managment of Acute Graft-Versus-Host Disease

Acute GvHD is often approached as if it were either a malignancy or an autoimmune disorder. Despite the undeniable mortality and morbidity associated with high grade GvHD, it is neither of the above. Acute GvHD is an exaggerated and dysregulated response of a normal, albeit inadequate, immune system to tissue damage that is intrinsic to the BMT procedure. The donor's immune system is put into a setting where its sensors tell it that there is a massive and uncontrolled infection, and its efforts to deal with this injury result in clinical acute GvHD. Our thinking about this problem revolves around the notion that tissue injury intrinsic to the high dose conditioning regimen results in the breakdown of mucosal barriers, allowing endotoxin into the tissues. Toll-like receptors (TLR) on dendritic cells (DC) bind to endotoxin and activate pathways that lead to DC maturation and induce inflammation [33]. The up-regulation of costimulatory molecules, MHC molecules, adhesion molecules, cytokines, chemokines, prostanoids, and other inflammatory mediators prime and trigger T-cell mediated attack on target tissues. It is likely that there are components of both adaptive immunity and innate immunity involved in the process, thus linking together hypotheses of the cytokine storm [34], the danger hypothesis [35], and more traditional notions of adaptive and innate immunity [36]. Moreover, there is probably failure of regulatory/inhibitory pathways that ordinarily would have limited the tissue damage.

One must put strategies for the management and therapy of acute GvHD into the framework of dysregulation of a normal inflammatory response, rather than approaching acute GvHD as if it were a malignancy. High doses of multiple immunosuppressive agents will often control the inflammation, but if the immune response is paralyzed to the degree that the donor's immune system cannot function, one must reasonably expect that there will be opportunistic infections, lymphoproliferative disorders, and/or relapse of the underlying malignancy. Most studies of therapy for acute GvHD show substantial response rates with a rather characteristically poor survival due to infection. Although T cells are intrinsic to the development and maintenance of GvHD, the T cell has monopolized our thinking about strategies to control GvHD. The objective of prophylaxis and therapy should be to reduce the nonspecific tissue damage associated with GvHD, with the restoration of regulatory circuits and allowing the recovery of effective immunity.

Finally, most of the conceptual framework underpinning current regimens for acute GvHD prophylaxis implicitly accepts that control of acute GvHD is tantamount to control of chronic GvHD. This approach needs to be reconsidered in the light of the risk of chronic GvHD despite adequate control of acute GvHD and of accumulating evidence that chronic GvHD is pathophysiologically distinct from acute GvHD.

11.3.1 Prophylaxis Strategies: Reducing Nonspecific Tissue Injury

If indeed the nonspecific tissue injury inflicted by the conditioning regimen contributes to acute GvHD, it follows that less toxic conditioning regimens would be associated with less acute GvHD. It has been known since the early era of BMT that both acute GvHD and death from GvHD could be prevented with appropriate gut decontamination and transplantation in a protected environment [37–40]. Much of this reduction may reflect less recruitment of innate immunity through TLRs as well as less nonspecific stimulation of inflammation through endotoxin. Thus, an important corollary to pharmacologic or cellular approaches to GvHD prevention is maintenance of normal barriers to microorganisms, manipulating the flora by eliminating gram negative rods, and prevention of infection through antibacterial and antiviral therapy.

The demonstration of less than expected acute GvHD was initially observed after donor lymphocyte infusions. The T cells are typically administered without pharmacologic GvHD prophylaxis, and the observed frequency of acute GvHD is lower and less severe than would be expected after transplantation without immunosuppressive drugs. This reduction may be multifactorial but one important component of this effect is likely to be less activation of inflammatory mediators as well as less stimulation of the innate immune system due to the lower level of tissue injury. One might reasonably also infer less systemic endotoxin exposure. The overall rate of GvHD after reduced-intensity conditioning (RIC) regimens is actually similar to what is observed after ablative conditioning [41, 42]; however, the onset of GvHD is delayed [43], and it is more likely to manifest as an overlap syndrome of acute and chronic GvHD. Thus, the initial tissue injury of high dose regimens accelerates the development of GvHD, but it does not eliminate the T cell recognition of miHA. Consequently, there appears to be little effect on overlap and chronic GvHD. Thus, while data on reducing both colonization with bacteria and reducing tissue injury with less intense regimens are suggestive and support the basic concepts described above, the effect is insufficient to control GvHD adequately in human transplantation. Prevention of mucositis could contribute to GvHD control, but studies with palifermin [44] did not discern a notable affect in this regard.

11.3.2 Inhibition of T-cell Proliferation

The workhorse of GvHD prophylaxis has traditionally been methotrexate (MTX) (Table 11.1). It was developed by E. Donnell Thomas and colleagues [45] and became the principle drug used in GvHD prevention. Initially there were no useful alternatives. Azathioprine and corticosteroids were available at the time, but single agent MTX became the predominant regimen until the advent of cyclosporine (CSP). MTX was associated with delay of count recovery, higher risk of mucositis and respiratory complications, and incomplete GvHD control. However, it was highly effective compared with no prophylaxis [46]. George Santos developed a cyclophosphamide-based regimen [47] that was not widely adopted. The principle of either approach is to administer a cell-cycle specific chemotherapeutic agent immediately after the transplant. The idea is to kill the T cells after they enter the cell cycle as part of their response to antigenic

Table 11.1 Acute GvHD prophylaxis

Modality	GvHD rate	Graft failure	Relapse	Regimen-related toxicity
MTX	+ + +	+	+	+ + +
Cyclosporine alone	+ + +	+	+	+ + +
T cell depletion	+	+ +	+ + +	+
MTX + calcineurin inhibitor	+ +	+	+	+ +
Calcineurin inhibitor + MMF	+ +	+	+	+ +
Tacrolimus + sirolimus	+	+	+	+

stimulation by host miHA. The addition of ATG and/or prednisone resulted in improvement in the GvHD rate but no improvement in survival [48]. Recently, the Santos approach using cyclophosphamide immediately after the BMT has been applied again with promising results in both matched related donor and haploidentical transplantation [49, 50].

While MTX has proven quite useful over the years, its intrinsic toxicity has prompted the search for alternative agents. Mycophenolate mofetil (MMF) is the prodrug of mycophenolic acid (MPA), a selective inhibitor of inosine monophosphate dehydrogenase. MMF inhibits the de novo pathway of guanosine nucleotide synthesis. Since de novo synthesis of purines is required in T cells, inhibition of this pathway prevents T cell proliferation [51]. Myeloid and mucosal cells can utilize salvage pathways, so the drug is less toxic to mucosa and myeloid recovery than MTX. A second useful effect of MPA is that it prevents the glycosylation of glycoproteins that are intrinsic to T cell trafficking into inflammatory sites. There are no studies of single agent MMF but in combination with a calcineurin inhibitor, either CSP or tacrolimus, there is reliable but incomplete control of GvHD [52–54].

11.3.3 Graft-Engineering—Reducing T-cell Numbers

Ever since we became able to recognize T cells and T cell subsets with monoclonal antibodies, there have been efforts to engineer the graft to prevent GvHD. A major flaw in our thinking was failing to realize the importance of T cells in important aspects of BMT, namely graft-versus-leukemia, engraftment, and immunological recovery. Thus, T cell depletion has never realized its imagined potential. Ex vivo graft manipulation with monoclonal antibodies plus rabbit complement, immunotoxins, lectins, CD34 columns, and physical techniques, such as centrifugal elutriation, all have been evaluated [55]. When marrow is collected from the iliac crest, it typically contains approximately 10^7 T cells/kg of recipient weight. Surprisingly, despite the infusion of 10-fold more T cells with a peripheral blood stem cell product, the risk of acute GvHD does not increase. The risk of chronic GvHD does increase with PBSC products [56, 57]. Thus, there may be a threshold above which additional T cells do not appear to be acutely harmful. On the other hand, the establishment of a clear dose-response relationship has been problematic, since the risk of acute GvHD depends on variables that are independent of the dose. Some of these include the number of miHA differences, virus exposure/reactivation, disease and stage, donor gender and age, recipient age, and conditioning regimen intensity. Studies of counterflow elutriation showed that 10^6 T cells/kg plus CSP resulted in a GvHD rate similar to CSP alone, but 5×10^5 T cells/kg plus CSP resulted in an overall rate of 22% – primarily limited to skin involvement [58]. Lectin depletion of T cells to a T cell dose approximately 10^5/kg without additional immunosuppression results in complete control of GvHD [59]. Similarly, donor lymphocyte infusions containing less than or equal to 10^7 $CD3^+$ cells/kg of recipient weight rarely results in GvHD. Very low numbers of T cells ($<3 \times 10^4$ CD3 T cells/kg) plus a large dose of $CD34^+$ cells can be associated with myeloid engraftment and little GvHD [60].

Early efforts to remove essentially all T cells using a broad panel of monoclonal antibodies resulted in graft failure and this approach has been abandoned [61]. However, subset depletion of $CD5^+$ or $CD6^+$ T cells seems to be associated with a low graft failure rate [62, 63] but problems with persistent disease and relapse. Depletion of $CD25^+$ T cells or $CD8^+$ T cells can be associated with a high graft failure rate [64, 65]. This observation probably reflects the removal of Treg ($CD4^+CD25^+FoxP3^+$). To some degree the higher graft failure rates may be controlled by increasing the intensity of the conditioning regimen [66], adding back T cells [58, 64, 67], infusing specific T cell lines [68], or with additional immunosuppressants [69]. However, these strategies typically do not overcome the observed higher incidence of Epstein-Barr virus induced lymphoproliferative disorders, loss of the GvT effect, and delayed recovery of protective immunity. A large multicenter study of unrelated donor BMT similarly showed no improvement in outcomes after TCD [70].

A novel approach is to establish a large scale mixed lymphocyte culture followed by removal of only the activated T cells that are generated in the reaction. This technique might abrogate some of the problems of nonspecific T cell depletion [71, 72]. However, these approaches have not undergone definitive clinical evaluations.

Finally, it is possible to deplete T cells in vivo rather than ex vivo using anti-thymocyte globulin [73, 74] or anti-CD52 therapy (alemtuzumab, Campath) [75]. Antithymocyte globulin appears to have interesting systemic effects beyond its intrinsic anti-T cell activity. Clearly, when given to the recipient proximate to the stem cell infusion it not only depletes T cells from the blood and lymphoid tissues of the host but also from the donor cell inoculum. It may also affect lymphocyte trafficking, DC function, B-cell function, and natural killer (NK) cell and Treg activity [76]. Alemtuzumab has effects on both T cells and DC that reduce acute and chronic GvHD at the expense of high relapse rates, graft failure, and opportunistic infections [75, 77–80]. Typically alemtuzumab containing regimens must be followed by donor lymphocyte infusions. Host DC that persist after conditioning are intrinsic to the development of acute GvHD [20, 81]. Donor DC may take over later in a mechanism called cross presentation. Thus, it is possible that DC depletion prior to stem cell infusion would prevent acute GvHD. The promiscuity of CD52 allows alemtuzumab to target B cells, T cells, monocytes, DC and other cells, thus raising the possibility that DC depletion prior to BMT could prevent GvHD [77]. However, the sensitivity of Langerhans cells to depletion is controversial [78], and the technique and role of pretransplant DC depletion remains to be established.

11.3.4 Inhibition of T-cell Activation and Function

The two calcineurin inhibitors (CNI) in common use are CSP and tacrolimus. Both drugs work indirectly by binding to intracellular proteins called immunophilins. CSP binds cyclophilin, and tacrolimus binds to FKBP12. The CNI/immunophillin complex further binds calmodulin and calcium, which then inhibits calcineurin phosphatase activity. This effect prevents the dephosphorylation and translocation of nuclear factor of activated T cells (NF-AT), which then goes on to inhibit lymphokines production as well as prevent the expression of cell surface IL-2R. The net result is the inhibition of T-lymphocyte activation and a block in the $G_0 \rightarrow G_1$ transition of mitosis.

Single agent CSP is similar in its ability to prevent acute GvHD to long course MTX [82]. The study that provided the framework for the next 15–20 years of GvHD prophylaxis demonstrated that CSP in combination with MTX significantly reduced the risk of acute GvHD and survival [83]. In general it is fair to say that the CSP-containing regimens had more renal insufficiency than CSP-free regimens but that careful monitoring of blood levels made the use of CSP manageable. Subsequent randomized trials of tacrolimus plus MTX compared with CSP plus MTX showed no advantage for either combination in related or unrelated donor BMT [84, 85]. Tacrolimus is associated with less tremor and hirsutism and may result in slightly better prevention of acute GvHD, but overall the outcomes were comparable. The addition of prednisone to CSP plus MTX regimen resulted in similar rates of GvHD and no improvement in survival, probably due to increased risk of infection [86].

Another effective agent for GvHD prevention is sirolimus. This drug is another natural product that is similar in structure to tacrolimus and CSP. All three drugs bind to immunophilins. In contrast to CSP and tacrolimus, sirolimus complexed with FKBP12 binds to mTOR. Ultimately mTOR inhibition blocks IL-2 mediated signal transduction that blocks mitosis in the $G_1 \rightarrow S$ phase transition. This effect is mediated through a complex pathway involving inhibition of ribosomal protein synthesis at several levels, as well as effects on transcription and translation [87]. The drug has similar effects on proliferation of T cells induced by IL-2, IL-4, IL-7, IL-12 and IL-15. Sirolimus affects lymphocyte activation at a later stage than either CSP or tacrolimus, and activation stimuli that resist inhibition to the latter agents have been shown to be sensitive to sirolimus. Since it acts through a separate mechanism from the tacrolimus-FKBP12 complex (and CSP-cyclophilin complex), sirolimus is synergistic with both tacrolimus and CSP. Since the sirolimus:mTOR complex does not bind to calcineurin, sirolimus also is free of nephrotoxicity and neurotoxicity, making combination therapy appealing. Clinical trials indicate that sirolimus is a promising addition to the GvHD armamentarium in both related and unrelated donor HSCT [88]. The elimination of MTX from the regimen results in faster engraftment, less mucositis, and less idiopathic pneumonia syndrome. Interestingly, sirolimus also has anti-CMV activity and the risk of CMV reactivation appears to be reduced by as much as 50% [89]. Finally, sirolimus has anticancer activity in several neoplasms, most pertinently ALL [90–92]. This drug has the potential advantage of controlling GvHD, preventing CMV reactivation, and simultaneously providing some anti-cancer activity.

11.3.5 Blockade of Inflammatory Stimulation and Effectors

A number of inflammatory cytokines (e.g., TNF-α, IL-1, IFN-γ) play important roles in clinical acute GvHD [93]. Elevated levels of TNF-α can be detected in the serum of patients with acute GvHD and other endothelial complications such as veno-occlusve disease (VOD) [94]. Moreover, as described below, both infliximab and etanercept can control acute GvHD that is resistant to corticosteroids, but neither drug has been useful in GvHD prophylaxis. Despite the observation that IL-1 levels are elevated in patients with acute GvHD, a randomized trial of IL-1 receptor antagonist did not demonstrate a reduction in GvHD rate [95].

An appealing strategy would be to prevent the recruitment localization and activation of lymphocytes during GvHD through blockade or inhibition of chemokines. Prevention of lymphocyte entry into secondary lymphoid organs, acquisition of appropriate homing and adhesion molecules, or modification of their entry into target tissues could all reduce GvHD [96–98]. Such molecules as FTY720 [99, 100] and alefacept [101] as well as new chemokine inhibitors may allow selective targeting of organ specific lymphocytes, although as yet little clinical experience has accumulated. None of these approaches has been subject to rigorous testing in clinical trials.

11.3.6 Therapy of Acute GvHD

Adrenal corticosteroids are the accepted primary therapy for acute GvHD that requires therapy [102] (Table 11.2). Surprisingly, there is no real consensus on whether to treat early stage acute GvHD (Stage 1 skin, overall grade I (IBMTR A)). Many experts feel that these patients do not need to be treated with systemic therapy, but recent clinical experience of the Blood and Marrow Transplantation Clinical Trials Network (BMT-CTN) indicates that many clinicians do indeed treat early grade acute GvHD. Typically, publications address therapy of Grade II-IV GvHD and indicate complete response rates of 25–40% [103]. Efforts to use higher doses have been associated with good early responses but excessive mortality from opportunistic infections. Several agents have been added to corticosteroids for refractory or resistant acute GvHD with what appeared to be promising results, e.g., ATG [104], anti-CD5 immunotoxin (XomaZyme) [105, 106], interleukin-1 receptor antagonist (IL-1RA) [95], infliximab (Remicade) [107, 108], soluble interleukin-1 receptor [109], and

Table 11.2 Therapy of acute GvHD

Modality	CR/PR rate	Survival (%)	comment
Primary therapy			
Corticosteroids	40	30	Doses >2 mg/kg/day can be harmful if sustained
ATG	50	30	
Daclizumab	50	30	Worse than steroids alone when used in combination for primary therapy
Calcineurin inhibitors	50	30	When used in patients who have not previously received CNI
Steroid-resistant acute GvHD			
Sirolimus	50	30	High blood levels associated with a risk of thrombotic microangiopathy
Anti-TNFα	60–70	30	High risk of invasive fungal infections
MMF	50	30	
Denileukin diftitox	50–70	30	
Pentostatin	50–70	30	
Daclizumab	50–70	30	

anti-CD147 therapy [110]. Randomized trials of corticosteroids plus daclizumab or ATG compared with corticosteroids alone resulted in similar or worse outcomes in the combination therapy group [111, 112], despite promising data in phase II studies [104, 113–115]. To date there have been no completed randomized control trials to establish a regimen that improves on corticosteroids. Moreover, there has not even been a study to determine the most efficacious dose of corticosteroids for initial therapy. The conventional starting dose is prednisone 2 mg/kg daily. The drug is tapered when GvHD manifestations come under control, often approximately 10% per week, although this regimen is closely personalized.

Several additional agents that function through distinct mechanisms of action have activity in phase II trials but have not been demonstrated to be superior to prednisone. Denileukin diftitox (Ontak) is a recombinant protein composed of the diphtheria toxin fragments A and B linked to IL-2. This is a Trojan horse approach that targets activated T cells through the IL-2 receptor. It is associated with a complete remission rate of about 45–50% [116, 117]. It has the potential advantage of only intoxicating activated T cells while leaving resting T cells alone to contribute to the homeostatic reconstitution of cellular immunity. Pentostatin (deoxycoformycin, Nipent) is a potent inhibitor of the enzyme adenosine deaminase that is critical for T cell function. It has relatively mild hematologic toxicity. Although experience is limited, the reported complete remission rate is 60% [118]. A drug with similar selectivity for lymphocytes described above is MMF. An improvement rate of about 65% has been reported [119]. Another approach is cytokine inhibition with etanercept

(Enbrel). This drug is a dimeric fusion protein consisting of the extracellular ligand-binding portion of the human TNF receptor linked to the Fc portion of human IgG1. It can bind to two TNF molecules (either TNFα or TNFβ), preventing them from binding to the cell surface TNF receptor. In contrast infliximab is a monoclonal anti-TNFR antibody that only binds to TNFα. A complete response rate as high as 77% to etanercept was reported in a very small number of patients [120]. A similar response rate to infliximab has been noted although the risk of fungal infection was very high [107, 108]. Sirolimus has activity in therapy as well as prophylaxis as noted previously. The initial studies used high doses that were associated with a high risk of thrombotic microangiopathy. Nevertheless, response rates of approximately 65% were observed [121]. Extracorporeal photopheresis (ECP) has been assessed primarily in Europe. It can be challenging to apply ECP to very sick patients with skin and gut GvHD, but published results suggest excellent responses particularly in patients with grades II/III disease [122]. Finally, an interesting approach has been the use of mesenchymal stem cells. These cells apparently do not need to be histocompatible, nor do they need to be obtained from the donor who donated the primary transplant. They are grown from the adherent layer of a short-term marrow culture and can be infused intravenously without causing GvHD. In a recent report on 40 patients with grades III–IV acute GvHD receiving a modest dose of cells [median 1.0 (range 0.4–9) 10^6 cells/kg], 47% of recipients had complete responses [123, 124]. The mechanism of activation of this effect is unclear, and these results will have to be confirmed; however, the approach is intriguing. All of these interesting approaches will ultimately need to be validated in well-designed controlled trials.

11.4 Summary

Acute GvHD is a multifactorial complex pathophysiology that integrates adaptive and innate immunity in a maladaptive fashion. It is best considered an exaggeration of normal physiologic mechanisms wherein the donor immune system attempts to rid the donor of antigens that are intrinsic to the donor. The inflammatory process that follows has the benefit of providing an anti-cancer effect for many diseases, but unfortunately the nonspecific nature of the inflammation can result in disability and death. As we understand the physiology of GvHD more completely, it behooves us to develop strategies to control it that are more subtle than massive doses of corticosteroids. By identifying completely the elements of the immune response that are responsible for GvHD, the challenge of the next decade will be to adjust our therapy to provide adequate control of the underlying malignancy without making the patient subject either to the damaging effects of GvHD per se or the ravages of immunologic failure.

References

1. Tan JT, Ha J, Cho HR, et al. Analysis of expression and function of the costimulatory molecule 4-1bb in alloimmune responses. Transplantation 2000;70:175–83.
2. Williams MA, Bevan MJ. Effector and memory CTL differentiation. Annu Rev Immunol. 2007;25:171–92.
3. Golding H, Munitz TI, Singer A. Characterization of antigen-specific, Ia-restricted, l3t4+ cytolytic T lymphocytes and assessment of thymic influence on their self specificity. J Exp Med. 1985;162:943–61.
4. Sun Y, Tawara I, Toubai T, Reddy P. Pathophysiology of acute graft-versus-host disease: recent advances. Transl Res. 2007;150:197–214.
5. Sprent J, Boehmer HV, Nabholz M. Association of immunity and tolerance to host H-2 determinants in irradiated F1 hybrid mice reconstituted with bone marrow cells from one parental strain. J Exp Med. 1975;142:321–31.
6. Bortin MM. A compendium of reported human bone marrow transplants. Transplantation 1970;9:571–87.
7. Korngold B, Sprent J. Lethal graft-versus-host disease after bone marrow transplantation across minor histocompatibility barriers in mice. Prevention by removing mature T cells from marrow. J Exp Med. 1978;148:1687–98.
8. Hamilton BL, Bevan MJ, Parkman R. Anti-recipient cytotoxic T lymphocyte precursors are present in the spleens of mice with acute graft versus host disease due to minor histocompatibility antigens. J Immunol. 1981;126:621–5.
9. Goulmy E, Gratama JW, Blokland E, Zwaan FE, van Rood JJ. A minor transplantation antigen detected by MHC-restricted cytotoxic T lymphocytes during graft-versus-host disease. Nature 1983;302:159–61.
10. Goulmy E, Voogt P, van Els C, de Bueger M, van Rood J. The role of minor histocompatibility antigens in GvHD and rejection: a mini-review. Bone Marrow Transplant. 1991;7 Suppl 1:49–51.
11. Simpson E, Scott D, James E, et al. Minor H antigens: genes and peptides. Eur J Immunogenet. 2001;28:505–13.
12. Wang W, Meadows LR, den Haan JM, et al. Human H-Y: a male-specific histocompatibility antigen derived from the SMCY protein. Science 1995;269:1588–90.
13. Bertinetto FE, Dall'Omo AM, Mazzola GA, et al. Role of non-HLA genetic polymorphisms in graft-versus-host disease after haematopoietic stem cell transplantation. Int J Immunogenet. 2006;33:375–84.
14. O'Reilly R. T-cell depletion and allogeneic bone marrow transplantation. Semin Hematol. 1992;29 Suppl 1:20–6.
15. Keever CA, Small TN, Flomenberg N, et al. Immune reconstitution following bone marrow transplantation: comparison of recipients of T-cell depleted marrow with recipients of conventional marrow grafts. Blood 1989;73:1340–50.
16. Korngold R, Sprent J. Variable capacity of l3t4+ T cells to cause lethal graft-versus-host disease across minor histocompatibility barriers in mice. J Exp Med. 1987;165:1552–64.
17. Berger M, Wettstein PJ, Korngold R. T cell subsets involved in lethal graft-versus-host disease directed to immunodominant minor histocompatibility antigens. Transplantation 1994;57:1095–102.
18. Murphy GF, Sueki H, Teuscher C, Whitaker D, Korngold R. Role of mast cells in early epithelial target cell injury in experimental acute graft-versus-host disease. J Invest Dermatol. 1994;102:451–61.
19. Jones SC, Friedman TM, Murphy GF, Korngold R. Specific donor vbeta-associated CD4 T-cell responses correlate with severe acute graft-versus-host disease directed to multiple minor histocompatibility antigens. Biol Blood Marrow Transplant. 2004;10:91–105.

20. Shlomchik WD, Couzens MS, Tang CB, et al. Prevention of graft versus host disease by inactivation of host antigen-presenting cells. Science 1999;285:412–5.
21. Matte CC, Liu J, Cormier J, et al. Donor APCs are required for maximal GVHD but not for GVL. Nat Med. 2004;10:987–92.
22. Ferrara JL, Levy R, Chao NJ. Pathophysiologic mechanisms of acute graft-vs.-host disease. Biol Blood Marrow Transplant. 1999;5:347–56.
23. Korngold R, Sprent J. Features of T cells causing H-2-restricted lethal graft-vs.-host disease across minor histocompatibility barriers. J Exp Med. 1982;155:872–83.
24. Jones SC, Murphy GF, Friedman TM, Korngold R. Importance of minor histocompatibility antigen expression by nonhematopoietic tissues in a CD4^{+} T cell-mediated graft-versus-host disease model. J Clin Invest. 2003;112:1880–6.
25. Asano M, Toda M, Sakaguchi N, Sakaguchi S. Autoimmune disease as a consequence of developmental abnormality of a T cell subpopulation. J Exp Med. 1996;184:387–96.
26. Kuniyasu Y, Takahashi T, Itoh M, Shimizu J, Toda G, Sakaguchi S. Naturally anergic and suppressive CD4+CD25+ T cells as a functionally and phenotypically distinct immunoregulatory T cell subpopulation. Int Immunol. 2000;12:1145–55.
27. Taylor P, Noelle R, Blazar B. CD4+CD25+ immune regulatory cells are required for induction of tolerance to alloantigens via costimulatory blockade. J Exp Med. 2001;193:1311–7.
28. Johnson B, Becker E, LaBelle J, Truitt R. Role of immunoregulatory donor T cells in suppression of graft-versus-host disease following donor leukocyte infusion therapy. J Immunol. 1999;163:6479–87.
29. Taylor P, Lees C, Blazar B. The infusion of ex vivo activated and expanded CD4+CD25+ immune regulatory cells inhibits graft-versus-host disease lethality. Blood 2002;99:3493–9.
30. Ermann J, Hoffmann P, Edinger M, et al. Only the CD62L+ subpopulation of CD4+CD25+ regulatory T cells protects from lethal acute GvHD. Blood 2005;105:2220–6.
31. Albert M, Liu Y, Anasetti C, Yu X. Antigen-dependent suppression of alloresponses by Foxp3-induced regulatory T cells in transplantation. Eur J Immunol. 2005;35:2598–607.
32. Jones S, Murphy G, Korngold R. Post-hematopoietic cell transplantation control of graft-versus-host disease by donor CD4+25+ T cells to allow an effective graft-versus-leukemia response. Biol Blood Marrow Transplant. 2003;9:243–56.
33. Schnare M, Barton GM, Holt AC, Takeda K, Akira S, Medzhitov R. Toll-like receptors control activation of adaptive immune responses. Nat Immunol. 2001;2(10):947–50.
34. Antin JH, Ferrara JLM. Cytokine dysregulation and acute graft-versus-host disease. Blood 1992;80:2964–8.
35. Matzinger P. The danger model: a renewed sense of self. Science 2002;296:301–5.
36. Medzhitov R, Janeway CA Jr. Decoding the patterns of self and nonself by the innate immune system. Science 2002;296:298–300.
37. van Bekkum DW, Roodenburg J, Heidt PJ, van der Waaij D. Mitigation of secondary disease of allogeneic mouse radiation chimeras by modification of the intestinal microflora. J Natl Cancer Inst. 1974;52:401–4.
38. Storb R, Prentice RL, Buckner CD, et al. Graft-versus-host disease and survival in patients with aplastic anemia treated by marrow grafts from HLA-identical siblings. Beneficial effects of a protective environment. N Engl J Med. 1983;308:302–7.
39. Beelen DW, Haralambie E, Brandt H, et al. Evidence that sustained growth suppression of intestinal anaerobic bacteria reduces the risk of acute graft-versus-host disease after sibling marrow transplantation. Blood 1992;80:2668–76.
40. Beelen D, Elmaagacli A, Muller K, Hirche H, Schaefer U. Influence of intestinal bacterial decontamination using metronidazole and ciprofloxacin or ciprofloxacin alone on the development of acute graft-versus-host disease after marrow transplantation in patients

with hematologic malignancies: final results and long-term follow-up of an open-label prospective randomized trial. Blood 1999;93:3267–75.
41. Slavin S, Nagler A, Naparstek E, et al. Nonmyeloablative stem cell transplantation and cell therapy as an alternative to conventional bone marrow transplantation with lethal cytoreduction for the treatment of malignant and nonmalignant hematologic diseases. Blood 1998;91:756–63.
42. Badros A, Barlogie B, Siegel E, et al. Improved outcome of allogeneic transplantation in high-risk multiple myeloma patients after nonmyeloablative conditioning. J Clin Oncol. 2002;20:1295–303.
43. Flowers ME, Traina F, Storer B, et al. Serious graft-versus-host disease after hematopoietic cell transplantation following nonmyeloablative conditioning. Bone Marrow Transplant. 2005;35:277–82.
44. Blazar BR, Weisdorf DJ, Defor T, et al. Phase 1/2 randomized, placebo-control trial of palifermin to prevent graft-versus-host disease (GVHD) after allogeneic hematopoietic stem cell transplantation (HSCT). Blood 2006;108:3216–22.
45. Storb R, Epstein R, Graham T, Thomas E. Methotrexate regimens for control of graft-versus-host disease in dogs with allogeneic marrow grafts. Transplantation 1970;9:240–6.
46. Lazarus HM, Coccia PF, Herzig RH, et al. Incidence of acute graft-versus-host disease with and without methotrexate prophylaxis in allogeneic bone marrow transplant patients. Blood 1984;64:215–20.
47. Santos GW, Sensenbrenner LL, Burke PJ, et al. Marrow transplanation in man following cyclophosphamide. Transplant Proc. 1971;3:400–4.
48. Ramsay NK, Kersey JH, Robison LL, et al. A randomized study of the prevention of acute graft-versus-host disease. N Engl J Med. 1982;306:392–7.
49. Luznik L, Fuchs E, Chen A, et al. Post-transplantation high-dose cyclophosphamide (Cy) is effective single agent GVHD prophylaxis that permits prompt immune reconstitution after myeloablative HLA matched related and unrelated bone marrow transplantation (BMT). Biol Blood Marrow Transplant. 2007;13 Suppl:4.
50. O'Donnell PV, Luznik L, Jones RJ, et al. Nonmyeloablative bone marrow transplantation from partially HLA-mismatched related donors using posttransplantation cyclophosphamide. Biol Blood Marrow Transplant. 2002;8:377–86.
51. Allison AC, Eugui EM. Mycophenolate mofetil and its mechanisms of action. Immunopharmacology 2000;47(2-3):85–118.
52. McSweeney PA, Niederwieser D, Shizuru JA, et al. Hematopoietic cell transplantation in older patients with hematologic malignancies: replacing high-dose cytotoxic therapy with graft-versus-tumor effects. Blood 2001;97:3390–400.
53. Niederwieser D, Maris M, Shizuru JA, et al. Low-dose total body irradiation (TBI) and fludarabine followed by hematopoietic cell transplantation (HCT) from HLA-matched or mismatched unrelated donors and postgrafting immunosuppression with cyclosporine and mycophenolate mofetil (MMF) can induce durable complete chimerism and sustained remissions in patients with hematological diseases. Blood 2003;101:1620–9.
54. Basara N, Blau WI, Kiehl MG, et al. Mycophenolate mofetil for the prophylaxis of acute GVHD in HLA-mismatched bone marrow transplant patients. Clin Transplant. 2000;14:121–6.
55. Ho VT, Soiffer RJ. The history and future of T-cell depletion as graft-versus-host disease prophylaxis for allogeneic hematopoietic stem cell transplantation. Blood 2001;98:3192–204.
56. Cutler C, Giri S, Jeyapalan S, Paniagua D, Viswanathan A, Antin JH. Acute and chronic graft-versus-host disease after allogeneic peripheral-blood stem-cell and bone marrow transplantation: a meta-analysis. J Clin Oncol. 2001;19:3685–91.
57. Allogeneic peripheral blood stem-cell compared with bone marrow transplantation in the management of hematologic malignancies: An individual patient data meta-analysis of nine randomized trials. J Clin Oncol. 2005;23:5074–87.

58. Wagner J, Santos G, Noga S, et al. Bone marrow graft engineering by counterflow centrifugal elutriation: results of a phase I-II clinical trial. Blood 1990;75:1370–7.
59. Kernan NA, Collins NH, Juliano L, Cartagena T, Dupont B, O'Reilly RJ. Clonable T lymphocytes in T cell-depleted bone marrow transplants correlate with development of graft-v-host disease. Blood 1986;68:770–3.
60. Aversa F, Tabilio A, Velardi A, et al. Treatment of high-risk acute leukemia with T-cell-depleted stem cells from related donors with one fully mismatched HLA haplotype. N Engl J Med. 1998;339:1186–93.
61. Martin PJ, Hansen JA, Buckner CD, et al. Effects of in vitro depletion of T cells in HLA-identical allogeneic marrow grafts. Blood 1985;66:664–72.
62. Antin JH, Bierer BE, Smith BR, et al. Selective depletion of bone marrow T lymphocytes with anti-CD5 monoclonal antibodies: effective prophylaxis for graft-versus-host disease in patients with hematologic malignancies. Blood 1991;78:2139–49.
63. Soiffer RJ, Weller E, Alyea EP, et al. CD6+ donor marrow T-cell depletion as the sole form of graft-versus-host disease prophylaxis in patients undergoing allogeneic bone marrow transplant from unrelated donors. J Clin Oncol. 2001;19:1152–9.
64. Martin PJ, Rowley SD, Anasetti C, et al. A phase I-II clinical trial to evaluate removal of CD4 cells and partial depletion of CD8 cells from donor marrow for HLA-mismatched unrelated recipients. Blood 1999;94:2192–9.
65. Martin PJ, Pei J, Gooley T, et al. Evaluation of a CD25-specific immunotoxin for prevention of graft-versus-host disease after unrelated marrow transplantation. Biol Blood Marrow Transplant. 2004;10:552–60.
66. Papadopoulos EB, Carabasi MH, Castro-Malaspina H, et al. T-cell-depleted allogeneic bone marrow transplantation as postremission therapy for acute myelogenous leukemia: Freedom from relapse in the absence of graft-versus-host disease. Blood 1998;91:1083–90.
67. Montero A, Savani BN, Kurlander R, et al. Lineage-specific engraftment and outcomes after T-cell-depleted peripheral blood stem cell transplant with Flu/Cy/TBI conditioning. Br J Haematol. 2005;130:733–9.
68. Greenberg PD, Riddell SR. Deficient cellular immunity—finding and fixing the defects. Science 1999;285:546–51.
69. Champlin R, Ho W, Gajewski J, et al. Selective depletion of CD8+ T lymphocytes for prevention of graft-versus-host disease after allogeneic bone marrow transplantation. Blood 1990;76:418–23.
70. Wagner JE, Thompson JS, Carter SL, Kernan NA. Effect of graft-versus-host disease prophylaxis on 3-year disease-free survival in recipients of unrelated donor bone marrow (T-cell depletion trial): a multi-centre, randomised phase II-III trial. Lancet 2005;366:733–41.
71. Andre-Schmutz I, Le Deist F, Hacein-Bey-Abina S, et al. Immune reconstitution without graft-versus-host disease after haemopoietic stem-cell transplantation: a phase 1/2 study. Lancet 2002;360:130–7.
72. Koh MB, Prentice HG, Corbo M, Morgan M, Cotter FE, Lowdell MW. Alloantigen-specific T-cell depletion in a major histocompatibility complex fully mismatched murine model provides effective graft-versus-host disease prophylaxis in the presence of lymphoid engraftment. Br J Haematol. 2002;118:108–16.
73. Bacigalupo A, Lamparelli T, Barisione G, et al. Thymoglobulin prevents chronic graft-versus-host disease, chronic lung dysfunction, and late transplant-related mortality: long-term follow-up of a randomized trial in patients undergoing unrelated donor transplantation. Biol Blood Marrow Transplant. 2006;12:560–5.
74. Bacigalupo A, Lamparelli T, Bruzzi P, et al. Antithymocyte globulin for graft-versus-host disease prophylaxis in transplants from unrelated donors: 2 randomized studies from gruppo italiano trapianti midollo osseo (GITMO). Blood 2001;98:2942–7.
75. Morris E, Thomson K, Craddock C, et al. Outcomes after alemtuzumab-containing reduced-intensity allogeneic transplantation regimen for relapsed and refractory non-Hodgkin lymphoma. Blood 2004;104:3865–71.

76. Mohty M. Mechanisms of action of antithymocyte globulin: T-cell depletion and beyond. Leukemia 2007;21:1387–94.
77. Klangsinsirikul P, Carter GI, Byrne JL, Hale G, Russell NH. Campath-1G causes rapid depletion of circulating host dendritic cells (DCs) before allogeneic transplantation but does not delay donor dc reconstitution. Blood 2002;99:2586–91.
78. Auffermann-Gretzinger S, Eger L, Schetelig J, Bornhauser M, Heidenreich F, Ehninger G. Alemtuzumab depletes dendritic cells more effectively in blood than in skin: a pilot study in patients with chronic lymphocytic leukemia. Transplantation 2007;83:1268–72.
79. Delgado J, Thomson K, Russell N, et al. Results of alemtuzumab-based reduced-intensity allogeneic transplantation for chronic lymphocytic leukemia: a British Society of Blood and Marrow Transplantation Study. Blood 2006;107:1724–30.
80. Tauro S, Craddock C, Peggs K, et al. Allogeneic stem-cell transplantation using a reduced-intensity conditioning regimen has the capacity to produce durable remissions and long-term disease-free survival in patients with high-risk acute myeloid leukemia and myelodysplasia. J Clin Oncol. 2005;23:9387–93.
81. Chakraverty R, Sykes M. The role of antigen-presenting cells in triggering graft-versus-host disease and graft-versus-leukemia. Blood 2007;110:9–17.
82. Storb R, Deeg HJ, Thomas ED, et al. Marrow transplantation for chronic myelocytic leukemia: a controlled trial of cyclosporine versus methotrexate for prophylaxis of graft-versus-host disease. Blood 1985;66:698–702.
83. Storb R, Deeg HJ, Pepe M, et al. Methotrexate and cyclosporine versus cyclosporine alone for prophylaxis of graft versus host disease in patients given HLA-identical marrow grafts for leukemia: long term followup of a controlled trial. Blood 1989;73:1729–34.
84. Ratanatharathorn V, Nash RA, Przepiorka D, et al. Phase III study comparing methotrexate and tacrolimus (prograf, FK506) with methotrexate and cyclosporine for graft-versus-host disease prophylaxis after HLA-identical sibling bone marrow transplantation. Blood 1998;92:2303–14.
85. Nash R, Antin J, Karanes C, et al. A phase III study comparing methotrexate and tacrolimus with methotrexate and cyclosporine for prophylaxis of acute graft-versus-host disease after marrow transplantation from unrelated donors. Blood 2000;96:2062–8.
86. Chao NJ, Snyder DS, Jain M, et al. Equivalence of 2 effective graft-versus-host disease prophylaxis regimens: results of a prospective double-blind randomized trial. Biol Blood Marrow Transplant. 2000;6:254–61.
87. Sehgal S. Rapamune (RAPA, rapamycin, sirolimus): mechanism of action immunosuppressive effect results from blockade of signal transduction and inhibition of cell cycle progression. Clin Biochem. 1998;31:335–40.
88. Cutler C, Li S, Ho VT, et al. Extended follow-up of methotrexate-free immunosuppression using sirolimus and tacrolimus in related and unrelated donor peripheral blood stem cell transplantation. Blood 2007;109:3108–14.
89. Marty FM, Bryar J, Browne SK, et al. Sirolimus-based graft-versus-host disease prophylaxis protects against cytomegalovirus reactivation after allogeneic hematopoietic stem cell transplantation: a cohort analysis. Blood 2007;110:490–500.
90. Teachey DT, Obzut DA, Cooperman J, et al. The mTOR inhibitor CCI-779 induces apoptosis and inhibits growth in preclinical models of primary adult human ALL. Blood 2006;107:1149–55.
91. Wei G, Twomey D, Lamb J, et al. Gene expression-based chemical genomics identifies rapamycin as a modulator of MCL1 and glucocorticoid resistance. Cancer Cell. 2006;10:331–42.
92. Lamb J, Crawford ED, Peck D, et al. The connectivity map: using gene-expression signatures to connect small molecules, genes, and disease. Science 2006;313:1929–35.
93. Ferrara JL, Reddy P. Pathophysiology of graft-versus-host disease. Semin Hematol. 2006;43:3–10.

94. Holler E, Kolb HJ, Moller A, et al. Increased serum levels of tumor necrosis factor alpha precede major complications of bone marrow transplantation. Blood 1990;75:1011–6.
95. Antin JH, Weinstein HJ, Guinan EC, et al. Recombinant human interleukin-1 receptor antagonist in the treatment of steroid-resistant graft-versus-host disease. Blood 1994;84:1342–8.
96. Sackstein R. A revision of Billingham's tenets: the central role of lymphocyte migration in acute graft-versus-host disease. Biol Blood Marrow Transplant. 2006;12 Suppl 1:2–8.
97. Waldman E, Lu SX, Hubbard VM, et al. Absence of beta7 integrin results in less graft-versus-host disease because of decreased homing of alloreactive T cells to intestine. Blood 2006;107:1703–11.
98. Dutt S, Ermann J, Tseng D, et al. L-selectin and beta7 integrin on donor CD4 T cells are required for the early migration to host mesenteric lymph nodes and acute colitis of graft-versus-host disease. Blood 2005;106:4009–15.
99. Hashimoto D, Asakura S, Matsuoka K, et al. FTY720 enhances the activation-induced apoptosis of donor T cells and modulates graft-versus-host disease. Eur J Immunol. 2007;37:271–81.
100. Kim YM, Sachs T, Asavaroengchai W, Bronson R, Sykes M. Graft-versus-host disease can be separated from graft-versus-lymphoma effects by control of lymphocyte trafficking with FTY720. J Clin Invest. 2003;111:659–69.
101. Shapira MY, Resnick IB, Bitan M, et al. Rapid response to alefacept given to patients with steroid resistant or steroid dependent acute graft-versus-host disease: a preliminary report. Bone Marrow Transplant. 2005;36:1097–101.
102. Van Lint MT, Milone G, Leotta S, et al. Treatment of acute graft-versus-host disease with prednisolone: significant survival advantage for day + 5 responders and no advantage for nonresponders receiving anti-thymocyte globulin. Blood 2006;107:4177–81.
103. MacMillan ML, Weisdorf DJ, Wagner JE, et al. Response of 443 patients to steroids as primary therapy for acute graft-versus-host disease: Comparison of grading systems. Biol Blood Marrow Transplant. 2002;8:387–94.
104. MacMillan ML, Weisdorf DJ, Davies SM, et al. Early antithymocyte globulin therapy improves survival in patients with steroid-resistant acute graft-versus-host disease. Biol Blood Marrow Transplant. 2002;8:40–6.
105. Byers VS, Henslee PJ, Kernan NA, et al. Use of an anti-pan T-lymphocyte ricin a chain immunotoxin in steroid-resistant acute graft-versus-host disease. Blood 1990;75:1426–32.
106. Martin PJ, Nelson BJ, Appelbaum FR, et al. Evaluation of a CD5-specific immunotoxin for treatment of acute graft-versus-host disease after allogeneic marrow transplantation. Blood 1996;88:824–30.
107. Marty FM, Lee SJ, Fahey MM, et al. Infliximab use in patients with severe graft-versus-host disease and other emerging risk factors of non-candida invasive fungal infections in allogeneic hematopoietic stem cell transplant recipients: a cohort study. Blood 2003;102:2768–76.
108. Couriel D, Saliba R, Hicks K, et al. Tumor necrosis factor-alpha blockade for the treatment of acute GVHD. Blood 2004;104:649–54.
109. McCarthy PL Jr, Williams L, Harris-Bacile M, et al. A clinical phase I/II study of recombinant human interleukin-1 receptor in glucocorticoid-resistant graft-versus-host disease. Transplantation 1996;62:626–31.
110. Macmillan ML, Couriel D, Weisdorf DJ, et al. A phase 2/3 multicenter randomized clinical trial of ABX-CBL versus ATG as secondary therapy for steroid-resistant acute graft-versus-host disease. Blood 2007;109:2657–62.
111. Lee SJ, Zahrieh D, Agura E, et al. Effect of up-front daclizumab when combined with steroids for the treatment of acute graft-versus-host disease: results of a randomized trial. Blood 2004;104:1559–64.

112. Cragg L, Blazar BR, Defor T, et al. A randomized trial comparing prednisone with antithymocyte globulin/prednisone as an initial systemic therapy for moderately severe acute graft-versus-host disease. Biol Blood Marrow Transplant. 2000;6:441–7.
113. Teachey DT, Bickert B, Bunin N. Daclizumab for children with corticosteroid refractory graft-versus-host disease. Bone Marrow Transplant. 2006;37:95–9.
114. Bordigoni P, Dimicoli S, Clement L, et al. Daclizumab, an efficient treatment for steroid-refractory acute graft-versus-host disease. Br J Haematol. 2006;135:382–5.
115. Przepiorka D, Kernan NA, Ippoliti C, et al. Daclizumab, a humanized anti-interleukin-2 receptor alpha chain antibody, for treatment of acute graft-versus-host disease. Blood 2000;95:83–9.
116. Ho VT, Zahrieh D, Hochberg E, et al. Safety and efficacy of denileukin diftitox in patients with steroid-refractory acute graft-versus-host disease after allogeneic hematopoietic stem cell transplantation. Blood 2004;104:1224–6.
117. Shaughnessy PJ, Bachier C, Grimley M, et al. Denileukin diftitox for the treatment of steroid-resistant acute graft-versus-host disease. Biol Blood Marrow Transplant. 2005;11:188–93.
118. Bolanos-Meade J, Jacobsohn DA, Margolis J, et al. Pentostatin in steroid-refractory acute graft-versus-host disease. J Clin Oncol. 2005;23:2661–8.
119. Basara N, Blau WI, Romer E, et al. Mycophenolate mofetil for the treatment of acute and chronic GVHD in bone marrow transplant patients. Bone Marrow Transplant. 1998;22:61–5.
120. Uberti JP, Ayash L, Ratanatharathorn V, et al. Pilot trial on the use of etanercept and methylprednisolone as primary treatment for acute graft-versus-host disease. Biol Blood Marrow Transplant. 2005;11:680–7.
121. Benito AI, Furlong T, Martin PJ, et al. Sirolimus (rapamycin) for the treatment of steroid-refractory acute graft-versus-host disease. Transplantation 2001;72:1924–9.
122. Greinix HT, Volc-Platzer B, Kalhs P, et al. Extracorporeal photochemotherapy in the treatment of severe steroid-refractory acute graft-versus-host disease: a pilot study. Blood 2000;96:2426–31.
123. Ringden O, Uzunel M, Rasmusson I, et al. Mesenchymal stem cells for treatment of therapy-resistant graft-versus-host disease. Transplantation 2006;81:1390–7.
124. Le Blanc K, Frassoni F, Ball L, et al. Mesenchymal stem cells for treatment of severe acute graft-versus-host disease. Blood 2006;108 Suppl 1:5304a.

Chapter 12
Biology and Management of Chronic Graft-Versus-Host Disease

Paul J. Martin and Steven Z. Pavletic

12.1 Clinical Presentation and Significance of Chronic GvHD

Chronic graft-versus-host disease (GvHD) is a pleiomorphic autoimmune and alloimune syndrome with onset generally occurring between 3 and 24 months after allogeneic hematopoietic stem cell transplantation (HSCT) [1]. The highly variable clinical manifestations of chronic GvHD frequently involve the skin, liver, eyes, mouth, respiratory tract, esophagus, and less frequently involve serosal surfaces, lower gastrointestinal tract, female genitalia, and fascia [2]. The biological mechanisms leading to chronic GvHD are not as well understood as those leading to acute GvHD. Although acute GvHD has been recognized as a risk factor for chronic GvHD, not all cases of acute GvHD evolve into chronic GvHD, and chronic GvHD can develop in the absence of any prior overt acute GvHD. In the skin, the initial phase of chronic GvHD is characterized by an intense mononuclear inflammatory infiltrate with destructive changes at the dermal–epidermal junction, accompanied by irregular acanthosis, hyperkeratosis or atrophy, progressing to dermal fibrosis and sclerosis [3]. Other hallmarks include destruction of tubuloalveolar glands and ducts in the skin, salivary and lacrimal glands and respiratory epithelium, and destruction of bile ducts in the liver.

It is estimated that about 3500 new cases of chronic GvHD are diagnosed each year in North America, but the prevalence of chronic GvHD is much higher, since the disease has a protracted clinical course [2]. Incidence and prevalence estimates are compromised by protean nature of the disease and the lack of standardized diagnostic criteria, and also by variability in observer experience, limited expert follow-up, and differences in statistical methods among studies.

The lack of standardized criteria and definitions for diagnosis and measurement of outcomes in clinical trials has hampered advances in the prevention and treatment of chronic GvHD. Consequently, no product has been approved by the US Food and Drug Administration for these indications. These problems

P.J. Martin (✉)
Fred Hutchinson Cancer Research Center, Seattle, WA, USA
e-mail: pmartin@fhcrc.org

M.R. Bishop (ed.), *Hematopoietic Stem Cell Transplantation*,
Cancer Treatment and Research 144, DOI 10.1007/978-0-387-78580-6_12,

have recently gained attention from the international transplant community, as demonstrated by a recent consensus development project sponsored by the National Institutes of Health [3–8]. The recommendations of the consensus development project should advance the standards and uniformity of chronic GvHD clinical research, although many of these newer criteria still need to be validated and refined.

12.2 Diagnosis of Chronic GvHD

The diagnosis of chronic GvHD requires at least one *diagnostic* sign that is found only in chronic GvHD and not in acute GvHD (e.g., poikiloderma, sclerotic skin features, oral lichen-planus like changes) or at least one *distinctive* sign that is highly suggestive of chronic GvHD (e.g., nail dystrophy, vitiligo-like depigmentation, or bronchiolitis obliterans with diagnosis based on pulmonary function tests and computerized tomography findings) together with laboratory or biopsy confirmation in the same or another organ (Table 12.1) [3]. Biopsies are also needed to rule out other potential diagnoses such as infection, drug toxicity and second cancers and to confirm the diagnosis when clinical signs are confined to internal organs or when clinical assessment is made difficult by concomitant medical conditions [3].

In the past, the presence of any manifestation of GvHD beyond 100 days after HSCT was called chronic GvHD, even if the manifestation was indistinguishable from acute GvHD. It has been observed, however, that acute GvHD may persist, recur or present more than 3 months after transplantation, particularly in patients who have received reduced-intensity conditioning. The current consensus recommends that acute and chronic GvHD should be distinguished by clinical manifestations and not by time after transplantation [3]. Two main categories of GvHD are now recognized, each with two subcategories (Table 12.2). The broad category of acute GvHD includes *classic* acute GvHD (maculopapular erythematous rash, gastrointestinal symptoms, or cholestatic hepatitis) occurring within 100 days after HSCT or donor leukocyte infusion (DLI), while *persistent, recurrent or late acute GvHD* (usually seen after withdrawal of immunosuppression) occurs more than 100 days after transplantation or DLI. The presence of GvHD without diagnostic or distinctive chronic GvHD manifestations defines these two categories. A second broad

Table 12.1 Requirements for chronic GvHD diagnosis

I	Presence of at least one *diagnostic*[a] clinical manifestation OR at least one *distinct*[a] manifestation confirmed by pertinent biopsy or other relevant clinical tests.
II	Distinction from acute GvHD (maculo-papular erythematous rash, elevated liver function tests, diarrhea-nausea-vomiting).
III	Exclusion of other possible diagnosis causing the clinical manifestation (i.e., infection, drug effect, second cancer).

[a]As defined in the reference by Filipovich et al. [3]

Table 12.2 Categories of GvHD according to the NIH consensus criteria

Category	Time of symptoms after HSCT or DLI	Presence of acute GvHD features[a]	Presence of chronic GvHD features
Acute GvHD			
Classic acute GvHD	≤100 days	Yes	No
Persistent, recurrent, or late-onset acute GvHD	>100 days	Yes	No
Chronic GvHD			
Classic chronic GvHD	No time limit	No	Yes
Overlap syndrome	No time limit	Yes	Yes

[a]Maculopapular erythematous rash, gastrointestinal symptoms, elevated liver function tests

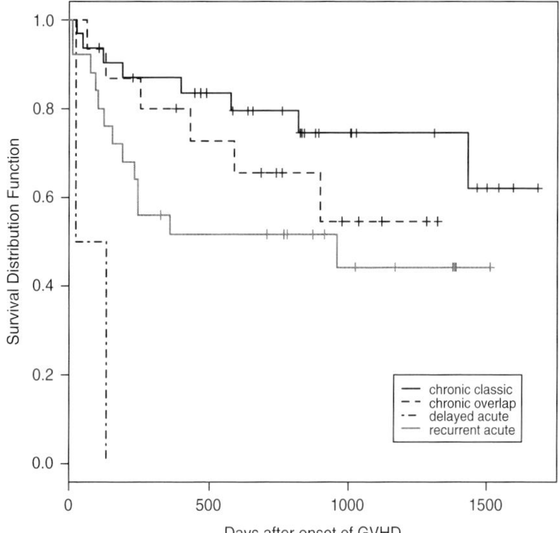

Fig. 12.1 Overall survival stratified by the GvHD type. The figure is reproduced with permission from the reference by Jagasia et al. [10]

GvHD category encompasses *classic* chronic GvHD with manifestations that can be ascribed only to chronic GvHD and an *overlap syndrome* with features of both acute and chronic GvHD. The newly defined entity of persistent, recurrent or late acute GvHD has been associated with poor survival when chronic GvHD patients were reclassified according to the new definition (Fig. 12.1) [9, 10].

12.3 Classification and Staging

Chronic GvHD has been classified according to the type of onset, need for systemic immunosuppressive therapy and mortality risk. The disease may evolve directly from acute GvHD ("progressive") or after resolution of acute

GvHD ("quiescent"), and also may develop without prior acute GvHD ("de novo" onset). Progressive onset has been most consistently associated with decreased survival. Historically, chronic GvHD was classified as limited (localized skin involvement and or liver dysfunction) or extensive (generalized skin involvement, liver histology showing aggressive hepatitis or involvement of any other target organ) [11]. This classification was formulated on the basis of results from a retrospective analysis of 20 patients who were diagnosed with chronic GvHD in an era before cyclosporine was used for post-transplant immunosuppression. This classification was intended to identify patients who needed systemic immunosuppressive therapy. More recent analysis has suggested that this classification system may have poor reproducibility and limited prognostic value [12].

Several investigators have developed scales and categorization systems designed to predict nonrelapse mortality (NRM) based on a variety of clinical factors at the onset of chronic GvHD [12–15]. The NIH consensus has recommended a system for scoring chronic GvHD manifestations in eight sites on a 0–3 scale. This system was not designed to predict NRM but was intended to assess the severity of and functional impact of chronic GvHD [3]. The eight organs include the skin, mouth, eyes, GI tract, liver, lungs, joints and fascia, and genital tract. A global staging of severity (none, mild, moderate, severe) is derived by combining organ-specific scores and is intended to replace the current "limited-extensive" scoring system [3, 11]. Mild chronic GvHD stage involves only one or two organs with maximum score of 1. Moderate chronic GvHD involves at least one organ with a maximum score or 2, or 3 or more organs with maximum scores of 1. A lung score of 1 is also considered as moderate stage chronic GvHD. Severe chronic GvHD involves at least one organ with a score of 3 or a lung score of 2. This staging system is not intended to be used for monitoring of therapeutic response in intervention trials [16].

12.4 Pathophysiology and Immunobiology of Chronic GvHD

Insight regarding the pathophysiology and immunobiology of chronic GvHD is limited. A wide variety of experimental models have indicated an association between type-2 polarized immune responses and the development of fibrosis [17], and donor type 2 immune responses are required for induction of skin GvHD in mice [18]. Complement factor 5 (C5) has been identified as a quantitative trait that modifies liver fibrosis in mice and humans [19], and C5b-9 complexes are deposited in the skin, liver, lung and kidney in mice with GvHD [20]. C3 is deposited at the dermal-epidermal junction in humans with chronic GvHD, but deposition of C5b-9 complexes has not been described.

12.4.1 Experimental Studies of Chronic GvHD

At least four different hypotheses regarding the pathogenesis of chronic GvHD have emerged from studies with animal models. One hypothesis posits that chronic GvHD results from thymic damage caused by acute GvHD, resulting in failure to delete nascent T cells that recognize antigens on donor cells. A second hypothesis implicates a central role for TGF-β in the pathogenesis of the disease. A third hypothesis implicates B cells and antibody-mediated mechanisms in certain manifestations of the disease. The fourth hypothesis posits that chronic GvHD results from insufficiency of T regulatory cells. The literature is confusing because the term "chronic GvHD" has been used to describe a syndrome of antibody-mediated glomerulonephritis that occurs when recipient B cells are activated by donor $CD4^+$ cells after transplantation of spleen cells from certain parental strains into nonirradiated F1 mice. The resulting nephrotic syndrome is more characteristic of lupus nephritis as opposed to chronic GvHD, although case reports have occasionally described nephrotic syndrome in patients with chronic GvHD.

12.4.1.1 Failure of Negative Selection in the Thymus

Cutaneous changes of acute and chronic GvHD occur in $H\text{-}2^b$ MHC-identical transplants between LP and C57BL/6 (B6) mice. Parkman [21] showed that clones from B6 recipients with chronic GvHD were all $CD4^+$ and all showed IL-2-dependent proliferative responses specific for MHC class II $I\text{-}A^b$ antigens expressed by both the donor and recipient. The observation that $CD4^+$ clones from recipients with chronic GvHD showed specificity for $I\text{-}A^b$ suggested that these cells had emerged from marrow progenitors that escaped negative selection in the thymus, and the observation that similar clones could be detected in mice with acute GvHD suggested that the processes responsible for generating such autoimmune clones begin early after transplantation.

Acute GvHD causes severe histopathological damage in the thymus, including injury to medullary epithelial cells, effacement of the corticomedullary junction, disappearance of Hassal's corpuscles and depletion of $CD4^+CD8^+$ cells [22]. In the thymus, developing T cells that express receptors with high affinity for peptide-MHC complexes or "self"-antigens on adjacent cells are deleted. This process of negative selection occurs in the medulla and is mediated most efficiently by marrow-derived dendritic cells and also by thymic medullary epithelium. Negative thymic selection among T cells developing in mice with GvHD is impaired [23], and the T cells developing in mice with GvHD are pathogenic. Zhang et al. [24] showed that dendritic cells were depleted in the thymus of B6 mice with acute GvHD caused by donor C3H.SW CD8 cells. The resulting absence of MHC-class II-positive dendritic cells in the thymic medulla allowed the development of $CD4^+$ cells that responded vigorously to B6 alloantigens. These $CD4^+$ cells caused chronic

GvHD when they were adoptively transferred into irradiated secondary B6 recipients. Administration of keratinocyte growth factor (KGF) at the time of the transplant enhanced reconstitution of dendritic cells in the thymus, and the $CD4^+$ cells that emerged from KGF-treated recipients did not cause GvHD in secondary B6 recipients [24].

Several groups have shown that transplantation of MHC-class II-deficient marrow into wild-type recipients of the same strain causes autoimmune damage in the skin [25, 26], liver and intestines [26]. Thymectomy prevented the disease, and adoptive transfer of $CD4^+$ cells caused acute GvHD in irradiated secondary recipients of the same strain. In a variation of the same approach, Sakoda et al. [27] found that irradiated C3H ($H\text{-}2^k$) recipients reconstituted with T cell-depleted marrow from MHC-class II-deficient B6 ($H\text{-}2^b$) donors developed a disease with clinical and histopathological features characteristic of chronic GvHD, including epidermal atrophy, follicular dropout, fat loss, dermal fibrosis, bile duct loss, with inflammation, atrophy and fibrosis of acinar tissue in the salivary glands. As was the case in B6 recipients, thymectomy prevented the disease. The chimeric $CD4^+$ cells proliferated in response to donor-type B6 antigen-presenting cells (APCs) but not in response to recipient-type C3H APCs. Adoptive transfer of chimeric $CD4^+$ cells in the presence of B6 APCs caused chronic GvHD in irradiated secondary C3H recipients. In irradiated secondary B6 recipients, however, the adoptively transferred $CD4^+$ cells caused acute GvHD.

Taken together, the results suggest that $CD4^+$ cells cause acute GvHD when they recognize antigens expressed by recipient epithelial tissues but cause chronic GvHD when they recognize antigens on donor marrow-derived cells but not on recipient cells. In this model, the acute or chronic nature of GvHD appears to be dictated respectively by the presence or absence of the recognized antigens on epithelial cells of the secondary recipient. Similar experiments have been done with B6 donors and MHC-mismatched BALB/c or MHC-matched BALB.B recipients. Irradiated secondary BALB/c recipients developed acute GvHD [27], while secondary BALB.B recipients developed chronic GvHD [27] after adoptive transfer of $CD4^+$ cells from chimeric donors with GvHD. Hence, an absence of the recognized antigens on recipient epithelial cells does not entirely explain the development of chronic GvHD in secondary recipients.

Further work is needed to define the B6 antigens that stimulate proliferation of donor $CD4^+$ cells in the model described by Sakoda et al. [27] In principle, the $CD4^+$ cells that develop in the chimeras are positively selected by thymic cortical epithelial cells of the C3H recipient and negatively selected by MHC class I-positive B6 APCs and also, to some extent, by recipient C3H epithelial cells in the thymic medulla. Although the donor-derived $CD4^+$ cells that escape MHC-class II-specific negative selection respond to wild type B6 APCs in vitro, the B6-derived APCs in the primary recipients do not express MHC-class II molecules and would not be expected to stimulate donor-derived $CD4^+$ cells in vivo.

Taken together, experiments with mice demonstrate that acute GvHD impairs negative selection of T cells in the thymus and that $CD4^{+}$ cells recognizing donor alloantigens can cause a syndrome with remarkable similarity to chronic GvHD. Further work is needed to determine whether these observations have relevance for chronic GvHD in humans. A report by Tsoi et al. in 1980 showed that T cells from transplant recipients showed proliferative responses after stimulation with donor cells in 7 of 22 cases (32%) with chronic GvHD and in only 1 of 12 cases without chronic GvHD. These findings are consistent with defective negative selection by donor derived [28] APCs in the thymus. In 8 of 22 (36%) chronic GvHD cases, however, responses were observed only after stimulation with recipient cells and not with donor cells, and in seven cases (32%), no response was observed after stimulation with either donor or recipient cells. These results suggest that although impaired negative selection by APCs in the thymus might contribute to the pathogenesis of chronic GvHD in some cases, it seems unlikely that this mechanism can account for all cases.

Role of TGF-β

A syndrome characteristic of chronic GvHD develops after transplantation of B10.D2 lymphoid cells into irradiated BALB/c recipients [29]. Skin changes include a mononuclear infiltrate deep in the dermis, loss of dermal fat, increased collagen deposition, and "dropout" of dermal appendages such as hair follicles, but in distinction to findings in acute GvHD, apoptosis of basal epithelial cells at the dermal-epidermal junction does not occur. Skin changes begin as early as day 11, and cutaneous fibrosis is apparent as early as day 21. Deposits of IgG, IgA and IgM appear at the dermal epidermal junction in this model [30]. Additional features of the disease in this model include inflammation and fibrosis in salivary and lacrimal glands, sclerosing cholangitis, progressive renal and gastrointestinal fibrosis, and development of anti-Scl-70 antibody [31].

Naïve donor $CD4^{+}$ cells initiate the disease in this strain combination [32, 33], and the dermal infiltrate comprises T cells, monocytes and macrophages [34]. APCs of either the donor or recipient are sufficient to initiate the disease, and costimulation of donor T cells through CD80 or CD86 on APCs is necessary in order to induce chronic GvHD [35]. In this model, costimulation of donor $CD4^{+}$ cells through CD40 on APCs is necessary to induce intestinal disease but not skin disease. T cells and macrophages in the skin express TGF-β1 but not TGF-β2 or TGF-β3 mRNA [36]. Microarray analysis also showed upregulated expression of type 1 (interferon-γ) and type 2 (IL-6, IL-10 and IL-13) cytokines, chemokines, and a variety of growth factors and cell adhesion molecules in recipients with chronic GvHD as compared to recipients without chronic GvHD [37]. Administration of a neutralizing antibody against TGF-β prevented or reduced virtually all cutaneous manifestations of chronic GvHD, including cellular infiltration, immune cell activation, thickening and fibrosis [34]. In contrast, neutralization of TGF-β by administration of latency-associated peptide prevented thickening and fibrosis, but did not prevent influx of T cells and monocytes or immune cell activation in the skin [38].

Cutaneous manifestations of chronic GvHD develop after transplantation of B10.D2 spleen cells into MHC-matched (H-2^d) BALB/c recipients but not after transplantation of B10 spleen cells into MHC-matched (H-2^b) BALB.B recipients or after transplantation of B10.BR spleen cells into MHC-matched (H-2^k) BALB.K recipients [38]. In each of these combinations, the background genes of the donor are of B10 origin, while those of the recipient are of BALB origin, and the combinations differ from each other only in the MHC. These observations were interpreted as indicating that H-2^d MHC class II molecules (I-A^d or I-E^d) could present minor antigen peptides derived from BALB skin to $CD4^+$ cells of B10 donors, while H-2^b and H-2^k class II molecules could not. Another explanation for this observation could be related to a polymorphism in the TNF-α gene, which is located in the MHC [39]. Expression of TNF-α is reduced in H-2^d mice as compared to H-2^b or H-2^k mice. Since TNF-α is a potent inhibitor of fibrosis induced by TGF-β, it has been proposed that the fibrosis observed with B10.D2 donors and BALB/c recipients might be related to an inability of cutaneous $CD4^+$ cells to produce TNF-α [39].

Attempts to prevent or treat chronic GvHD through direct or indirect manipulation of TGF-β may encounter unexpected complexity. For example, Asai et al. [39] showed that activated donor NK cells could attenuate the severity of acute GvHD through a TGF-β-dependent mechanism. TGF-β has a nonredundant, essential role in limiting T cell and NK cell responses, and TGF-β-deficient mice develop an early onset lethal autoimmune disease [40]. Since TGF-β induces Foxp3 expression and T-regulatory function in $CD4^+CD25^-$ precursors [41], TGF-β neutralization could exacerbate GvHD by interfering with development of T regulatory cells.

The ability of TGF-β neutralization to prevent or treat chronic GvHD may depend on the context in which the disease develops. Treatment of B10.D2 donors with G-CSF exacerbates the severity of skin GvHD in sublethally irradiated BALB/c recipients. Donor T cells are required for the development of GvHD, but the severity of cutaneous sclerosis is determined by the non-T cell fraction of grafts from G-CSF-treated donors [42, 43]. In this model, neutralization of TGF-β from day 0–42 had no effect on manifestations of GvHD in the skin, liver or gastrointestinal tract, but neutralization of TGF-β beginning on day 14 appeared to attenuate progression of the disease to some extent in the skin and gastrointestinal tract, but not the liver [43]. Neutralization of TGF-β early after transplantation exacerbated acute GvHD by interfering with the regulatory effects of TGF-β on proliferation of donor T cells stimulated by recipient alloantigens.

The role of TGF-β in human chronic GvHD has not been defined. Results of one study showed elevated serum levels of TGF-β in patients with chronic GvHD as compared to patients without chronic GvHD [44]. The interpretation of these results is complicated, since assays were carried out not with plasma, but with serum, which contains large amounts of TGF-β released from platelets during clotting. Gene expression studies have shown that increased TGF-β signaling in $CD4^+$ cells and $CD8^+$ cells was associated with a reduced risk of chronic GvHD in humans [45]. These data might appear to conflict with results from experiments with BD.D2 donors and BALB/c recipients, but four of the five TGF-β pathway genes that were examined also showed increased expression associated with a decreased risk of acute GvHD. The association of increased TGF-β activity with a reduced risk of chronic GvHD might result from a decreased risk of acute GvHD, since acute GvHD is a well-recognized risk factor for chronic GvHD.

Experiments with B10.D2 donors and BALB/c recipients have suggested an alternative approach toward prevention or treatment of chronic GvHD in humans. Established chronic GvHD in this model can be reversed by administration of a CD137-specific antibody [46], an approach that has been used successfully to treat $CD4^+$-mediated experimental autoimmune diseases.

Role of B Cells

Deposition of antibody at the junction between the dermis and epidermis has been demonstrated in both murine models [30] and in humans [47] with chronic GvHD. Studies by Zhang et al. [48] showed that both euthymic and athymic BALB/c recipients developed high levels of double strand DNA-specific IgG1 and IgG2a autoantibodies in the serum, cutaneous sclerosis, and glomerulonephritis with proteinuria, beginning within the first 2 weeks after transplantation of spleen cells from DBA/2 (H-2^d) donors. Induction of disease required both donor $CD4^+CD25^-$ T cells and donor B cells, while donor $CD4^+CD25^+$ cells prevented the disease. In the absence of donor B cells, donor $CD4^+$ cells caused acute GvHD without cutaneous sclerosis or glomerulonephritis. The relevance of this model for human chronic GvHD could be questioned, since double-strand DNA-specific autoantibodies, immune complex glomerulonephritis, and proteinuria are characteristic of systemic lupus but rarely occur in patients with chronic GvHD [49].

Several lines of evidence suggest that B cells are likely to have some role in the pathogenesis of chronic GvHD in humans. First, anecdotal experience and phase 2 studies have shown clinical improvement in some patients with chronic GvHD after administration of a CD20-specific antibody [50]. Second, biomarker studies have shown enhanced CD86 expression after TLR9 stimulation of B cells from patients with chronic GvHD, as compared to those from controls [51]. Third, agonistic antibodies against platelet-derived growth factor receptor (PDGFR) were detected in serum from each of 22 patients with clinical extensive chronic GvHD but not in serum from any of 17 patients without chronic GvHD [52]. These antibodies induce tyrosine phosphorylation of PDGFR, accumulation of reactive oxygen species, and stimulation of type 1 collagen gene expression by fibroblasts, through a Ras and ERK1/2-dependent signaling pathway. These results suggest novel approaches for treatment of chronic

GvHD, since ligand-induced phosphorylation of the PDGFR is susceptible to inhibition by certain tyrosine-kinase inhibitors, including imatinib.

12.4.1.2 Role of T Regulatory Cells

Anderson et al. [53] showed that radiation-resistant recipient $CD4^+CD25^+$ T regulatory cells can protect against severe chronic GvHD in experiments with B10.D2 donors and BALB/c recipients. Similar attenuation of chronic GvHD manifestations could also be produced by administration of donor-derived T regulatory cells [48, 53]. Recent results have suggested that acute GvHD interferes with development of T regulatory cells after the transplant, thereby creating conditions that are permissive for development of autoimmunity [54, 55]. In these experiments, spleen cells from B6 → BALB/c chimeras with GvHD were adoptively transferred into nonirradiated secondary immunodeficient B6 or BALB/c recipients. Cells from the chimeras caused colitis in secondary B6 recipients but not in BALB/c recipients [54]. T regulatory cells did not develop in mice with acute GvHD, and T regulatory cells added to the secondary graft prevented GvHD in secondary recipients [55]. Taken together, results from several animal models suggest that T regulatory cells [48, 53, 55] or regulatory dendritic cells [56] could be used to control chronic GvHD, although conflicting results have been reported with respect to the role of T-regulatory cells in preventing the development of chronic GvHD in humans [57–61].

12.5 Management of Chronic GvHD in Humans

Chronic GvHD contributes to late post-transplant morbidity and mortality, but pathophysiologic processes associated with chronic GvHD also produce important therapeutic graft-versus-tumor (GvT) effects in patients with malignant disease. Due to insufficient understanding of chronic GvHD biology, current treatments are typically based on nonspecific global immunosuppression. How to gain clinical advantage by separating beneficial effects (i.e., GvT) from harmful effects (i.e., GvHD) poses a major challenge [62].

12.5.1 Prevention of Chronic GvHD

Although acute GvHD is the best predictor for the development of chronic GvHD, a number of strategies that successfully decreased the incidence of acute GvHD have not decreased the risk of chronic GvHD [16, 63–68]. Other unsuccessful attempts to prevent chronic GvHD include administration of thalidomide, intravenous immunoglobulin, or hydroxychloroquine, or preemptive treatment of sub-clinical chronic GvHD diagnosed by skin or lip biopsy [69–72]. Addition of anti-thymocyte globulin or anti-CD52 monoclonal antibody to preparative regimens appears to provide protection against extensive chronic GvHD but increases the risk of infection and attenuates GvT effects [73, 74].

12.5.2 Treatment of Chronic GvHD

The aims of chronic GvHD treatment are to stop the destructive immunological process, alleviate symptoms, and prevent disease progression that may lead to irreversible disability or death. The ultimate goal is to establish immunological tolerance and withdraw immunosuppressive therapy. The typical course of chronic GvHD is protracted, lasting on average 2–3 years. Approximately 85% of patients who survive beyond 5 years after diagnosis are able to discontinue systemic therapy [75]. The principal components of chronic GvHD therapy include systemic treatment with agents that suppress or modulate immune responses, integrated with ancillary therapy and supportive care (see below). Symptomatic mild chronic GvHD is often effectively treated with local therapies alone (e.g., topical steroids to the skin or cyclosporine eye drops), but systemic therapy should be considered for patients who meet criteria for moderate-severe global severity [3]. Some experts incorporate the presence or absence of high-risk features (e.g., thrombocytopenia or progressive onset) and the underlying reason for transplantation (e.g., malignant versus nonmalignant disease) or current comorbid conditions (e.g., infection) in assessing the indications for systemic treatment of chronic GvHD.

12.5.2.1 Primary Therapy

The most widely used initial systemic treatment of chronic GvHD relies on prednisone alone in conjunction with cyclosporine or tacrolimus [2, 76-79]. In contrast to acute GvHD where a more fulminant presentation and high frequency of gastrointestinal symptoms require parenteral treatment, chronic GvHD can usually be managed by oral treatment. Treatment typically begins with prednisone at 1 mg/kg/day in a single oral dose in the morning to mimic the normal circadian rhythm of adrenal corticosteroid secretion. Cyclosporine or tacrolimus are dosed twice a day to keep blood concentrations within the therapeutic range. If this treatment produces clinical improvement, the dose of prednisone is tapered (e.g., 25% per week) to a target of 1 mg/kg every other day. Responses are evaluated every 3 months during alternate day prednisone administration. The 3-month time frame for evaluation of response to a given therapy is based on the observation that 90% of patients who ultimately respond to therapy will show signs of response at that point [80]. If response is observed at 3 months, therapy is continued until chronic GvHD manifestations resolve, when weaning of prednisone doses can be resumed. If there is no response by the 3-month time point, or if disease manifestations progress at any time, secondary treatment should be started [76, 77].

Very few studies have attempted to improve outcomes of primary therapy for chronic GvHD. An early study showed harm when azathioprine was added to prednisone [76], and a subsequent trial [77] showed only limited benefit when cyclosporine was added to prednisone for treatment of patients with platelet counts above 100,000/μL at the onset of chronic GvHD. Two randomized trials testing the addition of thalidomide as part of initial therapy showed no clinical benefit [81, 82]. Currently two multi-centered randomized phase III trials are testing whether adding mycophenolate mofetil (USA trial: ClinicalTrials.gov Identifier NCT00089141) or enteric coated mycophenolic acid (European trial: ClinicalTrials.gov Identifier NCT00298324) as part of the initial immunosuppressive regimen improves the success rate of primary therapy.

12.5.2.2 Secondary Therapy

Initial treatment fails to produce a partial or complete response within the first year in approximately 50% of patients with chronic GvHD [15]. Indications for secondary treatment include progression of chronic GvHD manifestations in a previously affected organ or site, development of new manifestations in a previously unaffected organ or site, stable persistence of chronic GvHD despite 4–12 weeks of sustained therapy, or inability to taper immunosuppression without recurrence of clinical manifestations. Earlier initiation of secondary therapy would be appropriate in patients with more severe chronic GvHD, while a longer trial of initial therapy would be appropriate in patients with sclerotic skin changes or other slowly reversible manifestations.

The recalcitrant nature of bronchiolitis obliterans (BO) represents a special situation where full steroid doses of 1 mg/kg/day are typically administered for many months, and stabilization of disease progression may be considered as success. A delay in initiating secondary therapy might also be appropriate when the next agent to be used has a high risk of toxicity. Inability to tolerate therapy (e.g., steroid myopathy or calcineurin and/or sirolimus induced thrombotic microangopathy) may also be considered an indication for secondary treatment.

There is no current standard of care for secondary treatment of chronic GvHD. Many phase II studies of secondary treatment have been published, with response rates ranging between 25% and 75%. Responses are frequently incomplete and not durable [9, 50, 83–105]. Agents that have been used for secondary treatment of chronic GvHD are summarized in Table 12.3. Most of these agents have been tested in small numbers of patients with marginal success and with poor clinical satisfaction [106]. Agents that are currently in vogue for treatment of steroid-resistance chronic GvHD include extracorporeal photopheresis, rituximab, and pentostatin.

Since there is no therapeutic standard, the selection of agents for secondary treatment of chronic GvHD is typically made after reviewing the agents used for prior treatment, considering the compatibility of new agents with any continuing concurrent treatment, evaluating the overall risks and benefits,

Table 12.3 Second line agents used for the treatment of chronic GvHD

Commonly used	Sometimes used	Rarely used	Case reports
Mycophenolate	PUVA	Azathioprine	Daclizumab
Steroid pulse	Thalidomide	ATG	Infliximab
ECP	Ursodiol	TLI	Etarnecept
Sirolimus	Clofazimine	Low dose MTX	Imatinib
Pentostatin	Acitretin	Cytoxan	Montelukast
Rituximab			Bortezomib
Plaquenil			

ECP extracorporeal photopheresis, *PUVA* psoralen-ultraviolet A light, *ATG* anti-thymocyte globulin, *TLI* total lymphoid irradiation, *MTX* methotrexate

and assessing patient preferences. Physicians must be also be mindful of the distinction between active disease and irreversible organ damage, since the former may respond to treatment, but the latter cannot.

12.5.3 Ancillary Therapy and Supportive Care

Clinical manifestations of chronic GvHD can persist for prolonged periods of time, causing significant morbidity. Hence, ancillary therapy and supportive care to prevent infections, optimize nutrition, ameliorate morbidity and optimize functional performance and capacity are critical components of management [7]. As used in the NIH consensus recommendations, the term "ancillary therapy" refers to any intervention such as topical corticosteroids, cyclosporine eye drops or any other nonsystemic therapeutic intervention directed at control of symptoms. The term "supportive care" includes a broad spectrum of interventions that are directed at control of organ specific or systemic symptoms. Supportive care includes antibiotics for prevention of infections, management of osteoporosis, metabolic problems, physical therapy, as well as a number of educational, preventive and psychosocial measures. Occasionally, their use may circumvent the need for systemic treatment or allow doses of systemic agents to be reduced [7].

In general, close serial monitoring of all organ systems is recommended to promote early detection and intervention. Especially challenging cases should be considered for consultation referral at one of the major national centers with multidisciplinary expertise in studying chronic GvHD. Infection is the most common cause of mortality in patients with chronic GvHD and prophylaxis of infections requires special emphasis. The immune defects in chronic GvHD are broad, encompassing macrophage function, antibody production and T cell function. All patients with chronic GvHD are considered at risk for infection with encapsulated bacteria, particularly *Streptococcus pneumoniae*, but also *H. influenzae* and *Neisseria meningitides*. Prophylactic antibiotics should be given to all patients with chronic GvHD as long as systemic immunosuppressive treatment is being administered [7].

12.5.4 Prognosis and Outcomes

The characteristics most consistently associated with an increased risk of late NRM among patients with chronic GvHD are thrombocytopenia ($<100 \times 10^9$/L) and progressive onset of chronic GvHD from acute GvHD. A number of other factors associated with increased NRM in patients with chronic GvHD have been reported and include elevated serum total bilirubin concentration, generalized or lichen planus-like skin involvement, poor Karnofsky performance status, steroid therapy at the time of onset, diarrhea, weight loss, GI involvement, lack of oral involvement, history of prior acute GvHD grades II-IV, HLA mismatch, increased age, or lack of therapeutic response to chronic GvHD treatment [12–15, 75, 80, 107]. Studies evaluating prognostic factors for NRM all have retrospective designs. These studies frequently included patients from various treatment eras and patient populations that were heterogeneous with respect to the hematopoietic cell source (bone marrow versus peripheral blood), donor type (related versus unrelated), patient age (inclusion of pediatric patients), intensity of the pretransplant conditioning regimen (myeloablative versus reduced-intensity), and treatment for chronic GvHD. These factors could potentially affect the reproducibility of results in different patient populations [107].

Stewart et al. identified prognostic factors associated with time to permanent discontinuation of systemic immunosuppression, which is considered a surrogate endpoint for cure of chronic GvHD. Factors associated with poor prognosis included peripheral blood hematopoietic cell source, female donor for male recipient, recipient HLA mismatch, elevated serum total bilirubin concentration, and involvement of multiple organ sites at the onset of chronic GvHD [75]. Arora et al. identified the attainment of complete therapeutic response as an important predictive factor for permanent withdrawal of immunosuppression [15]. Prospective validation and refinement of risk factors for NRM among patients with chronic GvHD should be a major goal of future research so that patients receive appropriate risk-adjusted treatment.

12.6 Future Prospects

Clinical interest in chronic GvHD has increased recently, but the basic research needed for clinical translation remains scant. No animal model fully replicates all of the features of chronic GvHD in humans, and it appears likely that multiple biological mechanisms account for the diverse features the disease. The disease is clearly initiated by donor T cells that recognize recipient alloantigens, since the incidence of chronic GvHD can be decreased by exhaustive depletion of T cell from the graft. On the other hand, experimental studies have clearly demonstrated that "autoreactive" T cells and B cells, together with deficiency of T regulatory cells, can contribute to pathogenesis of the disease through mechanisms that do not necessarily depend on prior acute GvHD or thymic dysfunction. In reality, chronic GvHD may represent a "syndrome" with diverse causes among individual patients. In the future, it might become possible to tailor specific therapeutic interventions for patients as individually needed for each distinct pathophysiologic mechanism involved in development of the disease.

References

1. Shulman HM, Sale GE, Lerner KG, et al. Chronic cutaneous graft-versus-host disease in man. Am J Pathol. 1978;91:545–70.
2. Lee SJ, Vogelsang G, Flowers ME. Chronic graft-versus-host disease. Biol Blood Marrow Transplant. 2003;9:215–33.
3. Filipovich AH, Weisdorf D, Pavletic S, et al. National Institutes of Health Consensus Development Project on Criteria for Clinical Trials in Chronic Graft-versus-Host Disease: I. Diagnosis and Staging Working Group Report. Biol Blood Marrow Transplant. 2005;11:945–56.
4. Shulman HM, Kleiner D, Lee SJ, Morton T, Pavletic SZ, Farmer E, Moresi JM, Greenson J, Janin A, Martin PJ, McDonald G, Flowers ME, Turner M, Atkinson J, Lefkowitch J, Washington MK, Prieto VG, Kim SK, Argenyi Z, Diwan AH, Rashid A, Hiatt K, Couriel D, Schultz K, Hymes S, Vogelsang GB. Histopathologic diagnosis of chronic graft-versus-host disease: National Institutes of Health Consensus Development Project on Criteria for Clinical Trials in Chronic Graft-versus-Host Disease: II. Pathology Working Group Report. Biol Blood Marrow Transplant. 2006;12:31–47.
5. Schultz KR, Miklos DB, Fowler D, Cooke K, Shizuru J, Zorn E, Holler E, Ferrara J, Shulman H, Lee SJ, Martin P, Filipovich AH, Flowers ME, Weisdorf D, Couriel D, Lachenbruch PA, Mittleman B, Vogelsang GB, Pavletic SZ. Toward biomarkers for chronic graft-versus-host disease: National Institutes of Health Consensus Development Project on Criteria for Clinical Trials in Chronic Graft-versus-Host Disease: III. Biomarker Working Group Report. Biol Blood Marrow Transplant. 2006; 12:126–37.
6. Pavletic SZ, Martin P, Lee SJ, Mitchell S, Jacobsohn D, Cowen EW, Turner ML, Akpek G, Gilman A, McDonald G, Schubert M, Berger A, Bross P, Chien JW, Couriel D, Dunn JP, Fall-Dickson J, Farrell A, Flowers ME, Greinix H, Hirschfeld S, Gerber L, Kim S, Knobler R, Lachenbruch PA, Miller FW, Mittleman B, Papadopoulos E, Parsons SK, Przepiorka D, Robinson M, Ward M, Reeve B, Rider LG, Shulman H, Schultz KR, Weisdorf D, Vogelsang GB. Measuring therapeutic response in chronic graft-versus-host disease: National Institutes of Health Consensus Development Project on Criteria for Clinical Trials in Chronic Graft-versus-Host Disease: IV. Response Criteria Working Group report. Biol Blood Marrow Transplant. 2006;12:252–66.
7. Couriel D, Carpenter PA, Cutler C, Bolanos-Meade J, Treister NS, Gea-Banacloche J, Shaughnessy P, Hymes S, Kim S, Wayne AS, Chien JW, Neumann J, Mitchell S, Syrjala K, Moravec CK, Abramovitz L, Liebermann J, Berger A, Gerber L, Schubert M, Filipovich AH, Weisdorf D, Schubert MM, Shulman H, Schultz K, Mittelman B, Pavletic S, Vogelsang GB, Martin PJ, Lee SJ, Flowers ME. Ancillary therapy and supportive care of chronic graft-versus-host disease: National Institutes of Health Consensus Development Project on Criteria for Clinical Trials in Chronic Graft-versus-Host Disease: V. Ancillary Therapy and Supportive Care Working Group Report. Biol Blood Marrow Transplant. 2006;12:375–96.

8. Martin PJ, Weisdorf D, Przepiorka D, Hirschfeld S, Farrell A, Rizzo JD, Foley R, Socie G, Carter S, Couriel D, Schultz KR, Flowers ME, Filipovich AH, Saliba R, Vogelsang GB, Pavletic SZ, Lee SJ. National Institutes of Health Consensus Development Project on Criteria for Clinical Trials in Chronic Graft-versus-Host Disease: VI. Design of Clinical Trials Working Group report. Biol Blood Marrow Transplant. 2006; 12:491–505.
9. Couriel DR, Saliba R, Escalon MP, Hsu Y, Ghosh S, Ippoliti C, Hicks K, Donato M, Giralt S, Khouri IF, Hosing C, de Lima MJ, Andersson B, Neumann J, Champlin R. Sirolimus in combination with tacrolimus and corticosteroids for the treatment of resistant chronic graft-versus-host disease. Br J Haematol. 2005;130:409–17.
10. Jagasia M, Giglia J, Chinratanalab W, Dixon S, Chen H, Frangoul H, et al. Incidence and outcome of chronic graft-versus-host disease using National Institutes of Health consensus criteria. Biol Blood Marrow Transplant 2007;13:1207–15.
11. Shulman HM, Sullivan KM, Weiden PL, McDonald GB, Striker GE, Sale GE, Hackman R, Tsoi MS, Storb R, Thomas ED. Chronic graft-versus-host syndrome in man. A long-term clinicopathologic study of 20 Seattle patients. Am J Med. 1980;69: 204–17.
12. Lee SJ, Klein JP, Barrett AJ, Ringden O, Antin JH, Cahn JY, Carabasi MH, Gale RP, Giralt S, Hale GA, Ilhan O, McCarthy PL, Socie G, Verdonck LF, Weisdorf DJ, Horowitz MM. Severity of chronic graft-versus-host disease: association with treatment-related mortality and relapse. Blood 2002;100:406–14.
13. Akpek G, Zahurak ML, Piantadosi S, Margolis J, Doherty J, Davidson R, Vogelsang GB. Development of a prognostic model for grading chronic graft-versus-host disease. Blood 2001;97:1219–26.
14. Akpek G, Lee SJ, Flowers ME, Pavletic SZ, Arora M, Lee S, Piantadosi S, Guthrie KA, Lynch JC, Takatu A, Horowitz MM, Antin JH, Weisdorf DJ, Martin PJ, Vogelsang GB. Performance of a new clinical grading system for chronic graft-versus-host disease: a multicenter study. Blood 2003;102:802–9.
15. Arora M, Burns LJ, Davies SM, Macmillan ML, Defor TE, Miller WJ, Weisdorf DJ. Chronic graft-versus-host disease: a prospective cohort study. Biol Blood Marrow Transplant. 2003;9:38–45.
16. Pavletic SZ, Carter SL, Kernan NA, Henslee-Downey J, Mendizabal AM, Papadopoulos E, Gingrich R, Casper J, Yanovich S, Weisdorf D. Influence of T-cell depletion on chronic graft-versus-host disease: results of a multicenter randomized trial in unrelated marrow donor transplantation. Blood 2005;106:3308–13.
17. Wynn TA. Fibrotic disease and the T(H)1/T(H)2 paradigm. Nat Rev Immunol. 2004;4:583–94.
18. Nikolic B, Lee S, Bronson RT, Grusby MJ, Sykes M. Th1 and Th2 mediate acute graft-versus-host disease, each with distinct end-organ targets. J Clin Invest. 2000;105: 1289–98.
19. Hillebrandt S, Wasmuth HE, Weiskirchen R, Hellerbrand C, Keppeler H, Werth A, Schirin-Sokhan R, Wilkens G, Geier A, Lorenzen J, Kohl J, Gressner AM, Matern S, Lammert F. Complement factor 5 is a quantitative trait gene that modifies liver fibrogenesis in mice and humans. Nat Genet. 2005;37:835–43.
20. Niculescu F, Niculescu T, Nguyen P, Puliaev R, Papadimitriou JC, Gaspari A, Rus H, Via CS. Both apoptosis and complement membrane attack complex deposition are major features of murine acute graft-vs.-host disease. Exp Mol Pathol. 2005;79: 136–45.
21. Parkman R. Clonal analysis of murine graft-vs-host disease. I. Phenotypic and functional analysis of T lymphocyte clones. J Immunol. 1986;136:3543–8.
22. Ghayur T, Seemayer TA, Xenocostas A, Lapp WS. Complete sequential regeneration of graft-vs.-host-induced severely dysplastic thymuses. Implications for the pathogenesis of chronic graft-vs.-host disease. Am J Pathol. 1988;133:39–46.

23. Morohashi T, Ogasawara K, Kitaichi N, Iwabuchi K, Onoe K. Abrogation of negative selection by GvHR induced by minor histocompatibility antigens or H-2D antigen alone. Immunobiology 2000;202:268–79.
24. Zhang Y, Hexner E, Frank D, Emerson SG. CD4+ T cells generated de novo from donor hemopoietic stem cells mediate the evolution from acute to chronic graft-versus-host disease. J Immunol. 2007;179:3305–14.
25. Marguerat S, MacDonald HR, Kraehenbuhl JP, van Meerwijk JP. Protection from radiation-induced colitis requires MHC class II antigen expression by cells of hemopoietic origin. J Immunol. 1999;163:4033–40.
26. Teshima T, Reddy P, Liu C, Williams D, Cooke KR, Ferrara JL. Impaired thymic negative selection causes autoimmune graft-versus-host disease. Blood 2003;102:429–35.
27. Sakoda Y, Hashimoto D, Asakura S, Takeuchi K, Harada M, Tanimoto M, Teshima T. Donor-derived thymic-dependent T cells cause chronic graft-versus-host disease. Blood 2007;109:1756–64.
28. Tsoi MS, Storb R, Dobbs S, Medill L, Thomas ED. Cell-mediated immunity to non-HLA antigens of the host by donor lymphocytes in patients with chronic graft-vs-host disease. J Immunol. 1980;125:2258–62.
29. Jaffee BD, Claman HN. Chronic graft-versus-host disease (GvHD) as a model for scleroderma. I. Description of model systems. Cell Immunol. 1983;77:1–12.
30. Claman HN, Jaffee BD, Huff JC, Clark RA. Chronic graft-versus-host disease as a model for scleroderma. II. Mast cell depletion with deposition of immunoglobulins in the skin and fibrosis. Cell Immunol. 1985;94:73–84.
31. Ruzek MC, Jha S, Ledbetter S, Richards SM, Garman RD. A modified model of graft-versus-host-induced systemic sclerosis (scleroderma) exhibits all major aspects of the human disease. Arthritis Rheum. 2004;50:1319–31.
32. Korngold B, Sprent J. Lethal graft-versus-host disease after bone marrow transplantation across minor histocompatibility barriers in mice. Prevention by removing mature T cells from marrow. J Exp Med. 1978;148:1687–98.
33. Anderson BE, McNiff J, Yan J, Doyle H, Mamula M, Shlomchik MJ, Shlomchik WD. Memory CD4+ T cells do not induce graft-versus-host disease. J Clin Invest. 2003;112:101–8.
34. McCormick LL, Zhang Y, Tootell E, Gilliam AC. Anti-TGF-beta treatment prevents skin and lung fibrosis in murine sclerodermatous graft-versus-host disease: a model for human scleroderma. J Immunol. 1999;163:5693–9.
35. Anderson BE, McNiff JM, Jain D, Blazar BR, Shlomchik WD, Shlomchik MJ. Distinct roles for donor- and host-derived antigen-presenting cells and costimulatory molecules in murine chronic graft-versus-host disease: requirements depend on target organ. Blood 2005;105:2227–34.
36. Zhang Y, McCormick LL, Desai SR, Wu C, Gilliam AC. Murine sclerodermatous graft-versus-host disease, a model for human scleroderma: cutaneous cytokines, chemokines, and immune cell activation. J Immunol. 2002;168:3088–98.
37. Zhou L, Askew D, Wu C, Gilliam AC. Cutaneous gene expression by DNA microarray in murine sclerodermatous graft-versus-host disease, a model for human scleroderma. J Invest Dermatol. 2007;127:281–92.
38. Zhang Y, McCormick LL, Gilliam AC. Latency-associated peptide prevents skin fibrosis in murine sclerodermatous graft-versus-host disease, a model for human scleroderma. J Invest Dermatol. 2003;121:713–9.
39. Freund YR, Sgarlato G, Jacob CO, Suzuki Y, Remington JS. Polymorphisms in the tumor necrosis factor alpha (TNF-alpha) gene correlate with murine resistance to development of toxoplasmic encephalitis and with levels of TNF-alpha mRNA in infected brain tissue. J Exp Med. 1992;175:683–8.
40. Rubtsov YP, Rudensky AY. TGFbeta signalling in control of T-cell-mediated self-reactivity. Nat Rev Immunol. 2007;7:443–53.

41. Fu S, Zhang N, Yopp AC, Chen D, Mao M, Chen D, Zhang H, Ding Y, Bromberg JS. TGF-beta induces Foxp3+ T-regulatory cells from CD4+CD25– precursors. Am J Transplant. 2004;4:1614–27.
42. MacDonald KP, Rowe V, Filippich C, Johnson D, Morris ES, Clouston AD, Ferrara JL, Hill GR. Chronic graft-versus-host disease after granulocyte colony-stimulating factor-mobilized allogeneic stem cell transplantation: the role of donor T-cell dose and differentiation. Biol Blood Marrow Transplant. 2004;10:373–85.
43. Banovic T, MacDonald KP, Morris ES, Rowe V, Kuns R, Don A, Kelly J, Ledbetter S, Clouston AD, Hill GR. TGF-beta in allogeneic stem cell transplantation: friend or foe? Blood. 2005;106:2206–14.
44. Liem LM, Fibbe WE, van Houwelingen HC, Goulmy E. Serum transforming growth factor-beta1 levels in bone marrow transplant recipients correlate with blood cell counts and chronic graft-versus-host disease. Transplantation 1999;67:59–65.
45. Baron C, Somogyi R, Greller LD, Rineau V, Wilkinson P, Cho CR, Cameron MJ, Kelvin DJ, Chagnon P, Roy DC, Busque L, Sekaly RP, Perreault C. Prediction of graft-versus-host disease in humans by donor gene-expression profiling. PLoS Med. 2007;4:e23.
46. Kim J, Kim HJ, Park K, Kim J, Choi HJ, Yagita H, Nam SH, Cho HR, Kwon B. Costimulatory molecule-targeted immunotherapy of cutaneous graft-versus-host disease. Blood 2007;110:776–82.
47. Tsoi MS, Storb R, Jones E, Weiden PL, Shulman H, Witherspoon R, Atkinson K, Thomas ED. Deposition of IgM and complement at the dermoepidermal junction in acute and chronic cutaneous graft-vs-host disease in man. J Immunol. 1978;120:1485–92.
48. Zhang C, Todorov I, Zhang Z, Liu Y, Kandeel F, Forman S, Strober S, Zeng D. Donor CD4+ T and B cells in transplants induce chronic graft-versus-host disease with autoimmune manifestations. Blood 2006;107:2993–3001.
49. Rouquette-Gally AM, Boyeldieu D, Prost AC, Gluckman E. Autoimmunity after allogeneic bone marrow transplantation. A study of 53 long-term-surviving patients. Transplantation 1988;46:238–40.
50. Cutler C, Miklos D, Kim HT, Treister N, Woo SB, Bienfang D, Klickstein LB, Levin J, Miller K, Reynolds C, Macdonell R, Pasek M, Lee SJ, Ho V, Soiffer R, Antin JH, Ritz J, Alyea E. Rituximab for steroid-refractory chronic graft-versus-host disease. Blood 2006;108:756–62.
51. She K, Gilman AL, Aslanian S, Shimizu H, Krailo M, Chen Z, Reid GS, Wall D, Goldman F, Schultz KR. Altered toll-like receptor 9 responses in circulating B cells at the onset of extensive chronic graft-versus-host disease. Biol Blood Marrow Transplant. 2007;13:386–97.
52. Svegliati S, Olivieri A, Campelli N, Luchetti M, Poloni A, Trappolini S, Moroncini G, Bacigalupo A, Leoni P, Avvedimento EV, Gabrielli A. Stimulatory autoantibodies to PDGF receptor in patients with extensive chronic graft-versus-host disease. Blood 2007;110:237–41.
53. Anderson BE, McNiff JM, Matte C, Athanasiadis I, Shlomchik WD, Shlomchik MJ. Recipient CD4+ T cells that survive irradiation regulate chronic graft-versus-host disease. Blood 2004;104:1565–73.
54. Tivol E, Komorowski R, Drobyski WR. Emergent autoimmunity in graft-versus-host disease. Blood 2005;105:4885–91.
55. Chen X, Vodanovic-Jankovic S, Johnson B, Keller M, Komorowski R, Drobyski WR. Absence of regulatory T-cell control of TH1 and TH17 cells is responsible for the autoimmune-mediated pathology in chronic graft-versus-host disease. Blood 2007;110:3804–13.
56. Fujita S, Sato Y, Sato K, Eizumi K, Fukaya T, Kubo M, Yamashita N, Sato K. Regulatory dendritic cells protect against cutaneous chronic graft-versus-host disease mediated through CD4+CD25+Foxp3+ regulatory T cells. Blood 2007;110:3793–803.
57. Miura Y, Thoburn CJ, Bright EC, Phelps ML, Shin T, Matsui EC, Matsui WH, Arai S, Fuchs EJ, Vogelsang GB, Jones RJ, Hess AD. Association of Foxp3 regulatory gene expression with graft-versus-host disease. Blood 2004;104:2187–93.

58. Zorn E, Kim HT, Lee SJ, Floyd BH, Litsa D, Arumugarajah S, Bellucci R, Alyea EP, Antin JH, Soiffer RJ, Ritz J. Reduced frequency of FOXP3+ CD4+CD25+ regulatory T cells in patients with chronic graft-versus-host disease. Blood 2005;106:2903–11.
59. Rieger K, Loddenkemper C, Maul J, Fietz T, Wolff D, Terpe H, Steiner B, Berg E, Miehlke S, Bornhauser M, Schneider T, Zeitz M, Stein H, Thiel E, Duchmann R, Uharek L. Mucosal FOXP3+ regulatory T cells are numerically deficient in acute and chronic GvHD. Blood 2006;107:1717–23.
60. Meignin V, Peffault de Latour R, Zuber J, Regnault A, Mounier N, Lemaitre F, Dastot H, Itzykson R, Devergie A, Cumano A, Gluckman E, Janin A, Bandeira A, Socie G. Numbers of Foxp3-expressing CD4+CD25high T cells do not correlate with the establishment of long-term tolerance after allogeneic stem cell transplantation. Exp Hematol. 2005;33: 894–900.
61. Arimoto K, Kadowaki N, Ishikawa T, Ichinohe T, Uchiyama T. FOXP3 expression in peripheral blood rapidly recovers and lacks correlation with the occurrence of graft-versus-host disease after allogeneic stem cell transplantation. Int J Hematol. 2007;85: 154–62.
62. Ferrara JL, Anasetti C, Stadtmauer E, Antin J, Wingard J, Lee S, Levine J, Schultz K, Appelbaum F, Negrin R, Giralt S, Bredeson C, Heslop H, Horowitz M. Blood and marrow transplant clinical trials network state of the science symposium 2007. Biol Blood Marrow Transplant. 2007;13:1268–85.
63. Storb R, Deeg HJ, Pepe M, Doney K, Appelbaum F, Beatty P, Bensinger W, Buckner CD, Clift R, Hansen J, et al. Graft-versus-host disease prevention by methotrexate combined with cyclosporin compared to methotrexate alone in patients given marrow grafts for severe aplastic anaemia: long-term follow-up of a controlled trial. Br J Haematol. 1989;72:567–72.
64. Storb R, Pepe M, Anasetti C, Appelbaum FR, Beatty P, Doney K, Martin P, Stewart P, Sullivan KM, Witherspoon R, et al. What role for prednisone in prevention of acute graft-versus-host disease in patients undergoing marrow transplants? Blood. 1990;76: 1037–45.
65. Ross M, Schmidt GM, Niland JC, Amylon MD, Dagis AC, Long GD, Nademanee AP, Negrin RS, O'Donnell MR, Parker PM, Smith EP, Snyder DS, Stein AS, Wong RM, Forman SJ, Blume KG, Chao NJ. Cyclosporine, methotrexate, and prednisone compared with cyclosporine and prednisone for prevention of acute graft-vs.-host disease: effect on chronic graft-vs.-host disease and long-term survival. Biol Blood Marrow Transplant. 1999;5:285–91.
66. Ringden O, Paulin T, Lonnqvist B, Nilsson B. An analysis of factors predisposing to chronic graft-versus-host disease. Exp Hematol. 1985;13:1062–7.
67. Ratanatharathorn V, Nash RA, Przepiorka D, Devine SM, Klein JL, Weisdorf D, Fay JW, Nademanee A, Antin JH, Christiansen NP, van der Jagt R, Herzig RH, Litzow MR, Wolff SN, Longo WL, Petersen FB, Karanes C, Avalos B, Storb R, Buell DN, Maher RM, Fitzsimmons WE, Wingard JR. Phase III study comparing methotrexate and tacrolimus (prograf, FK506) with methotrexate and cyclosporine for graft-versus-host disease prophylaxis after HLA-identical sibling bone marrow transplantation. Blood 1998; 92:2303–14.
68. Kansu E, Gooley T, Flowers ME, Anasetti C, Deeg HJ, Nash RA, Sanders JE, Witherspoon RP, Appelbaum FR, Storb R, Martin PJ. Administration of cyclosporine for 24 months compared with 6 months for prevention of chronic graft-versus-host disease: a prospective randomized clinical trial. Blood 2001;98:3868–70.
69. Chao NJ, Parker PM, Niland JC, Wong RM, Dagis A, Long GD, Nademanee AP, Negrin RS, Snyder DS, Hu WW, Gould KA, Tierney DK, Zwingenberger K, Forman SJ, Blume KG. Paradoxical effect of thalidomide prophylaxis on chronic graft-vs.-host disease. Biol Blood Marrow Transplant. 1996;2:86–92.
70. Sullivan KM, Storek J, Kopecky KJ, Jocom J, Longton G, Flowers M, Siadak M, Nims J, Witherspoon RP, Anasetti C, Appelbaum FR, Bowden RA, Buckner CD, Crawford SW,

Deeg HJ, Hansen JA, McDonald GB, Sanders JE, Storb R. A controlled trial of long-term administration of intravenous immunoglobulin to prevent late infection and chronic graft-vs.-host disease after marrow transplantation: clinical outcome and effect on subsequent immune recovery. Biol Blood Marrow Transplant. 1996;2:44–53.

71. Loughran TP Jr, Sullivan K, Morton T, Beckham C, Schubert M, Witherspoon R, Sale G, Sanders J, Fisher L, Shulman H, et al. Value of day 100 screening studies for predicting the development of chronic graft-versus-host disease after allogeneic bone marrow transplantation. Blood 1990;76:228–34.
72. Fong T, Trinkaus K, Adkins D, Vij R, Devine SM, Tomasson M, Goodnough LT, Lopez S, Graubert T, Shenoy S, Dipersio JF, Khoury HJ. A randomized double-blind trial of hydroxychloroquine for the prevention of chronic graft-versus-host disease after allogeneic peripheral blood stem cell transplantation. Biol Blood Marrow Transplant. 2007;13:1201–6.
73. Hale G, Zhang MJ, Bunjes D, Prentice HG, Spence D, Horowitz MM, Barrett AJ, Waldmann H. Improving the outcome of bone marrow transplantation by using CD52 monoclonal antibodies to prevent graft-versus-host disease and graft rejection. Blood 1998;92:4581–90.
74. Bacigalupo A. Antithymocyte globulin for prevention of graft-versus-host disease. Curr Opin Hematol. 2005;12:457–62.
75. Stewart BL, Storer B, Storek J, Deeg HJ, Storb R, Hansen JA, Appelbaum FR, Carpenter PA, Sanders JE, Kiem HP, Nash RA, Petersdorf EW, Moravec C, Morton AJ, Anasetti C, Flowers ME, Martin PJ. Duration of immunosuppressive treatment for chronic graft-versus-host disease. Blood 2004;104:3501–6.
76. Sullivan KM, Witherspoon RP, Storb R, Weiden P, Flournoy N, Dahlberg S, Deeg HJ, Sanders JE, Doney KC, Appelbaum FR, et al. Prednisone and azathioprine compared with prednisone and placebo for treatment of chronic graft-v-host disease: prognostic influence of prolonged thrombocytopenia after allogeneic marrow transplantation. Blood 1988;72:546–54.
77. Sullivan KM, Witherspoon RP, Storb R, Deeg HJ, Dahlberg S, Sanders JE, Appelbaum FR, Doney KC, Weiden P, Anasetti C, et al. Alternating-day cyclosporine and prednisone for treatment of high-risk chronic graft-v-host disease. Blood 1988;72: 555–61.
78. Koc S, Leisenring W, Flowers ME, Anasetti C, Deeg HJ, Nash RA, Sanders JE, Witherspoon RP, Storb R, Appelbaum FR, Martin PJ. Therapy for chronic graft-versus-host disease: a randomized trial comparing cyclosporine plus prednisone versus prednisone alone. Blood 2002;100:48–51.
79. Flowers ME, Lee S, Vogelsang G. An update on how to treat chronic GVHD. Blood 2003;102:2312.
80. Wingard JR, Piantadosi S, Vogelsang GB, Farmer ER, Jabs DA, Levin LS, Beschorner WE, Cahill RA, Miller DF, Harrison D, et al. Predictors of death from chronic graft-versus-host disease after bone marrow transplantation. Blood 1989;74:1428–35.
81. Koc S, Leisenring W, Flowers ME, Anasetti C, Deeg HJ, Nash RA, Sanders JE, Witherspoon RP, Appelbaum FR, Storb R, Martin PJ. Thalidomide for treatment of patients with chronic graft-versus-host disease. Blood 2000;96:3995–6.
82. Arora M, Wagner JE, Davies SM, Blazar BR, Defor T, Enright H, Miller WJ, Weisdorf DF. Randomized clinical trial of thalidomide, cyclosporine, and prednisone versus cyclosporine and prednisone as initial therapy for chronic graft-versus-host disease. Biol Blood Marrow Transplant. 2001;7:265–73.
83. Giaccone L, Martin P, Carpenter P, Moravec C, Hooper H, Funke VA, Storb R, Flowers ME. Safety and potential efficacy of low-dose methotrexate for treatment of chronic graft-versus-host disease. Bone Marrow Transplant. 2005;36:337–41.
84. Teachey DT, Bickert B, Bunin N. Daclizumab for children with corticosteroid refractory graft-versus-host disease. Bone Marrow Transplant. 2006;37:95–9.

85. Vogelsang GB, Farmer ER, Hess AD, Altamonte V, Beschorner WE, Jabs DA, Corio RL, Levin LS, Colvin OM, Wingard JR, et al. Thalidomide for the treatment of chronic graft-versus-host disease. N Engl J Med. 1992;326:1055–8.
86. Mookerjee B, Altomonte V, Vogelsang G. Salvage therapy for refractory chronic graft-versus-host disease with mycophenolate mofetil and tacrolimus. Bone Marrow Transplant. 1999;24:517–20.
87. Lopez F, Parker P, Nademanee A, Rodriguez R, Al-Kadhimi Z, Bhatia R, Cohen S, Falk P, Fung H, Kirschbaum M, Krishnan A, Kogut N, Molina A, Nakamura R, O'Donnell M, Popplewell L, Pullarkat V, Rosenthal J, Sahebi F, Smith E, Snyder D, Somlo G, Spielberger R, Stein A, Sweetman R, Zain J, Forman S. Efficacy of mycophenolate mofetil in the treatment of chronic graft-versus-host disease. Biol Blood Marrow Transplant. 2005;11:307–13.
88. Carnevale-Schianca F, Martin P, Sullivan K, Flowers M, Gooley T, Anasetti C, Deeg J, Furlong T, McSweeney P, Storb R, Nash RA. Changing from cyclosporine to tacrolimus as salvage therapy for chronic graft-versus-host disease. Biol Blood Marrow Transplant. 2000;6:613–20.
89. Couriel D, Hosing C, Saliba R, Shpall EJ, Andelini P, Popat U, Donato M, Champlin R. Extracorporeal photopheresis for acute and chronic graft-versus-host disease: does it work? Biol Blood Marrow Transplant. 2006;12:37–40.
90. Jacobsohn DA, Chen AR, Zahurak M, Piantadosi S, Anders V, Bolanos-Meade J, et al. A phase II study of pentostatin in patiens with steroid-refractory shronic graft-versus-host disease. J Clin Oncol. 2007;25:4255–61.
91. Zaja F, Bacigalupo A, Patriarca F, Stanzani M, Van Lint MT, Fili C, Scime R, Milone G, Falda M, Vener C, Laszlo D, Alessandrino PE, Narni F, Sica S, Olivieri A, Sperotto A, Bosi A, Bonifazi F, Fanin R. Treatment of refractory chronic GvHD with rituximab: a GITMO study. Bone Marrow Transplant. 2007;40:273–7.
92. Gilman AL, Chan KW, Mogul A, Morris C, Goldman FD, Boyer M, Cirenza E, Mazumder A, Gehan E, Cahill R, Frankel S, Schultz K. Hydroxychloroquine for the treatment of chronic graft-versus-host disease. Biol Blood Marrow Transplant. 2000;6:327–34.
93. Akpek G, Lee SM, Anders V, Vogelsang GB. A high-dose pulse steroid regimen for controlling active chronic graft-versus-host disease. Biol Blood Marrow Transplant. 2001;7:495–502.
94. Vogelsang GB, Wolff D, Altomonte V, Farmer E, Morison WL, Corio R, Horn T. Treatment of chronic graft-versus-host disease with ultraviolet irradiation and psoralen (PUVA). Bone Marrow Transplant. 1996;17:1061–7.
95. Parker PM, Chao N, Nademanee A, O'Donnell MR, Schmidt GM, Snyder DS, Stein AS, Smith EP, Molina A, Stepan DE, Kashyap A, Planas I, Spielberger R, Somlo G, Margolin K, Zwingenberger K, Wilsman K, Negrin RS, Long GD, Niland JC, Blume KG, Forman SJ. Thalidomide as salvage therapy for chronic graft-versus-host disease. Blood 1995;86:3604–9.
96. Fried RH, Murakami CS, Fisher LD, Willson RA, Sullivan KM, McDonald GB. Ursodeoxycholic acid treatment of refractory chronic graft-versus-host disease of the liver. Ann Intern Med. 1992;116:624–9.
97. Lee SJ, Wegner SA, McGarigle CJ, Bierer BE, Antin JH. Treatment of chronic graft-versus-host disease with clofazimine. Blood 1997;89:2298–302.
98. Marcellus DC, Altomonte VL, Farmer ER, Horn TD, Freemer CS, Grant J, Vogelsang GB. Etretinate therapy for refractory sclerodermatous chronic graft-versus-host disease. Blood 1999;93:66–70.
99. Robin M, Guardiola P, Girinsky T, Hernandez G, Esperou H, Ribaud P, Rocha V, Garnier F, Socie G, Gluckman E, Devergie A. Low-dose thoracoabdominal irradiation for the treatment of refractory chronic graft-versus-host disease. Transplantation 2005;80:634–42.

100. Rodriguez V, Anderson PM, Trotz BA, Arndt CA, Allen JA, Khan SP. Use of infliximab-daclizumab combination for the treatment of acute and chronic graft-versus-host disease of the liver and gut. Pediatr Blood Cancer. 2007;49:212–5.
101. Busca A, Locatelli F, Marmont F, Ceretto C, Falda M. Recombinant human soluble tumor necrosis factor receptor fusion protein as treatment for steroid refractory graft-versus-host disease following allogeneic hematopoietic stem cell transplantation. Am J Hematol. 2007;82:45–52.
102. Arat M, Ilhan O, Iayan EA, Celebi H, Koc H, Akan H. Treatment of extensive chronic sclerodermatous graft-versus-host disease with high-dose immunosuppressive therapy and CD34+ autologous stem cell rescue. Blood 2001;98:892–3.
103. Mayer J, Krejci M, Doubek M, Pospisil Z, Brychtova Y, Tomiska M, Racil Z. Pulse cyclophosphamide for corticosteroid-refractory graft-versus-host disease. Bone Marrow Transplant. 2005;35:699–705.
104. Majhail NS, Schiffer CA, Weisdorf DJ. Improvement of pulmonary function with imatinib mesylate in bronchiolitis obliterans following allogeneic hematopoietic cell transplantation. Biol Blood Marrow Transplant. 2006;12:789–91.
105. Or R, Gesundheit B, Resnick I, Bitan M, Avraham A, Avgil M, Sacks Z, Shapira MY. Sparing effect by montelukast treatment for chronic graft versus host disease: a pilot study. Transplantation 2007;83:577–81.
106. Lee SJ, Vogelsang G, Gilman A, Weisdorf DJ, Pavletic S, Antin JH, Horowitz MM, Akpek G, Flowers ME, Couriel D, Martin PJ. A survey of diagnosis, management, and grading of chronic GVHD. Biol Blood Marrow Transplant. 2002;8:32–9.
107. Pavletic SZ, Smith LM, Bishop MR, Lynch JC, Tarantolo SR, Vose JM, Bierman PJ, Hadi A, Armitage JO, Kessinger A. Prognostic factors of chronic graft-versus-host disease after allogeneic blood stem-cell transplantation. Am J Hematol. 2005;78:265–74.

Chapter 13
Radioimmunoconjugates in Hematopoietic Stem Cell Transplantation

Ajay K. Gopal and Jane N. Winter

13.1 Introduction

Hematopoietic stem cell transplantation (HSCT) has offered the promise of prolonged disease control and the potential for cure to patients with a variety of high-risk or relapsed hematologic malignancies including those with leukemia and lymphoma [1–7]. The rationale for administering high-dose therapy prior to HSCT is derived from the steep dose-response relationship between chemo-radiotherapy and tumor cell kill in the hematologic malignancies with the hypothesis that escalation of the dose beyond the marrow ablative threshold to the toxicity limits of nonhematopoietic organs can result in improved responses and longer remissions. This relationship of dose and response has been shown to be particularly striking with the use of radiation therapy. Data suggest that localized external beam radiation for the treatment of lymphoma in doses over 44 Gy yielded in-field relapses of 6% as compared to disease recurrence rates of 63% when doses less than 27 Gy were utilized [8]. Based on these kinds of data demonstrating the exquisite radiosensitivity of lymphomas and leukemias, total body irradiation (TBI) has been incorporated into HSCT conditioning regimens [1, 9]. Further evidence for a radiation-dose disease-response relationship came from a randomized phase III trial comparing 12 Gy versus 15.75 Gy TBI in 71 AML patients in first remission [6]. The relapse rates of patients receiving the higher and standard TBI dose were 12% and 35% ($p = 0.06$), respectively, though nonrelapse mortality rates were 32% and 12% ($p = 0.04$), respectively. These outcomes resulted in identical relapse-free survivals for each group, but implied that if one could safely escalate the radiation dose to tumor sites, disease free survival could be improved.

A.K. Gopal (✉)
Division of Medical Oncology, Department of Medicine, University of Washington and Clinical Research Division, Fred Hutchinson Cancer Research Center, Seattle, WA 98 109, USA
e-mail: agopal@u.washington.edu

M.R. Bishop (ed.), *Hematopoietic Stem Cell Transplantation*,
Cancer Treatment and Research 144, DOI 10.1007/978-0-387-78580-6_13,

Table 13.1 Comparison of ^{131}I and ^{90}Y

	^{131}I	^{90}Y
Emission	Beta, gamma	Beta
Mean beta energy	0.192 MeV	0.934 MeV
Mean path length	0.8 mm	5.3 mm
Half-life	8 days	2.7 days
Nonspecific uptake	Thyroid	Bone, liver
Advantages	Inexpensive, simple labeling chemistry, imaging possible due to gamma emission	Few radiation safety precautions
Limitations	Radiation safety precautions due to high-energy gamma	Surrogate isotope required for imaging (^{111}In), expensive, more complex labeling chemistry

Radioimmunotherapy (RIT) represents a novel means to potentially achieve this goal by amplifying the radiation dose to tumor sites while relatively sparing toxicity to normal nontarget tissues. This strategy has been predominantly applied to the treatment of indolent non-Hodgkin's lymphoma (NHL) in the nontransplant setting with the FDA approval of two radioimmunoconjugates, iodine-131 (I-131) tositumomab (Bexxar®) and (Y-90) ibritumomab tiuxetan (Zevalin®) [10–16]. These antibodies both target CD20, a pan-B-cell antigen that is expressed on the majority of B-cell NHL [17, 18]. CD20 is an attractive target that has been employed by a variety of investigators as it is not thought to readily internalize, modulate, or shed and is only thought to be expressed on mature B cells and B-cell NHL [19, 20]. Most nontransplant and transplant studies of RIT have utilized either I-131 or Y-90 as the therapeutic radionuclide. The specific characteristics with theoretical advantages and limitations of these isotopes are summarized in Table 13.1.

Two basic RIT-based transplant strategies have emerged. The first approach maximizes the therapeutic potential of RIT by escalating the dose to the nonhematopoietic toxicity threshold either with or without high-dose chemotherapy much akin to the use of high-dose TBI. A second tactic adds standard nonmyeloablative doses of RIT to a maximized myeloablative chemotherapy conditioning regimen.

13.2 High-Dose ^{131}I-RIT and Autologous HSCT

The Seattle group, led by Dr. Oliver Press, was the first to use high-dose radioiodinated anti-B-cell antibodies followed by autologous HSCT (Table 13.2). These initial studies evaluated a variety of anti-B-cell antibodies including 1F5 (anti-CD20), tositumomab (anti-CD20), and MB-1 (anti-CD37) using precise individualized dosimetry confirming that tumor sites received on average 10 times the radiation exposure as the whole body and on average 1.5–2 times the radiation exposure as the highest normal organ (Table 13.3) [21, 22]. The studies

Table 13.2 Results from selected I-131-radioimmunotherapy based stem cell transplant conditioning regimens for lymphomas

Author	Dose (Gy)	Drug/target	Chemo	Lymphoma type/setting	n	Results
Press et al. [21]	10–30.75[a]	MB1/CD37, tositumomab/CD20, 1F5/CD20	–	B-cell NHL/relapsed	19	95% OR (84% CR)
Press et al. [24]	20–27[a]	Tositumomab/CD20	CY. VP-16	B-cell NHL/relapsed	52	83%/68% 2-year OS/PFS
Behr et al. [25]	27[a]	Rituximab/CD20	–	Mantle cell/relapsed	7	100% OR (86% CR)
Gopal et al. [26]	17–31[a]	Tositumomab/CD20	–	Follicular/relapsed	27	67%/48% 5-year OS/PFS
Vose et al. [27]	0.75[b]	Tositumoab/CD20	BEAM	B-cell NHL/relapsed or refractory	23	55%/39% 3-year OS/PFS
Vose et al. [28]	0.75[b]	Tositumomab/CD20	BEAM	Chemosensitive DLBCL	40	3-year PFS 70%
Gopal et al. [29]	25–27[a]	Tositumomab/CD20	–	B-cell NHL/relapsed, ≥60 years old	24	3-year PFS 51%

B-cell NHL B-cell non-Hodgkin's lymphoma, *DLBCL* diffuse large B cell lymphoma, *MCL* mantle cell lymphoma, *FL* follicular lymphoma, *OR* overall response, *CR* complete response, *OS* overall survival, *PFS* progression free survival, *RFS* relapse free survival, *CY* cyclophosphamide, *VP-16* etoposide, *BEAM* carmustine, etoposide, cytarabine, melphalan

[a]Dose to highest critical nontarget organ

[b]whole body dose

Table 13.3 Estimated absorbed radiation doses of tumors and normal organs

Site	Absorbed radiation dose range (Gy)	Tumor to organ ratio*	
		Mean ± SE	Range
Lungs	6.5–31.0	1.8 ± 0.2	1.1–4.2
Liver	3.8–19.3	3.0 ± 0.3	1.4–5.1
Kidneys	5.4–21.6	3.4 ± 0.3	1.7–7.0
Marrow	1.0–6.4	10.2 ± 1.1	3.6–22.4
Whole Body	1.0–5.7	10.4 ± 1.0	4.5–20.2
Tumor	10.1–91.5	–	–

*The ratio of absorbed radiation dose by the tumor to that absorbed by the organ. (Adapted from Press et al. [21])

also revealed that inferior biodistributions were observed in the setting of splenomegaly and tumor bulk over 500 cc. This trial established the maximally tolerated dose (MTD) of ^{131}I that could be administered via anti-B-cell antibodies to be 27 Gy to the critical normal organ receiving the highest radiation exposure (typically the lungs) suggesting that at this dose level tumor sites would receive on average greater than or equal to 40 Gy. This approach also yielded overall and complete response rates of 95% and 84%, respectively, in patients with relapsed B-cell NHL. Other important observations from this myeloablative RIT regimen included low rates of nonhematologic toxicity and confirming that stem cell infusion could safely occur at residual radiation exposure levels of less than 2 mR/h at 1 m. These studies also supported the dose-response relationship of radiation and tumor control with patients that received greater than or equal to 20 Gy to critical organs experiencing a 70% progression-free survival (PFS) as compared to 20% PFS in those that received less than 20 Gy ($p = 0.045$) [23].

The relative long-term efficacy of this high-dose RIT strategy was evaluated via a multivariable cohort analysis of 125 patients with relapsed or refractory follicular lymphoma treated with either myeloablative I-131 tositumomab followed by autologous HSCT or conventional high-dose therapy followed by autologous HSCT [26]. In this study, the estimated 5-year overall survival (OS) for high-dose RIT was 67% and for conventional high-dose therapy was 53% ($p = 0.004$). Similarly, 5-year PFS was estimated to be 48% for the high-dose RIT group and 29% for the conventional transplant group ($p = 0.03$) (Fig. 13.1). The authors concluded that some of the improvement in outcome was due to the reduced 100-day treatment-related mortality in the high-dose-RIT group (3.7%) as compared to the control arm (11.2%), emphasizing the tolerability of this strategy. This study also addressed the concerns radiation-induced leukemogenesis by noting that the estimated incidence of acute myeloid leukemia and myelodysplastic syndromes in the high-dose RIT group was 0.076 at 8 years, as compared to 0.086 at 7 years in the standard transplant group.

Building on the observations in younger patients that high-dose RIT and autologous HSCT was both tolerable and efficacious, this strategy was applied

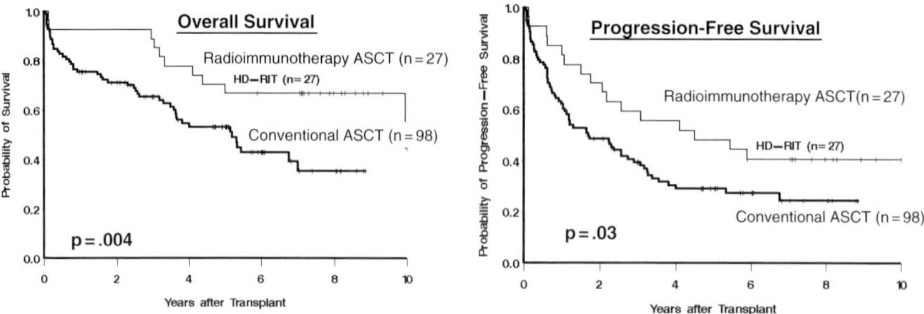

Fig. 13.1 Overall survival (**a**) and progression-free survival (**b**) of follicular lymphoma patients treated either with HD-RIT using ^{131}I-tositumomab and autologous HSCT or C-HDT and autologous HSCT (Adapted from Gopal et al. [26])

to older adults with relapsed B-cell NHL who may have otherwise been denied high-dose therapy [29]. Twenty-four patients over the age of 60 were treated with high-dose ^{131}I-tositumomab designed to deliver $\leq$25–27 Gy to critical normal organs followed by autologous HSCT. The patients on this study had received a median of four prior regimens, and 54% had chemotherapy resistant disease. Nevertheless, there were no treatment-related deaths and grade 4 nonhematologic toxicities occurred in less than 10% of patients yielding a 3-year OS and PFS of 59% and 51%, respectively.

Other groups have also utilized myeloablative doses of I-131 conjugated antibodies as part of autologous HSCT conditioning regimens. Behr and colleagues published a series of seven heavily pretreated mantle cell lymphoma patients who received high dose I-131 labeled rituximab following the identical dosimetry as the Seattle group to deliver less than 27 Gy to the lung followed by autologous HSCT [25]. In this series, all patients responded, with six of seven achieving a CR despite only moderate toxicity.

13.3 High-Dose ^{131}I-RIT Plus Chemotherapy and Autologous HSCT

In order to further improve on the efficacy seen with single-agent high-dose ^{131}I-RIT, investigators have evaluated adding high-dose chemotherapy to transplant conditioning regimens. This approach was first evaluated utilizing a regimen including high-dose cyclophosphamide and etoposide (VP-16), but where TBI would be supplanted by RIT [24]. The initial phase I data evaluating this strategy demonstrated that I-131 doses delivering less than 25 Gy to critical organs could be administered along with full doses of cyclophosphamide (100 mg/kg) and VP-16 (60 mg/kg). Toxicities were comparable to TBI-containing regimens and comparisons with adjusted nonrandomized controls suggested the RIT-based approach produced improved OS and PFS compared to a comparable TBI containing regimen (Fig. 13.2). This strategy has more recently been evaluated in a subset of 16 heavily pretreated patients with mantle cell lymphoma resulting in an estimated 3-year OS and PFS of 93% and 61%, respectively [30]. Extended phase II studies using this combined high-dose chemo-radioimmunotherapy regimen in various B-cell NHL histologies are ongoing to better define the safety and efficacy of this regimen.

13.4 Standard-Dose ^{131}I-RIT Plus High-Dose Chemotherapy and Autologous HSCT

An alternative strategy to myeloablative RIT is to add standard outpatient doses of RIT to full-dose myeloablative chemotherapy, allowing for further intensification of a maximal chemotherapeutic regimen and obviating some of

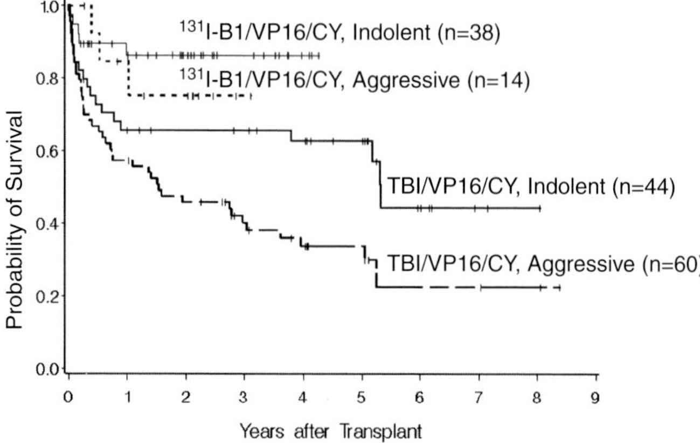

Fig. 13.2 Survival analyses according to type of lymphoma. Overall survival in 38 patients with relapsed indolent lymphomas (*thin solid line*) and 14 patients with relapsed aggressive lymphomas (*short dashes*) treated with ^{131}I-tositumomab, etoposide, cyclophosphamide, and ASCT and in 44 patients with relapsed indolent lymphomas (*thick solid line*) and 60 patients with relapsed aggressive lymphomas (*long thick dashes*) treated with external-beam TBI (1.5 Gy twice a day for 4 days), etoposide (60 mg/kg), cyclophosphamide (100 mg/kg), and ASCT

the technical and safety concerns of high-doses of radioisotopes. Vose and colleagues first assessed this approach in a phase I trial of 23 patients with relapsed or refractory B-cell NHL who were treated with escalating doses of standard I-131 tositumomab (Bexxar®) up to 0.75 Gy plus high-dose carmustine, etoposide, cytarabine, and melphalan (BEAM) followed by autologous HSCT (Fig. 13.3) [27]. This study demonstrated that the full 0.75 Gy whole body dose of I-131 tositumomab could be safely administered 7 days prior to initiating full-dose BEAM chemotherapy and 12 days prior to autologous

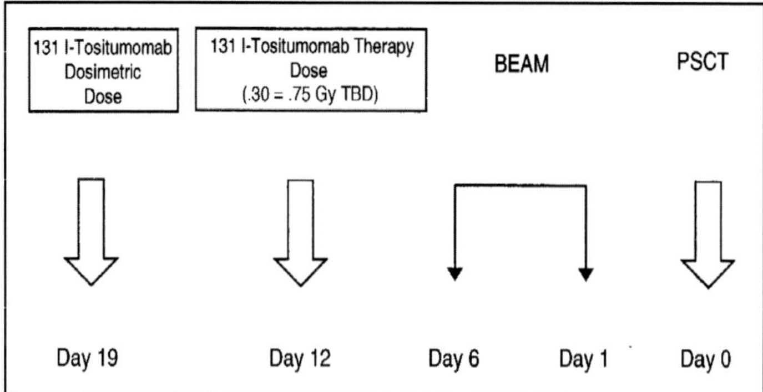

Fig. 13.3 Schema for iodine-131 tositumomab/carmustine, etoposide, cytarabine, and melphalan (BEAM) transplantation program. *TBD* total-body dose, *PSCT* peripheral-blood stem-cell transplantation (Vose et al. [27])

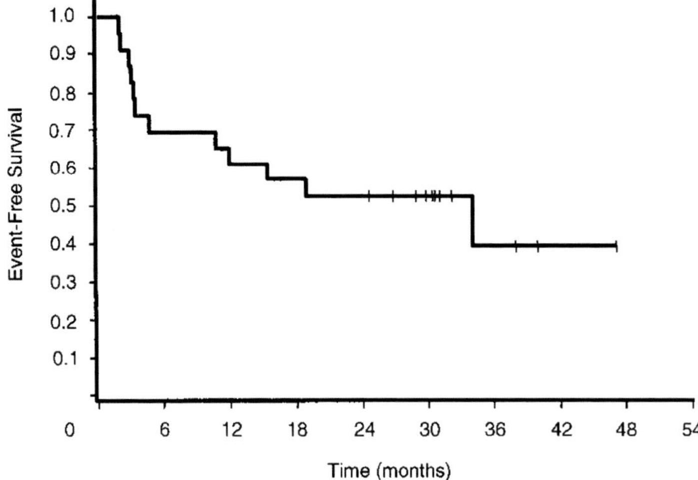

Fig. 13.4 Event-free survival for patients in the phase I iodine-131 tositumomab/carmustine, etoposide, cytarabine, and melphalan transplantation program (Vose et al. [27])

HSCT with no appreciable increase in toxicities or delay in engraftment. This regimen also achieved a CR rate of 57% and event free survival of 39% at a median follow-up of 38 months in a group of heavily pretreated (median 3 prior regimens, 51% chemotherapy-resistant) patients (Fig. 13.4). A follow up phase II study of 40 chemotherapy-sensitive diffuse large B-cell lymphoma patients by the Nebraska group confirmed the feasibility of this regimen and yielded an estimated 3-year PFS of 70% and OS of 81% [28]. These encouraging preliminary data have led to an ongoing national phase III trial comparing I-131 tositumomab-BEAM to rituximab-BEAM in patients with relapsed, chemotherapy-sensitive diffuse large B-cell lymphoma.

13.5 Dose-Escalated Yttrium-90 Ibritumomab Tiuxetan with HSCT Support

The anti-CD20 radioimmunoconjugate Yttrium-90 ibritumomab tiuxetan (Zevalin®) has been evaluated as a single agent at escalated doses with autologous stem cell support and in combination with chemotherapy where it has either replaced TBI or intensified a standard high-dose chemotherapy regimen in the context of either autologous or allogeneic HSCT (Table 13.4). Three groups have investigated dose-escalated Yttrium-90 ibritumomab tiuxetan as a single agent, using peripheral blood progenitor cells to circumvent the dose-limiting toxicity of RIT. Ferrucci and colleagues have dose-escalated Yttrium-90 ibritumomab tiuxetan based on weight, using three predefined dose levels (0.8, 1.2, and 1.5 mCi/kg) [31]. Patient-specific dosimetry was performed in all cases to evaluate

Table 13.4 Results from selected Y-90 radioimmunotherapy-based autologous stem cell transplant trials for CD20+ nonHodgkin lymphoma

Author	Dose	Chemo	Disease status	*n*	Results
RIT alone					
Ferrucci et al. [31], Vanazzi et al. [32]	0.8–1.5 mCi/kg	–	Resistant or refractory	25	CR 40%
Devizzi et al. [33]	0.8 or 1.2 mCi/kg	–	Relapsed or refractory	29	Indolent: 87%/55% 2-year OS/PFS; Aggressive: 85%/77% OS/PFS
Flinn et al. [34]	14–28 Gy[a]	–	Relapsed or refractory	22	CR 45%
Escalated RIT and chemotherapy					
Nademanee et al. [35, 36]	10 Gy[a]	Cy/etoposide	1st PR/CR relapsed or refractory	31	81%/65% 4-year OS/DFS
Winter [37]	1–17 Gy[a]	BEAM	Relapsed or refractory	44	52%/37% 3-year OS/PFS
Standard dose RIT and chemotherapy					
Shimoni et al. [41]	0.4 mCi/kg	BEAM	Primary refractory or refractory relapse	23	67%/52% 2-year OS/EFS
Gisselbrecht et al. [38]	0.4 mCi/kg	BEAM	Relapsed or refractory (all FL)	77	93% 1-year EFS
Krishnan et al. [39]	0.4 mCi/kg	BEAM	1st CR/PR, relapsed or refractory	41	89%/70% 2-year OS/PFS
Khouri et al. [40]	0.4 mCi/kg	BEAM	–	26	92%/83% 2-year OS/DFS

PFS progression-free survival, *DFS* disease-free survival, *OS* overall survival, *EFS* event-free survival, *CR* complete remission, *BEAM* carmustine, etoposide, cytarabine, melphalan
[a]Dose to highest critical nontarget organ

the distribution of activity in critical organs. Absorbed doses to target organs were highly variable for any of the cohorts. At the 2007 Annual Meeting of the American Society of Hematology, this group updated their experience, now with 17 patients at the highest dose level of 1.5 mCi/kg [32]. The histologies were varied, and all patients had refractory or transformed disease. The median activity of

90-Y was 100 mCi. All patients engrafted promptly. Significant toxicities included one patient with transient acute grade 3 liver toxicity, one patient who died 4 months after treatment due to hepatitis C virus reactivation, one patient who died 2 months after treatment because of cerebral ischemia and a fourth patient who developed a myelodysplastic syndrome 2 years post-therapy. The authors recommend an activity of 1.2 mCi/kg, three times the standard dose, for heavily pretreated patients. Similarly, Devizzi and colleagues from Milan have reported on 29 patients, also representative of a variety of histologic subtypes, who received either 0.8 mCi/kg ($n = 13$) or 1.2 mCi/kg ($n = 16$) followed by tandem re-infusions of mobilized peripheral blood progenitor cells on days +7 and +14 post-transplant in an attempt to reduce the duration of cytopenias [33]. No significant nonhematologic toxicities were reported, and engraftment was rapid, although it cannot be concluded that the tandem infusions were of benefit over the conventional approach. Given the heterogeneity of the patient population and short duration of follow-up, no conclusions can be drawn regarding efficacy. Flinn et al. have also dose-escalated Yttrium-90 ibritumomab tiuxetan with mobilized peripheral blood progenitor cell support in patients with relapsed or refractory B-cell NHL [34], but dose escalation was cohort defined based on absorbed dose to the critical organ, not patient weight. Thus far, five patients have received a cohort defined dose of 14–18 Gy to the critical organ, six patients have received 24 Gy, and two patients have received 28 Gy, Up to 143.1 mCi has been administered without significant nonhematologic toxicity, with the exception of one death from pneumonia occurring 27 days post-transplant. These three series show that dose escalation of Yttrium-90 ibritumomab tiuxetan is possible, but whether dose escalation should be performed using dosimetry to define a specific absorbed dose to the critical organ or by weight remains to be established. If dosed according to weight, 1.2 mCi/kg would appear to be the preferred dose, at least for more heavily pretreated patients.

In other studies investigating dose-escalated Yttrium-90 ibritumomab tiuxetan in the autologous transplant setting, increasing doses of RIT replaced TBI in combination with etoposide and cyclophosphamide [35]. Nademanee and colleagues from The City of Hope conducted a phase I/II trial combining high-dose Yttrium-90 ibritumomab tiuxetan with high-dose etoposide (40–60 mg/kg) and cyclophosphamide (100 mg/kg). The radioimmunotherapy was dosed to achieve an absorbed dose of 10 Gy to any normal organ excluding the spleen or bone marrow. Thirty-one patients with follicular, diffuse large B-cell, and mantle cell lymphomas, including seven patients in first CR or PR, were treated with Yttrium-90 ibritumomab tiuxetan (median = 71.6; range: 37–105 mCi) and cyclophosphamide and etoposide. This series has recently been updated [36]. At a median follow up of 55 months, the 4-year estimated overall survival was 81%, and the disease-free survival was 65%. One patient failed to engraft, but otherwise toxicities were similar to those associated with standard transplant regimens. These results are also comparable to data presented by Press et al using I-131 tositumomab with the same doses of etoposide and cyclophosphamide [24], but with a much higher absorbed dose to critical organs (25 Gy).

In an attempt to improve on outcomes with high-dose chemotherapy and autologous HSCT, Winter and colleagues enrolled 44 patients with relapsed or refractory CD20^{+} B-cell NHL on a phase I trial of dose-escalated Yttrium-90 ibritumomab tiuxetan followed by high-dose BEAM and autologous HSCT in which the doses were calculated to deliver cohort-defined radiation doses (100–1700 cGy) to critical organs (liver, lung or kidney) with three to six patients per cohort [37]. Unlike other reported series, the patient population was mostly aggressive lymphomas (16% mantle cell, 57% diffuse aggressive, and 16% transformed) with only 11% indolent histologies, and all patients had relapsed or proven refractory disease. The toxicity profile was similar to that associated with high-dose BEAM. Two dose-limiting toxicities occurred at the 17Gy dose level: one patient with grade 4 stomatitis died of pneumonia and sepsis on day + 10 post-transplant, and one patient experienced septic emboli to the lung on day + 13 post-transplant. One heavily pretreated patient developed myelodysplasia on day + 291 post-transplant and expired of sepsis on day + 483 post-transplant. With a median follow-up of 21 months, the 3-year overall and progression-free survivals were 52% and 37%, respectively.

For dosimetry-based trials, 15Gy to the critical organ (nearly always liver) was the dose recommended by the investigators. Although patient-specific doses calculated to deliver a cohort-prescribed absorbed radiation dose to the critical organ were highly variable, the two dose-limiting toxicities occurred at nearly identical doses (1.14 and 1.20 mCi/kg, respectively) when calculated according to weight. Whereas eight other patients safely received at least twice the conventional 0.4-mCi/kg dose, 0.8 mCi/kg was the dose recommended for phase II studies, if dosing is to be based on weight and not dosimetry. Outcomes are encouraging given the high-risk patient population, but a phase III trial will be required to establish whether or not the addition of dose-escalated Yttrium-90 ibritumomab tiuxetan to high-dose BEAM improves outcomes in NHL patients undergoing autologous HSCT.

13.6 Standard Dose Yttrium-90 Ibritumomab Tiuxetan with HSCT Support

Whereas individualized dosing based on dosimetry requires experienced nuclear medicine physicians and a significant time commitment, weight-based dosing at the standard nontransplant dose of 0.4 mCi/kg combined with high-dose BEAM has been investigated (Table 13.4). Gisselbrecht et al., representing Groupe d'Etude des Lymphomes de l'Adulte (GELA), recently reported the results of a phase II trial consisting of 77 patients, the majority (90%) with relapsed or refractory follicular lymphoma, treated with a combination of standard dose Yttrium-90 ibritumomab tiuxetan and high-dose BEAM with HSCT [38]. Toxicity was similar to that observed with high-dose BEAM alone. First-line therapy had included rituximab in only 29 cases. After a minimum follow-up of 1 year for all patients, the estimated 2-year event-free survival is 93%. Two other series of relapsed and refractory lymphomas, 33 patients from the City of Hope and 26 patients from the M.D. Anderson Cancer Center, have been reported; both used the standard dose of 0.4 mCi/kg of Yttrium-90 ibritumomab tiuxetan and high-dose BEAM [39,40]. This dose is very easy to combine with Yttrium-90 ibritumomab tiuxetan and does not appear to increase the risk of toxicities. In chemotherapy-refractory patients with either primary refractory or refractory an Israeli trial in relapse and with positive [18] fluorodeoxyglucose positron emission tomography (FDG-PET) at the time of transplant, the estimated 2-year overall and progression-free survival rates were 67% and 52%, respectively (median follow-up = 17 months; range: 6–27 months) [41] Again, whether RIT added to high-dose BEAM improves outcomes over BEAM alone, must be established in a phase III randomized trial.

13.7 RIT and Allogeneic HSCT for NonHodgkin Lymphoma

There has been limited experience incorporating radioimmunotherapy into preparative regimens for allogeneic HSCT in patients with lymphoma. In hopes of providing better disease control for patients undergoing nonmyeloablative allogeneic HSCT, Gopal and colleagues treated 14 patients with chemotherapy-refractory lymphoma with standard-dose Yttrium-90 ibritumomab tiuxetan in addition to fludarabine and low-dose TBI followed by allogeneic HSCT [42]. Although follow-up was short (median follow-up for surviving patients = 6 months), half of these high-risk patients remain disease-free. Twelve patients with multiply relapsed lymphoma received standard-dose Yttrium-90 ibritumomab tiuxetan in addition to fludarabine and either busulfan or melphalan followed by allogeneic HSCT in a study reported by Shimoni and colleagues [43]. Immunosuprression was tapered rapidly in an effort to enhance the graft-versus-leukemia effect, but resulted in severe acute graft-versus-host disease. The nonrelapse mortality was high (42%), but only three patients have relapsed suggesting that this strategy may enhance disease control. At the MD Anderson, seven patients received reduced doses of Yttrium-90 ibritumomab tiuxetan (0.3 or 0.4 mCi/kg) in addition to nonmyeloablative conditioning, and five remain in complete remission with a median follow-up of 16 months [40]. Further investigation is required to better define the role of radioimmunotherapy in allogeneic HSCT for lymphoma.

13.8 RIT Based Transplant Conditioning Regimens Transplants for Leukemia (Table 13.5)

Historical data also emphasize the radiosensitivity of leukemias [44]. Expectedly, TBI has been an effective component of many transplant conditioning regimens in part to maximize the anti-leukemic effect. A variety of radioimmunoconjugates

Table 13.5 Selected trials utilizing RIT preparative regimens prior to allogeneic transplantation for AML

Author	Isotope	Dose	Target	Additional therapy	Leukemia type/setting	*n*	Results
Appelbaum et al. [46]	I-131	110–330 mCi	CD33	Cy/TBI	AML	4	75% CR
Jurcic et al. [52]	I-131	50–70 mCi/m^2	CD33	Bu/Cy	AML	19	95% CR, 53% TRM
Matthews et al. [53]	I-131	3.5–12.25 Gy[a]	CD45	Cy/TBI	AML/MDS/ALL	34	65-month DFS (AML)
Bunjes et al. [54]	Re-188	7.4 Gy[a]	CD66	Cy/TBI or Bu/Cy	AML/MDS	36	45% DFS at 18 months
Burke et al. [55]	I-131	122–437 mCi	CD33	Bu/Cy	AML/CML/MDS	31	Median OS = 4.9 months
Pagel et al. [56]	I-131	12–24 Gy[a]	CD45	Flu, TBI (2 Gy)	AML/AML	33	55% DFS at 10 months
Ringhoffer et al. [57]	Re-188/Y-90	9.7 ± 5.3 Gy[a]	CD66	Flu/ATG = Mel	AML/MDS	20	52% 2-year OS
Pagel et al. [51]	I-131	5.25 Gy[a]	CD45	Bu/Cy	AML-CR1	46	61% DFS at 3 years

AML acute myeloid leukemia, *MDS* myelodysplastic syndrome, *ALL* acute lymphocytic leukemia, *CML* chronic myeloid leukemia, *CR* complete response, *DFS* disease free survival, *OS* overall survival, *TRM* treatment related mortality, *Bu* Busulfan, *Cy* cyclophosphamide, *Flu* fludarabine, *ATG* Anti-thymocyte globulin, *Mel* melphalan, *TBI* total body irradiation, *Gy* gray, *I-131* iodine-131, *Y-90* Yttrium-90, *Re-188* rhenium-188

[a]Dose to highest critical nontarget organ

have been employed for the purpose of further escalating the radiation dose to hemato-lymphoid tissues (Table 13.2), and again, two basic strategies have emerged. The first approach utilized the addition of RIT to full dose preparative regimens either with or without TBI [9, 45]. The initial projects targeted the myeloid antigen CD33 and demonstrated that marrow and spleen could be preferentially targeted in most patients; however, it was noted that the short residence time of I-131 in some patients rendered a lower radiation exposure to hemato-lymphoid organs than to nontarget sites [46]. It was hypothesized that this short residence time could be attributed to the internalizing properties of the CD33 antigen and the observation that internalized I-131-conjugates were rapidly dehalogenated, resulting in release of the isotope from the cell [47]. In an attempt to overcome this limitation, investigators focused on the noninternalizing antigen, CD45. CD45 is expressed on the majority of hematopoietic cells and approximately 90% of acute leukemias; CD45 is not known to be expressed on nonhematopoietic tissues [48, 49]. Initial studies by the Seattle group indicated that the use of this strategy could deliver a median of 24 and 50 Gy of additional radiation to marrow and spleen, respectively, along with a full-dose conditioning regimen of cyclophosphamide (120 mg/kg) and TBI (12 Gy) [50]. More recently, a phase II study evaluated the use of this regimen along with busulfan (16 mg/kg) and cyclophosphamide (120 mg/kg) for high-risk AML patients in first complete remission [51]. These data demonstrated that mean of 11.3 and 29.7 Gy of additional radiation could safely be delivered to the marrow and spleen without an increase in nonrelapse mortality and an estimated 61% 3-year disease-free survival.

The more recently-developed RIT transplant strategy for leukemia is to add intensified radiation to reduced intensity preparative regimens, allowing the bulk of therapy to be targeted and maximally intensified. Preliminary results of this approach were reported by Pagel and colleagues, indicating that escalating doses of I-131 anti-CD45 therapy could be safely added to the Seattle fludarabine/2 Gy TBI regimen [56]. Thus far an additional 24 Gy has been delivered to liver resulting in up to an added 46 Gy to marrow and 81 Gy to spleen without incurring an increase in early mortality. Dose escalation of this study continues. A second group also followed this strategy by combining either Y-90 or Re-188 labeled anti-CD66 antibodies followed by the reduced-intensity regimen of fludarabine and antithymocyte globulin with or without melphalan [57]. This study illustrated that a median of 21.9 Gy could be delivered to the marrow space and improved marrow delivery was noted with Y-90 over Re-188. Importantly, treatment-related mortality (TRM) was not observed to be higher than historical controls and overall survival at 2 years was 52%.

13.9 Conclusions

As evidenced by the many studies cited above, the addition of radioimmunotherapy to conventional transplant regimens or its use as a single modality is not associated with significant nonhematologic toxicity. The cumulative data suggest that radioimmunotherapy has the potential to improve disease control and to increase cure rates with both autologous and allogeneic HSCT. The possibility of an increase in the incidence of secondary acute myeloid leukemia and myelodysplasia associated with RIT and autologous HSCT must be considered, especially in patients who have been heavily pretreated with chemotherapy. Whereas the risk of secondary leukemia and myelodysplasia may be as high as 10–15% following a conventional autologous HSCT for NHL, the addition of RIT has the potential to further increase the risk, and thus will need to be monitored closely. It is encouraging that investigators from the City of Hope have not found an increased risk of secondary leukemia or myelodysplasia when comparing patients receiving RIT as part of their transplant regimen to other transplant patients with the same risk factors [58]. Clinicians and researchers enthusiastically await phase III studies comparing standard regimens and RIT in a randomized head-to-head comparison. A multi-center trial comparing rituximab plus BEAM to I-131 tositumomab plus BEAM prior to autologous HSCT in patients with persistent or recurrent diffuse large B-cell NHL is underway.

Acknowledgments Grant support: Lymphoma Research Foundation Mantle Cell Lymphoma Research Initiative, SCOR Grant 7040 from the Leukemia and Lymphoma Society, NIH grants P01CA44991 and CA060553.

References

1. Gulati S, Yahalom J, Acaba L, et al. Treatment of patients with relapsed and resistant non-Hodgkin's lymphoma using total body irradiation, etoposide, and cyclophosphamide and autologous bone marrow transplantation. J Clin Oncol. 1992;10:936–41.
2. Philip T, Guglielmi C, Hagenbeek A, et al. Autologous bone marrow transplantation as compared with salvage chemotherapy in relapses of chemotherapy-sensitive non-Hodgkin's lymphoma (see comments). N Engl J Med. 1995;333:1540–5.
3. Schouten HC, Qian W, Kvaloy S, et al. High-dose therapy improves progression-free survival and survival in relapsed follicular non-Hodgkin's lymphoma: results from the randomized European CUP trial. J Clin Oncol. 2003;21:3918–27.
4. Dreyling M, Lenz G, Hoster E, et al. Early consolidation by myeloablative radiochemotherapy followed by autologous stem cell transplantation in first remission significantly prolongs progression-free survival in mantle-cell lymphoma: results of a prospective randomized trial of the European MCL Network. Blood 2005;105:2677–84.
5. Burnett AK, Goldstone AH, Stevens RM, et al. Randomised comparison of addition of autologous bone-marrow transplantation to intensive chemotherapy for acute myeloid leukaemia in first remission: results of MRC AML 10 trial. UK Medical Research Council Adult and Children's Leukaemia Working Parties. Lancet 1998;351:700–8.
6. Clift RA, Buckner CD, Appelbaum FR, et al. Allogeneic marrow transplantation in patients with acute myeloid leukemia in first remission: a randomized trial of two irradiation regimens. Blood 1990;76:1867–71.
7. Bensinger WI, Clift R, Martin P, et al. Allogeneic peripheral blood stem cell transplantation in patients with advanced hematologic malignancies: a retrospective comparison with marrow transplantation. Blood 1996;88:2794–800.
8. Fuks Z, Kaplan HS. Recurrence rates following radiation therapy of nodular and diffuse malignant lymphomas. Radiology 1973;108:675–84.

9. Bordigoni P, Vernant JP, Souillet G, et al. Allogeneic bone marrow transplantation for children with acute lymphoblastic leukemia in first remission: a cooperative study of the Groupe d'Etude de la Greffe de Moelle Osseuse. J Clin Oncol. 1989;7:747–53.
10. Kaminski MS, Zasadny KR, Francis IR, et al. Radioimmunotherapy of B-cell lymphoma with [131I]anti-B1 (anti-CD20) antibody. N Engl J Med. 1993;329:459–65.
11. Kaminski MS, Zelenetz AD, Press OW, et al. Pivotal study of iodine I 131 tositumomab for chemotherapy-refractory low-grade or transformed low-grade B-cell non-Hodgkin's lymphomas. J Clin Oncol. 2001;19:3918–28.
12. Kaminski MS, Tuck M, Estes J, et al. 131I-tositumomab therapy as initial treatment for follicular lymphoma. N Engl J Med. 2005;352:441–9.
13. Press OW, Unger JM, Braziel RM, et al. A phase 2 trial of CHOP chemotherapy followed by tositumomab/iodine I 131 tositumomab for previously untreated follicular non-Hodgkin lymphoma: Southwest Oncology Group Protocol S9911. Blood 2003;102: 1606–12.
14. Witzig TE, White CA, Wiseman GA, et al. Phase I/II trial of IDEC-Y2B8 radioimmunotherapy for treatment of relapsed or refractory CD20(+) B-cell non-Hodgkin's lymphoma. J Clin Oncol. 1999;17:3793–803.
15. Witzig TE, White CA, Gordon LI, et al. Safety of yttrium-90 ibritumomab tiuxetan radioimmunotherapy for relapsed low-grade, follicular, or transformed non-Hodgkin's lymphoma. J Clin Oncol. 2003;21:1263–70.
16. Witzig TE, Gordon LI, Cabanillas F, et al. Randomized controlled trial of yttrium-90-labeled ibritumomab tiuxetan radioimmunotherapy versus rituximab immunotherapy for patients with relapsed or refractory low-grade, follicular, or transformed B-cell non-Hodgkin's lymphoma. J Clin Oncol. 2002;20:2453–63.
17. Tedder TF, Streuli M, Schlossman SF, Saito H. Isolation and structure of a cDNA encoding the B1 (CD20) cell-surface antigen of human B lymphocytes. Proc Natl Acad Sci USA. 1988;85:208–12.
18. Tedder TF, Engel P. CD20: a regulator of cell-cycle progression of B lymphocytes. Immunol Today. 1994;15:450–4.
19. Press OW, Howell-Clark J, Anderson S, Bernstein I. Retention of B-cell-specific monoclonal antibodies by human lymphoma cells. Blood 1994;83:1390–7.
20. Press OW, Farr AG, Borroz KI, Anderson SK, Martin PJ. Endocytosis and degradation of monoclonal antibodies targeting human B-cell malignancies. Cancer Res. 1989;49: 4906–12.
21. Press OW, Eary JF, Appelbaum FR, et al. Radiolabeled-antibody therapy of B-cell lymphoma with autologous bone marrow support (see comments). N Engl J Med. 1993;329:1219–24.
22. Eary JF, Krohn KA, Press OW, Durack L, Bernstein ID. Importance of pre-treatment radiation absorbed dose estimation for radioimmunotherapy of non-Hodgkin's lymphoma. Nucl Med Biol. 1997;24:635–8.
23. Press OW, Eary JF, Appelbaum FR, et al. Phase II trial of 131I-B1 (anti-CD20) antibody therapy with autologous stem cell transplantation for relapsed B cell lymphomas. Lancet 1995;346:336–40.
24. Press OW, Eary JF, Gooley T, et al. A phase I/II trial of iodine-131-tositumomab (anti-CD20), etoposide, cyclophosphamide, and autologous stem cell transplantation for relapsed B-cell lymphomas. Blood 2000;96:2934–42.
25. Behr TM, Griesinger F, Riggert J, et al. High-dose myeloablative radioimmunotherapy of mantle cell non-Hodgkin lymphoma with the iodine-131-labeled chimeric anti-CD20 antibody C2B8 and autologous stem cell support. Results of a pilot study. Cancer 2002;94:1363–72.
26. Gopal AK, Gooley TA, Maloney DG, et al. High-dose radioimmunotherapy versus conventional high-dose therapy and autologous hematopoietic stem cell transplantation for relapsed follicular non-Hodgkin lymphoma: a multivariable cohort analysis. Blood 2003;102:2351–7.

27. Vose JM, Bierman PJ, Enke C, et al. Phase I trial of iodine-131 tositumomab with high-dose chemotherapy and autologous stem-cell transplantation for relapsed non-Hodgkin's lymphoma. J Clin Oncol. 2005;23:461–7.
28. Vose J, Bierman P, Bociek G, et al. Radioimmunotherapy with 131-I tositumomab enhanced survival in good prognosis relapsed and high-risk diffuse large B-cell lymphoma (DLBCL) patients receiving high-dose chemotherapy and autologous stem cell transplantation. American Society of Clinical Oncology. Chicago: ASCO. J Clin Oncol. (Abstract 8013) 2007:18s.
29. Gopal AK, Rajendran JG, Gooley TA, et al. High-dose [131I]tositumomab (anti-CD20) radioimmunotherapy and autologous hematopoietic stem-cell transplantation for adults ≥60 years old with relapsed or refractory B-cell lymphoma. J Clin Oncol. 2007;25:1396–402.
30. Gopal AK, Rajendran JG, Petersdorf SH, et al. High-dose chemo-radioimmunotherapy with autologous stem cell support for relapsed mantle cell lymphoma. Blood 2002;99: 3158–62.
31. Ferrucci PF, Vanazzi A, Grana CM, et al. High activity 90Y-ibritumomab tiuxetan (Zevalin) with peripheral blood progenitor cells support in patients with refractory/resistant B-cell non-Hodgkin lymphomas. Br J Haematol. 2007;139:590–9.
32. Vanazzi A, Ferrucci PF, Grana CM, et al. High dose 90yttrium ibritumomab tiuxetan with PBSC support in refractory-resistant NHL patients. Blood 2007;118:560a.
33. Devizzi L, Seregni E, Guidetti A, Forni C, et al. High-dose myeloablative Zevalin radioimmunotherapy with tandem stem-cell autografting has promising activity, minimal toxicity and full feasibility in an out-patient setting. Blood (ASH Annual Meeting Abstracts). 2006;108:3047.
34. Flinn IW, KB, Frey E, Bianco JA, Hammes RJ, Webb J, et al. Dose finding trial of yttrium 90 (^{90}Y) ibritumomab tiuxetan with autologous stem cell transplantation (ASCT) in patients with relapsed or refractory B-cell non-Hodgkin's lymphoma (NHL). J Clin Oncol (Suppl; ASCO Meeting Proceedings, Part 1, June 20, No. 185, Abstract 7535). 2006;24:7535.
35. Nademanee A, Forman S, Molina A, et al. A phase 1/2 trial of high-dose yttrium-90-ibritumomab tiuxetan in combination with high-dose etoposide and cyclophosphamide followed by autologous stem cell transplantation in patients with poor-risk or relapsed non-Hodgkin lymphoma. Blood 2005;106:2896–902.
36. Nademanee A, Raubitschek A, Molina A, et al. Updated results of high-dose yttriun 90 (^{90}Y) ibritumomab tiuxetan with high-dose etoposide (VP-16) and cyclophosphamide (CY) followed by autologous hematopoietic cell transplant (AHSCT) for poor-risk or refractory B-cell non-Hodgkin's lymphoma. Blood (ASH Annual Meeting Abstracts), Nov 2007;110:1891.
37. Winter JN, Inwards D, Spies S, et al. 90-Y Ibritumumab tiuxetan (Zevalin®, 90YZ) Doses Calculated to deliver up to 1500cGY to critical organs may be safely combined with high-dose BEAM and autotransplant in NHL. Blood (ASH Annual Meeting Abstracts, 2006;330).
38. Gisselbrecht C, Decaudin D, Mounier N, Tilly H, et al. 90Yttrium ibritumomab tiuxetan (Zevalin) combined with BEAM (Z-BEAM) conditioning regimen plus autologous stem cell transplantation in relapsed or refractory follicular lymphoma. GELA Phase II Study. Blood (ASH Annual Meeting Abstracts), Nov 2007;110:22.
39. Krishnan A, Nademanee A, Fung HC, et al. Phase II trial of a transplantation regimen of yttrium-90 ibritumomab tiuxetan and high-dose chemotherapy in patients with non-Hodgkin's lymphoma. J Clin Oncol. 2008;26:90–5.
40. Khouri IF, Saliba RM, Hosing C, Valverde R, et al. Efficacy and safety of yttrium 90 (90Y) ibritumomab tiuxetan in autologous and nonmyeloablative stem cell transplantation (NST) for relapsed non-Hodgkin's lymphoma (NHL). Blood (ASH Annual Meeting Abstracts), Nov 2006;108:315.
41. Shimoni A, Zwas ST, Oksman Y, et al. Yttrium-90-ibritumomab tiuxetan (Zevalin) combined with high-dose BEAM chemotherapy and autologous stem cell transplantation for chemo-refractory aggressive non-Hodgkin's lymphoma. Exp Hematol. 2007;35:534–40.

42. Gopal AK, Rajendran JG, Pagel JM, et al. A phase II trial of 90Y-ibritumomab tiuxetan-based reduced intensity allogeneic peripheral blood stem cell (PBSC) transplantation for relapsed CD20+ B-cell non-Hodgkin's lymphoma (NHL). Blood (ASH Annual Meeting Abstracts), Nov 2006; 108:316.
43. Shimoni A, Zwas ST, Oksman Y, et al. Ibritumomab tiuxetan (Zevalin) combined with reduced-intensity conditioning and allogeneic stem-cell transplantation (SCT) in patients with chemorefractory non-Hodgkin's lymphoma. Bone Marrow Transplant. 2008 Feb, 41(4):355–361. Epub 2007 Nov 19.
44. Atkinson JB, Mahoney FJ, Schwartz IR, Hesch JA. Therapy of acute leukemia by whole-body irradiation and bone marrow transplantation from an identical normal twin. Blood 1959;14:228–34.
45. Ringden O, Ruutu T, Remberger M, et al. A randomized trial comparing busulfan with total body irradiation as conditioning in allogeneic marrow transplant recipients with leukemia: a report from the Nordic Bone Marrow Transplantation Group. Blood 1994;83:2723–30.
46. Appelbaum FR, Matthews DC, Eary JF, et al. The use of radiolabeled anti-CD33 antibody to augment marrow irradiation prior to marrow transplantation for acute myelogenous leukemia. Transplantation 1992;54:829–33.
47. Press OW, Shan D, Howell-Clark J, et al. Comparative metabolism and retention of iodine-125, yttrium-90, and indium-111 radioimmunoconjugates by cancer cells. Cancer Res. 1996;56:2123–9.
48. Poppema S, Lai R, Visser L, Yan XJ. CD45 (leucocyte common antigen) expression in T and B lymphocyte subsets. Leuk Lymphoma. 1996;20:217–22.
49. Nakano A, Harada T, Morikawa S, Kato Y. Expression of leukocyte common antigen (CD45) on various human leukemia/lymphoma cell lines. Acta Pathol Jpn. 1990;40:107–15.
50. Matthews DC, Appelbaum FR, Eary JF, et al. Phase I study of (131)I-anti-CD45 antibody plus cyclophosphamide and total body irradiation for advanced acute leukemia and myelodysplastic syndrome. Blood 1999;94:1237–47.
51. Pagel JM, Appelbaum FR, Eary JF, et al. 131I-anti-CD45 antibody plus busulfan and cyclophosphamide before allogeneic hematopoietic cell transplantation for treatment of acute myeloid leukemia in first remission. Blood 2006;107:2184–91.
52. Jurcic JG, Caron PC, Nikula TK, et al. Radiolabeled anti-CD33 monoclonal antibody M195 for myeloid leukemias. Cancer Res. 1995;55:5908s–10s.
53. Matthews DC, Martin PJ, Nourigat C, Appelbaum FR, Fisher DR, Bernstein ID. Marrow ablative and immunosuppressive effects of 131I-anti-CD45 antibody in congenic and H2-mismatched murine transplant models. Blood 1999;93:737–45.
54. Bunjes D, Buchmann I, Duncker C, et al. Rhenium 188-labeled anti-CD66 (a, b, c, e) monoclonal antibody to intensify the conditioning regimen prior to stem cell transplantation for patients with high-risk acute myeloid leukemia or myelodysplastic syndrome: results of a phase I–II study. Blood 2001;98:565–72.
55. Burke JM, Caron PC, Papadopoulos EB, et al. Cytoreduction with iodine-131-anti-CD33 antibodies before bone marrow transplantation for advanced myeloid leukemias. Bone Marrow Transplant. 2003;32:549–56.
56. Pagel J, Appelbaum F, Rajendran J, et al. 131I-anti-CD45 antibody plus fludarabine, low-dose TBI and PBSC infusion for elderly patients with advanced acute myeloid leukemia or high-risk myelodysplastic syndrome. Blood 2005;106:119a.
57. Ringhoffer M, Blumstein N, Neumaier B, et al. 188Re or 90Y-labelled anti-CD66 antibody as part of a dose-reduced conditioning regimen for patients with acute leukaemia or myelodysplastic syndrome over the age of 55: results of a phase I–II study. Br J Haematol. 2005;130:604–13.
58. Krishnan AY, Palmer JM, Bhatia SC, et al. The impact of incorporating targeted radioimmunotherapy (RIT) into transplant preparative regimens on the incidence of therapy related myelodysplasia (t-MDS) or AML (t-AML) following autologous stem cell transplant (ASCT) for lymphoma. Blood (ASH Annual Meeting Abstracts). 2007;110:1082.

Chapter 14
Evolving Indications for Hematopoietic Stem Cell Transplantation in Multiple Myeloma and Other Plasma Cell Disorders

Guido Tricot, Maurizio Zangari, Roberto Sorasio, and Benedetto Bruno

14.1 Introduction

Multiple myeloma is a differentiated clonal B-cell tumor, consisting in the early stages of the disease of slowly proliferating malignant plasma cells (myeloma cells). It is the second most common hematologic malignancy after non-Hodgkin's lymphoma. Normal plasma cells are very hardy cells and usually the only type of cell to survive the effects of myelosuppressive chemotherapy and radiation. The plasma cells have abnormal cytogenetics even at the stage of monoclonal gammopathy of undetermined significance, as evidenced by fluorescence in-situ hybridization (FISH) or cIg/DNA content [1–3]. Before it transforms to an aggressive disease, which is typically associated with extramedullary disease, immature morphology of the myeloma cells, rapid proliferation, and increase in LDH, the disease is entirely bone marrow stroma-dependent and, therefore, contained within the active hematopoietic bone marrow, although breakout lesions from the bone can be seen. The myeloma cell displays on its membrane a multitude of receptors, the ligands of which are present in the micro-environment. Such receptors are the IL-6 receptor, the IL-15 receptor, the IGF (insulin-like growth factor) receptor, CD38, and Notch [4–7]. Binding of these receptors by their ligands results in the activation of four major pathways: STAT-3, RAS, Akt and NF-kB, which promote growth and survival of the myeloma cells and also result in the secretion by the plasma cells of angiogenic factors [8–11]. There is a tremendous redundancy in this system so that blocking one of these pathways will have little effect on the survival and growth of myeloma cells. This is in contrast to chronic myeloid leukemia where blocking of a single pathway (BCR-ABL) will have a major effect on the disease. In addition to supporting growth and survival, the micro-environment also places most of myeloma cells in a deep G1 phase by up-regulation of p21 and p27. This is accomplished by binding of fibronectin and

G. Tricot (✉)
Professor of Medicine, University of Utah School of Medicine, Salt Lake City, UT, USA
e-mail: Guido.Tricot@hsc.utah.edu

M.R. Bishop (ed.), *Hematopoietic Stem Cell Transplantation*,
Cancer Treatment and Research 144, DOI 10.1007/978-0-387-78580-6_14,

V-CAM present in the micro-environment to VLA-4 (CD49d) expressed on the membrane of myeloma cells, as well as by Jagged-1 induced Notch signaling [8, 12]. Cells in the G1 phase of the cell cycle are very poor targets for conventional dose chemotherapy.

It is very likely that in myeloma, just as in many other cancers, a cancer stem cell population exists. It is estimated that one in 10,000 to one in 20,000 malignant cells is a cancer stem cell. Based on the extensive somatic mutations in the complementarity regions of the gene coding for the heavy chain, it is very likely that this cancer stem cell arises from a B-cell that has had extensive exposure to antigen in the germinal center and therefore most likely is either a memory B-cell or a plasmablast [13, 14]. It has been proposed that the myeloma cancer stem cell is CD138-negative and CD19-positive, based on the observation that this population, whether derived from myeloma cell lines or primary myeloma samples, has an increased clonogenic potential [15]. The clonogenic potential of myeloma cells is increased by dendritic cells, leading to loss of CD138 and expression of bcl-6 [16]. Hedgehog signaling, which determines the fate of progenitor cells, promotes the expansion of the myeloma stem cell [17]. The small subset of myeloma cells that manifests hedgehog pathway activation is markedly concentrated in the tumor stem cell compartment. If there is indeed a myeloma stem cell, such a cell will have many characteristics in common with a hematopoietic stem cell in that it is resistant to conventional doses of chemotherapy, and that such doses of chemotherapy will be necessary, which can at least eradicate hematopoietic stem cells, and therefore such therapy will require stem cell support. The agents most toxic to hematopoietic stem cells are alkylators such as melphalan, busulfan and BCNU, agents found to be very effective in myeloma, while other alkylators such as cyclophosphamide and platinum compounds, which spare hematopoietic stem cells, are much less effective in myeloma even at higher doses. The difficulty in myeloma is not to eradicate the more differentiated myeloma compartment, which comprises more than 99.9% of the tumor mass, but to also kill the myeloma stem cells. Consequently, achieving a hematologic remission, as currently defined, will have a poor correlation with long-term outcome and should not be used as an early substitute for survival estimates.

14.2 Autologous Hematopoietic Stem Cell Transplantation in Multiple Myeloma

14.2.1 Autologous Transplantation for Recently Diagnosed Myeloma Patients

It has been more than 25 years since the late Tim McElwain and colleagues introduced high-dose melphalan for the treatment of multiple myeloma. Administration of melphalan 100–140 mg/m^2 without stem cell support induced biochemical and bone marrow remissions in three (all previously untreated) of the nine myeloma patients, which was much higher than the 3–5% complete response typically seen with conventional therapy [18]. The efficacy of high dose melphalan in myeloma was subsequently confirmed in larger studies [19, 20]. However, high-dose melphalan induced prolonged aplasia of 5–8 weeks and was therefore associated with high morbidity and mortality rates in a disease with a median age of 67 years [18, 21]. This led other investigators to the concept of stem cell rescue, which allowed further dose escalation of melphalan to 200 mg/m^2. Stem cell support was initially provided with autologous bone marrow, which could contain up to 30% plasma cells [22], and subsequently with peripheral blood stem cells, containing more CD34$^+$ cells/kg and therefore resulting in more prompt bone marrow recovery and less morbidity and mortality. Indeed, with a dose of 5×10^6 CD34$^+$ cells/kg or more, the median time of severe neutropenia and thrombocytopenia is not much longer than 1 week [23]. This made application of autologous hematopoietic stem cell transplantation (HSCT) feasible in patients 60–75 years old, who were in otherwise good clinical condition, and it reduced procedure-related mortality to 2–5% [21], which is not higher than that seen with 6 months of conventional chemotherapy and/ or the novel agents, such as bortezomib, thalidomide and lenalidomide [24–27]. In an attempt to minimize toxicity and to maximize myeloma cell kill, the concept of tandem autologous transplantation was introduced by Barlogie and colleagues in Total Therapy I [28]. The underlying hypothesis was that rather than giving a single very intensive preparative regimen prior to stem cell rescue, providing effective, but less toxic high-dose chemotherapy twice would be better tolerated in older patients and equally effective. Total Therapy I was designed to include all active agents available at that time for the treatment of myeloma to increase the complete remission rate as a first important step to improve overall survival. A total of 231 patients were enrolled from 1990 to 1994. With a median follow up of 12 years, 62 patients are still alive and 31 have not progressed. Patients still alive more likely had normal cytogenetics, a normal C-reactive protein (CRP), hemoglobin and lactate dehydrogenase (LDH) level, and had completed two transplants within a 12-month period. The 10-year event-free and overall survivals were 15% and 33%, respectively. The superiority of Total Therapy I over conventional treatment was established by using historical controls, matched for all-important available prognostic markers, were treated on Southwest Oncology trials during the same period [29]. Autotransplantation induced a higher response rate (85% vs. 52%; $p < 0.001$) and significantly extended event-free (49 months vs. 22 months; $p = 0.001$) and overall survival (62+ months vs. 48 months; $p = 0.01$). The superiority of autologous HSCT over conventional therapy was subsequently confirmed in prospective randomized trials. The IFM-90 study by the Intergroupe Francais Du Myelome (IFM) included 200 patients under the age of 65. Stem cell rescue was performed with bone marrow. Data were analyzed on intent to treat basis [30]. More than one-quarter of patients randomized to the transplant arm never received a transplant. Nevertheless, response rates (81% vs. 57%), complete remission rates (22% vs. 5%), and 5-year event-free (28% vs.

10%) and overall survival (52% vs. 12%) were significantly better in the transplant arm. This study was criticized because of the small number of patients and the poor response rate in the control arm. In another randomized study performed in the United Kingdom, the Medical Research Council Myeloma VII Trial enrolled 407 previously untreated myeloma patients younger than 65; 401 could be evaluated. Also in this study with a median follow up of surviving patients of 42 months, the complete response rate (44% vs. 8%; $p < 0.001$), progression-free (28 months vs. 20 months; $p < 0.001$) and overall survival (54 months vs. 42 months; $p = 0.04$) were superior in the transplant arm [31]. There was a trend toward a greater survival benefit of HSCT in patients with poor prognosis, defined as a high $\beta 2$ microglobulin level of greater than 8 mg/L. On the other hand, three studies using either high-dose total body irradiation (TBI) or oral busulfan, failed to show a benefit for the transplant arm when compared to standard chemotherapy [32–34]. In one of these studies [33] patients failing to respond to induction treatment were excluded from randomization, although it is especially in this group of patients that autologous HSCT shows the most benefit compared to conventional chemotherapy (see below). Excellent outcomes were also reported by the Royal Marsden Hospital group. A total of 451 myeloma patients, 51% previously untreated, received a single autotransplant between 1985 and 2001 [35]. The treatment-related mortality was 6%, which is somewhat higher than in most other studies. Fifty-nine percent of the patients achieved a complete or near-complete remission. The 10-year progression-free and overall survivals were 16.5% and 31.4%, respectively. Better overall survival was seen in patients with low $\beta 2$-microglobulin, age less than 60 years and normal albumin levels. In its evidence-based review, the American Society for Blood and Marrow Transplantation concluded that autologous HSCT is the preferred treatment modality for myeloma and that its application is recommended as de novo rather than as salvage therapy [36]. Yet, less than half of the patients aged 65 or less with myeloma actually proceeds to transplantation [37]. Between October 1998 and February 2004, 668 newly diagnosed myeloma patients were randomized upfront to intensive therapy including tandem autologous transplants with or without thalidomide during the whole treatment. With a median of 42 months of follow-up for surviving patients, the complete remission rate (62% vs. 43%; $p < 0.001$) and the 5-year event-free survival (56% vs. 44%; $p = 0.01$) were superior in the thalidomide arm. However, the 5-year overall survival was similar, approximately 65% in both arms ($p = 0.9$). Median survival after relapse was significantly shorter in the thalidomide arm (1.1 years vs. 2.7 years; $p = 0.001$). Toxicity was also higher in the thalidomide arm, especially deep vein thrombosis and peripheral neuropathy [38]. When comparing the nonthalidomide arm of Total Therapy 2 (more intensive induction, consolidation, and maintenance therapy) to Total Therapy 1, the complete remission rates were similar (43% vs. 41%). However, the 5-year event-free survival was better on Total Therapy 2 (43% vs. 28%; $p < 0.001$) with also a trend for better overall survival (62% vs. 57%; $p = 0.11$). Superior event-free and overall survivals were seen in the two-thirds of patients with normal metaphase cytogenetics [38].

14.2.2 The Preparative Regimen for Autologous Hematopoietic Stem Cell Transplantation

Most preparative regimens are based on either melphalan alone or a combination of melphalan and TBI. Other alkylating agents such as busulfan, carmustine, thiotepa and cyclophosphamide have been used less often. The IFM study 9502, which included 282 newly diagnosed and evaluable myeloma patients under the age of 65, compared in a prospective randomized trial melphalan 140 mg/m^2 with 8 Gy of TBI to melphalan 200 mg/m^2 [39]. Patients randomized to the melphalan arm only showed significantly faster recovery of neutrophils and platelets and required fewer transfusions, and the median duration of hospitalization was significantly shorter. There was a trend toward a better complete and very good partial remission rate in the melphalan only arm (55% vs. 43%; $p = 0.06$). The median event-free survival was identical, but the 45-month overall survival was superior in the melphalan only arm (65.8% vs. 45.5%; $p = 0.05$), probably due to more effective salvage treatment in the melphalan only patients. Two additional nonrandomized studies confirm the superiority of melphalan 200 mg/m^2 over TBI-containing preparative regimens. In the University of Arkansas experience, TBI-containing regimens were associated with a higher treatment-related mortality and inferior event-free and overall survival, despite similar complete remission rates [40]. These investigators speculated that a more profound and prolonged immunosuppression after TBI was responsible for the inferior outcome. The European Group for Blood and Marrow Transplantation (EBMT) analysis on prognostic factors for outcome after autologous transplantation in myeloma also demonstrated that non-TBI preparative regimens were independently associated with a superior outcome [41]. In a study from the M.D. Anderson Cancer Center, which included 186 newly diagnosed patients, a preparative regimen with thiotepa, busulfan and cyclophosphamide was compared to melphalan 200 mg/m^2 in a retrospective analysis. The response rate (66% vs. 69%), progression-free (21 months vs. 20 months) and overall survival (46 months vs. not reached) were similar in both groups. The authors concluded that a more intensive regimen did not improve outcome and that melphalan 200 mg/m^2 should be the standard preparative regimen [42]. Based on all these data, melphalan 200 mg/m^2 has become the preferred preparative regimen.

14.2.3 Graft Contamination with Myeloma Cells

There is ample and convincing evidence that not only bone marrow, but also peripheral blood stem cells are contaminated with myeloma cells [43, 44]. Applying quantitative PCR amplification assays of patient-specific CDR3 DNA sequences on peripheral blood mononuclear cell samples, myeloma cells can be detected in virtually all myeloma patients [44, 45]. The re-infusion of contaminated peripheral blood stem cell collections may contribute to disease relapse as has been demonstrated for other malignancies such as acute and chronic myeloid leukemia, and neuroblastoma [46, 47]. Additionally, an inverse correlation has been established between plasma cell contamination of the peripheral blood stem cell product and disease-free survival, although this was a small study that included only 33 patients [48]. This may be more a reflection of the higher tumor burden than contribution of contaminated myeloma cells to relapse. Indirect evidence of the potential importance of a clean graft comes from an EBMT study, comparing outcomes of 25 myeloma patients receiving bone marrow or peripheral blood stem cells from an identical twin to 125 case-matched controls who received autologous and thus contaminated transplants [49]. The overall survival tended to be better (73 months vs. 44 months; $p = 0.1$) and progression-free survival was significantly better (72 months vs. 25 months; $p = 0.009$) for the syngeneic transplants. The risk of relapse at 48 months was significantly lower (36% vs. 78%; $p = 0.009$). Different ex vivo purging techniques, based on chemical and immunologic approaches, have been applied to obtain “tumor-free” grafts. Delayed hematologic recovery and increased infectious complications have compromised the applicability of these strategies, despite their success in substantially reducing myeloma cell contamination of the graft. In a multi-center Phase III randomized trial, hematologic recovery and toxicity after autologous transplantation were compared between patients receiving CD34$^+$ cell-selected grafts versus unselected grafts [50]. Time to platelet recovery was slightly delayed in patients receiving CD34$^+$ cell-selected grafts with less than 2×10^6 CD34$^+$ cells/kg. There was no difference in event-free and overall survival between the two arms. Moreover, salvage therapy may be more difficult in patients who have received CD34$^+$ cell-selected grafts. Because of the high cost and the lack of benefit of tumor cell-reduced grafts, this area of research is no longer pursued.

14.2.4 Single Versus Tandem Autologous Transplants

Despite the superiority of autologous transplantation over conventional chemotherapy, the 7-year event-free survival in the IFM 90 trial was only 16% with no plateau on the survival curve. Achievement of a very good partial response (VGPR; i.e., more than 90% reduction in M-protein) or better was associated with a significantly better overall survival. Therefore, the same French group tested in a prospective randomized trial (IFM 94) whether outcome could be improved by the application of tandem transplants [51]. In that study 399 newly diagnosed myeloma patients under the age of 60 years were randomly assigned to a single versus tandem transplants. Patients in the single transplant arm received melphalan 140 mg/m^2 with 8 Gy of TBI, while those in the tandem transplant arm received a first transplant with melphalan 140 mg/m^2, followed by melphalan 140 mg/m^2 with 8 Gy of TBI for the second transplant. No difference was observed in the VGPR or better rate between the two arms (50% vs. 42%;

$p = 0.1$). However, the event-free (20% vs. 10%; $p = 0.03$) and overall survival at 7 years (42% vs. 21%; $p = 0.01$) was superior in the tandem transplant arm. For patients in the single transplant arm who did not achieve at least a VGPR within 3 months after transplant, the 7-year survival was only 11% vs. 43% in the tandem transplant arm ($p < 0.001$). However, patients achieving at least a VGPR after a single transplant did not appear to benefit significantly from a second transplant ($p = 0.7$). On multivariate analysis, $\beta 2$ microglobulin, LDH, and the treatment arm were all independent prognostic markers associated with survival (all $p < 0.01$). In another prospective randomized study, the Bologna 96 clinical study of single versus double autologous HSCT for myeloma, 321 patients were randomly assigned to receive either melphalan 200 mg/m^2 alone or melphalan 200 mg/m^2 followed by melphalan 120 mg/m^2 plus busulfan 12 mg/kg [52]. A higher percentage of patients in the double transplant arm achieved at least a near complete remission in the tandem transplant arm (47% vs. 33%; $p = 0.008$) and these patients had a longer relapse-free (42 months vs. 28 months; $p < 0.001$) and event-free survival (35 months vs. 23 months; $p = 0.001$). Benefits offered by tandem transplantation were particularly evident among patients failing to achieve at least a near complete remission after the first transplant. Transplant-related mortality was 3% in the single and 4% in the tandem transplant arm. The administration of a second transplant and the introduction of novel agents in the treatment of myeloma for patients relapsing in the single transplant arm resulted in a failure to see a benefit in overall survival for the double transplant group. Therefore, the available data favor tandem transplants in younger myeloma patients at least in those not achieving an excellent response after the first transplant. The issue of benefit and timing of a second autologous HSCT has been addressed in a retrospective analysis of the EBMT, which included approximately 7500 patients [53]. Since this was not a prospective randomized study, there may be major biases related to differences in prognostic factors and to the multiple centers who had contributed to the patient database. On the other hand, the large number of patients analyzed probably compensated for many of these biases. In this study, the hazard ratio (HR) of relapse was clearly lower if a second transplant was performed within 12 months after the first transplant (HR compared to no second transplant was 0.43 for second transplants performed <6 months after the first and 0.51 between 6 and 12 months). A second transplant more than 12 months after the first transplant still had a significantly lower relapse rate compared to no second transplant before relapse (HR = 0.64), but its benefit was not as pronounced as with a second transplant within 12 months. Moreover, the transplant-related mortality was clearly higher if the second transplant was performed more than 12 months after the first. When in this retrospective analysis an elective second transplant was compared to a second transplant at relapse, an elective second transplant clearly improved overall survival (HR for survival 1.7; $p < 0.0001$), while a second transplant at relapse did not confer any survival benefit over salvage treatment with nontransplant modalities (HR = 1.06; $p = 0.55$).

14.2.5 Autologous Transplantation for Primary Refractory Myeloma

High dose therapy has consistently increased tumor cytoreduction and has extended event-free and overall survival in patients with primary refractory myeloma (<50% reduction in M-protein). Alexanian and colleagues reported on 27 patients with primary refractory myeloma who received an autologous transplant and compared their outcome to 60 control patients receiving conventional chemotherapy [54]. The transplanted patients had a median survival of 83 months compared to 38 months for patients receiving standard treatments for primary refractory myeloma ($p = 0.03$). Autologous transplantation for primary refractory myeloma later in the disease (>1 year) resulted in significantly lower response rates and shorter progression-free survival. In a study from the Royal Marsden Hospital, Surrey, UK, patients with primary refractory myeloma to induction therapy had a similar event-free survival compared to those with chemotherapy-sensitive patients ($p = 0.2$) with an early difference in outcome in favor of the chemotherapy-sensitive patients, mainly due to the higher transplant-related mortality in the primary refractory patients [55]. The time to relapse was also identical in the two groups ($p = 0.6$). The authors concluded that myeloma patients should not be excluded from autologous HSCT based upon lack of response to induction chemotherapy. The Mayo Clinic reported its experience with outcome of stem cell transplantation in 50 patients with primary refractory myeloma to induction therapy and compared it to that of 101 patients with chemotherapy-sensitive disease [56]. The 1-year progression-free survival for refractory patients was 70% compared to 83% for chemotherapy-sensitive patients ($p = 0.65$). The authors recommended early stem cell transplantation for patients with primary refractory myeloma.

14.2.6 Autotransplantation for Elderly Patients

Most high dose therapy trials have only included relatively young patients with good organ function. However, the median age of myeloma patients is 67 years. If a major impact of autologous HSCT on outcome is to be achieved, it will have to be performed also in patients over the age of 65. Age per se should not be a contra-indication for transplantation, but comorbidities can be. It is obvious that comorbidities increase in older patients, and therefore, more elderly myeloma patients may not be candidates for autologous HSCT. Several studies have reported contradictory findings on the impact of age on the ability to collect stem cells. In a retrospective analysis including 984 patients with 106 over the age of 70 years, increasing age correlated inversely with $CD34^+$ cell yield [57]. However, the overwhelming majority (85%) of elderly patients were able to collect greater than 4×10^6 $CD34^+$ cells/kg provided that the duration of preceding therapy was 12 months or less and the platelet count was 200,000/

μL or more. With the introduction of peripheral blood stem cell transplants, shortening the duration of severe cytopenias, and improved supportive care, the toxicity of autologous HSCT has clearly decreased. The Arkansas group has compared the outcome of 49 previously treated and untreated myeloma patients over the age of 65 to that of pair mates matched for important prognostic factors [58]. No significant difference was seen in percentage of patients completing two transplants (65% vs. 76%; $p = 0.3$). Time to hematopoietic recovery after first and second transplant was comparable in both groups. Treatment-related mortality was 8% in the older and 2% in the younger patients. The frequency of complete remission was lower in older patients (20% vs. 43%; $p = 0.02$). Median durations of event-free ($p = 0.2$) and overall survival ($p = 0.4$) were not significantly different. The safety of autologous HSCT in older patients was subsequently confirmed in other studies [59, 60]. The role of autologous HSCT in older patients has recently been challenged by the IFM 99-06 trial comparing melphalan-prednisone to melphalan-prednisone plus thalidomide and to twice melphalan 100 mg/m^2 with stem cell support [61]. A total of 436 patients between the ages of 65 and 75 were enrolled. Median follow-up was 32 months. Progression-free and overall survivals were significantly better for patients randomized to the melphalan-prednisone plus thalidomide. The authors concluded that melphalan-prednisone plus thalidomide is effective treatment for older myeloma patients, probably superior to autologous HSCT. It should be noted, however, that 30% of patients randomized to transplantation never received a transplant and that the dose of melphalan was suboptimal even for older patients. In older patients in good general health, tandem autotransplants probably still is the preferred treatment, but the dose of melphalan should be reduced to 140 mg/m^2 instead of 200 mg/m^2 to minimize toxicity and to maximize the chance that a second transplant can be administered in a timely fashion.

14.2.7 Autotransplantation in Patients with Renal Failure

Pharmacokinetic studies performed in 20 patients, including six with severe renal failure, five of which were on dialysis, showed that melphalan levels and metabolism were not different in patients with renal failure [62]. However, high dose melphalan was associated with more toxicity ($p = 0.0005$) and longer hospitalizations ($p = 0.004$) in renal failure patients. The Arkansas group reported data on 81 consecutive myeloma patients with renal failure (creatinine of >2 mg/dL or >176.8 μmol/L) at the time of transplantation [63]. Thirty-eight patients were dialysis dependent. The median age was 53 years and one-quarter had received >12 months of preceding therapy. The first 60 patients received melphalan 200 mg/m^2; the dose of melphalan was reduced to 140 mg/m^2 for the last 21 patients. A complete remission of 26% and 38%, respectively, was observed after the first and second transplant. Median overall survival was

52+ months. Melphalan 140 mg/m^2 was better tolerated and appeared equally effective as melphalan 200 mg/m^2. It should be mentioned that only 40% received their planned second transplant. In another study from the same group of investigators, the outcome of 59 patients on dialysis at the time of first transplant was analyzed. Of 54 patients evaluable for renal function improvement, 13(24%) became dialysis independent at a median of 4 months after AT (range: 1–16) [64]; 37 had been on dialysis for 6 months or less. The 5-year event-free and overall survivals were 24% and 36%, respectively. One-quarter of patients became dialysis-independent. Shorter duration of dialysis-dependency and a pretransplant creatinine clearance of greater than 10 mL/min predicted for a significantly higher probability of becoming dialysis-independent post-transplantation. These data suggest that autologous HSCT should be performed early in the disease course to maximize the probability of reversing end-stage renal failure. Raab et al. compared outcome of 17 patients with dialysis-dependent renal failure who received melphalan 100 mg/m^2 to that of 17 matched pairs without renal failure, treated with melphalan 200 mg/m^2 [65]. No significant difference in hematologic toxicity, transplant-related mortality or disease response was observed, and event-free and overall survivals were comparable. However, dialysis-dependent patients required more extensive intravenous antibiotic administration and longer hospitalizations. Similar observations were made by Knudsen et al. [66]. They did observe a significantly higher transplant-related mortality (17% vs. 1%) in patients with severe renal failure. The dose of melphalan in renal failure patients varied between 100 and 200 mg/m^2. These data clearly indicate that autologous HSCT in patients with renal failure is feasible and can reverse dialysis-dependency. However, it is more toxic and requires better supportive care skills. The dose of melphalan should be reduced to 100–140 mg/m^2 dependent on age and comorbidities.

14.2.8 Prognostic Factors with Autotransplantation

Myeloma is a highly heterogeneous disease with survival ranging from a few months to more than 15 years. The Durie-Salmon staging system, which is based on renal function and estimates of tumor burden, clearly has prognostic significance and has allowed better interpretation of clinical trials, but has major shortcomings such as assessment of lytic lesions and the lack of attention to proliferation characteristics [67]. The International Staging System was introduced recently and is based on data of more than 10,000 patients [68]. It only uses albumin and β2-microglobulin levels, which are readily available to practicing oncologists. It clearly separates patients into good, intermediate and high risk myeloma. Although this classification is now widely applied, it does not include any genetic information about the cancer cells. The importance of cytogenetics was first demonstrated by metaphase cytogenetics and subsequently by FISH. Patients with cytogenetic abnormalities on metaphase analysis have an inferior prognosis [69, 70]. Finding abnormal metaphase cytogenetics is probably the best surrogate marker available at this time for stroma-independent and, therefore, aggressive myeloma [71]. The worst outcome is seen in patients with a hypodiploid karyotype and/or complete deletion of chromosome 13 or partial deletion of its long arm [72]. Patients with a hyperdiploid karyotype and no deletion 13 have a somewhat better outcome. Chromosome 14q32 translocations, involving the gene coding for the immunoglobulin heavy chain are frequent in myeloma and probably represent an important early event in its pathogenesis, since these translocations are found with almost the same frequency in monoclonal gammopathy of undetermined significance. Multiple partners have been identified for the 14q32 translocations, some associated with good, others with poor prognosis. The t(11;14)(q13;q32), which results in a high expression of cyclin D1 and present in 20% of myeloma patients, is associated with a good prognosis [73, 74]. These patients have myeloma cells with more lymphoplasmacytic morphology and a pseudo-diploid karyotype. The plasma cells are often CD20-positive. This translocation is also common in primary amyloidosis [75]. Although many patients with this translocation relapse, they remain relatively sensitive to therapy. The t(6;14)(p21;q32), present in 5% of myeloma patients, results in over-expression of cyclin D3 [76]. It shares the same good prognosis with the t(11;14). On the other hand, the t(14;16)(q32;q23), present in 5% of patients and resulting in over-expression of *c-MAF,* t(14;20)(q32;q11), present in <5% and resulting in high *MAF-B* and the t(4;14)(p16;q32), present in 15% and resulting in high expression of *FGFR3* in the majority of patients, are associated with a poor prognosis also with stem cell transplantation [77–80]. These poor prognosis translocations can only be detected by FISH and not by conventional cytogenetics. They are often associated with deletion 13 on conventional cytogenetics. Deletion of 17p, involving the p53 gene is usually a mono-allelic deletion. It also has a poor prognosis and is present in 10–33% of myeloma patients [81, 82]. Metaphase and FISH chromosomal analysis represent only a crude way to assess DNA changes and provide no clues of which genes are either over- or under-expressed. Gene expression profiling permits quantitation of RNA expression of more than 30,000 genes with many of those related to cancer biology such as proliferation, apoptosis, DNA repair, and drug resistance. Applying unsupervised hierarchical clustering to highly purified plasma cells of newly diagnosed patients, seven subgroups of myeloma have been identified, based on either spiked gene expression as a consequence of a translocation involving 14q32, hyperdiploidy, or proliferation characteristics [80]. This biological classification also had major prognostic significance with inferior outcome for patients with a proliferative signature or with spikes of *MMSET, c-MAF,* or *MAF-B,* thus confirming and adding to the FISH data. To molecularly define high risk myeloma, 70 either highly over- or under-expressed genes were identified that were linked to early myeloma-related death [83]. A high proportion of up-regulated genes mapped to chromosome 1q, while a high proportion of down-regulated genes mapped to chromosome 1p. The ratio of mean expression levels of up-regulated to down-regulated genes defined a group of high-risk patients, which constituted 13% of the entire myeloma population with a short event-free and overall survival. Multivariate discriminant analysis showed that a subset of only 17 genes predicted outcome equally well as the 70 gene model. On multivariate analysis of outcomes of 220 newly diagnosed myeloma patients entered on Total Therapy 2, including standard prognostic variables, metaphase cytogenetics, magnetic resonance imaging, FISH, and gene expression profiling (GEP), the hazard ratio for overall survival was highest for GEP (3.07; $p < 0.001$), followed by amplification of 1q21 (1.71; $p = 0.05$) (see below). The 3-year survival decreased progressively from 92% to 78% to 43%, according to the presence of none (49% of patients), one (35%), or both (16%) of these unfavorable variables [84]. One of the genes mapping to 1q21 is *CKS1B*. Overexpression of this gene is associated by itself with a poor prognosis [85]. Overexpression of 1q21 can also be assessed by FISH. Amplification of 1q21 (amp1q21) heralds a poor prognosis and remains an independent factor on multivariate analysis with an inferior event-free and overall survival [86]. In the absence of GEP, much of the prognostic value can be assessed by combining metaphase cytogenetics with FISH for t(11;14) and amp1q21 with a significantly inferior event-free survival for patients with cytogenetic abnormalities and amp1q21 but no t(11;14) (Fig. 14.1).

14.2.9 Autotransplantation for Relapsed/Refractory Myeloma

Although curative in only a minority of myeloma patients, the introduction of high-dose treatment (HDT) with autologous HSCT has led to a significantly longer event-free and overall survival, and to a better quality of life when compared to standard-dose therapy (SDT).

The optimal time of the application of HDT in MM patients, i.e., early in the course of the disease versus at relapse following conventional chemotherapy, is still controversial. Fermand et al. compared, in a randomized fashion, the outcome of the disease in two groups of relatively young (<56 years) patients; 91 patients received HDT and autologous HSCT after a short induction treatment (early transplant) and 94 patients received HDT and HDT and autologous HSCT as rescue procedure (i.e., in case of primary resistance to conventional chemotherapy or at relapse; late transplant) [87]. With a median follow-up of 58 months, the overall survival was identical (64.6 months vs. 64 months) in the two groups. In 1993, three North American cooperative groups launched a prospective randomized trial (S9321) comparing HDT (melphalan 140 mg/m^2 plus total-body irradiation 12 Gy) with SDT using the vincristine, carmustine, melphalan, cyclophosphamide, and prednisone (VBMCP) regimen. Responders on both arms ($\geq$75%) were randomly assigned to interferon (IFN) or no maintenance treatment. After induction therapy with four cycles of vincristine, adriamycin, and dexamethasone (VAD), patients were

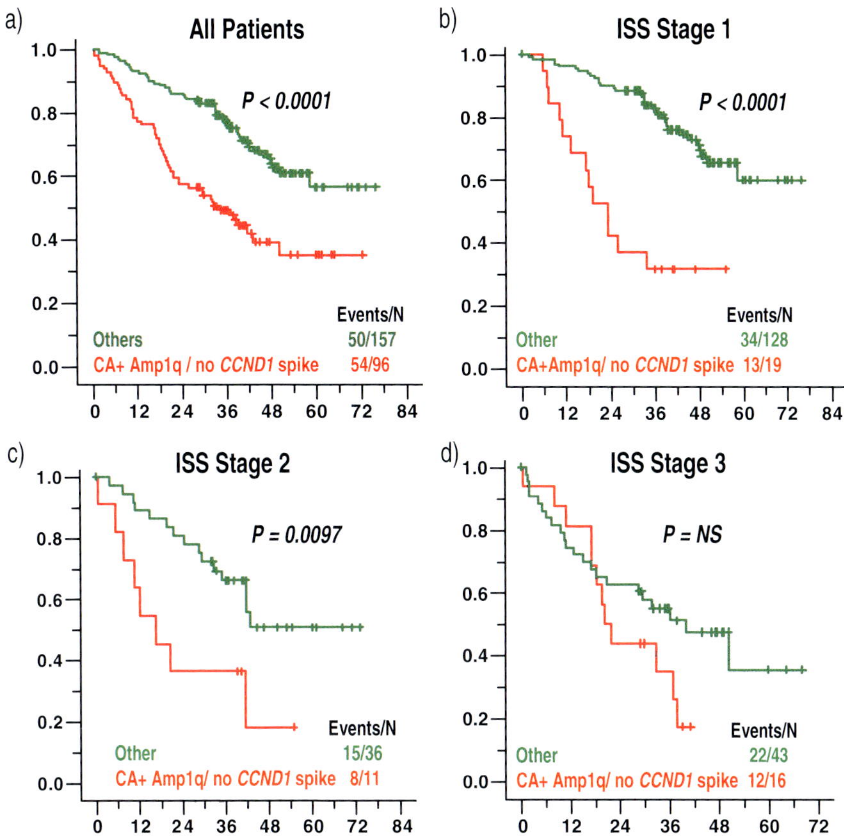

Fig. 14.1 In a subgroup of 253/351 patients FISH analysis for amplification of 1q21 was performed. An inferior event-free survival was observed in patients with CA and amplification of 1q21 in the overall group and in ISS stages 1 and 2. Patients with *CCND1* spikes were grouped with those lacking CA or amplification of 1q21 or both

randomly assigned to either HDT with melphalan plus TBI or to SDT with VBMCP for 1 year; all patients received high-dose cyclophosphamide, and except for allogeneic HSCT candidates, proceeded with peripheral blood stem cell collection. Patients were stratified according to Durie-Salmon stage, β2-microglobulin serum level, and response to VAD induction. Responding patients ($\geq$75% M-protein reduction) were randomly assigned to 4 years of maintenance therapy with interferon versus observation. Patients treated on the VBMCP arm were offered the option of salvage autologous HSCT at the time of disease progression or relapse. In the VBMCP arm, 87 of 157 patients with follow-up after relapse received a salvage autotransplant, resulting in a median survival time of 30 months (Fig. 14.2); this was slightly higher than the survival time of 23 months noted among the remaining patients receiving nontransplantation based salvage therapies (p = 0.13) [34].

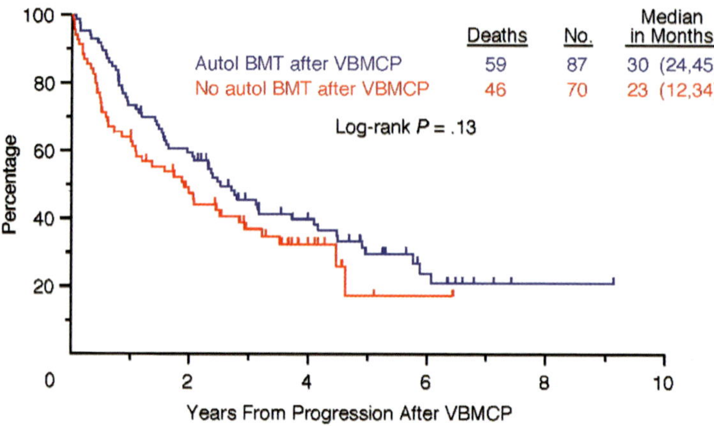

Fig. 14.2 Overall survival according to salvage therapy

Patients with primary refractory, progressive disease, or not achieving 50% monoclonal protein reduction with the initial standard-dose regimen respond differently to HDT than patients who relapse either while on conventional chemotherapy or after discontinuation of such treatment (see above). Vesole et al. reported the effect of HDT on 135 patients with refractory myeloma [88]. Either melphalan 100 mg/m^2 (47 patients), TBI with melphalan, or thiotepa (21 patients), melphalan 200 mg/m^2 $\times$ 1 (25 patients) and melphalan 200 mg/m^2 $\times$ 2 (45 patients) were applied as preparative regimens. When compared to historic controls, even among patients with resistant relapse and high β2-microglobulin levels, more intensive treatment resulted in superior event-free and overall survival durations. Primary refractory patients treated with TBI experienced significantly longer event-free and overall survival durations (32 and 66 months, respectively) than those with resistant relapse (4 and 7 months, respectively; $p = 0.007$, 0.007, respectively). Similar results were observed in melphalan 200 mg/m^2 recipients. Primary refractory patients experienced longer event-free and overall survival durations (4 and 7 months, respectively) than those with resistant relapse (17 and 21 months, respectively; $p = 0.006$, 0.01, respectively). In a subset analysis reported by the University of Arkansas, primary refractory status was also associated to superior event-free survival (23 months vs. 14 months; $p = 0.002$) and overall survival (39 months vs. 25 months; $p = 0.08$) compared to patients with resistant relapse [21]. The effectiveness of HDT in refractory MM (relapsed and primary refractory) was also evident in an Intergroup trial [89]. On an intent-to-treat basis from transplant registration, the median progression-free survival and overall survival duration in a group of 66 patients with refractory myeloma to alkylating agents, dexamethasone, or VAD was 11 and 19 months, respectively. Rajkumar et al. reported on 75 patients who received transplantation for relapsed or primary refractory myeloma; the OS for conventionally treated patients, relapsed myeloma after conventional therapy, and primary refractory individuals, differed significantly with median survivals of 12, 21 and 30 months, respectively [90]. Plasma cell labeling index was significantly lower in patients with primary refractory disease when compared with relapsed cases, suggesting that the low proliferative activity of the disease in the former group might partly explain the resistance to conventional chemotherapy. In contrast to the experience in other B-cell malignancies, primary refractory status does not negatively affect the anti-myeloma effect of HDT with autologous HSCT.

Pineda et al. recently reported on the effect of high dose melphalan-based autotransplant for multiple myeloma [91]. A total of 1064 previously treated patients enrolled on different HDT protocols was examined. Trials included, for previously treated patients, induction with DT-PACE (dexamethasone, thalidomide, cisplatin, adriamycin, cyclophosphamide, and etoposide) followed by intended tandem transplants either with MEL200 (melphalan 200 mg/m^2), or MEL140 (melphalan 140 mg/m^2) in case of renal insufficiency with creatinine greater than 3 mg/dL or advanced age greater than 70 years [92]. Others received a MEL-DT-PACE hybrid regimen (MEL140 plus DT-PACE). In case partial response (PR) was not achieved after the first transplant, second transplant regimens used MEL140 plus either TBI or high-dose cyclophosphamide or the BEAM regimen [carmustine (BCNU), etoposide, arabinosyl cytosine, melphalan] [93]. Myeloma responses were reported according to the Blade criteria. Median follow-up was 38 months (range 0.6–201). The Kaplan-Meier method was applied to estimate event-free and overall survival, and comparisons between different arms were made using the log-rank test (Fig. 14.3). Event-free survival (median = 24 months) and overall survival (median = 44 months) were measured from the first day of melphalan administration until disease recurrence or

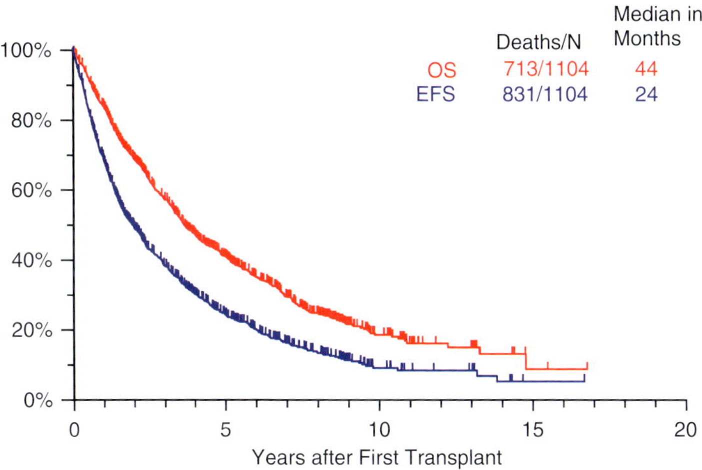

Fig. 14.3 This figure depicts Kaplan-Meier plots of the durations of OS and EFS

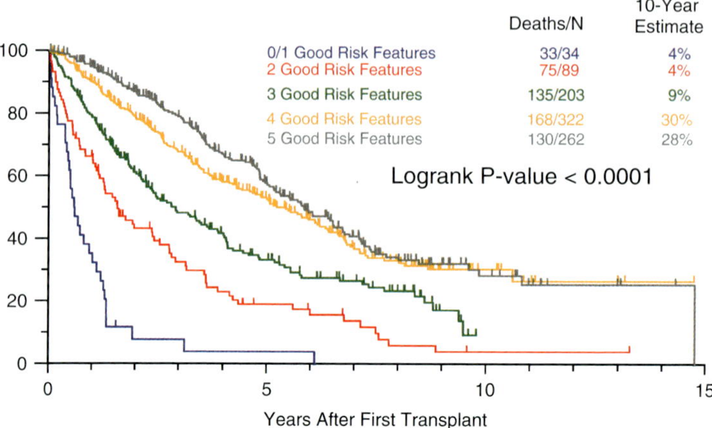

Fig. 14.4 Kaplan-Meier plots of overall survival (OS) according to the number of favorable prognostic factors. Five good-risk features include no cytogenetic abnormality (CA) 13/hypodiploidy, Beta-2-microglobulin <3 mg/L, albumin greater than or equal to 3 g/dL, platelet count greater than or equal to 100,000/(mu/L), and C-reactive protein <6 mg/L

death. Overall survival according to the number of favorable pretransplant parameters for all enrolled patients is shown in Fig. 14.4.

Significant differences were observed between the five subgroups: outcomes worsened progressively as the number of good-risk features declined from 5 to 4 to 3 to 2 to less than 2. Ten-year overall survival was 25% with the best and 2% in the worst constellation of prognostic factors. As most patients eventually relapse after one or two cycles of HDT, it is important to consider the issue of further treatment intensification as salvage approach. Resistance of the malignant clone and subclinical toxicity to vital organs may compromise long-term survival. Mansi et al. were the first to prove "continuing chemosensitivity" by reporting a response rate of 93% and a response duration of 17 months in a group of 29 patients who, after relapsing following a single course of melphalan 140 mg/m^2, were treated with re-induction therapy followed by melphalan 200 mg/m^2 and autologous bone marrow transplant [94]. At the University of Arkansas, the outcome of 196 patients who relapsed after a single or double transplant was evaluated [95]. Patients received standard-dose treatment or a further transplant. Multivariate analysis showed that patients who relapsed late (>1 year) after the previous HDT and had low β2-microglobulin levels at the time of relapse were the best candidates for further autotransplantation. Among a total of 1358 patients receiving two prior autologous transplants (median interval from first to second transplant = 4 months), 98 received a further autologous transplant at relapse. In a search for favorable features associated with post-third autotransplant survival, pretransplant 1, 2 and 3 features, especially the presence of metaphase cytogenetic abnormalities (CA) and standard laboratory features such as, β2-microglobulin, CRP, LDH, albumin, hemoglobin, and creatinine were examined as well as the time interval from second to third transplant and whether a third transplant was applied to rescue Total Therapy 1 or 2 (newly diagnosed) or other patients receiving tandem transplants after more extensive prior treatment [38, 96]. Remarkably, the presence of CA at any of the indicated time points had no impact on survival after a third autologous HSCT, typically with a melphalan 200 mg/m^2 preparative regimen. According to multivariate analysis, the second to third transplant interval (time-dependent covariate analysis) (HR 8.8, $p = 0.002$) and hypo-albuminemia <3.0 g/dL (HR 3.2, $p < 0.0001$) were independently important. Thus, post-third transplant survival was superior among the 41 patients with a post-second transplant event-free survival greater than 3 years and albumin greater than 3.0 gm/dL prior to the third transplant (median overall survival = 21 months; 5-year overall survival = 20%), with an intermediate outcome noted for the 34 patients with one of these favorable features present (median overall survival = 10 months; 3-year overall survival = 20%) while the worst outcome was noted in the 13 patients who were both hypo-albuminemic and had received their 3rd transplant within 3 years of the second transplant (median overall survival = 3 months, no survival beyond 12 months) [97]. Prolonged overall survival with second on-demand autologous transplant in multiple myeloma has been reported by Elice et al. [98]. A total of 130 consecutive multiple myeloma patients were treated with autologous HSCT after conditioning with melphalan 200 mg/m^2 followed by a second autologous HSCT at relapse or disease progression. A total of 107 (82%) patients completed the first autologous HSCT. The best response obtained after autologous HSCT was complete response (CR) in 23%, very good partial response (VGPR) in 28%, partial response (PR) in 42%, and minimal response (MR) in 7%. Median overall and event-free survivals were 65.4 and 27.7 months, respectively. Myeloma relapse or progression was observed in 70 patients; 26 received a second autologous HSCT (with a median time of 20.4 months from first autologous HSCT). A major response (partial remission or better) was obtained in 69% of these patients. Median overall and event-free survival rates after the second autologous HSCT were 38.1 and 14.8 months, respectively. Treatment-related mortality was 1.9% after the first autologous HSCT and no deaths occurred related to the second transplant, confirming that a second autologous HSCT at relapse or progression is a safe and effective strategy. Even in the era where new drugs such as thalidomide, lenalidomide and bortezomib alone or in combination have produced significant responses and may also have a positive effect on survival of myeloma patients, HDT remains a valuable option in the treatment of myeloma patients relapsing after transplantation, especially those with more durable responses after initial transplant(s). After the salvage transplant, a combination of newer drugs with dexamethasone can be applied to increase the response duration.

14.3 Allogeneic Hematopoietic Stem Cell Transplantation in Multiple Myeloma

Though new insights into its biology have identified molecular mechanisms that have become targets of recently developed agents with potent anti-tumor activity, multiple myeloma remains a fatal plasma cell malignancy [99, 100]. High-dose chemotherapy with autologous HSCT, after induction with chemotherapy or newer agents, is regarded as the standard of care for newly diagnosed myeloma patients younger than 65 years [28, 30, 31, 51, 52]. However, relapse is a continuous risk and only a few good-prognosis patients live disease-free for longer than 10 years [31, 51]. Constant recurrence following autologous HSCT is primarily due to their failure to eradicate all myeloma cells. Conversely, allogeneic HSCT remains the only potentially curative treatment for its well documented graft-versus-myeloma effects [101]. Given the high transplant mortality and morbidity related to the high-dose myeloablative preparative regimens used until recently, its application has primarily been limited to younger relapsed/refractory patients [102–104]. These limitations have lately been significantly reduced through reduced-intensity or nonmyeloablative conditioning regimens [105]. The introduction of less intense conditionings has led to at least two important clinical and biological implications: the increase of the eligible age for allogeneic HSCT up to 65–70 years even in medically unfit patients and the shift of the burden of tumor eradication from the chemotherapy of the conditioning to the immune attack of myeloma cells by donor T cells [106, 107]. Though the results of recent trials are promising, the subset of patients who may most benefit from an allograft remains to be defined. The clinical outcomes of myeloablative and reduce-intensity/nonmyeloablative allogeneic HSCT, the biological concepts of graft-versus-myeloma effects, and possible future developments are reported below.

14.3.1 Allografting After Myeloablative Conditioning Regimens

High treatment-related mortality (TRM) has restricted this approach to young, medically fit patients, and even here transplant-related mortality rates are of the order of 30-60% [102–104]. The recent shift from myeloablative, high-dose conditionings to reduced-intensity/nonmyeloablative regimens has further limited its clinical application. Most commonly used myeloablative conditioning regimens (Table 14.1) have included cyclophosphamide with TBI, or busulfan with cyclophosphamide, or melphalan and TBI [34, 102–104, 108–116].

Even though chemotherapy-sensitive disease has almost universally been reported as a prerequisite for higher response rates and post-transplant overall and disease-free survivals, the outcome of most trials of allogeneic HSCT for multiple myeloma has been strongly biased by patient selection and pretransplant characteristics. Comparing results reported in different studies is

Table 14.1 Myeloablative conditioning regimens utilized for allogeneic HSCT in multiple myeloma

Author	Patients	Median age (years)	Donor related/unrelated	Conditioning	Transplant-related mortality, %	Complete remission, %	Overall survival, %
Bensinger et al. [104,108]	136	43–48 (<60)	114/22	Bu, Cy, ±TBI	48 (at day 100), 63 (at 1 year)	34	22 (at 5 years)
Barlogie et al. [34]	36	≤55	36/0	Melphalan (100 mg/m^2), TBI (12 Gy)	53 (at 1 year)	–	39 (at 7 years)
Reece et al. [109]	26	43	22/4	Cy,TBI, Bu,Cy, melphalan (100 mg/m^2), TBI	19 (at day 100)	62	47 (at 3 years)
Alyea et al. [110]	24	46	24/0	Cy,TBI (14 Gy), Bu,Cy	10	–	55 (at 2 years)
Kulkarni et al. [111]	33	38	29/4	Melphalan (110 mg/m^2), TBI (10.5 Gy) Cy, TBI (9.5 Gy), Cy, melphalan, Bu,Cy	54	37	36 (at 3 years)
Le Blanc et al. [112]	37	47	37/0	Cy, TBI (12 Gy), melphalan (140 mg/m^2), TBI (10.5 Gy), Bu,Cy, Others	22	57	32 (at 40 months)
Couban et al. [113]	22	43	22/0	Melphalan (160 mg/m^2), TBI (12 Gy), Cy, TBI (12 Gy), Bu,Cy	59	50	32 (at 3 years)
Varterasian et al. [114]	24	43	–	Cy, TBI, melphalan, TBI, Bu,Cy, TMI, others	25	–	40 (at 3 years)

therefore extremely difficult and not very helpful to establish the curative potential of the procedure. Overall, clinical complete remissions (CCR) have been observed in 20–60% of patients though variable definitions of complete remission have been used [34, 102–104, 108–116]. Widely used criteria for CCR require negative immunofixation of both serum and urine monoclonal paraproteins with no evidence of myeloma cells on bone marrow biopsy and bone marrow aspirate by morphology and flow cytometry [117]. In most trials, approximately 50% of patients with chemotherapy-sensitive disease at the time of transplant have achieved a CCR with a median onset 3 months after transplant. Overall, despite these high rates of CCR, late relapses occur, and in most series, only 10–25% of patients remain disease-free after 10 years and possibly cured. Disease remission, in this subset of patients, is frequently detected by molecular methods. Molecular remissions, as a prelude to tumor eradication and eventual cure, are far more frequent after myeloablative allogeneic HSCT as compared to autologous HSCT and can occur in up to 50% of patients in CCR after allografting [118]. In a subset of patients, these remissions are prolonged, suggesting a complete eradication [119].

The majority of allogeneic HSCT trials have enrolled younger patients, usually in their fifth decade. Despite this, the reported early TRM ranges from 20% to 50% [34, 102–104, 108–116]. Causes of death are primarily regimen-related, graft-versus-host-disease (GvHD) and its treatment-related opportunistic infections. Overall, the reason of the high TRM observed in multiple myeloma rather than other hematological malignancies remains unknown. Possible explanations include myeloma effects on baseline organ functions and, importantly, a profound immunodeficiency predisposing to organ toxicities and opportunistic infections. Interestingly, the largest multicenter analysis by EBMT registry clearly suggested that survival improved in the late 1990s given a remarkable reduction in TRM through better supportive care and patient selection criteria [120]. In this retrospective study on 690 patients undergoing myeloablative allogeneic HSCT, patients who received a bone marrow allograft between 1983 and 1993 were compared to those transplanted between 1994 and 1998. In this latter cohort, a subset of patients also received granulocyte-colony-stimulating factor (G-CSF) mobilized peripheral blood stem cells (PBSC). TRM at 6 and 24 months was significantly lower in patients transplanted between 1994 and 1998 than between 1983 and 1993 (21% vs. 38% and 30% vs. 46%, respectively). However, the median age at transplant was only 44 years (range 18–57), whereas the median age of myeloma patients at diagnosis is approximately 65 years. The reduced toxicity was associated with better clinical outcome, and median overall and progression-free survivals at 3 years increased from 35% to 55% and from 7 to 19 months for patients transplanted between 1983–1993 and 1994–1998, respectively. No differences in outcomes were reported between patients who received marrow and those who received PBSC, though a slightly higher incidence of chronic GvHD was observed with the use of PBSC. More recently, Barlogie et al. reported on the randomized US Intergroup Trial S9321 [34]. Initially, the study design included myeloablative allografting for patients younger than 55 years with a suitable sibling donor. This arm was prematurely closed because of 53% TRM. However, 22% of the patients enrolled remain alive and progression-free at 7 years. Importantly, the authors show that both overall and event-free survival curves remain flat with follow-up extending to 10 years, consistent with a cured subgroup of patients.

The largest single-center experience so far reported is from the Seattle group [104, 108]. In total, 136 patients, all younger than 60 years (median ages, 43–48 years), underwent myeloablative allogeneic HSCT between 1987 and 1999 from related (84%) and unrelated donors (16%). Most patients were heavily pretreated, beyond first response, or with chemotherapy-resistant disease, and only 21% had chemotherapy-sensitive disease. Most patients received a combination of busulfan and cyclophosphamide with or without TBI. The study reported a currently unacceptable day-100 TRM of 48%. An additional 15% of patients died of transplant-related causes at 1 year, most commonly due to GvHD and infections. Overall, the 5-year survival was 22% with disease-free survival of 14%. However, in 34% of patients who achieved post-transplant CCR, overall and disease-free survivals at 5 years were 48% and 37%, respectively. Importantly, subgroup analyses showed that early TRM was lower, approximately 20%, for patients with responsive disease who were transplanted within 1 year from diagnosis.

No prospective randomized trials have compared allografting after myeloablative conditioning regimen with autografting. A retrospective case-matched analysis of 189 patients who underwent myeloablative allogeneic HSCT and 189 who were treated with autologous HSCT before 1995 and reported to the EBMT registry showed superior clinical outcomes with autografting [121]. A more recent single-center retrospective comparison of autologous HSCT versus allogeneic HSCT from HLA-identical siblings or unrelated donors has been reported [122]. One-hundred-fifty-eight patients younger than 55 years were transplanted through the Leukemia/Bone Marrow Transplantation Program of British Columbia between 1989 and 2002. Seventy-two patients received an allograft after myeloablative conditioning, 58 from a sibling donor and 14 from an unrelated donor, whereas 86 received an autograft. After a median follow up of 88 months, 61 patients of the entire series were alive. Twenty-eight patients were alive following allogeneic HSCT after a median follow-up of 102 months and 33 following autologous HSCT after a follow-up of 87 months. Twenty-one (75%) out of the 28 patients who received an allograft remained in continuous remission. However, no statistically significant differences were observed in either overall or event-free survivals between the two groups. Interestingly, neither acute nor chronic GvHD had an impact on overall or event-free survival. As the authors state, the lack of formal inclusion criteria led to inevitable selection bias. Patients with younger age and chemo-resistant disease were more likely to be offered allogeneic HSCT. Other confounding factors were different initial therapeutic strategies, conditioning regimens, prognostic factors, and comorbidities.

Overall, in the light of the current available data, it is important to point out that the retrospective nature and the heterogeneous inclusion criteria and treatment strategies of most studies inevitably reflect a substantial selection bias that reduces the statistical power and prevents researchers from determining the real role of myeloablative allogeneic HSCT in multiple myeloma. However, published reports almost unanimously conclude that better outcome is associated with chemo-sensitive disease at transplant and, importantly, that allografting at an earlier disease phase is associated with better clinical outcomes. Altogether, clinical trials also support the concept that, though long-term cure is possible in a subset of patients, allogeneic HSCT has so far benefited a minority of younger patients with matched sibling donors.

Acute and chronic GvHD (reviewed in Chap. 11 by Korngold and Antin and Chap. 12 by Martin and Pavletic, respectively) have been the most challenging transplant-related complications, occurring in up to 60% of T-replete allografts. The incidence of GvHD may further increase with patient age, with the use of unrelated or mismatched donors, and with female donors, especially if multiparous [123]. Though GvHD has also been associated with decreased risk of disease relapse [108], no recent changes in its treatment have yet translated into significant survival advantages. Most early clinical trials on myeloablative allografting included bone marrow grafts. G-CSF mobilized PBSC have recently been increasingly utilized as a source of stem cells, especially in patients with HLA-identical sibling donors. The biological differences of the graft composition may have an important clinical impact. In PBSC grafts, the content of T cells is significantly higher as well as their polarization toward a Th-2 cell phenotype more typically observed during active chronic GvHD. The EBMT analysis reported a trend toward higher chronic GvHD in PBSC recipients; however, the short follow-up did not allow researchers to draw conclusions on the ultimate impact on clinical outcome of the use of PBSC [120]. Though no higher incidence and severity of acute GvHD have been reported, it is still controversial if the use of PBSC is correlated with a higher incidence of extensive GvHD that may affect quality of life and clinical outcomes [124–126]. Currently, prospective randomized studies comparing bone marrow versus PBSC grafts in hematological malignancies are in progress.

Many laboratory parameters have been used to predict prognosis in myeloma patients undergoing allogeneic HSCT. Low albumin and high β2-microglobulin have been associated with worse clinical outcome after allografting [108, 120]. Newer biological parameters have recently been more helpful to categorize patients. Chromosome 13 deletion [del(13)], detected by standard cytogenetics or FISH, has been the genetic abnormality most commonly associated with worse prognosis in several studies [70, 127, 128]. However, a recent more comprehensive analysis failed to define del(13) as an independent prognostic factor. In fact, its prognostic significance appeared to be associated with the presence of other abnormalities such as t(4;14) and del(17p) [129]. In the near future, advanced technologies such as gene-expression profiling may allow researchers to correlate the genetic constitution and the biological behavior of the disease and determine how these factors influence prognosis [83, 84, 130]. However, these molecular technologies are not readily available at most institutions, and their translational role in clinical practice remains to be determined in future years.

14.3.2 Allografting After Nonmyeloablative/Reduced Intensity Conditioning Regimens

The association of allografting with long-term disease-free survival in a subset of patients suggested that graft-versus-myeloma effects may have potentially been curative for myeloma. This observation led to the exploration of less intense, highly immunosuppressive, though less myelosuppressive, conditioning regimens, aimed at establishing stable donor engraftment while drastically reducing organ toxicity. One of the most widely used conditionings was developed by the Seattle group based upon preclinical studies on the dog model, which showed that donor engraftment could be obtained after a nonmyeloablative regimen consisting of low dose of TBI of 200 cGy coupled with potent post-transplant immunosuppression with cyclosporine and mycophenolic acid (mycophenolate mofetil) [131]. This strategy was soon translated into clinical studies. However, in the first 18 myeloma patients treated with this approach, two rejections of the donor cells were observed, and only transient CCR and partial remission were achieved in two and three patients, respectively [132]. These results indicated that it would be imperative to explore the effects of more effective cytoreduction before nonmyeloablative allogeneic HSCT to improve responses. A new treatment modality, especially for newly diagnosed patients who had not been heavily pretreated, involved an autologous HSCT followed, 2–4 months later, by a TBI-based nonmyeloablative allogeneic HSCT [107]. As compared to myeloablative conditioning, designed to produce simultaneous cytoreduction and adequate immunosuppression to establish stable donor engraftment, the tandem autologous-allogeneic approach allows researchers to separate in time the high-dose cytoreduction and the graft-versus-myeloma effect with the potential of reducing treatment-related toxicity. The first multicenter experience with this approach included 54 stage II–III patients, median age 52 years (range 27–71), half of them with refractory or relapsed myeloma [107]. Fifty-two patients completed the tandem autologous-allogeneic HSCT procedure. CCR was reported in 57%, and overall TRM was 22%. Overall chronic GvHD developed in 60%. After a median follow-up of 60 months, overall and progression free survivals were 69% and 38%, respectively.

Overall, in recent years, a number of reduced-intensity regimens (Table 14.2) have been introduced into phase II clinical trials including intermediate-dose melphalan (100–140 mg/m^2), with or without fludarabine, 200 cGy TBI 200 alone or with fludarabine, and intermediate-dose busulfan [133–141].

Table 14.2 Nonmyeloablative and reduced intensity conditioning regimens utilized for allogeneic HSCT in multiple myeloma

Author	Patients	Donor related/ unrelated	Conditioning	Transplant-related mortality, %	Chronic GVHD, %	Complete remission, %	Overall survival, %
Mohty et al. [133]	41	41/0	Bu, Fluda, ATG	17	41	24	62 (at 2 years)
Peggs et al. [134]	20	12/8	TBI, Fluda, alemtuzumab	15	–	10	71 (at 2 years)
Einsele et al. [135]	22	7/15	TBI (2 Gy), Fluda, Cy	23	32	27	26 (at 2 years)
Giralt et al. [136]	22	11/9	Fluda, melphalan (90/ 140 mg/m^2)	41	27	32	30 (at 2 years)
Gerull et al. [137]	52	32/20	TBI (2 Gy), Fluda	17	70	27	41 (at 1.5 years)
Bruno et al. [138]	22	0/22	TBI (2 Gy), Fluda	18	61	20	79 (at 2 year)
Maloney et al. [107]	54	52/0	TBI (2 Gy)/(2 Gy)TBI, Fluda	22	60	57	69 (at 5 years)
Lee et al. [139]	45	33/12	Melphalan (100 mg/m^2), TBI (2 Gy), Fluda	38	13	64	36 (at 3 years)
Kroger et al. [106]	17	9/8	Melphalan (100 mg/m^2), Flu, ATG	18	7	73	74 (at 2 years)
Kroger et al. [140]	21	0/21	Melphalan (100–140 mg/ m^2), Flu, ATG	24	12	40	74 (at 2 years)
Galimberti et al. [141]	20	20/0	TBI (2 Gy), Fluda /Cy, Fluda	20	30	35	58 (at 2 years)

Anti-thymocyte globulin or the anti-CD52 antibody alemtuzumab have also been included in some studies to reduce GvHD [134, 140]. Even though there is no consensus on which regimen is superior in terms of toxicity and efficacy, a planned autologous HSCT followed by a nonmyeloablative or reduced-intensity allogeneic HSCT with G-CSF mobilized PBSC to reduce the risk of graft rejection and, possibly, determine higher graft-versus-myeloma effects appears to be the most widely used approach [106, 107].

Recently, an EBMT study has retrospectively compared the clinical outcomes of allogeneic HSCT after either reduced-intensity or myeloablative conditioning regimens in patients transplanted between 1998 and 2002 [142]. One-hundred-ninety-six patients conditioned with myeloablative regimens were compared with 321 patients conditioned with nonmyeloablative or reduced-intensity regimens between 1998 and 2002. Though TRM was significantly lower in the reduced-intensity group (24% vs. 37% at 2 years, $p = 0.002$), no statistical differences in overall and progression-free survivals were observed between the two groups by multivariate analysis. This finding was due to significantly higher relapse rate in the reduced-intensity group ($p = 0.0001$). The use of less intense regimens can indeed come at the cost of higher relapse rates; however, the conclusions of this study should be considered with some caution as many selection biases are evident between the two cohorts of patients. In the reduced-intensity group, there was a remarkably higher number of patients who failed one or more autologous transplants, more patients with refractory disease, more T-cell depleted allografts, and higher use of unrelated donors.

The concept of "Mendelian or genetic randomization" has recently been applied to assess clinical outcomes between patients with hematological malignancies treated with allografting or other therapies [143–146]. Though not universally accepted, this method relies on the biological process, described by Mendel, through which offspring randomly inherit genetic traits half from the mother and half from the father. One in four siblings is then expected to have a potential HLA-identical sibling donor. The comparison by the intention-to-treat principle between patients with HLA-identical siblings who can be assigned to allografting and those without, who cannot receive an allograft, is used as a surrogate for an unbiased randomization. Only a formal statistical randomization, however, between patients with suitable donors could provide stronger evidence. A French study initially compared two protocols that enrolled high risk myeloma patients in the light of elevated serum $\beta 2$-microglobulin and del(13) [147]. All patients underwent a first autologous transplant after high dose melphalan at 200 mg/m^2. Sixty-five patients with HLA-identical sibling donors received an allograft after a reduced intensity conditioning with busulfan, fludarabine, and high-dose anti-thymocyte globulin at 12.5 mg/kg. These patients were compared with 219 patients without a suitable sibling donor who were treated with a second autograft after melphalan at 220 mg/m^2. TRM and response rates were not statistically different. After a median follow-up of 2 years, overall and event free survivals were 35% and 25%, and 41% and 30% for the double autologous and the autologous-allogeneic groups, respectively. These findings may indicate that patients with poor prognostic factors such as del(13) and high $\beta 2$-microglobulin may not benefit from reduced-intensity allogeneic HSCT. Though a remarkably low 7% incidence of chronic GvHD was reported, the high dose of anti-thymocyte globulin is a matter of concern as it may have highly prevented a strong graft-versus-myeloma effect. However, another report by Kroger et al. showed that del(13) was an independent, poor-risk factor for overall and progression-free survival after reduced-intensity allogeneic HSCT, given a higher risk of relapse [148]. A recent study reported on 245 consecutive myeloma patients, up to the age of 65 years, who were newly diagnosed between 1998 and 2004. One-hundred-sixty-two of 199 patients with at least one sibling were HLA-typed with their potential sibling donors. All patients received induction with two to three cycles of VAD-based regimens, cyclophosphamide, and G-CSF for PBSC mobilization followed by autologous HSCT after melphalan at 200 mg/m^2 [149]. Eighty patients with an HLA-identical sibling were offered TBI-based nonmyeloablative conditioning followed by allogeneic HSCT with G-CSF mobilized PBSC, whereas 82 patients without an HLA-identical sibling were assigned to receive a second autologous transplant after high-dose (140–200 mg/m^2) or intermediate-dose (100 mg/m^2) melphalan-based conditioning regimens. The new feature of this study was the assignment of treatment in function of a single criterion: presence/absence of an HLA-identical sibling donor, regardless of disease stage and prognostic factors. By intent-to-treat analysis, after a median follow up of 45 months, overall and event-free survivals were significantly longer in patients with donors: 80 months vs. 54 months ($p = 0.01$) and 35 months vs. 29 months ($p = 0.02$), respectively. By multivariate analysis, the presence of HLA-identical siblings was an independent variable significantly associated with longer overall and event-free survivals. Fifty-eight and 46 patients completed the tandem autologous-allogeneic and the tandem autologous HSCT programs, respectively. CCR rates were 55% and 26% with the tandem autologous-allogeneic and the tandem autologous ($p = 0.004$), whereas TRM was 10% and 2%, respectively (p = nonsignificant). Median overall survival was not reached in the tandem autologous-allogeneic group and was 58 months in the tandem autologous group ($p = 0.03$). Event-free survival was 43 and 33 months, respectively ($p = 0.07$). Given that cytogenetic information was available in only a third of the patients registered in the study, the impact of del(13) after the tandem autologous-allogeneic HSCT approach could not be determined. However, though exploratory with low statistical power, a stratified analysis on the intent-to-treat population that defined high risk patients in the light of high $\beta 2$-microglobulin levels or del(13) reported adjusted hazard ratios of 0.34 and 0.52 for overall and event-free survivals, respectively, similar to those obtained in the whole series. This finding suggests that patients with an HLA-identical sibling have better overall and event-free survivals as compared to those without an HLA-identical sibling.

Large prospective studies, based on the Mendelian randomization principle, such as the BMT-CTN-0102 trial in the USA and the Dutch-Belgian Hemato-Oncology Cooperative Group (HOVON) trial in Europe are currently in progress and will offer helpful information to determine the role of the tandem autologous-allogeneic HSCT approach using a TBI-based nonmyeloablative conditioning regimen in the next few years. An extended phase II trial of 106 newly diagnosed myeloma patients transplanted with the Seattle regimen was recently presented by the Italian Group for Bone Marrow Transplantation (GITMO) [150]. After a median follow-up of 54 months, overall survival was not reached and event-free survival was 35 months. Overall response, defined as combined CCR and partial remission, was 91% with 53 patients achieving CCR after allografting. Response prior to allogeneic HSCT was significantly associated with the achievement of post-transplant CCR and longer event-free survival. Interestingly, chronic GvHD was not correlated with either the achievement of CCR or response duration.

14.3.3 Graft-Versus-Myeloma Effects and Graft-Versus-Host Disease

The unique and potentially eradicating effect of allografting relies on the immune attack of donor T cells against disease-specific antigens capable of inducing a potent graft-versus-myeloma effect. Initial evidence for the existence of such an effect was the transfer of myeloma idiotype-specific immunity from an actively immunized marrow donor to the recipient [151]. Anecdotal observations of complete responses after the infusion of donor lymphocytes or withdrawal of immunosuppression in patients with persistent or relapsed disease after allografting were further evidence [152–155]. Subsequent larger studies showed that, though donor lymphocyte infusions (DLI) could induce response rates up to 50%, durable complete responses were, however, achieved in only a minority of patients [101, 156, 157]. Furthermore, this cell therapy was often associated with clinical GvHD. Lokhorst et al. reported on 27 relapsed patients who received 52 DLI at a median of 30 months after allogeneic HSCT [158, 159]. Debulking therapy was administered to 13 patients before DLI. Overall 14 patients (52%) responded, including six (22%) who achieved CCR. Major toxicity was acute and chronic GvHD present in 55% and 26% of patients respectively. Median overall survival was 18 months, 11 for patients who did not respond and not yet reached for responding patients. Other studies reported that the strongest predictors for response following DLI were acute and chronic GvHD [160, 161]. The authors concluded that both GvHD and graft-versus-myeloma shared the same antigenic targets.

GvHD and its treatment-related complications have always been a matter of concern for clinicians. Moreover, chronic GvHD can highly affect the patient's quality of life. GvHD can indeed be almost completely eliminated by T-cell depletion of the donor graft. However, this manipulation has invariably been associated with higher risk of relapse of the underlying hematological malignancies [162]. Though the experience is limited in myeloma, partial T-cell depletion to allow donor engraftment and limit the risk of GvHD has also been investigated. Alyea et al. used a myeloablative conditioning regimen followed by a CD6-depleted donor bone marrow graft. Selected CD4$^+$-donor lymphocytes were infused later to evoke graft-versus-myeloma effect [110]. The incidence of grade II–III GvHD was 21%, and TRM was 10%. Only one patient achieved a CCR at 6 months without the addition of donor lymphocytes. Fourteen out of 24 patients received donor lymphocytes and response was observed in 10 patients, with seven developing acute or chronic GvHD. Two-year overall and progression-free survivals were 55% and 42%, respectively. Importantly, donor lymphocytes could not be given as scheduled to 42% of patients, either as a result of GvHD or other transplant-related complications. The use of alemtuzumab (a.k.a. Campath), a monoclonal anti-CD52 antibody, has also been explored to reduce the incidence of GvHD, either by treatment "in the bag" or by systemic infusion prior to the conditioning regimen [134, 163]. Though the incidence of GvHD was significantly reduced, the use of alemtuzumab clearly affected disease responses and their duration [134]. All these observations clearly indicate the important role of donor T cells in providing efficient graft-versus-myeloma activity. Lokhorst et al. recently reported on a prospective phase III study by the HOVON group [164, 165]. Fifty-three patients with an HLA-identical sibling underwent a partially T-cell-depleted allograft as part of their initial treatment plan. The overall response was 89%, including 19% CCR. After a median follow-up of 38 months post-transplant, 20 patients were alive and 33 dead, 14 from progressive disease and 18 from TRM. Median overall and progression-free survivals after allografting were 17 and 25 months respectively. Only three patients were in continuous CCR. This prospective multi-center study did not support the use of T-cell-depleted myeloablative allogeneic HSCT in myeloma. The strategy of pre-emptive DLI after partially T-cell depleted allografting has also been evaluated. Levenga et al. reported on 24 myeloma patients treated with a partially T-cell-depleted myeloablative allogeneic HSCT [166]. Patients enrolled in the study were intended to receive subsequent pre-emptive DLI. Twenty of 24 patients responded with 10 patients (42%) reaching complete remission. One-year TRM was 29%. Overall, 13 patients (54%) received pre-emptive lymphocyte infusions. GvHD higher than grade I following the infusion developed in four (30%). After a median follow-up of 67 months, 11 patients (46%) were alive, seven of whom (29%) in continuous CCR including four in molecular remission. All these patients had received pre-emptive lymphocytes.

Though GvHD was associated with disease response in the majority of clinical trials, it is encouraging that more recent studies employing nonmyeloablative conditionings did not correlate disease response and its duration with the development of chronic GvHD [149, 150]. In a recent evaluation of 106 patients enrolled in a prospective phase II study, the development of both acute or chronic GvHD was not significantly associated with either the achievement of complete remission or its duration post transplant [150]. This is consistent with the notion that GvHD may not be essential for graft-versus-myeloma, though the relationship between the two phenomena appeared strong in studies employing myeloablative conditioning. New methods to augment graft-versus-myeloma effects to allow long-term disease control and possibly decrease toxicity are presented below.

14.4 Future Developments

Tandem autologous-allogeneic HSCT approaches are currently widely used in clinical trials. The rationale of the tandem approach is to separate temporally the high-dose chemotherapy from allografting, to combine the benefits of autologous HSCT (higher disease response and prolonged survival compared to conventional chemotherapy) and allogeneic HSCT (graft-versus-myeloma effects) while reducing transplant-related toxicities. Drastic reduction in early TRM and CCR rates of over 50% including molecular remissions have been reported. However, the risk of relapse is not negligible. New methods to augment graft-versus-myeloma effects should be explored to allow better long-term disease control. For this purpose, allogeneic HSCT and new drugs with molecular targets, such as thalidomide, lenalidomide, and bortezomib, should not be viewed as mutually exclusive. Bortezomib and thalidomide re-induce responses in relapsed patients following allografting and may also be employed to achieve profound cytoreduction and reduce myeloma to a minimal residual state before allografts [167–170]. Thus, it is imperative to thoroughly explore their roles in increasing the efficacy of tandem autologous-allogeneic HSCT. Major improvements will also lie in the separation of the potentially eradicating graft-versus-myeloma effects from the detrimental GvHD. New insights into the pathophysiology of acute GvHD have led to the development of conditioning regimens with total-lymphoid irradiation that reduce its incidence but appear to preserve the anti-tumor effects of donor T cells [171]. Furthermore, the identification of disease-specific antigens may trigger more potent myeloma-specific immune responses of donor cytotoxic T cells [172]. The recurrent observation that allografting at an earlier phase of the disease is associated with more effective GVM may also be related to an expression profile of potential antigenic targets for T cells that varies through the various disease phases. Siegel et al. recently identified HLA-A*0201-presented T cell epitopes derived from the oncofetal antigen-immature laminin receptor protein in hematological cancers, which include myeloma [173]. However, the expression of these antigens on myeloma cells is lost when the disease is advanced. In conclusion, the therapeutic role of allogeneic HSCT will ultimately be determined in control studies where patients are allocated treatment in the light of prognostic factors and groups are confronted in a randomized fashion.

References

1. Drach J, Angerler J, Schuster J, et al. Interphase fluorescence in situ hybridization identifies chromosomal abnormalities in plasma cells from patients with monoclonal gammopathy of undetermined significance. Blood 1995;86:3915.
2. Zandecki M, Obein V, Bernardi F, et al. Monoclonal gammopathy of undetermined significance: chromosome changes are a common finding within bone marrow plasma cells. Br J Haematol. 1995;90:693.
3. Latreille J, Barlogie B, Johnston D, et al. Ploidy and proliferative characteristics in monoclonal gammopathies. Blood 1982;59:43.
4. Klein B, Zhang XG, Lu ZY, et al. Interleukin-6 in human multiple myeloma. Blood 1995;85:863.
5. Tinhofer I, Marschitz I, Henn T, et al. Expression of functional interleukin-15 receptor and autocrine production of interleukin-15 as mechanisms of tumor propagation in multiple myeloma. Blood 2000;95:610.
6. Ge NL, Rudikoff S. Insulin-like growth factor I is a dual effector of multiple myeloma cell growth. Blood 2000;96:2856.
7. Jundt F, Probsting K, Anagnostopoulos I, et al. Jagged 1-Notch signaling drives proliferation of multiple myeloma cells. Blood 2004;103:3511.
8. Nefedova Y, Cheng P, Alsina M, et al. Involvement of Notch-1 signaling in bone marrow stroma-mediated de novo drug resistance of myeloma and other malignant lymphoid cell lines. Blood 2004;103:3503.
9. Rebollo A, Martinez AC. Ras proteins: recent advances and new functions. Blood 1999;94:2971.
10. Pene F, Claessens YE, Muller O, et al. Role of the phosphatidylinositol 3-kinase/Akt and mTOR/P70S6-kinase pathways in the proliferation and apoptosis in multiple myeloma. Oncogene 2002;21:6587.
11. Wang CY, Mayo MW, Korneluk RG, et al. NF-kappaB antiapoptosis: Induction of TRAF1 and TRAF2 and c-IAP1 and c-IAP2 to suppress caspase-8 activation. Science 1998;281:1680.
12. Damiano JS, Cress AE, Hazlehurst LA, et al. Cell adhesion mediated drug resistance (CAM-DR): role of integrins and resistance to apoptosis in human myeloma cell lines. Blood 1999;93:1658.
13. Bakkus MH, Van Riet I, De Greef C, et al. The clonogenic precursor cell in multiple myeloma. Leuk Lymphoma. 1995;18:221.
14. Vescio RA, Cao J, Hong CH, et al. Myeloma Ig heavy chain V region sequences reveal prior antigenic selection and marked somatic mutation but no intraclonal diversity. J Immunol. 1995;155:2487.
15. Matsui W, Huff CA, Wang Q, et al. Characterization of clonogenic multiple myeloma cells. Blood 2004;103(6):2332–6.
16. Kukreja A, Hutchinson A, Dhodapkar K, et al. Enhancement of clonogenicity of human multiple myeloma by dendritic cells. J Exp Med. 2006;203(8):1859–65.
17. Peacock CD, Wang Q, Gesell GS, et al. Hedgehog signaling maintains a tumor stem cell compartment in multiple myeloma. Proc Natl Acad Sci USA. 2007;104(10):4048–53.
18. McElwain TJ, Powles RL. High-dose intravenous melphalan for plasma-cell leukaemia and myeloma. Lancet 1983;2:822.
19. Moreau P, Fiere D, Bezwoda WR, et al. Prospective randomized placebo-controlled study of granulocyte-macrophage colony-stimulating factor without stem-cell transplantation after high-dose melphalan in patients with multiple myeloma. J Clin Oncol. 1997;15:660–6.
20. Sirohi B, Kulkarni S, Powles R. Some early phase II trials in previously untreated multiple myeloma: The Royal Marsden experience. Semin Hematol. 2001;38:209–18.
21. Vesole DH, Tricot G, Jagannath S, et al. Autotransplants in multiple myeloma: what have we learned? Blood 1996;88:838.

22. Barlogie B, Hall R, Zander A, et al. High-dose melphalan with autologous bone marrow transplantation for multiple myeloma. Blood 1986;67:1298.
23. Tricot G, Jagannath S, Vesole D, et al. Peripheral blood stem cell transplants for multiple myeloma: identification of favorable variables for rapid engraftment in 225 patients. Blood 1995;85:588–96.
24. Alexanian R, Barlogie B, Tucker S. VAD-based regimens as primary treatment for multiple myeloma. Am J Hematol. 1990;33:86–9.
25. Monconduit M, Menard JF, Michaux JL, et al. VAD or VMBCP in severe multiple myeloma. The Groupe d'Etudes et de Recherche sur le Myélome (GERM). Br J Haematol. 1992;80:199–204.
26. Rajkumar SV, Blood E, Vesole D, et al. Eastern Cooperative Oncology Group. Phase III clinical trial of thalidomide plus dexamethasone compared with dexamethasone alone in newly diagnosed multiple myeloma: a clinical trial coordinated by the Eastern Cooperative Oncology Group. J Clin Oncol. 2006;24:431–6.
27. Mateos MV, Hernández JM, Hernández MT, et al. Bortezomib plus melphalan and prednisone in elderly untreated patients with multiple myeloma: results of a multicenter phase 1/2 study. Blood 2006;108:2165–72.
28. Barlogie B, Tricot GJ, van Rhee F, et al. Long-term outcome results of the first tandem autotransplant trial for multiple myeloma. Br J Haematol. 2006;135:158–64.
29. Barlogie B, Jagannath S, Vesole DH, et al. Superiority of tandem autologous transplantation over standard therapy for previously untreated multiple myeloma. Blood 1997;89:789.
30. Attal M, Harousseau JL, Stoppa AM, et al. A prospective, randomized trial of autologous bone marrow transplantation and chemotherapy in multiple myeloma. Intergroupe Francais du Myelome. N Engl J Med. 1996;335:91–7.
31. Child JA, Morgan GJ, Davies FE, et al. Medical Research Council Adult Leukaemia Working Party. High-dose chemotherapy with hematopoietic stem-cell rescue for multiple myeloma. N Engl J Med. 2003;348:1875–83.
32. Fermand JP, Katsahian S, Divine M, et al. Group Myelome-Autogreffe. High-dose therapy and autologous blood stem-cell transplantation compared with conventional treatment in myeloma patients aged 55 to 65 years: long-term results of a randomized control trial from the Group Myelome-Autogreffe. J Clin Oncol. 2005;23:9227–33.
33. Richardson PG, Sonneveld P, Schuster MW, et al. Assessment of proteasome inhibition for extending remissions (APEX) investigators. Bortezomib or high-dose dexamethasone for relapsed multiple myeloma. N Engl J Med. 2005;352:2487–98.
34. Barlogie B, Kyle RA, Anderson KC, et al. Standard chemotherapy compared with high-dose chemoradiotherapy for multiple myeloma: final results of phase III US Intergroup Trial S9321. J Clin Oncol. 2006;24:929–36.
35. Sirohi B, Powles R, Mehta J, et al. An elective single autograft with high-dose melphalan: single-center study of 451 patients. Bone Marrow Transplant. 2005;36:19–24.
36. Hahn T, Wolff SN, Czuczman M, et al. American Society for Blood and Marrow Transplantation (ASBMT). The role of cytotoxic therapy with hematopoietic stem cell transplantation in the treatment of diffuse large cell B-cell non-Hodgkin's lymphoma. Biol Blood Marrow Transplant. 2003;9:667.
37. Morris TC, Velangi M, Jackson G, et al. Northern Ireland Regional Haematology Group; Northern Regional Haematologists Group; Clinical Trials Committee of The British Scoiety for Blood and Marrow Transplantation. Less than half of patients aged 65 years or under with myeloma proceed to transplantation: results of a two region population-based survey. Br J Haematol. 2005;128:510–2.
38. Barlogie B, Tricot G, Anaissie E, et al. Thalidomide and hematopoietic-cell transplantation for multiple myeloma. N Engl J Med. 2006;354:1021–30.
39. Moreau P, Facon T, Attal M, et al. Comparison of 200 mg/m(2) melphalan and 8 Gy total body irradiation plus 140 mg/m(2) melphalan as conditioning regimens for peripheral blood

stem cell transplantation in patients with newly diagnosed multiple myeloma: final analysis of the Intergroupe Francophone du Myelome 9502 randomized trial. Blood 2002;99:731.
40. Desikan KR, Tricot G, Dhodapkar M, et al. Melphalan plus total body irradiation (MEL-TBI) or cyclophosphamide (MEL-CY) as a conditioning regimen with second autotransplant in responding patients with myeloma is inferior compared to historical controls receiving tandem transplants with melphalan alone. Bone Marrow Transplant. 2000;25:483.
41. Björkstrand B, Svensson H, Ljungmand P, et al. 2522 autotransplants in multiple myeloma: a registry study from the European Group for Blood and Marrow Transplantation (EBMT). Blood 1997; (Abstract no. 1862).
42. Anagnostopoulos A, Aleman A, Ayers G, et al. Comparison of high-dose melphalan with a more intensive regimen of thiotepa, busulfan, and cyclophosphamide for patients with multiple myeloma. Cancer 2004;100:2607–12.
43. Corradini P, Voena C, Astolfi M, et al. High-dose sequential chemoradiotherapy in multiple myeloma: residual tumor cells are detectable in bone marrow and peripheral blood cell harvests and after autografting. Blood 1995;85:1596.
44. Gazitt Y, Tian E, Barlogie B, et al. Differential mobilization of myeloma cells and normal hematopoietic stem cells in multiple myeloma after treatment with cyclophosphamide and granulocyte-macrophage colony-stimulating factor. Blood 1996;87:805.
45. Billadeau D, Quam L, Thomas W, et al. Detection and quantitation of malignant cells in the peripheral blood of multiple myeloma patients. Blood 1992;80:1818.
46. Brenner MK, Rill DR, Moen RC, et al. Gene-marking to trace origin of relapse after autologous bone-marrow transplantation. Lancet 1993;341:85.
47. Deisseroth AB, Zu Z, Claxton D, et al. Genetic marking shows that Ph+ cells present in autologous transplants of chronic myelogenous leukemia (CML) contribute to relapse after autologous bone marrow in CML. Blood 1994;83:3068.
48. Gertz MA, Witzig TE, Pineda AA, et al. Monoclonal plasma cells in the blood stem cell harvest from patients with multiple myeloma are associated with shortened relapse-free survival after transplantation. Bone Marrow Transplant. 1997;19:337.
49. Gahrton G, Svensson H, Björkstrand B, et al. Syngeneic transplantation in multiple myeloma—a case-matched comparison with autologous and allogeneic transplantation. European Group for Blood and Marrow Transplantation. Bone Marrow Transplant. 1999;24:741–5.
50. Vescio R, Schiller G, Stewart AK, et al. Multicenter phase III trial to evaluate CD34(+) selected versus unselected autologous peripheral blood progenitor cell transplantation in multiple myeloma. Blood 1999;93:1858.
51. Attal M, Harousseau JL, Facon T, et al. InterGroupe Francophone du Myélome. Single versus double autologous stem-cell transplantation for multiple myeloma. N Engl J Med. 2003;349:2495–502.
52. Cavo M, Tosi P, Zamagni E, et al. Prospective, randomized study of single compared with double autologous stem-cell transplantation for multiple myeloma: Bologna 96 clinical study. J Clin Oncol. 2007;25:2434–41.
53. Morris C, Iacobelli S, Brand R, et al. Chronic Leukaemia Working Party Myeloma Subcommittee, European Group for Blood and Marrow Transplantation. Benefit and timing of second transplantations in multiple myeloma: clinical findings and methodological limitations in a European Group for Blood and Marrow Transplantation registry study. J Clin Oncol. 2004;22:1674–81.
54. Alexanian R, Dimopoulos MA, Hester J, et al. Early myeloablative therapy for multiple myeloma. Blood 1994;84:4278–82.
55. Greipp PR, Leong T, Bennett JM, et al. Plasmablastic morphology – an independent prognostic factor with clinical and laboratory correlates: Eastern Cooperative Oncology Group (ECOG) myeloma trial E9486 report by the ECOG Myeloma Laboratory Group. Blood 1998;91:2501.

56. Kumar S, Lacy MQ, Dispenzieri A, et al. High-dose therapy and autologous stem cell transplantation for multiple myeloma poorly responsive to initial therapy. Bone Marrow Transplant. 2004;34:161.
57. Morris CL, Siegel E, Barlogie B, et al. Mobilization of CD34+ cells in elderly patients (≥70 years) with multiple myeloma: influence of age, prior therapy, platelet count and mobilization regimen. Br J Haematol. 2003;120:413.
58. Siegel DS, Desikan KR, Mehta J, et al. Age is not a prognostic variable with autotransplants for multiple myeloma. Blood 1999;93:51–4.
59. Reece DE, Bredeson C, Perez WS, et al. Autologous stem cell transplantation in multiple myeloma patients <60 vs ≥60 years of age. Bone Marrow Transplant. 2003;32:1135–43.
60. Jantunen E, Kuittinen T, Penttila K, et al. High-dose melphalan (200 mg/m^2) supported by autologous stem cell transplantation is safe and effective in elderly (≥65 years) myeloma patients: comparison with younger patients treated on the same protocol. Bone Marrow Transplant. 2006;37:917–22.
61. Facon T, Mary J, Harousseau J, et al. Superiority of melphalan-prednisone (MP) + thalidomide (THAL) over MP and autlogous stem cell transplantation in the treatment of newly diagnosed elderly patients with multiple myeloma. J Clin Oncol. 2006;24: (Abstract).
62. Tricot G, Alberts DS, Johnson C, et al. Safety of autotransplants with high-dose melphalan in renal failure: a pharmacokinetic and toxicity study. Clin Cancer Res. 1996;2:947–52.
63. Badros A, Barlogie B, Siegel E, et al. Results of autologous stem cell transplant in multiple myeloma patients with renal failure. Br J Haematol. 2001;114:822–9.
64. Lee CK, Zangari M, Barlogie B, et al. Dialysis-dependent renal failure in patients with myeloma can be reversed by high-dose myeloablative therapy and autotransplant. Bone Marrow Transplant. 2004;33:823–8.
65. Raab MS, Breitkreutz I, Hundemer M, et al. The outcome of autologous stem cell transplantation in patients with plasma cell disorders and dialysis-dependent renal failure. Haematologica 2006;91:1555–8.
66. Knudsen LM, Nielsen B, Gimsing P, et al. Autologous stem cell transplantation in multiple myeloma: outcome in patients with renal failure. Eur J Haematol. 2005;75:27–33.
67. Durie BG, Salmon SE. A clinical staging system for multiple myeloma. Correlation of measured myeloma cell mass with presenting clinical features, response to treatment, and survival. Cancer 1975;36:842–54.
68. Greipp P, San Miguel J, Durie B, et al. International staging system for multiple myeloma. J Clin Oncol. 2005;23:3412.
69. Tricot G, Barlogie B, Jagannath S, et al. Poor prognosis in multiple myeloma is associated only with partial or complete deletions of chromosome 13 or abnormalities involving 11q and not with other karyotype abnormalities. Blood 1995;86:4250.
70. Desikan R, Barlogie B, Sawyer J, et al. Results of high-dose therapy for 1000 patients with multiple myeloma: durable complete remissions and superior survival in the absence of chromosome 13 abnormalities. Blood 2000;95:4008.
71. Tricot G, Barlogie B, Van Rhee F. Treatment advances in multiple myeloma. Br J Haematol. 2004;125:24–30.
72. Fassas AB, Spencer T, Sawyer J, et al. Both hypodiploidy and deletion of chromosome 13 independently confer poor prognosis in multiple myeloma. Br J Haematol. 2002;118:1041.
73. Fonseca R, Blood E, Rue M, et al. Clinical and biologic implications of recurrent genomic aberrations in myeloma. Blood 2003;101:4569.
74. Moreau P, Facon T, Leleu X, et al. Recurrent 14q32 translocations determine the prognosis of multiple myeloma, especially in patients receiving intensive chemotherapy. Blood 2002;100:1579.

75. Hayman SR, Bailey RJ, Jalal SM, et al. Translocations involving the immunoglobulin heavy-chain locus are possible early genetic events in patients with primary systemic amyloidosis. Blood 2001;98:2266.
76. Shaughnessy J Jr, Gabrea A, Qi Y, et al. Cyclin D3 at 6p21 is dysregulated by recurrent chromosomal translocations to immunoglobulin loci in multiple myeloma. Blood 2001;98:217.
77. Cavo M, Terragna C, Renzulli M, et al. Poor outcome with front-line autologous transplantation in t(4;14) multiple myeloma: low complete remission rate and short duration of remission. J Clin Oncol. 2006;24:e4–5.
78. Bergsagel PL, Kuehl WM. Molecular pathogenesis and a consequent classification of multiple myeloma. J Clin Oncol. 2005;23:6333–8.
79. Gertz MA, Lacy MQ, Dispenzieri A, et al. Clinical implications of t(11;14)(q13;q32), t(4;14)(p16.3;q32), and −17p13 in myeloma patients treated with high-dose therapy. Blood 2005;106:2837–40.
80. Zhan F, Huang Y, Colla S, et al. The molecular classification of multiple myeloma. Blood 2006;108:2020–8.
81. Drach J, Ackermann J, Fritz E, et al. Presence of a p53 gene deletion in patients with multiple myeloma predicts for short survival after conventional-dose chemotherapy. Blood 1998;92:802.
82. Chang H, Qi C, Yi QL, et al. p53 gene deletion detected by fluorescence in situ hybridization is an adverse prognostic factor for patients with multiple myeloma following autologous stem cell transplantation. Blood 2005;105:358.
83. Shaughnessy JD Jr, Zhan F, Burington BE, et al. A validated gene expression model of high-risk multiple myeloma is defined by deregulated expression of genes mapping to chromosome 1. Blood 2007;109:2276–84.
84. Shaughnessy JD, Haessler J, van Rhee F, et al. Testing standard and genetic parameters in 220 patients with multiple myeloma with complete data sets: superiority of molecular genetics. Br J Haematol. 2007;137:530–6.
85. Zhan F, Colla S, Wu X, et al. CKS1B, overexpressed in aggressive disease, regulates multiple myeloma growth and survival through SKP2- and p27Kip1-dependent and -independent mechanisms. Blood 2007;109:4995–5001.
86. Hanamura I, Stewart JP, Huang Y, et al. Frequent gain of chromosome band 1q21 in plasma-cell dyscrasias detected by fluorescence in situ hybridization: incidence increases from MGUS to relapsed myeloma and is related to prognosis and disease progression following tandem stem-cell transplantation. Blood 2006;108:1724–32.
87. Fermand JP, Ravaud P, Chevret S, et al. High dose therapy and autologous blood stem cell transplantation in multiple myeloma: upfront or rescue treatment? Results of a multicenter sequential randomized clinical trial. Blood 1998;92:3191–6.
88. Vesole DH, Barlogie B, Jagannath S, et al. High-dose therapy for refractory multiple myeloma: improved prognosis with better support care and double transplants. Blood 1994;84:950–6.
89. Vesole D, Crowley J, Catchatourian R, et al. High-dose melphalan with autotransplantation for refractory multiple myeloma: results of a Southwest Oncology Group phase II trial. J Clinic Oncol. 1999;17:2173–9.
90. Rajkumar SV, Fonseca R, Lacy MQ, et al. Autologous stem cell transplantation for relapsed and primary refractory myeloma. Bone Marrow Transplant. 1999; 23:1267–72.
91. Pineda-Roman M, Haessler J, Hollmig K, et al. High-dose melphalan (MEL) based autotransplants (AT) for multiple myeloma (MM): the Arkansas experience since 1989 in more than 2,800 patients. J Clin Oncol. 2007;25: (Abstract 8043).
92. Lee CK, Barlogie B, Munshi N, et al. DTPACE: an effective, novel combination chemotherapy with thalidomide for previously treated patients with myeloma. J Clinic Oncol. 2003;21:2723–9.

93. Tricot G, Reiner M, Zangari M, et al. Melphalan 200 mg/m^2 (MEL 200) and MEL 140/DT-PACE are equally effective in multiple myeloma (MM), while the latter is less toxic. Blood 2005;106: (Abstract 839).
94. Mansi JL, Cunningham D, Viner C, et al. Repeat administration of high dose melphalan in relapsed myeloma. Br J Cancer. 1993;68:983–7.
95. Tricot G, Jagannath S, Vesole DH, et al. Relapse of multiple myeloma after autologous transplantation: survival after salvage therapy. Bone Marrow Transplant. 1995;16:7–11.
96. Barlogie B, Anaissie E, van Rhee F, et al. Incorporating bortezomib into upfront treatment for multiple myeloma: early results of total therapy 3. Br J Haematol. 2007;138:176–85.
97. Lee CK, Barlogie B, Fassas A, et al. Third Autotransplant for the management of 98 patients among 1358 who had received prior tandem autotransplants: benefit apparent when 2nd to 3rd transplant interval exceeds 3 years. Blood 104: (Abstract 540).
98. Elice F, Raimondi R, Tosetto A, et al. Prolonged overall survival with second on-demand autologous transplant in multiple myeloma. Am J Hematol. 2006;81:426–31.
99. Hideshima T, Mitsiades C, Tonon G, et al. Understanding multiple myeloma pathogenesis in the bone marrow to identify new therapeutic targets. Nat Rev Cancer. 2007;7:585–98.
100. Bruno B, Giaccone L, Rotta M, et al. Novel targeted drugs for the treatment of multiple myeloma: from bench to bedside. Leukemia 2005;19:1729–38 (Review).
101. Mehta J, Singhal S. Graft-versus-myeloma. Bone Marrow Transplant. 1998;22:835–43 (Review).
102. Gahrton G, Tura S, Ljungman P, et al. Allogeneic bone marrow transplantation in multiple myeloma. N Engl J Med. 1991;325:1267–73.
103. Gahrton G, Tura S, Ljungman P, et al. Prognostic factors in allogeneic bone marrow transplantation for multiple myeloma. J Clin Oncol. 1995;13:1312–22.
104. Bensinger WI, Buckner CD, Anasetti C, et al. Allogeneic marrow transplantation for multiple myeloma: an analysis of risk factors on outcome. Blood 1996;88:2787–93.
105. Bensinger WI. Reduced intensity allogeneic stem cell transplantation in multiple myeloma. Front Biosci. 2007;12:4384–92.
106. Kroger N, Schwerdtfeger R, Kiehl M, et al. Autologous stem cell transplantation followed by a dose-reduced allograft induces high complete remission rate in multiple myeloma. Blood 2002;100:755–60.
107. Maloney DG, Molina AJ, Sahebi F, et al. Allografting with nonmyeloablative conditioning following cytoreductive autografts for the treatment of patients with multiple myeloma. Blood 2003;102:3447–54.
108. Bensinger WI, Maloney D, Storb R. Allogeneic hematopoietic cell transplantation for multiple myeloma. Semin Hematol. 2001;38:243–9.
109. Reece DE, Shepherd JD, Klingemann HO, et al. Treatment of myeloma using intensive therapy and allogeneic bone marrow transplantation. Bone Marrow Transplant. 1995;15:117–23.
110. Alyea E, Weller E, Schlossman R, et al. T-cell-depleted allogeneic bone marrow transplantation followed by donor lymphocyte infusion in patients with multiple myeloma: induction of graft-versus-myeloma effect. Blood 2001;98:934–9.
111. Kulkarni S, Powles RL, Treleaven JO, et al. Impact of previous high-dose therapy on outcome after allografting for multiple myeloma. Bone Marrow Transplant. 1999;23:675–80.
112. Le Blanc R, Montminy-Metivier S, Belanger R, et al. Allogeneic transplantation for multiple myeloma: further evidence for a GVHD-associated graft-versus-myeloma effect. Bone Marrow Transplant. 2001;28:841–8.
113. Couban S, Stewart AK, Loach D, et al. Autologous and allogeneic transplantation for multiple myeloma at a single centre. Bone Marrow Transplant. 1997;19:783–9.

114. Varterasian M, Janakiraman N, Karanes C, et al. Transplantation in patients with multiple myeloma: a multicenter comparative analysis of peripheral blood stem cell and allogeneic transplant. Am J Clin Oncol. 1997;20:462–6.
115. Russell NH, Miflin G, Stainer C, et al. Allogeneic bone marrow transplant for multiple myeloma. Blood 1997;89:2610–1 (Letter).
116. Cavo M, Bandini G, Benni M, et al. High-dose busulfan and cyclophosphamide are an effective conditioning regimen for allogeneic bone marrow transplantation in chemosensitive multiple myeloma. Bone Marrow Transplant. 1998;22:27–32.
117. Blade J, Samson D, Reece D, et al. Criteria for evaluating disease response and progression in patients with multiple myeloma treated by high-dose therapy and haemopoietic stem cell transplantation. Myeloma Subcommittee of the European Group for Blood Marrow Transplantation. Br J Haematol. 1998;102:1115–23.
118. Corradini P, Voena C, Tarella C, et al. Molecular and clinical remissions in multiple myeloma: role of autologous and allogeneic transplantation of hematopoietic cells. J Clin Oncol. 1999;17:208–15.
119. Corradini P, Cavo M, Lokhorst H, et al. Molecular remission after myeloablative allogeneic stem cell transplantation predicts a better relapse-free survival in patients with multiple myeloma. Blood 2003;102:1927–9.
120. Gahrton G, Svensson H, Cavo M, et al. Progress in allogenic bone marrow and peripheral blood stem cell transplantation for multiple myeloma: a comparison between transplants performed 1983–1993 and 1994–1998 at European Group for Blood and Marrow Transplantation centres. Br J Haematol. 2001;113:209–16.
121. Bjorkstrand BB, Ljungman P, Svensson H, et al. Allogeneic bone marrow transplantation versus autologous stem cell transplantation in multiple myeloma: a retrospective case-matched study from the European Group for Blood and Marrow Transplantation. Blood 1996;88:4711–8.
122. Kuruvilla J, Shepherd JD, Sutherland HJ, et al. Long-term outcome of myeloablative allogeneic stem cell transplantation for multiple myeloma. Biol Blood Marrow Transplant. 2007;13:925–31.
123. Gahrton G. Risk assessment in haematopoietic stem cell transplantation: impact of donor-recipient sex combination in allogeneic transplantation. Best Pract Res Clin Haematol. 2007;20:219–29 (Review).
124. Schrezenmeier H, Passweg JR, Marsh JC, et al. Worse outcome and more chronic GvHD with peripheral blood progenitor cells than bone marrow in HLA-matched sibling donor transplants for young patients with severe acquired aplastic anemia. Blood 2007;110:1397–400.
125. Oehler VG, Radich JP, Storer B, et al. Randomized trial of allogeneic related bone marrow transplantation versus peripheral blood stem cell transplantation for chronic myeloid leukemia. Biol Blood Marrow Transplant. 2005;11:85–92.
126. Flowers ME, Parker PM, Johnston LJ, et al. Comparison of chronic graft-versus-host disease after transplantation of peripheral blood stem cells versus bone marrow in allogeneic recipients: long-term follow-up of a randomized trial. Blood 2002;100:415–9.
127. Shaughnessy J Jr, Tian E, Sawyer J, et al. Prognostic impact of cytogenetic and interphase fluorescence in situ hybridization-defined chromosome 13 deletion in multiple myeloma: early results of total therapy II. Br J Haematol. 2003;120:44–52.
128. Barlogie B Jr, Shaughnessy JD. Early results of total therapy II in multiple myeloma: implications of cytogenetics and FISH. Int J Hematol. 2002;76 Suppl 1:337–9.
129. Avet-Loiseau H, Attal M, Moreau P, et al. Genetic abnormalities and survival in multiple myeloma: the experience of the Intergroupe Francophone du Myelome. Blood 2007;109:3489–95.
130. Matsui S, Yamanaka T, Barlogie B, et al. Clustering of significant genes in prognostic studies with microarrays: application to a clinical study for multiple myeloma. Stat Med. 2008;27:1106–20.

131. Storb R, Yu C, Wagner JL, et al. Stable mixed hematopoietic chimerism in DLA-identical littermate dogs given sublethal total body irradiation before and pharmacological immunosuppression after marrow transplantation. Blood 1997; 89:3048–54.
132. McSweeney PA, Niederwieser D, Shizuru JA, et al. Hematopoietic cell transplantation in older patients with hematologic malignancies: replacing high-dose cytotoxic therapy with graft-versus-tumor effects. Blood 2001;97:3390–400.
133. Mohty M, Boiron JM, Damaj G, et al. Graft-versus-myeloma effect following antithymocyte globulin-based reduced intensity conditioning allogeneic stem cell transplantation. Bone Marrow Transplant. 2004;34:77–84.
134. Peggs KS, Mackinnon S, Williams CD, et al. Reduced-intensity transplantation with *in vivo* T-cell depletion and adjuvant dose-escalating donor lymphocyte infusions for chemotherapy-sensitive myeloma: limited efficacy of graft-versus-tumor activity. Biol Blood Marrow Transplant. 2003:9;257–265.
135. Einsele H, Schafer HJ, Hebart HP, et al. Follow-up of patients with progressive multiple myeloma undergoing allografts after reduced-intensity conditioning. Br J Haematol. 2003;121:411–8.
136. Giralt S, Aleman A, Anagnostopoulos A, et al. Fludarabine/melphalan conditioning for allogeneic transplantation in patients with multiple myeloma. Bone Marrow Transplant. 2002:30;367–73.
137. Gerull S, Goerner M, Benner A, et al. Long-term outcome of nonmyeloablative allogeneic transplantation in patients with high-risk multiple myeloma. Bone Marrow Transplant. 2005:36;963–9.
138. Bruno B, Sorasio R, Patriarca F, et al. Unrelated donor haematopoietic cell transplantation after non-myeloablative conditioning for patients with high-risk multiple myeloma. Eur J Haematol. 2007;78:330–7.
139. Lee CK, Badros A, Barlogie B, et al. Prognostic factors in allogeneic transplantation for patients with high-risk multiple myeloma after reduced intensity conditioning. Exp Hematol. 2003;31:73–80.
140. Kroger N, Sayer HG, Schwerdtfeger R, et al. Unrelated stem cell transplantation in multiple myeloma after a reduced-intensity conditioning with pretransplantation antithymocyte globulin is highly effective with low transplantation-related mortality. Blood 2002;100:3919–24.
141. Galimberti S, Benedetti E, Morabito F, et al. Prognostic role of minimal residual disease in multiple myeloma patients after non-myeloablative allogeneic transplantation. Leuk Res. 2005;29:961–6.
142. Crawley C, Iacobelli S, Bjorkstrand B, et al. Reduced-intensity conditioning for myeloma: lower nonrelapse mortality but higher relapse rates compared with myeloablative conditioning. Blood 2007;109:3588–94.
143. Wheatley K, Gray R. Commentary: Mendelian randomization—an update on its use to evaluate allogeneic stem cell transplantation in leukaemia. Int J Epidemiol. 2004;33:15–7.
144. Balduzzi A, Valsecchi MG, Uderzo C, et al. Chemotherapy versus allogeneic transplantation for very-high-risk childhood acute lymphoblastic leukaemia in first complete remission: comparison by genetic randomisation in an international prospective study. Lancet 2005;366:635–42.
145. Woods WG, Neudorf S, Gold S, et al. A comparison of allogeneic bone marrow transplantation, autologous bone marrow transplantation, and aggressive chemotherapy in children with acute myeloid leukemia in remission. Blood 2001;97:56–62.
146. Suciu S, Mandelli F, de Witte T, et al. Allogeneic compared with autologous stem cell transplantation in the treatment of patients younger than 46 years with acute myeloid leukemia (AML) in first complete remission (CR1): an intention-to-treat analysis of the EORTC/GIMEMAAML-10 trial. Blood 2003;102:1232–40.

147. Garban F, Attal M, Michallet M, et al. Prospective comparison of autologous stem cell transplantation followed by dose-reduced allograft (IFM99-03 trial) with tandem autologous stem cell transplantation (IFM99-04 trial) in high-risk de novo multiple myeloma. Blood 2006;107:3474–80.
148. Kroger N, Schilling G, Einsele H, et al. Deletion of chromosome band 13q14 as detected by fluorescence in situ hybridization is a prognostic factor in patients with multiple myeloma who are receiving allogeneic dose-reduced stem cell transplantation. Blood 2004;103:4056–61.
149. Bruno B, Rotta, F. Patriarca, et al. A comparison of allografting with autografting for newly-diagnosed myeloma. N Engl J Med. 2007;356:1110–20.
150. Giaccone L, Patriarca F, Rotta M, et al. Tandem autografting-nonmyeloablative allografting for newly diagnosed multiple myeloma: the GITMO (Gruppo Italiano Trapianto di Midollo) experience. Haematologica 2007;92(s1):s4 Abs 0403.
151. Kwak LW, Taub DD, Duffey PL, et al. Transfer of myeloma idiotype-specific immunity from an actively immunised marrow donor. Lancet 1995;345:1016–20.
152. Tricot G, Vesole DH, Jagannath S, et al. Graft-versus-myeloma effect: proof of principle. Blood 1996;87:1196–8.
153. Verdonck LF, Lokhorst HM, Dekker AW, et al. Graft-versus-myeloma effect in two cases. Lancet 1996;347:800–1.
154. Aschan J, Lonnqvist B, Ringden O, et al. Graft-versus-myeloma effect. Lancet 1996;348:346 (Letter).
155. Libura J, Hoffmann T, Passweg J, et al. Graft-versus-myeloma after withdrawal of immunosuppression following allogeneic peripheral stem cell transplantation. Bone Marrow Transplant. 1999;24:925–7.
156. Collins RH Jr, Shpilberg O, Drobyski WR, et al. Donor leukocyte infusions in 140 patients with relapsed malignancy after allogeneic bone marrow transplantation. J Clin Oncol. 1997;15:433–44.
157. Zeiser R, Bertz H, Spyridonidis A, et al. Donor lymphocyte infusions for multiple myeloma: clinical results and novel perspectives. Bone Marrow Transplant. 2004;34:923–8.
158. Lokhorst HM, Schattenberg A, Cornelissen JJ, et al. Donor leukocyte infusions are effective in relapsed multiple myeloma after allogeneic bone marrow transplantation. Blood 1997;90:4206–11.
159. Lokhorst HM, Schattenberg A, Cornelissen JJ, et al. Donor lymphocyte infusions for relapsed multiple myeloma after allogeneic stem-cell transplantation: predictive factors for response and long-term outcome. J Clin Oncol. 2000;18:3031–7.
160. Lokhorst HM, Wu K, Verdonck LF, Laterveer LL, et al. The occurrence of graft-versus-host disease is the major predictive factor for response to donor lymphocyte infusions in multiple myeloma. Blood 2004;103:4362–4.
161. van de Donk NW, Kroger N, Hegenbart U, et al. Prognostic factors for donor lymphocyte infusions following non-myeloablative allogeneic stem cell transplantation in multiple myeloma. Bone Marrow Transplant. 2006;37:1135–41.
162. Horowitz MM, Gale RP, Sondel PM, et al. Graft versus-leukemia reactions after bone marrow transplantation. Blood 1990;75:555–62.
163. Hale O, Jacobs P, Wood L, et al. CD52 antibodies for prevention of graft-versus-host disease and graft rejection following transplantation of allogeneic peripheral blood stem cells. Bone Marrow Transplant. 2000;26:69–76.
164. Lokhorst HM, Segeren CM, Verdonck LF, et al. Partially T-cell-depleted allogeneic stem-cell transplantation for first-line treatment of multiple myeloma: a prospective evaluation of patients treated in the phase III study HOVON 24 MM. J Clin Oncol. 2003;21:1728–33.
165. Preijers FWMB, van HennikPB, Schattenberg A, et al. Counterflow centrifugation allows addition of appropriate numbers of T cells to allogeneic marrow and blood

stem cell grafts to prevent severe GVHD without substantial loss of mature and immature progenitor cells. Bone Marrow Transplant. 1999;23:1061–70.

166. Levenga H, Levison-Keating S, Schattenberg AV, et al. Multiple myeloma patients receiving pre-emptive donor lymphocyte infusion after partial T-cell-depleted allogeneic stem cell transplantation show a long progression-free survival. Bone Marrow Transplant. 2007;40:355–9.
167. Bruno B, Patriarca F, Sorasio R, et al. Bortezomib with or without dexamethasone in relapsed multiple myeloma following allogeneic hematopoietic cell transplantation. Haematologica 2006;91:837–9.
168. van de Donk NW, Kroger N, Hegenbart U, et al. Remarkable activity of novel agents bortezomib and thalidomide in patients not responding to donor lymphocyte infusions following nonmyeloablative allogeneic stem cell transplantation in multiple myeloma. Blood 2006;107:3415–6.
169. Kroger N, Shimoni A, Zagrivnaja M, et al. Low-dose thalidomide and donor lymphocyte infusion as adoptive immunotherapy after allogeneic stem cell transplantation in patients with multiple myeloma. Blood 2004;104:3361–3.
170. Kroger N, Zabelina T, Ayuk F, et al. Bortezomib after dose-reduced allogeneic stem cell transplantation for multiple myeloma to enhance or maintain remission status. Exp Hematol. 2006;34:770–5.
171. Lowsky R, Takahashi T, Liu YP, et al. Protective conditioning for acute graft-versus-host disease. N Engl J Med. 2005;353:1321–31. Erratum in: N Engl J Med. 2006;354:884.
172. Atanackovic D, Arfsten J, Cao Y, et al. Cancer-testis antigens are commonly expressed in multiple myeloma and induce systemic immunity following allogeneic stem cell transplantation. Blood 2007;109:1103–12.
173. Siegel S, Wagner A, Friedrichs B, et al. Identification of HLA-A*0201-presented T cell epitopes derived from the oncofetal antigen-immature laminin receptor protein in patients with hematological malignancies. J Immunol. 2006;76:6935–44.

Chapter 15
Role of Hematopoietic Stem Cell Transplantation in the Treatment of Non-Hodgkin's Lymphoma

Philip J. Bierman and Gordon L. Phillips

15.1 Introduction

In 2007 it is estimated that there will be more than 63,000 new cases of non-Hodgkin's lymphoma (NHL) in the United States and that nearly 19,000 people will die from NHL. Non-Hodgkin's lymphoma accounts for approximately 4% of all new cancer diagnoses. The NHL incidence rate increased more than 50% between 1975 and the early 1990s, although this increase has reached a plateau recently. The reasons for this epidemic of NHL are largely unexplained but are partially related to improvements in diagnosis, the aging population, acquired immune deficiency syndrome (AIDS), and environmental exposures.

The etiology of NHL is unknown in most cases. However, the incidence of NHL is increased in the presence of congenital and acquired immune deficiency. Non-Hodgkin's lymphoma is associated with various viruses including the Epstein-Barr virus (EBV), the human T-cell lymphotropic virus type I, human herpesvirus 8, and the hepatitis C virus. In addition, infection with *Helicobacter pylori* and possibly other bacteria have been linked to the development of NHL. Environmental agents such as herbicides and hair dyes have been associated with an increased risk of NHL in some studies, and there appears to be an increased risk of NHL in first-degree relatives of people with hematopoietic malignancies.

The management of NHL has been improved by the adoption of the World Health Organization classification system which incorporates morphology, immunophenotype, genetic features, and clinical features to separate lymphomas into categories that represent distinct clinical entities. The classification of lymphoma, and subsequent management, will continue to improve as new technology, such as gene expression profiling, is used to identify subtypes with distinct characteristics [1].

P.J. Bierman (✉)
Department of Internal Medicine, Section of Oncology-Hematology, University of Nebraska Medical Center, 987680 Nebraska Medical Center, Omaha, NE 68198-7680, USA
e-mail: pjbierma@unmc.edu

M.R. Bishop (ed.), *Hematopoietic Stem Cell Transplantation*, Cancer Treatment and Research 144, DOI 10.1007/978-0-387-78580-6_15,

This chapter will focus on recent developments related to hematopoietic stem cell transplantation (HSCT) for NHL, and is not meant to be an exhaustive review of all recent references. Only results for the most common types of NHL will be discussed in detail.

15.2 Autologous Hematopoietic Stem Cell Transplantation

Forty years ago, the median survival of patients with diffuse aggressive NHL was measured in months after treatment with single-agent chemotherapy. It was subsequently shown that these patients could be cured with regimens developed for Hodgkin lymphoma (a.k.a. Hodgkin's disease; reviewed in Chap. 16 by Moskowitz and Sweetenham). Later, doxorubicin-containing regimens were introduced, and the 5-year survival rate for all types of NHL increased more than 30% between 1975 and 2000. Recently, NHL treatment has been revolutionized by the use of the anti-CD20 antibody, rituximab, which increases response rates and prolongs survival when combined with chemotherapy for diffuse large B-cell lymphoma (DLBCL) [2] and follicular lymphoma [3]. Nevertheless, some patients fail to attain an initial remission or subsequently relapse. New agents provide additional treatment options, although the prognosis for patients with relapsed and refractory NHL remains poor.

This situation has led to the use of high-dose therapy followed by autologous hematopoietic stem cell transplantation (HSCT) for patients with relapsed and refractory NHL. This approach is based upon steep dose–response curves exhibited by several agents, especially alkylating agents and radiation, whose dose-limiting toxicity is myelosuppression. Attempts at treating radiation- and chemotherapy induced myelosuppression date to the late 1950s. Later, techniques for bone marrow harvest and cryopreservation were perfected, and studies in the late 1970s showed that reinfusion of cryopreserved bone marrow stem cells could accelerate hematopoietic recovery following chemotherapy and cure patients with relapsed lymphoma.

Use of this therapy expanded rapidly and led to the landmark PARMA trial demonstrating the superiority of autologous HSCT over conventional salvage chemotherapy for patients with relapsed aggressive NHL [4], and autologous HSCT is now standard therapy for patients with relapsed chemotherapy-sensitive DLBCL. More than 2500 autologous HSCT procedures were registered with the Center for International Blood and Marrow Transplant Research (CIBMTR) in 2003 [5]. This value is felt to represent approximately 60% of the transplants being performed in North and South America. Non-Hodgkin's lymphoma is the second most common indication for autologous HSCT in North America and in Europe [5, 6]. The European Group for Blood and Marrow Transplantation (EBMT) recorded more than 4600 autologous HSCT procedures for NHL in 2005.

The use of peripheral blood as a source of hematopoietic stem cells has increased dramatically. More than 95% of autologous transplants are now performed with peripheral blood hematopoietic stem cells instead of marrow [5, 6]. Transplants are easier, safer, and less expensive; the 100-day mortality rate following autologous HSCT for NHL is below 5%. These advances are due to increased experience, better patient selection, the use of peripheral blood stem cells, and improvements in supportive care such as the use of hematopoietic growth factors. Autologous HSCT can be performed safely in older patients by community oncologists in the outpatient setting, and even without blood product support if need be. Autologous HSCT is now used for most NHL subtypes, and it is being used as part of primary therapy. Improvements in preparative regimens and post-transplant therapy are being explored. Efforts are being focused on prevention and management of late effects of autologous HSCT.

15.3 Allogeneic Hematopoietic Stem Cell Transplantation

For various reasons relating to patient selection, lack of matched donors, and physician bias, allogeneic HSCT is used much less frequently than autologous HSCT for NHL. Data from the CIBMTR and EBMT indicate that approximately 15–20% of transplants for NHL are allogeneic [5, 6]. That said, allogeneic HSCT has several potential advantages as compared to autologous HSCT. The first advantage is the near universal ability to collect adequate numbers reconstituting stem cells from normal donors, since a significant proportion of NHL patients cannot have adequate numbers of cells obtained for autologous HSCT. In addition to quantitative advantages, there is a qualitative advantage, reflected by a reduction in late hematological complications such as myelodysplastic syndromes (MDS) and acute myeloid leukemia (AML) [7]. Another advantage associated with allogeneic HSCT is that inadvertent re-inoculation of contaminating clonogeneic tumor cells is avoided. Finally, allogeneic HSCT permits the immunologic effect of graft-versus-lymphoma (GvLym) effect [8]. GvLym appears to be most potent in patients with indolent histology, and is modest in its ability to deal with bulky or rapidly progressive NHL [9]. Although the existence of a GvLym effect has been debated, studies have demonstrated the ability of GvLym effects to eradicate NHL cells to conventional chemotherapy and/or radiotherapy.

Despite these advantages, allogeneic HSCT is associated with disadvantages including limitations due to patient age, comorbidity and performance status, difficulties in identifying suitable donors, and higher rates of nonrelapse mortality.

Two relatively recent advances have allowed the use of allogeneic HSCT in a much wider range of NHL patients. First, the use of "nonmyeloablative" (NMA) or "reduced-intensity" conditioning (RIC) regimens has allowed allogeneic HSCT to be performed in patients that would ordinarily be excluded because of age, comorbidity, or prior autologous HSCT. The former (NMA) are often similar to conventional chemotherapy, while the latter (RIC) approach the intensity of a fully myeloablative regimen (However, this distinction is not always obvious, and for simplicity, both of these types of regimens will all be referred to as RIC unless specifically noted). These regimens are not designed to eradicate all NHL cells, rather to serve as a platform to reduce early transplant-related mortality so that patients can benefit from later GvLym effects [9].

The next advance is the use of "alternative donors" instead of HLA-related siblings. These include haploidentical family donors, unrelated donors, and unrelated (usually) umbilical cord blood that permits patients without matched siblings to undergo allogeneic HSCT with comparable outcomes.

Despite these advances, widespread use of allogeneic HSCT is limited by toxicity, and the use of this approach would be increased by the ability to augment GvLym effects and/or the ability to decrease the incidence of graft-versus-host-disease (GvHD).

15.4 Pretransplant Considerations

15.4.1 Patient Selection

Patients are selected for treatment with HSCT if they are predicted to have an unsatisfactory outcome with less aggressive conventional treatment. In addition, selection is also based upon the likelihood of a more favorable outcome with transplantation and the ability of the patient to tolerate autologous or allogeneic HSCT. The International Prognostic Index (IPI) [10] has been used to identify patients with aggressive NHL who are unlikely to experience a satisfactory outcome with initial therapy and who may be suitable candidates for upfront transplants (see below). Similar prognostic indices may be useful for patients with other types of NHL, although these indices may be less useful in rituximab-treated patients. New imaging technology and molecular techniques may also provide important information (see below).

Sensitivity to conventional salvage chemotherapy is the most important tool for identifying appropriate transplant candidates among patients with relapsed and refractory NHL. Other tools may be used to identify patients who are likely to do well following autologous HSCT including clinical prognostic factors [11] and newer imaging techniques (see below) [12].

Finally, an evaluation of comorbid conditions is essential to determine the risk of transplant-related mortality and suitability for HSCT, although it is difficult to quantify these conditions. While age is an important prognostic factor for both allogeneic and autologous HSCT, it appears to be of lesser importance for patients treated with autologous HSCT, although the influence of selection-bias cannot be ignored [13]. Other comorbid conditions related to general health status and organ function may exclude patients from HSCT.

The importance of comorbidity has become more obvious with the use of RIC allogeneic HSCT, which allows older patients to be treated with allogeneic HSCT. Investigators from Seattle developed a comorbidity index based upon cardiac, renal, hepatic, pulmonary, and other parameters to predict nonrelapse mortality following RIC-allo or myeloablative allogeneic HSCT. The impact of this comorbidity index was evaluated for patients treated with allogeneic HSCT for NHL and chronic lymphocytic leukemia [14]. The outcome for patients without comorbidity was similar when results of myeloablative allogeneic HSCT and RIC allogeneic HSCT were compared. However, among patients with comorbidity, nonrelapse mortality was lower ($p = 0.009$) and survival was prolonged ($p = 0.04$) following RIC conditioning (see Fig. 15.1).

15.4.2 Pretransplant Cytoreduction

Almost invariably, the outcome of patients transplanted without evidence of disease is better than those who have a significant tumor burden, and it is common practice to administer conventional chemotherapy prior to the high-dose preparative regimen for patients undergoing HSCT. This practice reduces tumor burden and establishes "chemotherapy sensitivity." Chemotherapy sensitivity has traditionally been measured with routine imaging studies such as computerized tomography (CT) scans, although 18-fluorodeoxyglucose positron emission tomography (FDG-PET) scanning is likely to increase our ability to determine responsiveness.

It is unknown whether patients who demonstrate partial chemotherapy sensitivity should proceed directly to HSCT or whether they should receive additional conventional therapy to achieve additional cytoreduction (i.e., complete response) prior to transplantation. The latter approach may improve outcome but may also lead to additional post-transplant toxicity. Nevertheless, it seems prudent to treat to maximum response as long as patients tolerate therapy. The selection of agents used for this purpose should be made after consideration of prior treatment and the planned high-dose therapy regimen. Regimens that contain carmustine and melphalan may impair the ability to mobilize peripheral stem cells.

In addition to chemotherapy, it is common practice to administer adjunctive pre or post-transplant radiation to sites of bulky disease. This is often difficult because of cumulative doses of prior radiation, poor performance status, or delayed engraftment following autologous HSCT. The use of involved-field radiation may lead to responses that allow some patients to proceed to transplant and provide better local control [15, 16]; however, randomized trials have not been reported. The use of peri-transplant irradiation has been associated with improved survival in some analyses [17], although this has been difficult to demonstrate conclusively. The use of pretransplant radiation may lead to an increased risk of secondary MDS (see below) and respiratory complications [18].

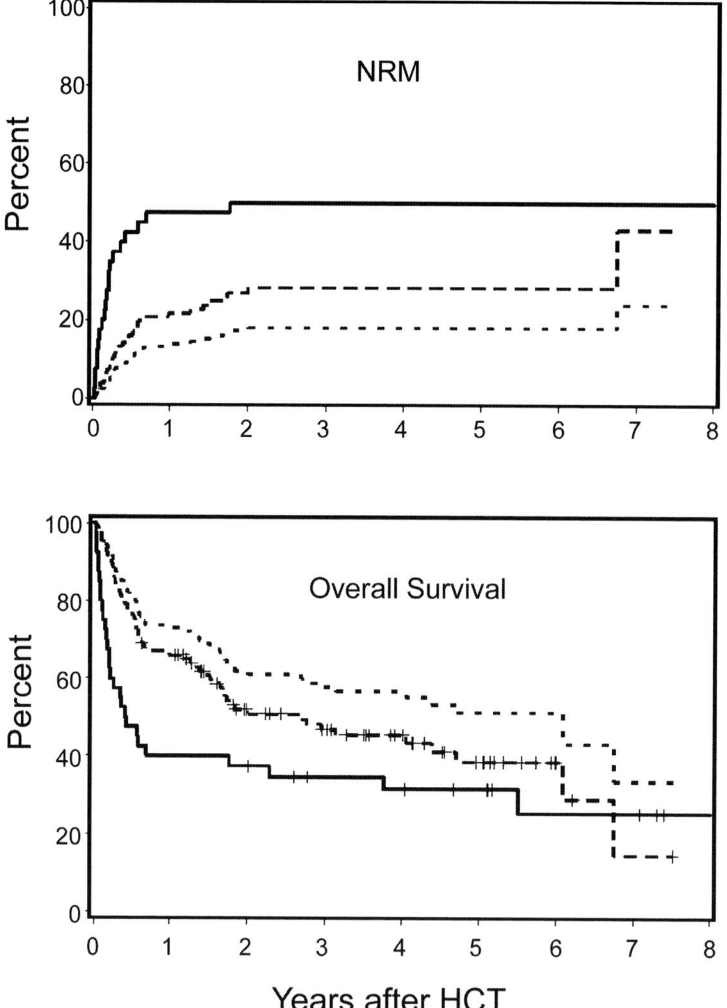

Fig. 15.1 Cumulative incidence of nonrelapse mortality (NRM) and actuarial survival following allogeneic hematopoietic stem cell transplantation for non-Hodgkin's lymphoma and chronic lymphocytic leukemia in patients with significant comorbidity. Solid line: myeloablative conditioning; Dashed line: nonmyeloablative conditioning; Dotted line: myeloablative conditioning-adjusted outcome (from Sorror et al. [14])

15.4.3 Stem Cell Mobilization and Collection

Cell dose is recognized as an important variable influencing outcome of autologous HSCT, despite the knowledge that this assay is only a crude surrogate for the reconstituting hematopoietic stem cell. This relationship has been improved somewhat with better assays for reconstituting stem cells such as the CD34 and CD133 antigens, and the widespread use of mobilized peripheral blood as a source of hematopoietic stem cells. Cell dose is also an important variable for those undergoing allogeneic HSCT, but is more complex, and this discussion will focus on considerations related to autologous HSCT for NHL.

A minimum of 2.0×10^6/kg of $CD34^+$ cells is usually collected to ensure prompt hematopoietic recovery, although a lower number may be adequate in some cases. For example, investigators from Stanford University compared outcomes of NHL patients who were transplanted with greater than or equal to 2.0×10^6/kg $CD34^+$ cells with those who had poorer collections [19]. No significant differences in event-free survival or overall survival were seen, although transplant-related mortality rates were 3.6% and 11.8%, respectively ($p = 0.08$).

A sufficient quantity of peripheral blood hematopoietic stem cells can be collected from the majority of patients. Several options exist for patients who do not achieve this goal, including simple repetition or the use of steady state or primed bone marrow. The agent plerixafor (AMD 3100) is also likely to be useful for "poor mobilizers." This drug increases the movement of hematopoietic stem cells into the circulation and appears to be more potent than granulocyte colony-stimulating factor (G-CSF, filgrastim) alone, for stem cell mobilization in both autologous and allogeneic donors [20].

15.5 Transplant Considerations

15.5.1 Conditioning Regimens

15.5.1.1 Autologous Hematopoietic Stem Cell Transplantation

In the past, early mortality caused a large fraction of treatment failures following autologous HSCT. Now, early mortality is less than 5%, and treatment failure is almost invariably from progressive NHL. A variety of approaches have been used to improve the results of both autologous and allogeneic HSCT for NHL; most involve improvements to the high-dose therapy regimen, although no regimens have been conclusively shown to be superior. Some groups have increased the dose of chemotherapy agents in common regimens such as CBV (cyclophosphamide, carmustine, etoposide) or BEAM (carmustine, etoposide, cytarabine, melphalan). This has not led to substantial improvements in outcome, and may lead to increased toxicity [21, 22]. At the University of Alabama, the role of pharmacokinetic (PK)-directed dosing of intravenous busulfan prior to autologous HSCT for NHL has been investigated [23]. When compared to historical controls who received regimens containing oral busulfan, the nonrelapse mortality decreased from 27% to 3% ($p = 0.01$). The actuarial 5-year survival was 28% for controls and 58% for those treated with PK-directed intravenous busulfan ($p = 0.01$).

Other groups have used high-dose sequential chemotherapy regimens in an attempt to improve the preparative regimen. These regimens consist of an initial induction or debulking phase. After this, non cross-resistant single agents are administered at high doses over intervals of 1–3 weeks to prevent the emergence of resistant clones. This phase is followed by hematopoietic stem cell collection and autologous HSCT. These regimens have been used for a variety of types of NHL in the relapse setting and as upfront treatment [24–27]. These regimens have been associated with improved outcomes in some randomized trials [26], but not in others [24, 27].

Another innovation in this area involves the use of double (tandem) autologous HSCT. Although phase II trials demonstrate that this is feasible, a substantial number of patients are not able proceed to the second transplant, and this approach has not been widely adopted [28, 29]. The use of autologous HSCT followed by RIC allogeneic HSCT has also been tested. Limited phase II data demonstrate the feasibility of this approach, but morbidity and mortality are high, and there is a high relapse rate [30, 31].

Several groups have incorporated radiolabeled antibodies as a replacement for total body irradiation (TBI) in high-dose therapy regimens (reviewed in Chap. 13 by Gopal and Winter). In theory, this tactic increases the dose of radiation that can be delivered to sites of disease while limiting exposure to healthy organs. The group from Seattle has used high doses of the radiolabled anti-CD20 antibody ^{131}I-tositumomab, followed by autologous HSCT for patients with relapsed and refractory NHL. A retrospective analysis compared patients with follicular NHL who were treated in this manner with results of similar patients who were treated with conventional high-dose therapy regimens followed by autologous HSCT [32]. The actuarial 5-year progression-free survival of patients treated with high-dose radio-immunotherapy was 48%, as compared with 29% for patients treated with conventional autologous HSCT ($p = 0.06$). The actuarial 5-year overall survival rates were 67% and 53%, respectively ($p = 0.02$).

Several other groups have combined radiolabeled antibodies with high-dose chemotherapy for NHL autologous HSCT [33, 34]. These trials have been conducted with ^{90}Y-ibritumomab-tiuxetan, as well as ^{131}I-tositumomab. Toxicity does not appear to be significantly increased compared with high-dose chemotherapy, alone. The Blood and Marrow Transplant Clinical Trials Network (BMT CTN) is conducting a randomized trial comparing high-dose BEAM versus BEAM plus ^{131}I-tositumomab for relapsed and refractory DLCBL. The combination of radiolabeled antibodies with chemotherapy is also being investigated for allo-HCT [35].

Rituximab has also been used with high-dose chemotherapy regimens prior to autologous HSCT. This agent may augment the efficacy of the high-dose therapy regimen itself, and can also be used as an in-vivo purging agent prior to stem cell collection (see below). Improved outcomes compared with historical controls have been reported [36, 37].

15.5.1.2 Allogeneic Hematopoietic Stem Cell Transplantation

In addition to cytotoxic effects, conditioning for allogeneic HSCT requires profound immunosuppressive effects to prevent graft rejection. Both of these functions are accomplished relatively well with the TBI- or busulfan-based regimens that usually include cyclophosphamide. When used for NHL, these regimens are identical to ones used for leukemia and other diseases.

Regimens used for RIC allogeneic HSCT de-emphasize the direct antineoplastic effects of conditioning so that GvLym effects may emerge. Most of these regimens utilize fludarabine or pentostatin, and are usually combined with cyclophosphamide, busulfan, thiotepa, or low doses of TBI (200–600 cGy). These regimens are almost always used with mobilized blood instead of bone marrow prior to HSCT.

15.5.2 Purging

A major concern associated with autologous HSCT involves the potential risk that reinoculation of clonogenic tumor cells may contribute to relapse following transplant. Most relapses occur at sites of prior disease, which suggests that relapse is usually due to failure of the high-dose therapy to eradicate residual NHL. Nevertheless, the risk of tumor contamination exists and methods of eliminating these cells (purging) have been developed.

Although conclusive data are lacking, several lines of evidence suggest that purging may be beneficial. For example, retrospective analyses have demonstrated improved survival of NHL patients who were treated with purged autologous HSCT, when compared with historical controls [38]. In addition, registry analyses of autologous HSCT for follicular or low-grade NHL have found lower rates of recurrence when recipients of purged autologous HSCT were compared with those receiving unpurged transplants [39, 40]. An analysis of patients who received antibody-complement purged autologous bone marrow transplantation (BMT) at Dana-Farber Cancer Institute also provides support for the value of purging [41]. The actuarial 12-year progression-free survival was 66.7% for patients who received grafts without molecular evidence of tumor cells, as compared with 26.3% for those with detectable tumor contamination ($p = 0.001$) (see Fig. 15.2). However, no significant difference in overall survival was observed, and these results may simply be a manifestation of chemotherapy sensitivity. Despite these results, other analyses have failed to show benefits from purging, including the only randomized trial evaluating autologous BMT for follicular lymphoma [42].

Several purging methods have been used to reduce tumor contamination. In the past, most methods used "ex-vivo" methods to eliminate contaminating after collection [43]. Positive selection techniques have also been used to isolate $CD34^+$ cells for transplantation. This method can reduce molecularly-detectable tumor cells and lead to rapid hematopoietic recovery [44], although

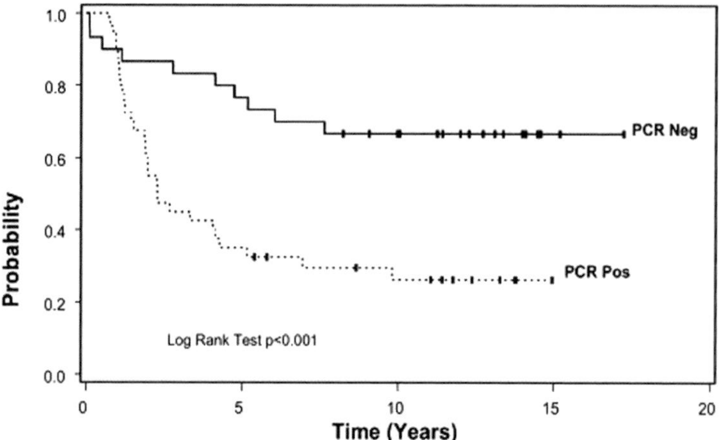

Fig. 15.2 Progression-free survival of patients receiving autologous bone marrow transplants from marrow with or without molecular evidence of tumor contamination (from Brown et al. [41])

impaired immune reconstitution and an increased risk of infectious complications has been reported [43, 44]. More recently "in-vivo" purging has been utilized. This refers to the use of systemic therapy to reduce tumor contamination in the peripheral blood prior to stem cell collection.

Several investigators have administered rituximab prior to stem cell harvest as a method of in-vivo purging. This can also eliminate detectable tumor cells from stem cell collections [45]. A randomized comparison of $CD34^+$ cell collection with rituximab in-vivo purging for patients with NHL has been reported [38]. The positive selection technique was associated with $CD34^+$ cell loss and slightly delayed myeloid recovery. Recovery of immunoglobulin levels were delayed in patients who received in-vivo purging.

The role of purging remains controversial, and its value may only be proven with a randomized trial or with gene-marking studies that conclusively demonstrate that cells from the autograft contribute to relapse. Nevertheless, there is evidence that purging may benefit patients with low-grade or follicular NHL, and use of this approach is reasonable even without definitive evidence of benefit.

15.6 Post-Transplant Considerations

In addition to peri-transplant radiation (see above), a variety of other approaches has been used to decrease the rate of progression after HSCT. Several groups have investigated the use of rituximab following autologous HSCT for NHL [46, 47]. This is capable of eliminating minimal residual disease following autologous HSCT, although late neutropenia and/or prolonged immunosuppression have been observed. The role of rituximab maintenance following autologous HSCT for aggressive NHL is being evaluated in separate phase III trials sponsored by the National Cancer Institute of Canada (NCIC) and Memorial Sloan-Kettering Cancer Center (MSKCC).

Other agents have also been administered following autologous HSCT to decrease the rate of disease progression. Examples include additional chemotherapy [15] and interleukin-2 (IL-2) [48], although benefits have not been established. IL-2 has been combined with cyclosporine and interferon to induce autologous GvHD effects following autologous HSCT for NHL, although benefits have not been clearly demonstrated [49].

15.7 Results of Autologous Hematopoietic Stem Cell Transplantation

15.7.1 Diffuse Large B-Cell/Aggressive Lymphoma

In the landmark PARMA trial, patients with chemotherapy-sensitive relapsed aggressive NHL were randomized to receive additional salvage chemotherapy or to treatment with autologous HSCT [4]. Both arms also received involved-field radiation therapy. The actuarial 5-year event-free survival was 46% following autologous HSCT, as compared to 12% for patients treated with salvage chemotherapy ($p = 0.001$). The overall survival rates were 53% and 32%, respectively ($p = 0.038$). Notably, only 58% of patients responded to salvage chemotherapy and were randomized. Furthermore, 11% of patients randomized to autologous HSCT were not transplanted. The potential influence of selection bias is also evident in a retrospective analysis from MSKCC [11]. This study evaluated patients with relapsed and refractory DLCBL who received salvage chemotherapy with ICE (ifosfamide, carboplatin, etoposide). Approximately 65% of patients underwent autologous HSCT. The actuarial 4-year progression-free survival and overall survival for all patients, including those who were not transplanted, was 28% and 34%, respectively. This type of intent-to-treat analysis is necessary to evaluate the true benefit of autologous HSCT in this situation.

Results from the PARMA trial led to generalized consensus that autologous HSCT is the standard of care for patients with chemotherapy-sensitive relapsed DLBCL, and other large registry series have shown comparable results [50, 51]. Nevertheless, conclusions derived from trials such as these that were performed in the "pre-rituximab" era may need to be reexamined. For example, the addition of rituximab may improve the results of salvage chemotherapy for DLBCL and allow more patients to be eligible for transplantation. This was demonstrated in another study from MSKCC where the addition of rituximab to the ICE salvage regimen increased the complete remission rate to 53%, as compared to 27% for historical controls treated with ICE, alone ($p = 0.01$) [52]. In a retrospective analysis from Washington University, disease-free survival ($p < 0.001$), and overall survival ($p < 0.001$) were significantly better in patients with intermediate-grade NHL who received rituximab as part of salvage chemotherapy within 3 months of autologous HSCT [53]. Conversely, patients treated with upfront chemotherapy plus rituximab may be harder to salvage. In the international CORAL study, some DLCBL patients were less likely to respond to rituximab-containing salvage chemotherapy and proceed to autologous HSCT if they had received rituximab previously [54]. Nevertheless, virtually all investigators would recommend using rituximab with pretransplant chemotherapy if this improves response rates.

Numerous prognostic factors are associated with outcomes following autologous HSCT for aggressive NHL. A PARMA follow-up study, showed that survival following autologous HSCT was not influenced by the age-adjusted IPI, applied at the time of relapse [55]. The overall survival following autologous HSCT for patients with IPI scores of 1–3 was significantly better than patients treated with conventional salvage chemotherapy. However, overall survival following autologous HSCT was not significantly better than salvage chemotherapy for patients with IPI scores of 0. The age-adjusted IPI score was predictive of outcome at MSKCC, however [11]. An analysis from the University of Minnesota also showed that the IPI at relapse correlated with survival following autologous HSCT for DLBCL [56], and the age-adjusted IPI at transplant correlated with survival in an analysis from the Grupo Español de Linformas/Transplante Autólogo de Médula Osea (GEL/TAMO) Spanish Registry [50].

Some of the ambiguities associated with the use of clinical prognostic factors may be overcome by using functional imaging with FDG-PET for predicting response to autologous HSCT for NHL. A retrospective analysis from Belgium found that a negative pretransplant FDG-PET scan for patients with aggressive NHL was associated with significantly better progression-free survival ($p < 0.004$) and overall survival ($p < 0.018$), whereas the IPI was not a significant factor [57]. In another analysis, FDG-PET scan findings were evaluated after conventional salvage chemotherapy prior to planned autologous HSCT [12]. The 2-year failure-free survival was estimated at 72% for FDG-PET-negative patients, 38% for those with partial FDG-PET response, and 10% for nonresponders ($p < 0.001$). A risk score using both FDG-PET response and age-adjusted IPI at relapse was developed. In another study, the actuarial 1-year event-free survival was 79% for patients with aggressive NHL with negative FDG-PET scans prior to autologous HSCT, as compared to 42% for patients with positive scans ($p = 0.007$) [58]. The corresponding 1-year overall survival rates were estimated to be 91% and 38%, respectively ($p < 0.001$).

Although most series of autologous HSCT for aggressive NHL have examined results in relapsed patients, others may also benefit. Transplantation is unlikely to benefit patients who are truly refractory to primary therapy, although registry results show that autologous HSCT may benefit some patients who do not attain a complete remission with initial therapy, especially if they respond to additional salvage therapy. A report from the North American registry examined results of autologous HSCT in patients who did not achieve a complete remission with initial therapy for aggressive lymphoma [17]. The actuarial 5-year progression-free survival and overall survival were 31% and 37%, respectively. A GEL/TAMO analysis showed that overall survival at 5 years was estimated to be 43% for patients with DLBCL who failed to enter complete remission with primary therapy [59]. These results demonstrate that not all patients with "primary refractory" disease have a poor outcome; those who attain a partial response with initial treatment can benefit from autologous HSCT. Conversely, transplantation (either auto- or allogeneic HSCT) of patients with truly chemoresistant NHL is usually not recommended.

15.7.1.1 Transplant in First Remission

Patient-related and tumor-related characteristics can be used to identify patients with DLBCL who are less likely to attain a remission with primary therapy and more likely to relapse [1, 10]. One method to improve results for these patients involves incorporating autologous HSCT into primary therapy or as consolidation therapy.

Phase II trials have demonstrated long-term progression-free survival rates of 60–80% with this approach. Unfortunately most of these trials only reported results for patients who actually underwent autologous HSCT. The outcome of all patients from the time of diagnosis, including those not transplanted (intent to treat), needs to be known to evaluate the merits of upfront transplantation, or else randomized trials must be performed.

Several prospective randomized trials have also evaluated the benefits of upfront or front-line autologous HSCT for patients with aggressive NHL. These trials differ with respect to inclusion criteria, time of randomization, and type of treatment and length of treatment prior to transplantation. In the LNH87-2 trial from Groupe d'Etude des Lymphomes de l'Adulte (GELA), patients with intermediate- and high-grade NHL who had a complete remission with an induction chemotherapy regimen were randomized to treatment with sequential consolidation chemotherapy or to treatment with autologous HSCT [60]. A retrospective subgroup analysis of patients in the high-intermediate and high-risk age-adjusted IPI groups showed that the actuarial 8-year overall survival rate was 49% for patients randomized to receive sequential chemotherapy and 64% for patients randomized to autologous HSCT ($p = 0.04$). Notably, only 61% of patients achieved a complete remission with initial therapy and were eligible for randomization, and only 69% of patients randomized to autologous HSCT underwent transplantation. The 072 trial from Groupe Ouest Est d'Etude des Leucémies et Autres Maladies du Sang (GOELAMS) also evaluated the use of a regimen utilizing autologous HSCT as part of primary therapy for patients with intermediate- and high-grade NHL with a maximum of two risk factors in the age-adjusted IPI [61]. Patients in one arm were randomized to treatment with eight cycles of CHOP (cyclophosphamide, doxorubicin, vincristine, prednisone). The other treatment arm consisted of a novel epirubicin-containing regimen, followed by treatment with methotrexate and cytarabine, followed by high-dose chemotherapy with autologous HSCT. The 5-year event-free survival was estimated at 37% for patients treated with CHOP and 55% for those treated with autologous HSCT ($p = 0.037$). The 5-year overall survival rates were estimated at 56% and 71%, respectively ($p = 0.076$). Among patients in the high-intermediate age-adjusted IPI risk group, the actuarial 5-year event-free survival (56% vs. 28%; $p = 0.003$) and overall survival (74% vs. 44%; $p = 0.001$) were higher in the transplant arm (see Fig. 15.3).

Other trials have failed to show benefits with upfront autologous HSCT, including the phase-III MISTRAL study which compared CHOP with high-dose sequential chemotherapy and autologous HSCT [24]. The role of front-line autologous HSCT in aggressive NHL has been examined in a meta-analysis [62]. Considerable heterogeneity and methodological flaws in the design of the randomized trials and an overall failure to show survival advantages with front-line transplantation were noted. While there is little evidence that this approach benefits good-risk patients, there is some evidence that upfront autologous HSCT may benefit poor-prognosis patients when treated with a full course of conventional chemotherapy, or regimens that yield a high rate of complete remission prior to autologous HSCT. Patients in first remission may be appropriate candidates for clinical trials involving autologous HSCT according to National Comprehensive Cancer Network (NCCN) guidelines. This approach is considered effective by members of the American Society for Blood and Marrow Transplantation (ASBMT) executive committee [63]. It must also be

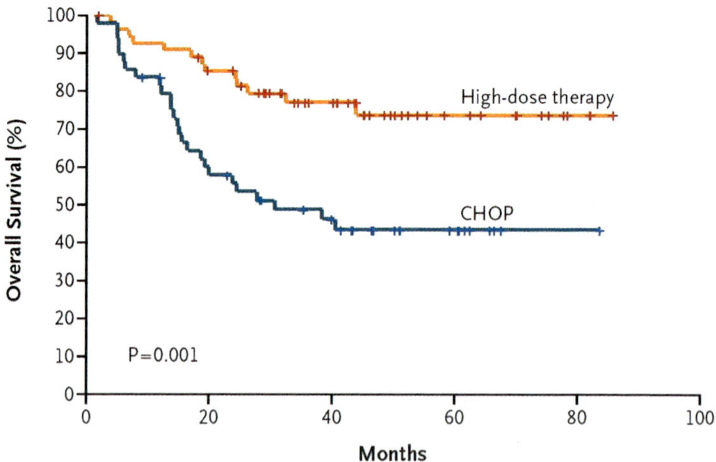

Fig. 15.3 Overall survival for aggressive histology NHL patients with high-intermediate age-adjusted International Prognostic Index (from Milpied et al. [61])

noted that it is now more difficult to identify a poor-prognosis group in rituximab-treated patients, and the results of the previous upfront transplant trials may no longer be valid. The North American Intergroup S9704 trial comparing CHOP plus rituximab (R-CHOP) with R-CHOP followed by autologous HSCT has completed accrual and results are pending. The German High-Grade non-Hodgkin's Lymphoma Study Group trial 2002-1 is also conducting a phase III upfront transplant trial utilizing three autologous HSCT procedures with the MegaCHOEP (rituximab plus cyclophosphamide, doxorubicin, vincristine, etoposide, prednisone) regimen.

15.7.1.2 Allogeneic Hematopoietic Stem Cell Transplantation

Retrospective analyses and phase II trials have examined the use of myeloablative allogeneic HSCT for DLBCL. It is often difficult to interpret results because of treatment heterogeneity and because most studies do not contain uniform populations of patients with DLBCL. Investigators from British Columbia reported that actuarial 5-year event-free survival and overall survival were 43% and 48%, respectively, following allogeneic HSCT for relapsed and refractory aggressive NHL [64]. Some patients had unrelated donors. The 1-year cumulative incidence of nonrelapse mortality was 25%. Patients who developed grade 3–4 acute GvHD and those with short initial remissions had significantly worse outcomes. The 5-year event-free survival for the subgroup with DLCBL was estimated to be 36%. The actuarial 5-year overall survival and progression-free survival were 39% and 36%, respectively, in patients from a nationwide Japanese survey who received myeloablative allogeneic HSCT [65]. This cohort also contained patients with unrelated donors and patients with a prior autologous HSCT. The transplant-related mortality was 42%. Overall survival was poorer in patients with chemotherapy-resistant disease, a prior transplant, and those with previous radiation. The actuarial 5-year survival was 33% (estimated from survival curve) for those with DLBCL.

An EBMT analysis examined results of allogeneic HSCT for patients with intermediate-grade NHL [66]. Approximately 10% of patients had unrelated donors. The 4-year overall survival, progression-free survival, and treatment-related mortality were estimated at 38.3%, 34.6%, and 41.8% respectively. A case-matching study with autologous HSCT recipients was performed and patients with intermediate-grade NHL undergoing allogeneic HSCT were found to have lower relapse rates, but higher transplant-related mortality and significantly worse overall survival. An analysis from Johns Hopkins University also compared results of auto- and allogeneic HSCT for relapsed DLBCL [67]. Patients under age 60 with matched siblings generally received allogeneic transplants. The actuarial 3-year event-free survival was 19.1% following allogeneic HSCT, as compared to 30.9% following autologous HSCT ($p = 0.2$). The actuarial 3-year overall survival rates were 23.7% and 33.1%, respectively ($p = 0.17$) (see Fig. 15.4). The transplant-related mortality rates were 51.1% and 23.9%, respectively ($p < 0.001$). The actuarial 3-year overall survival

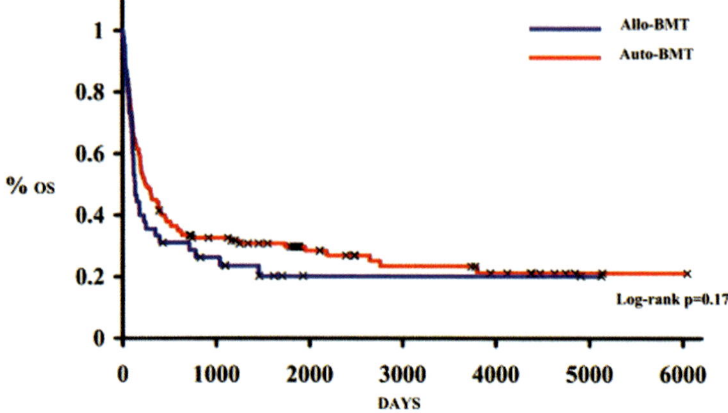

Fig. 15.4 Overall survival following hematopoietic stem cell transplantation for relapsed diffuse large B-cell lymphoma (from Aksentijevich et al. [67])

following allogeneic HSCT for patients with resistant disease was 12.1%, as compared to 19.1% following autologous HSCT ($p = 0.08$). This demonstrates that prognostic factors are similar for patients undergoing autologous HSCT or allogeneic HSCT, and that allogeneic HSCT for poor-risk patients is not necessarily better.

These studies demonstrate that myeloablative allogeneic HSCT can cure patients with relapsed and refractory aggressive NHL. Although relapse rates following allogeneic HSCT are lower than relapse rates following autologous HSCT, survival advantages have not been demonstrated in most cases because of increased transplant-related mortality due to regimen-related toxicity and GvHD. These results do not allow us to determine which patients with DLCBL are appropriate candidates for myeloablative allogeneic HSCT, and use of this approach is unlikely to increase greatly due to increased use of RIC allogeneic HSCT.

Reduced-intensity allogeneic HSCT for DLBCL has been examined in several series. The ability to exploit potential GvLym effects with this treatment is limited by the inability to avoid the complications of GvHD. In addition, GvLym effects are less potent in patients with aggressive histology, high tumor burdens, or rapid growth rates. In an EBMT analysis of RIC allogeneic HSCT, the 1-year overall survival, progression-free survival, and transplant-related mortality for patients with aggressive lymphomas were estimated at 52%, 32%, and 30%, respectively [68]. The 2-year progression-free survival was estimated at 12.9%. The risk of progressive disease was significantly higher in patients with aggressive histology when compared to patients with indolent NHL, and results were poorer in patients with resistant disease. An analysis of RIC allogeneic HSCT from Seattle also noted that relapse rates were higher if patients were not in remission at the time of transplant, although relapse rates were low for all histologic subtypes if patients were in complete remission prior

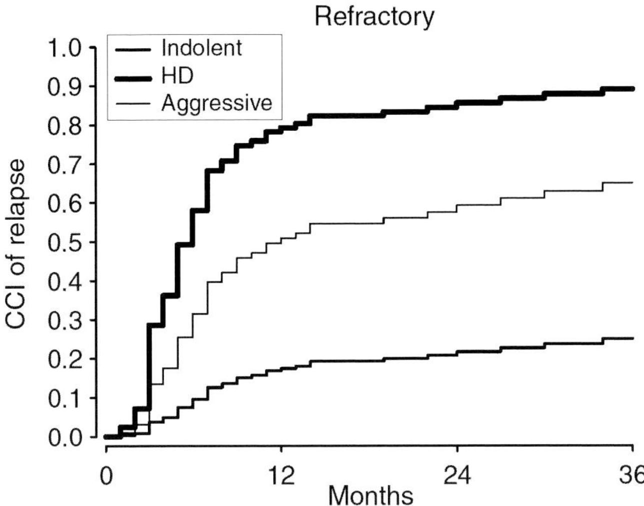

Fig. 15.5 Cumulative incidence of relapse following reduced-intensity allogeneic hematopoietic stem cell transplantation for lymphoma (from Corradini et al. [70])

to transplantation [69]. The 3-year cumulative incidence of relapse was 68% for patients with aggressive histology NHL in the Italian registry who received RIC allogeneic HSCT with refractory disease, suggesting that this treatment is less likely to benefit these patients (see Fig. 15.5) [70]. A report from the United Kingdom also noted that patients with aggressive histology had a significantly higher risk of relapse and lower event-free survival following RIC allogeneic HSCT [71].

A retrospective analysis from the City of Hope compared the results of RIC allogeneic HSCT and myeloablative allogeneic HSCT for NHL [72]. The 2-year relapse rate for patients with intermediate-grade NHL following RIC allogeneic HSCT was 44%, as compared with 12% following myeloablative conditioning ($p = 0.02$). However, the actuarial 2-year progression-free survival rates were 31% and 44% ($p = 0.83$), and overall survival was 36% and 50%, respectively ($p = 0.32$).

These results demonstrate that patients with DLCBL and other aggressive histologic subtypes may also benefit from RIC allogeneic HSCT. The best outcomes are in patients with chemotherapy-sensitive disease who are transplanted with low tumor burden. The relapse rate appears to be higher following RIC, as compared with myeloablative allogeneic HSCT. This suggests that despite the role of GvLym, the chemotherapy regimen itself must not be neglected as an important component of tumor eradication. There are some patients with aggressive NHL who are probably more likely to benefit from myeloablative conditioning, such as those with refractory disease or significant tumor burdens, although appropriate candidates are not clearly defined.

15.7.2 Follicular Lymphoma

A large number of reports have examined the results of autologous HSCT for relapsed and refractory follicular lymphoma. Other indolent NHL subtypes are often included in these analyses. A retrospective study examined the outcome of patients with follicular lymphoma who progressed following treatment on the GELA prospective GELF 86 protocol [73]. The 5-year freedom from treatment failure was estimated at 42% for patients treated with autologous HSCT, as compared to 16% for patients treated with conventional salvage therapy ($p = 0.0001$). The 5-year overall survival rates were 58% and 38%, respectively ($p = 0.0002$). A retrospective single-institution study from France used patients as their own controls to compare the event-free survival following autologous HSCT for follicular lymphoma with the event-free survival following treatment prior to transplantation [74]. There were fewer patients with recurrent disease within 5 years of transplant ($p < 0.01$), and the event-free survival following autologous HSCT was longer than the most recent conventional treatment ($p < 0.01$).

Several long-term follow-up studies of autologous HSCT for patients with relapsed and refractory follicular or low-grade lymphoma have been reported recently [75–79]. Although a continuous pattern of relapse typical of follicular lymphoma is noted in many of these trials, it appears that 20–50% of patients experience long-term progression-free survival. Outcome appears best in younger, chemotherapy-sensitive patients. The groups from Dana-Farber Cancer Institute and St. Bartholomew's Hospital recently reported long-term follow-up results of purged autologous BMT for follicular lymphoma patients in second or subsequent remission [78]. The actuarial 10-year progression-free survival and overall survival were 48% and 54%, respectively, and there also was evidence of a late plateau in remission (see Fig. 15.6). Remission duration ($p < 0.001$) and overall survival ($p = 0.02$) among patients transplanted in second remission were significantly better than historical controls treated with conventional chemotherapy. These results must be examined in light of the significant risk of secondary MDS/AML, particularly following TBI conditioning (see below).

The randomized European CUP trial compared the results of autologous HSCT and conventional salvage chemotherapy for patients with relapsed follicular lymphoma in a study design that was similar to the PARMA trial [42]. Patients with relapsed or progressive follicular lymphoma who were chemotherapy-sensitive were then randomized to continued treatment with salvage chemotherapy or to treatment with high-dose therapy followed by auto-BMT. Transplanted patients were also randomized to receive either purged or unpurged marrow. Although the trial was closed early, the 2-year progression-free survival was estimated to be 26% for patients receiving chemotherapy salvage, as compared to 58% for patients transplanted with purged marrow, and 55% for those receiving unpurged marrow. The actuarial 4-year overall survival rates were 46%, 71%, and 77%, respectively. Progression-free survival ($p = 0.0009$) and overall survival ($p = 0.026$) were higher

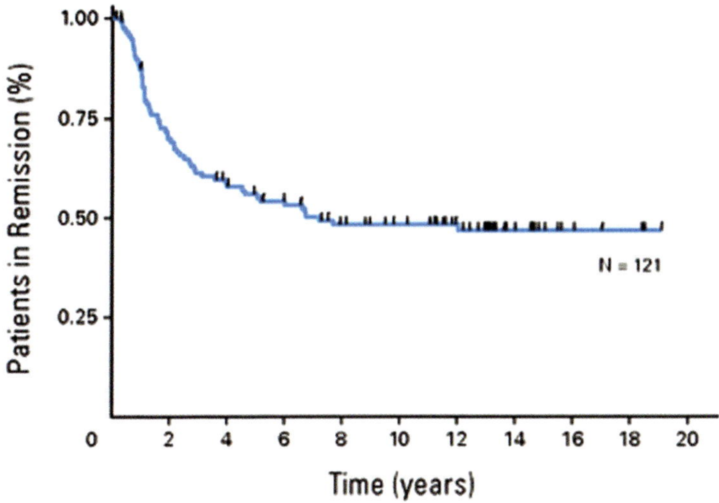

Fig. 15.6 Remission duration following autologous bone marrow transplantation for follicular lymphoma (from Rohatiner et al. [78])

in transplanted patients, although no benefits were associated with purging (see above).

These results demonstrate that autologous HSCT is a reasonable option for patients with relapsed follicular lymphoma, although the applicability of these results is confounded by the widespread use of rituximab with primary therapy and the introduction of new treatments such as radiolabeled antibodies.

Some trials of autologous HSCT for follicular lymphoma have included only follicular lymphoma grades 1 and 2. Other trials have included patients with follicular lymphoma grade 3, which may have a clinical behavior more closely related to DLBCL. In a retrospective analysis from the City of Hope, the actuarial 10-year disease-free survival following autologous HSCT for follicular large cell lymphoma was 27%, as compared to 38% for patients with DLBCL ($p = 0.70$) [80]. The actuarial 10-year overall survival rates were 58% and 46%, respectively ($p = 0.27$). Both survival curves had a similar appearance and displayed evidence of a plateau. At the University of Nebraska, the actuarial 5-year progression-free survival following autologous HSCT was 47%, 49%, and 36% for follicular lymphoma grades 1, 2, and 3, respectively [77]. The actuarial 5-year overall survival rates were 61%, 70%, and 57%, respectively. Follicular grade 3 histology was associated with poorer progression-free survival ($p = 0.004$) and overall survival ($p = 0.01$).

15.7.2.1 Transplant in First Remission

Like aggressive lymphomas, upfront autologous HSCT has also been investigated for patients with follicular lymphoma. Long-term follow-up of phase II studies investigating the role of upfront transplantation following CHOP or CHOP-like regimens demonstrate that long-term progression-free survival is possible [41]. Upfront autologous HSCT for follicular lymphoma has been evaluated in three randomized trials.

A German Low-Grade Lymphoma Study Group trial randomized patients who responded to four to six cycles of CHOP-like therapy to receive treatment with additional chemotherapy followed by autologous HSCT, or to treatment with additional CHOP-like chemotherapy followed by interferon maintenance [81]. The 5-year progression-free survival was estimated at 62% for patients randomized to autologous HSCT, as compared to 36% for those randomized to interferon maintenance ($p < 0.0001$). Overall survival results were not reported for each treatment arm. The GOELAMS conducted another trial in which patients in the standard treatment arm received six cycles of anthracycline-based therapy [82]. Responders received six additional cycles of chemotherapy with interferon. Patients in the experimental arm were treated with another anthracycline-based regimen and responders received additional conventional chemotherapy and then autologous HSCT. The 5-year event-free survival was estimated to be 48% in the standard treatment arm and 60% in the transplant arm ($p = 0.050$). The corresponding overall survival rates were 84% and 78%, respectively ($p = 0.49$). The lack of a difference in survival was attributed to an excess of secondary malignancies in the transplant arm. A third randomized trial was conducted by GELA [83]. In this trial patients were randomized between treatment with an anthracycline-based regimen plus interferon, or to treatment with CHOP followed by autologous HSCT. The actuarial 7-year event-free survival rate was 28% in the standard treatment arm and 38% in the transplant arm ($p = 0.11$). Actuarial overall survival was 71% and 76%, respectively ($p = 0.53$) (see Fig. 15.7).

All of these trials fail to show definite evidence of a plateau in progression-free survival or differences in overall survival associated with upfront autologous HSCT for follicular lymphoma. Furthermore, randomized trials have not

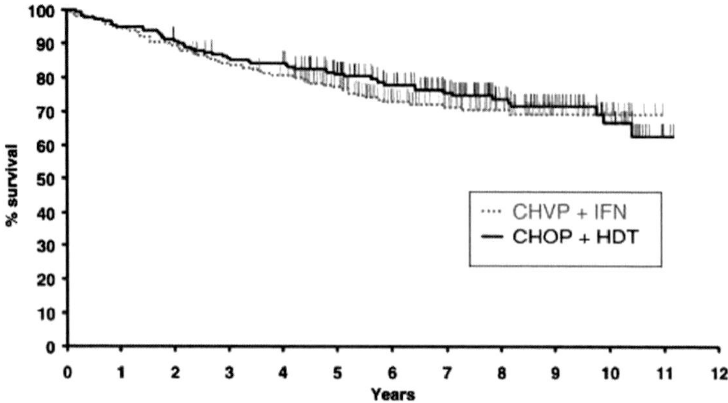

Fig. 15.7 Overall survival for follicular lymphoma (from Sebban et al. [83])

been performed in rituximab-treated patients, and interpretation of results is further complicated by the availability of new treatments. Thus, the use of autologous HSCT for follicular NHL in first remission cannot be considered standard therapy and should probably be performed only in the context of a clinical trial.

15.7.2.2 Transformed Lymphoma

The prognosis for patients with follicular lymphoma following histologic transformation is poor. Several reports have evaluated the results of autologous HSCT for transformed lymphomas and demonstrate that prolonged event-free survival can be observed. In a retrospective analysis from Ottawa, the actuarial 5-year progression-free survival following autologous HSCT was 25% for patients with transformed follicular lymphoma, as compared to 56% for patients that had not undergone transformation ($p = 0.007$) [76]. The actuarial 5-year overall survival rates were 56% and 72%, respectively ($p = 0.33$). A retrospective analysis from the Cleveland Clinic compared the results of autologous HSCT for patients with transformed and de-novo DLBCL [84]. No significant differences in 4-year event-free survival (38% vs. 37%), or overall survival (61% vs. 53%) were observed. A case-matching study from the EBMT also compared results of autologous HSCT for transformed and de-novo intermediate- and high-grade NHL [85]. No significant differences in progression-free survival or overall survival were observed. These results indicate that autologous HSCT is a reasonable option for patients with transformed follicular lymphoma, although ^{131}I-tositumomab and ^{90}Y-ibritumomab tiuxetan are approved for this indication. Allogeneic HSCT has also been used for patients with transformed NHL [86].

15.7.2.3 Allogeneic Hematopoietic Stem Cell Transplantation

There is little experience with allogeneic HSCT for follicular lymphoma in first remission; this modality has been used almost exclusively for patients with relapsed and refractory disease. An analysis from the International Bone Marrow Transplant Registry (IBMTR) examined the outcome of myeloablative allogeneic HSCT in patients with low-grade (mostly follicular) NHL [87]. The actuarial 3-year disease-free survival and overall survival were each 49%. The risk of recurrence was 16% and there was evidence of a plateau in disease-free survival. Similar results were observed in a series of patients from British Columbia who had myeloablative allogeneic HSCT for relapsed and refractory follicular lymphoma [88]. The 5-year overall survival and event-free survival were estimated to be 58% and 53%, respectively. The cumulative incidence of nonrelapse mortality and disease progression were 23% and 24%, respectively.

Several reports have compared the results of autologous and myeloablative allogeneic HSCT for follicular and low-grade NHL. In an EBMT analysis, the

4-year progression-free survival and overall survival following myeloablative allogeneic HSCT were estimated to be 42.7% and 51.1%, respectively [66]. The procedure-related mortality was 38%. Chemotherapy sensitivity was associated with a significantly lower relapse rate and longer survival. A case-matching study demonstrated that the risk of relapse was lower following allogeneic HSCT, although overall survival was better in patients treated with autologous HSCT. An analysis from the IBMTR/Autologous Blood and Marrow Transplant Registry also compared the results of autologous and myeloablative allogeneic HSCT for follicular lymphoma [40]. The risk of disease recurrence following allogeneic HSCT was 54% lower than those treated with unpurged autologous HSCT ($p < 0.001$). However, the risk of treatment-related mortality was 4.4-fold higher in allogeneic HSCT recipients ($p < 0.001$). The 5-year actuarial survival following allogeneic HSCT, purged autologous HSCT, and unpurged autologous HSCT were 51%, 62%, and 55% (see Fig. 15.8). There was evidence of a plateau following allogeneic HSCT, while recipients of autologous HSCT exhibited a continuous pattern of treatment failure. This suggests that patients may need to be followed for several years to demonstrate a survival advantage associated with allogeneic HSCT. It is also noteworthy that results of HSCT improved over time, and caution should be used when comparing any results to historical controls. A retrospective analysis from M.D. Anderson Cancer Center (MDACC) also compared results of autologous and allogeneic HSCT for indolent NHL [89]. The rate of disease progression was 74% in the autologous HSCT group, as compared with 19% in the allogeneic HSCT group ($p = 0.003$). The 100-day mortality was 34% and 6%, respectively, however ($p < 0.001$). The overall survival rate following allogeneic HSCT was 49%, as compared to 34% following autologous HSCT ($p > 0.05$). The survival curve following allogeneic HSCT reached a plateau, while a continuous pattern of progression was observed following autologous HSCT.

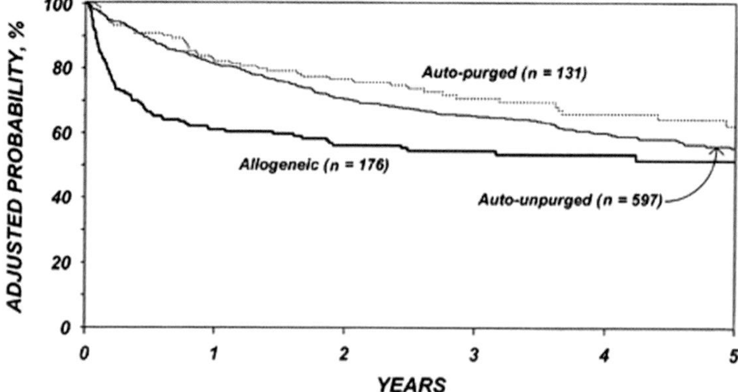

Fig. 15.8 Overall survival following hematopoietic stem cell transplantation for follicular lymphoma (from van Besien et al. [40])

Allogeneic HSCT following myeloablative conditioning is capable of curing follicular NHL, although this approach is associated with high rates of treatment-related mortality. These results provide a strong rationale for the use of RIC allogeneic HSCT for these patients, because of the high chemotherapy sensitivity and radiation sensitivity of these patients and the relatively modest growth rate of these tumors that allows GvLym effects to be realized.

A report from Seattle investigated the use of NMA allogeneic HSCT for patients with indolent NHL [86]. The 3-year progression-free survival and overall survival were estimated to be 52% and 43%, respectively. Somewhat surprisingly, the rate of relapse was not influenced by the pretransplant remission status. Similar results of RIC-allogeneic HSCT for follicular NHL have been reported by other groups [68, 70, 71]. A retrospective analysis from the French registry showed that 3-year event-free survival and overall survival following RIC allogeneic HSCT for low-grade NHL were 51% and 56%, respectively [90]. The treatment-related mortality was 40%. A CIBMTR analysis comparing myeloablative and RIC allogeneic HSCT for follicular lymphoma found no significant differences in transplant-related mortality, progression-free survival, or overall survival [91]. In this study, the 3-year progression/relapse rate was 9% following myeloablative conditioning, as compared with 21% for patients receiving reduced-intensity conditioning ($p = 0.03$).

These results, while encouraging, do not allow us to determine the optimal timing of allogeneic HSCT for follicular lymphoma and do not allow us to determine the role of myeloablative conditioning. The latter approach may still be warranted in many patients, especially those without comorbidities and those with substantial tumor burdens. The majority of trials are from the "pre-rituximab" era and management decisions are more difficult because of the large number of nontransplant options for these patients. The high non-relapse mortality suggests that allogeneic HSCT should probably not be used in first remission, although heavily-treated patients and those with large tumor burdens are also unlikely to benefit. The high early mortality associated with allogeneic HSCT suggests that patients will need to be observed for several years to demonstrate potential survival advantages when compared to autologous HSCT. A phase III trial from the BMT CTN comparing autologous HSCT with RIC allogeneic HSCT for relapsed and refractory follicular NHL is ongoing.

15.7.3 Mantle Cell Lymphoma

In general, the prognosis for patients with mantle cell lymphoma is poor. Although front-line chemotherapy regimens yield high response rates, there is a continuous pattern of relapse and median survival is 3–4 years. Response rates are improved by adding rituximab to standard chemotherapy regimens, although it is not known if survival is prolonged, and even patients who achieve complete remission are not considered to be cured.

The use of autologous HSCT for relapsed and refractory mantle cell lymphoma has been evaluated in phase II trials and retrospective analyses [92–94]. Results are better in chemotherapy-sensitive patients who are transplanted earlier in the course of the disease. However, overall results are disappointing and the majority of trials show a continuous pattern of relapse without evidence of a plateau in survival curves.

15.7.3.1 Transplant in First Remission

Because of the poor results of primary therapy for mantle cell lymphoma and the disappointing results of autologous HSCT for relapsed patients, attention has been directed at using transplantation for patients in first remission. Registry data and retrospective analyses show that results of autologous HSCT for patients with mantle cell lymphoma in first remission are better than results of autologous HSCT for relapsed and refractory patients [92, 93]. However, the results of any treatment are likely to be better if used early in the course of disease.

Investigators from MDACC reported the outcome of 25 mantle cell lymphoma patients who were treated with Hyper-CVAD (cyclophosphamide, doxorubicin, vincristine, dexamethasone alternating with cytarabine, methotrexate) followed by HSCT (four allogeneic) in first remission [95]. The actuarial 3-year event-free survival was 72%, as compared with 28% for historical controls treated with CHOP-like regimens ($p = 0.0001$). The actuarial overall survival rates were 92% and 56%, respectively ($p = 0.05$). A matched-pair analysis from Canada also analyzed results of a phase II trial incorporating autologous HSCT for newly-diagnosed patients with mantle cell lymphoma [96]. Results were remarkably similar to the MDACC results. The 3-year progression-free survival was estimated at 89% for patients transplanted in first remission, as compared with 29% for historical controls ($p < 0.00001$). The actuarial 3-year overall survival rates were 88% and 65%, respectively ($p = 0.052$). An Italian multi-center trial investigated the use of high-dose sequential chemotherapy with autologous HSCT for patients with newly-diagnosed mantle cell lymphoma [97]. The actuarial 54-month event-free survival was 79%, as compared to 18% for historical controls who were treated with CHOP-like therapy ($p = 0.027$). The actuarial overall survival rates were 89% and 42%, respectively ($p < 0.0001$).

The only prospective randomized trial of frontline autologous HSCT for mantle cell lymphoma was reported by the European Mantle Cell Lymphoma Network [98]. Patients who responded to CHOP-like induction therapy were randomized to maintenance treatment with interferon or to treatment with high-dose therapy followed by autologous HSCT. The median time to treatment failure was 29 months in patients randomized to autologous HSCT, as compared to 15 months for patients randomized to interferon maintenance

($p = 0.0023$). The actuarial 3-year progression-free survival rates were 62% and 27% respectively ($p = 0.019$). However, the actuarial 3-year overall survival rates were 76% and 68%, respectively ($p = 0.16$). No evidence of a survival plateau in progression-free survival was noted in either arm. No significant differences in progression-free survival were noted when patients who received initial therapy with CHOP were compared to those treated with R-CHOP.

The role of autologous HSCT for mantle cell lymphoma is unresolved. It is not clear that any patients are cured with this approach, even when utilized as part of primary therapy. The introduction of new agents, such as proteasome inhibitors, has increased therapeutic options.

15.7.3.2 Allogeneic Hematopoietic Stem Cell Transplantation

Although autologous HSCT may benefit selected patients with mantle cell lymphoma, it is not certain that any patients are cured. Most trials show a continuous pattern of relapse, especially for patients not transplanted in remission. These results provide a rationale for allogeneic HSCT for patients with mantle cell lymphoma.

Interpretation of results of myeloablative allogeneic HSCT is hampered by the fact that these cases are often grouped within larger series of "aggressive" or "high-grade" NHL. Nevertheless, several groups have reported results of series containing only patients with mantle cell lymphoma. In a series of mantle cell lymphoma patients from MDACC treated with allogeneic HSCT (including two with RIC), the 3-year overall survival and failure-from-progression were each estimated to be 55% [99]. Outcomes were significantly better in patients with chemotherapy-sensitive disease, and there was a trend toward improved survival in a subgroup of patients transplanted in first remission. Investigators from Johns Hopkins performed a retrospective comparison of results from auto- or allogeneic HSCT for mantle cell lymphoma [93]. Younger patients with matched sibling donors generally received allogeneic transplants, and most patients were transplanted in first complete or partial remission. The median event-free survival following autologous- and allogeneic HSCT was 43 months and 5.5 months, respectively ($p = 0.005$). A multivariate analysis revealed that the risk of treatment failure was significantly higher in patients transplanted with relapsed and refractory disease. The 3-year event-free survival was approximately 70% in each group when results of patients transplanted in first remission were examined ($p = 0.38$). A retrospective analysis from the University of Nebraska also compared results of auto- and myeloablative allogeneic HSCT for mantle cell lymphoma [94]. The 5-year event-free survival was estimated at 44% following allogeneic HSCT, as compared with 39% following autologous HSCT ($p = 0.85$). The corresponding relapse rates were 21% and 56%, respectively ($p = 0.11$). Overall survival was estimated to be 49% and 47%, respectively (see Fig. 15.9).

These small series fail to show definite survival advantages following myeloablative allogeneic HSCT for mantle cell lymphoma, although difference may

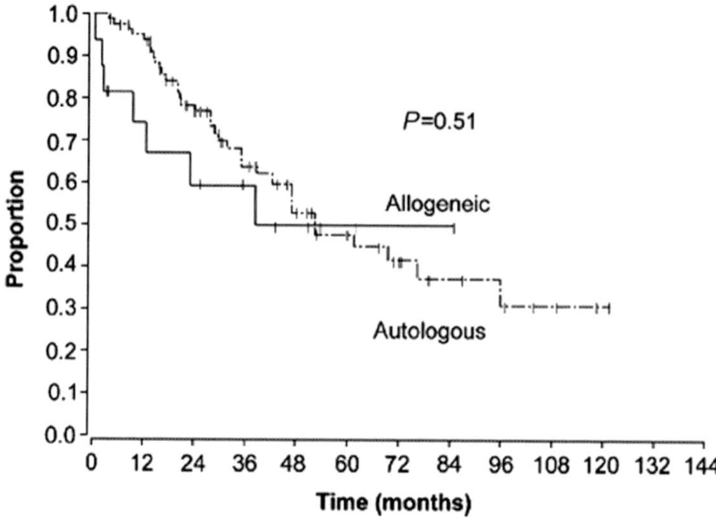

Fig. 15.9 Overall survival following hematopoietic stem cell transplantation for mantle cell lymphoma (from Ganti et al. [94])

be observed with longer follow-up. Many investigators are now examining the role of RIC allogeneic HSCT for these patients. The actuarial 2-year progression-free survival and overall survival in a series of mantle cell lymphoma patients undergoing NMA allogeneic HSCT from Seattle were 60% and 64%, respectively [100]. The actuarial 2-year nonrelapse mortality was 24% in this cohort, which included a high percentage of patients who had unrelated donors and those who had failed a prior autologous HSCT. The 2-year cumulative incidence of relapse was 16%. More recently, the same investigators analyzed relapse rates following RIC-allogeneic HSCT in patients with various hematological malignancies [69]. The relapse risk for patients with mantle cell lymphoma was similar to patients with low-grade NHL, and was not related to remission status. These results provide evidence for a GvLym effect in these patients. The group from MDACC has also reported results of RIC allogeneic HSCT for mantle cell lymphoma [101]. A large fraction of these patients also received transplants from unrelated donors and had progressed following autologous HSCT. The estimated 3-year survival was 85.5%. Some patients who progressed after transplantation attained another remission following donor lymphocyte infusion.

In contrast to these results, the 1-year probability of disease progression was estimated to be 48% for mantle cell lymphoma patients treated with RIC allogeneic HSCT in an EBMT registry analysis [68]. The actuarial 2-year progression-free survival and overall survival were 0% and 12.8%, respectively. The actuarial 3-year progression-free survival and overall survival were 33% and 45%, respectively among patients in the Italian registry who received RIC allogeneic HSCT for mantle cell lymphoma [70]. The risk of disease progression or death was approximately 2- to 2.5-fold higher than patients with indolent NHL.

In a retrospective City of Hope analysis, the 2-year relapse rate following RIC allogeneic HSCT for mantle cell lymphoma was 60%, as compared with 20% following myeloablative conditioning ($p = 0.05$) [72]. The actuarial 2-year progression-free survival was 20% and 40%, respectively ($p = 0.36$). Overall survival rates were 30% and 50%, respectively ($p = 0.6$).

These conflicting results make it difficult to make firm recommendations regarding the timing and type of transplantation for mantle cell lymphoma. The use of allogeneic HSCT may be reasonable in situations where autologous HSCT is unlikely to be beneficial, such as patients with relapsed disease. Although some reports have suggested that disease status is less important [69], it seems unlikely that RIC-allogeneic HSCT will cure a significant fraction of patients with advanced or refractory disease, and efforts should be made to produce a state of minimal tumor burden prior to transplantation. It is possible that these patients are more likely to benefit from myeloablative conditioning, although transplant-related mortality may be higher. There is a rationale for testing the role of RIC-allogeneic HSCT for patients in first remission, especially younger patients with adverse prognostic factors. Alternatively, autologous HSCT in first remission, followed by RIC-allogeneic HSCT at relapse may be a better strategy.

15.7.4 Peripheral T-Cell Lymphoma

Approximately 10–15% of lymphomas in western countries are classified as peripheral T-cell lymphoma (PTCL). These lymphomas comprise a heterogeneous group of lymphoid neoplasms. Some, such as anaplastic large cell lymphoma, have a prognosis that is comparable to DLBCL. The most common subtype of PTCL is peripheral T-cell lymphoma, unspecified (PTCL-U, PTCL-NOS). The prognosis for these patients is significantly worse than DLCBL. Interpretation of results of autologous HSCT for relapsed and refractory PTCL is often difficult because reports often contain various types of PTCL with different behaviors. In addition, series frequently contain large numbers of patients treated in first remission.

A retrospective registry analysis from the British Society of Bone Marrow Transplantation (BSBMT) and the Australasian Bone Marrow Transplant Recipient Registry (ABMTRR) reported results of autologous HSCT for PTCL [102]. The actuarial 3-year overall survival and progression-free survival were 53% and 50%, respectively, although 48% of patients were transplanted in first remission. Overall survival was significantly better in patients with chemotherapy-sensitive disease and in patients with anaplastic large cell histology. Patients with PTCL-NOS had a significantly worse outcome. The actuarial 5-year survival and progression-free survival were 54% and 44%, respectively, in a nationwide survey of autologous HSCT for PTCL from Finland [103]. In

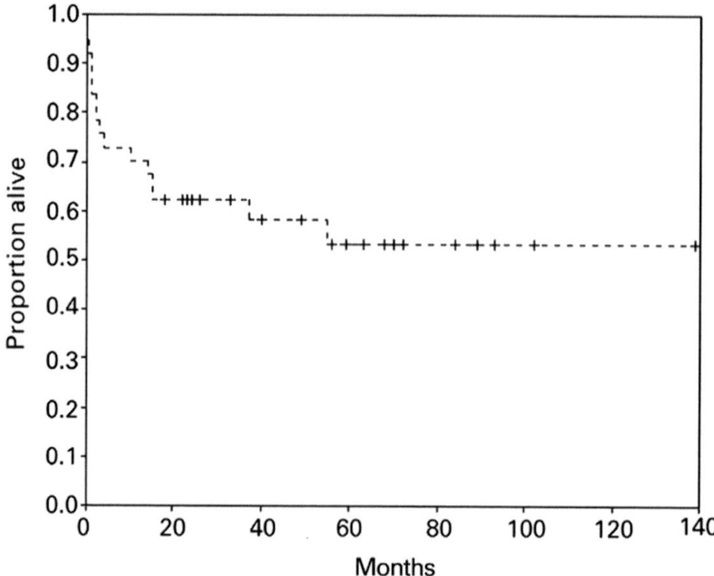

Fig. 15.10 Overall survival following autologous hematopoietic stem cell transplantation for anaplastic large cell lymphoma (solid line) and peripheral T-cell lymphoma, not otherwise specified (dashed line) (from Jantunen et al. [103])

this series, 49% of patients were transplanted in first complete or partial remission. The actuarial 5-year overall survival was 85% for patients with anaplastic large cell lymphoma, as compared to 35% for patients with other histologic subtypes ($p = 0.007$) (see Fig. 15.10). Another analysis of autologous HSCT for PTCL was reported from GEL/TAMO [104]. The actuarial 5-year survival and time to treatment failure for relapsed and refractory patients were 45% and 39%, respectively. A low IPI score was associated with longer time to treatment failure.

Results of autologous HSCT for patients with relapsed and refractory PTCL have been reported by other institutions [105–107]. Patients with anaplastic large cell histology appear to have a better prognosis than patients with other types of PTCL [105, 106]. The 10-year overall survival and progression-free survival following autologous HSCT for anaplastic large cell lymphoma was estimated to be 70% and 47%, respectively in an EBMT analysis [108]. Investigators from Toronto compared the results of autologous HSCT for patients with PTCL and patients with DLCBL [106]. The actuarial 3-year event-free survival for patients with anaplastic large cell lymphoma was 67%, as compared to 42% for patients with DLCBL ($p = 0.41$). The actuarial 3-year event-free survival for patients with PTCL-NOS was 23%, which was significantly worse than DLCBL ($p = 0.028$). In another analysis, the actuarial 3-year survival following autologous HSCT for patients with anaplastic large cell lymphoma was 79%, as compared to 44% for other types of PTCL ($p = 0.08$)

[105]. Investigators from Vanderbilt University also examined results of HSCT (autologous and allogeneic) for PTCL [109]. The actuarial 3-year overall survival for patients with anaplastic large cell lymphoma was 86%, as compared to 36% for historical controls with DLCBL ($p = 0.0034$). Patients with anaplastic large cell lymphoma that expressed anaplastic lymphoma kinase (ALK^+) had significantly better event-free survival and overall survival than ALK-negative patients. In contrast, an analysis from MSKCC showed no significant differences in progression-free survival and overall survival when the results of autologous HSCT for PTCL and DLCBL were compared in a cohort that excluded ALK^+ anaplastic large cell lymphomas [107].

15.7.4.1 Transplant in First Remission

The relatively poor prognosis following autologous HSCT for relapsed and refractory PTCL, especially nonanaplastic large cell histology, has led to use of transplantation for patients in first remission. It is not surprising that retrospective analyses have generally shown that results of autologous HSCT for PTCL patients in first remission are better than results for relapsed and refractory patients [102–104]. As noted before, these observations are biased and provide little information about the merits of upfront transplantation.

A GELA trial examined the prognostic factors of 52 patients with T-cell lymphomas in the LNH-87 trial [60] and the subsequent LNH93-3 trial who achieved complete remission with induction chemotherapy and were consolidated with autologous HSCT [110]. The actuarial 5-year disease-free survival and overall survival for patients with anaplastic T-cell lymphoma was 77%, and 91%, respectively. These results were not statistically different than the results from patients with DLCBL. However, the actuarial 5-year disease-free survival and overall survival for patients with nonanaplastic T-cell lymphomas transplanted in first remission were only 44% and 54%, respectively ($p = 0.0006$). In another trial, these same patients were compared with matched controls in the GELA database that were treated with chemotherapy alone [111]. The actuarial 5-year overall survival was estimated to be 78% for patients with B-cell lymphomas who had age-adjusted IPI scores of 2–3, as compared 72% for matched controls who received chemotherapy ($p = 0.04$). However, autologous HSCT in first remission did not benefit patients with nonanaplastic T-cell lymphomas (actuarial 5-year overall survival 49% vs. 44%; $p = 0.87$). Updated results of a retrospective GEL/TAMO analysis of autologous HSCT for patients with PTCL in first remission have been published [112]. The actuarial 5-year overall survival and progression-free survival were 68% and 63%, respectively. The actuarial 5-year survival was 84% for patients with anaplastic large cell lymphoma, as compared with 61% for others ($p = 0.058$). The actuarial 5-year progression-free survival was 80% and 55%, respectively ($p = 0.036$).

No randomized trials of autologous HSCT for PTCL in first remission have been reported, although preliminary results of a phase II trial from Germany have been updated [113]. In this trial, patients who responded to CHOP chemotherapy received additional induction therapy followed by high-dose therapy and autologous HSCT. With a 10-month median follow-up 22 of 33 transplanted patients (67%) were projected to be in continuous remission following transplantation. It must be noted that 39% of patients did not proceed to autologous HSCT because of toxicity or progressive disease. The results of upfront autologous HSCT in two Italian phase II trials have also been reported [25]. Overall, 46 of 62 patients (74%) were able to proceed to autologous HSCT. The actuarial 12-year overall survival and event-free survival were 34% and 30%, respectively. The 12-year overall survival was estimated at 62% for patients with ALK$^+$ anaplastic large cell lymphoma, as compared to 21% for others ($p = 0.005$). The event-free survival rates were 54% and 18%, respectively ($p = 0.006$). The outcome of patients with PTCL-U was similar to other non ALK$^+$ patients. A GEL-TAMO trial evaluated the use of a high-dose CHOP regimen followed by autologous HSCT [114]. Twenty-seven percent of patients did not proceed to autologous HSCT because of toxicity, disease progression, or refusal. The 3-year progression-free survival and overall survival for all patients was estimated to be 73% and 53%, respectively.

The conflicting results of these trials indicate that well designed trials are necessary to evaluate the role of autologous HSCT for PTCL. Results for patients with relapsed anaplastic large cell lymphoma, especially if ALK$^+$, appear comparable to results of DLBCL. The results for PTCL-U and other subtypes are worse and better treatments are needed. The results of upfront autologous HSCT are also disappointing for nonanaplastic subtypes and randomized trials must be performed to evaluate this type of treatment.

15.7.4.2 Allogeneic Hematopoietic Stem Cell Transplantation

The poor results of autologous HSCT for PTCL provide a rationale for the use of allogeneic HSCT for these patients. In a retrospective review from British Columbia four of five patients with PTCL were alive and free of disease between 90 and 135 months following myeloablative allogeneic HSCT [64]. A retrospective analysis from the BSBMT and ABMTRR examined the results of myeloablative allogeneic HSCT in 18 patients with T-cell lymphomas [102]. The 3-year transplant-related mortality was 39%, and median survival was only 2.5 months. The 3-year progression-free survival and overall survival were estimated to be 33% and 39%, respectively. The actuarial 3-year overall survival following myeloablative allogeneic HSCT was 69% (estimated from survival curve) for 22 patients with PTCL-U in a report from Japan [65]. The median survival was 10.6 months following allogeneic HSCT for PTCL in a small series from Germany [115]. The 1-year actuarial survival was 40%, as compared to 58% for patients treated with autologous HSCT ($p = 0.66$).

The use of RIC allogeneic HSCT for PTCL has also been investigated. Seventeen patients with relapsed and refractory disease were treated on a phase II trial of RIC allogeneic HSCT in Italy [116]. Approximately half had been treated previously with autologous HSCT. The actuarial 3-year progression-free survival and overall survival were 64% and 81%, respectively. The estimated 2-year probability of nonrelapse mortality was 6%. Some patients who progressed after transplant responded to donor lymphocyte infusions. The actuarial 2-year survival was 100% among five patients with PTCL who received RIC-allogeneic HSCT in a United Kingdom study [71], and 6 of 10 patients with T-cell lymphomas were reported to be in remission following RIC allogeneic HSCT in another report from Germany [117]. In an analysis of RIC-allogeneic HSCT from the Italian registry, no significant differences in relapse risk and overall survival were observed when results of patients with aggressive B-cell NHL and T-cell NHL were compared [70]. A retrospective analysis from the City of Hope found no significant differences in outcome among patients with T-cell lymphomas who were treated with myeloablative allogeneic HSCT and those who received RIC allogeneic HSCT [72].

The results of primary treatment for PTCL are disappointing. The results of autologous HSCT are also disappointing, especially for patients with nonanaplastic histology. It is hoped that well designed trials will evaluate the role of upfront autologous HSCT for these patients. The results of allogeneic HSCT are promising, particularly when RIC-allogeneic HSCT is used.

15.8 Late Complications of Hematopoietic Stem Cell Transplantation

A variety of nonrelapse late events may lead to compromises in the quality of life and increased mortality in long-term survivors of autologous HSCT and allogeneic HSCT for NHL [118, 119]. These problems are mostly related to treatment rather than a specific hematologic malignancy, although some of these problems may be more likely to occur in patients with NHL. The magnitude of these problems was recently examined in a nationwide analysis from Finland, which included 542 NHL patients treated with autologous HSCT between 1990 and 2003 [120]. Late nonrelapse mortality was observed in 4.8% of patients transplanted for NHL. The risk of dying from MDS/AML following autologous HSCT for NHL was 0.9%. These risks were less than for patients with Hodgkin lymphoma. The risk of late complications following allogeneic HSCT is greater because of the added burden of complications related to chronic GvHD [121], although this will not be discussed in detail (please refer to Chap. 12 by Martin and Pavletic).

Although treatment advances have allowed patients to survive long enough to be at risk for late complications, this should not lead to passive acceptance of these complications as the cost of cure. Measures to prevent or ameliorate these problems must assume an increasing role in the design of new treatment strategies. Comprehensive, long-term follow-up is a requirement for the proper care of the post-transplant patient, with NHL or any other diagnosis. Guidelines have recently been published for this population [122]. Numerous late complications of HSCT have been described, although only second malignancies will be discussed.

15.8.1 Autologous Hematopoietic Stem Cell Transplantation

There have been numerous reports of MDS/AML, or rarely acute lymphoid leukemia (ALL), following autologous HSCT for NHL. These events are felt to be related to prior exposure to conventional chemotherapy with alkylating agents, topoisomerase II inhibitors, and radiotherapy. Those related to alkylators are characterized by a prolonged latent phase before the development of MDS, a rapid progression to AML, abnormalities of chromosomes 5 and 7, and poor response to therapy. In contrast, those related to topoisomerase II drug exposure are characterized by a shorter latency, 11q chromosome abnormalities, and better short term response to therapy. There is wide variability among reports in the incidence of secondary MDS/AML, although this value may reach 10% at 10 years following autologous HSCT [123].

While cases of secondary MDS/AML are most likely caused by cytotoxic agents administered prior to treatment with high-dose therapy and autologous HSCT [124], components of the autologous HSCT regimen such as high-dose etoposide and TBI have also been implicated. It is also possible that other factors such as delayed immune recovery following transplantation may also play a role.

The prognosis of transplant-related MDS/AML is poor and efforts to reduce the incidence of this problem and to identify high-risk patients is warranted. It is likely that using autologous HSCT earlier in the course of disease may decrease the risk of secondary malignancies. Furthermore, examination of the bone marrow should be considered prior to autologous HSCT, since cytogenetic abnormalities, especially those identified with FISH analysis, may correlate with later development of MDS/AML [124].

There is less information regarding the development of solid tumors after autologous HSCT for NHL. A retrospective analysis from Dana-Farber Cancer Institute examined the risk of developing malignancies following treatment with a TBI-containing regimen and autologous HSCT for NHL [125]. The 10-year cumulative risk of developing a second malignancy was 21%, and approximately half of these cases were MDS/AML. Nonmelanoma skin cancers were the largest proportion of nonhematologic malignancies, although a large number of solid tumors involving breast, prostate, lung, and other sites were observed. The main risk factor for developing second malignancies was older age.

15.8.2 Allogeneic Hematopoietic Stem Cell Transplantation

Although the risk of secondary MDS/AML is relatively low following allogeneic HSCT, the risk of post-transplant lymphoproliferative disorders

(PTLD) is increased. These disorders are usually EBV-driven and usually occur early after allogeneic HSCT. The incidence is increased in patients who receive intensive immunosuppression because of GvHD and in those who receive T-cell depleted grafts. In one long-term follow-up study the relative risk of solid tumors following allogeneic HSCT was increased 8.3-fold for those who survived beyond 10 years [126]. Uncommon tumors were often seen, such as those involving bone, oral cavity, brain, liver, thyroid, and connective tissues.

Chronic GvHD is the major cause of late nonrelapse mortality following allogeneic HSCT and will not be discussed in detail. However, prolonged immune dysregulation may contribute to an increased risk of second malignancies [127].

15.9 Summary

Over the last 25 years the use of auto- and allogeneic HSCT for NHL increased dramatically. This therapy is being used for types of NHL that were not even defined when transplantation was first used. Although thousands of NHL patients have had their lives prolonged or have been cured with transplantation, the role of HSCT is still undefined in most situations.

Unfortunately, HSCT is often used simply because satisfactory nontransplant options are unavailable. Allogeneic HSCT is often used because of the perception that autologous HSCT will be ineffective. Reduced-intensity allogeneic HSCT is often utilized in situations when definite evidence of superiority over myeloablative allogeneic HSCT, and even autologous HSCT, do not exist. Treatment decisions are even more difficult today because of better primary treatments and because of the introduction of effective new agents and targeted therapies for relapsed and refractory disease. It is hoped that the role of HSCT for NHL will be refined when results of ongoing phase III trials are available.

References

1. Rosenwald A, Wright G, Chan WC, et al. The use of molecular profiling to predict survival after chemotherapy for diffuse large B-cell lymphoma. N Engl J Med. 2002;346:1937–47.
2. Feugier P, Van Hoof A, Sebban A, et al. Long-term results of the R-CHOP study in the treatment of elderly patients with diffuse large B-cell lymphoma: a study by the Groupe d'Etude des Lymphomes de l'Adulte. J Clin Oncol. 2005;23:4117–26.
3. Marcus R, Imrie K, Belch A, et al. CVP chemotherapy plus rituximab compared with CVP as first-line treatment for advanced follicular lymphoma. Blood 2005;105:1417–23.
4. Philip T, Guglielmi C, Hagenbeek A, et al. Autologous bone marrow transplantation as compared with salvage chemotherapy in relapses of chemotherapy-sensitive non-Hodgkin's lymphoma. N Engl J Med. 1995;333:1540–5.
5. Pasquini M. Part I-CIBMTR summary slides, 2005. CIBMTR Newsl. 2006;12:5–8.
6. Gratwohl A, Baldomero H, Frauendorfer K, et al. Results of the EBMT activity survey 2005 on haematopoietic stem cell transplantation: focus on increasing use of unrelated donors. Bone Marrow Transplant. 2007;39:71–87.

7. Leone G, Pagano L, Ben-Yehuda D, et al. Therapy-related leukemia and myelodysplasia: susceptibility and incidence. Haematologica 2007;92:1389–98.
8. Butcher BW, Collins RH. The graft-versus-lymphoma effect: clinical review and future opportunities. Bone Marrow Transplant. 2005;36:1–17.
9. Baron F, Storb R. The immune system as a foundation for immunologic therapy and hematologic malignancies: a historical perspective. Best Pract Res Clin Haematol. 2006;19:637–53.
10. Shipp MA. Prognostic factors in non-Hodgkin's lymphoma: who has "high-risk" disease? Blood 1994;83:1165–73.
11. Hamlin PA, Zelenetz AD, Kewalramani T, et al. Age-adjusted International Prognostic Index predicts autologous stem cell transplantation outcome for patients with relapsed or primary refractory diffuse large B-cell lymphoma. Blood 2003;102:1989–96.
12. Schot BW, Zijlstra JM, Sluiter WJ, et al. Early FDG-PET assessment in combination with clinical risk scores determines prognosis in recurring lymphoma. Blood 2007;109: 486–91.
13. Jantunen E. Autologous stem cell transplantation beyond 60 years of age. Bone Marrow Transplant. 2006;38:715–20.
14. Sorror ML, Storer BE, Maloney DG, et al. Outcomes after allogeneic hematopoietic cell transplantation with nonmyeloablative or myeloablative conditioning regimens for treatment of lymphoma and chronic lymphocytic leukemia. Blood 2008;111:446–52.
15. Rapoport AP, Meisenberg B, Sarkodee-Adoo C, et al. Autotransplantation for advanced lymphoma and Hodgkin's disease followed by post-transplant rituxan/GM-CSF or radiotherapy and consolidation chemotherapy. Bone Marrow Transplant. 2000;29: 303–12.
16. Oehler-Jänne C, Taverna C, Stanek N, et al. Consolidative involved field radiotherapy after high dose chemotherapy and autologous stem cell transplantation for non-Hodgkin's lymphoma: a case-control study. Hematol Oncol. 2007;Published Online Dec 17, 2007.
17. Vose JM, Zhang MJ, Rowlings PA, et al. Autologous transplantation for diffuse aggressive non-Hodgkin's lymphoma in patients never achieving remission: a report from the Autologous Blood and Marrow Transplant Registry. J Clin Oncol. 2001;19:406–13.
18. Friedberg JW, Neuberg D, Monson J, et al. The impact of external beam radiation therapy prior to autologous bone marrow transplantation in patients with non-Hodgkin's lymphoma. Biol Blood Marrow Transplant. 2001;7:446–53.
19. Stockerl-Goldstein KE, Reddy SA, Horning SF, et al. Favorable treatment outcome in non-Hodgkin's lymphoma patients with "poor" mobilization of peripheral blood progenitor cells. Biol Blood Marrow Transplant. 2000;6:506–12.
20. Cashen AF, Lazarus HM, Devine SM. Mobilizing stem cells from normal donors: is it possible to improve upon G-CSF? Bone Marrow Transplant. 2007;39:577–88.
21. Robertson MJ, Abonour R, Hromas R, et al. Augmented high-dose regimen of cyclophosphamide, carmustine, and etoposide with autologous hematopoietic stem cell transplantation for relapsed and refractory aggressive non-Hodgkin's lymphoma. Leuk Lymphoma. 2005;46:1477–87.
22. Puig N, de la Rubia J, Remigia MJ, et al. Morbidity and transplant-related mortality of CBV and BEAM preparative regimens for patients with lymphoid malignancies undergoing autologous stem-cell transplantation. Leuk Lymphoma. 2006;47:1488–94.
23. Aggarwal C, Gupta S, Vaughan WP, et al. Improved outcomes in intermediate- and high-risk aggressive non-Hodgkin lymphoma after autologous hematopoietic stem cell transplantation substituting intravenous for oral busulfan in a busulfan, cyclophosphamide, and etoposide preparative regimen. Biol Blood Marrow Transplant. 2006; 12:770–7.
24. Betticher DC, Martinelli G, Radford JA, et al. Sequential high dose chemotherapy as initial treatment for aggressive sub-types of non Hodgkin lymphoma: results of the international randomized phase III trial (MISTRAL). Ann Oncol. 2006;17:1546–52.

25. Corradini P, Tarella C, Zallio F, et al. Long-term follow-up of patients with peripheral T-cell lymphomas treated up-front with high-dose chemotherapy followed by autologous stem cell transplantation. Leukemia 2006;20:1533–8.
26. Gianni AM, Bregni M, Siena S, et al. High-dose chemotherapy and autologous bone marrow transplantation compared with MACOP-B in aggressive B-cell lymphoma. N Engl J Med. 1997;336:1290–7.
27. Olivieri A, Santini G, Patti C, et al. Upfront high-dose sequential therapy (HDS) versus VACOP-B with or without HDS in aggressive non-Hodgkin's lymphoma: long-term results by the NHLCSG. Ann Oncol. 2005;16:1941–8.
28. Haioun C, Mounier N, Quesnel B, et al. Tandem autotransplant as first-line consolidative treatment in poor-risk aggressive lymphoma: a pilot study of 36 patients. Ann Oncol. 2001;12:1749–55.
29. Ahmed T, Rashid K, Waheed F. Long-term survival of patients with resistant lymphoma treated with tandem stem cell transplant. Leuk Lymphoma. 2005;46:405–14.
30. Carella AM, Cavaliere M, Lerma E, et al. Autografting followed by nonmyeloablative immunosuppressive chemotherapy and allogeneic peripheral-blood hematopoietic stem-cell transplantation as treatment of resistant Hodgkin's disease and non-Hodgkin's lymphoma. J Clin Oncol. 2000;18:3918–24.
31. Gutman JA, Bearman SI, Nieto Y, et al. Autologous transplantation followed closely by reduced-intensity allogeneic transplantation as consolidative immunotherapy in advanced lymphoma patients: a feasibility study. Bone Marrow Transplant. 2005;36: 443–51.
32. Gopal AK, Gooley TA, Maloney DG, et al. High-dose radioimmunotherapy versus conventional high-dose therapy and autologous hematopoietic stem cell transplantation for relapsed follicular non-Hodgkin lymphoma: a multivariable cohort analysis. Blood 2003;102:2351–7.
33. Vose JM, Bierman PJ, Enke C, et al. Phase I trial of Iodine-131 tositumomab with high-dose chemotherapy and autologous stem-cell transplantation for relapsed non-Hodgkin's lymphoma. J Clin Oncol. 2005;23:461–7.
34. Krishnan A, Nademanee A, Fung HC, et al. Phase II trial of a transplantation regimen of yttrium-90 ibritumomab tiuxetan and high-dose chemotherapy in patients with non-Hodgkin's lymphoma. J Clin Oncol. 2008;26:90–5.
35. Gopal AK, Pagel JM, Rajendran JG, et al. Improving the efficacy of reduced intensity allogeneic transplantation for lymphoma using radioimmunotherapy. Biol Blood Marrow Transplant. 2006;12:697–702.
36. Sieniawski M, Staak O, Glossmann JP, et al. Rituximab added to an intensified salvage chemotherapy program followed by autologous stem cell transplantation improved the outcome in relapsed and refractory aggressive non-Hodgkin lymphoma. Ann Hematol. 2007;86:107–15.
37. Tarella C, Zanni M, Nicola MD, et al. Prolonged survival in poor-risk diffuse large B-cell lymphoma following front-line treatment with rituximab-supplemented, early-intensified chemotherapy with multiple autologous hematopoietic stem cell support: a multicenter study by GITIL (Gruppo Italiano Terapie Innovative nei Linfomi). Leukemia 2007; 21:1802–11.
38. van Heeckeren WJ, Wollweiler J, Fu P, et al. Randomized comparison of two B-cell purging protocols for patients with B-cell non-Hodgkin lymphoma: in vivo purging with rituximab versus ex vivo purging with CliniMACS $CD34^+$ cell enrichment device. Br J Haematol. 2005;132:42–55.
39. Bierman PJ, Sweetenham JW, Loberiza FR, et al. Syngeneic hematopoietic stem-cell transplantation for non-Hodgkin's lymphoma: a comparison with allogeneic and autologous transplantation—The Lymphoma Working Committee of the International Bone Marrow Transplant Registry and the European Group for Blood and Marrow Transplantation. J Clin Oncol. 2003:21:3744–53.

40. van Besien K, Loberiza FR, Bajorunaite R, et al. Comparison of autologous and allogeneic hematopoietic stem cell transplantation for follicular lymphoma. Blood 2003;102:3521–9.
41. Brown JR, Feng Y, Gribben JG, et al. Long-term survival after autologous bone marrow transplantation for follicular lymphoma in first remission. Biol Blood Marrow Transplant. 2007;13:1057–65.
42. Schouten HC, Qian W, Kvaloy S, et al. High-dose therapy improves progression-free survival and survival in relapsed follicular non-Hodgkin's lymphoma: results from the randomized European CUP trial. J Clin Oncol. 2003;21:3918–27.
43. Jacobsen E, Freedman A. B-cell purging in autologous stem-cell transplantation for non-Hodgkin lymphoma. Lancet Oncol. 2004;5:711–7.
44. Imai Y, Chou T, Kobinai K, et al. Isolation and transplantation of high purified $CD34^+$ progenitor cells: purging efficacy, hematopoietic reconstitution in non-Hodgkin's lymphoma (NHL): results of Japanese phase II study. Bone Marrow Transplant. 2005; 35:479–87.
45. Belhadj K, Delfau-Larue MH, Elgnaoui T, et al. Efficiency of in vivo purging with rituximab prior to autologous peripheral blood progenitor cell transplantation in B-cell non-Hodgkin's lymphoma: a single institution study. Ann Oncol. 2004;15:504–10.
46. Horwitz SM, Negrin RS, Blume KG, et al. Rituximab as adjuvant to high-dose therapy and autologous hematopoietic cell transplantation for aggressive non-Hodgkin lymphoma. Blood 2004;103:777–83.
47. Brugger W, Hirsch J, Grünebach F, et al. Rituximab consolidation after high-dose chemotherapy and autologous blood stem cell transplantation in follicular and mantle cell lymphoma: a prospective, multicenter phase II study. Ann Oncol. 2004;15:1691–8.
48. Holmberg LA, Maloney D, Bensinger W. Immunotherapy with rituximab/interleukin-2 after autologous stem cell transplantation as treatment for $CD20^+$ non-Hodgkin's lymphoma. Clin Lymphoma Myeloma. 2006;7:135–9.
49. Bolaños-Meade J, Garrett-Mayer E, Luznik L, et al. Induction of autologous graft-versus-host disease: results of a randomized prospective clinical trial in patients with poor risk lymphoma. Biol Blood Marrow Transplant. 2007;13:1185–91.
50. Caballero MD, Pérez-Simón JA, Iriondo A, et al. High-dose therapy in diffuse large cell lymphoma: results and prognostic factors in 452 patients from the GEL-TAMO Spanish Cooperative Group. Ann Oncol. 2003;14:140–51.
51. Vose JM, Rizzo DJ, Tao-Wu J, et al. Autologous transplantation for diffuse aggressive non-Hodgkin lymphoma in first relapse or second remission. Biol Blood Marrow Transplant. 2004;110:116–27.
52. Kewalramani T, Zelenetz AD, Nimer SD, et al. Rituximab and ICE as second-line therapy before autologous stem cell transplantation for relapsed or primary refractory diffuse large B-cell lymphoma. Blood 2004;103:3684–8.
53. Hoerr AL, Gao F, Hidalgo J, et al. Effects of pretransplantation treatment with rituximab on outcomes of autologous stem-cell transplantation for non-Hodgkin's lymphoma. J Clin Oncol. 2004;22:4561–6.
54. Hagberg H, Gisselbrecht C. Randomised phase III study of R-ICE versus R-DHAP in relapsed patients with CD20 diffuse large B-cell lymphoma (DLBCL) followed by high-dose therapy and a second randomization to maintenance treatment with rituximab or not: an update of the CORAL study. Ann Oncol. 2006;17 Suppl. 4:iv31–2.
55. Blay JY, Gomez F, Sebban C, et al. The International Prognostic Index correlates to survival in patients with aggressive lymphoma in relapse: analysis of the PARMA trial. Blood 1998;92:3562–68.
56. Lerner RE, Thomas W, DeFor TE, et al. The International Prognostic Index assessed at relapse predicts outcomes of autologous transplantation for diffuse large-cell non-Hodgkin's lymphoma in second complete or partial remission. Biol Blood Marrow Transplant. 2007;13:486–92.

57. Spaepen K, Stroobants S, Dupont P, et al. Prognostic value of pretransplantation positron emission tomography using fluorine 18-flurodeoxyglucose in patients with aggressive lymphoma treated with high-dose chemotherapy and stem cell transplantation. Blood 2003;102:53–59.
58. Filmont JE, Gisselbrecht C, Cuenca X, et al. The impact of pre- and post-transplantation positron emission tomography using 18-fluorodeoxyglucose on poor-prognosis lymphoma patients undergoing autologous stem cell transplantation. Cancer 2007;110: 1361–9.
59. Rodriguez J, Caballero MD, Gutierrez A, et al. Autologous stem-cell transplantation in diffuse large B-cell non-Hodgkin's lymphoma not achieving complete response after induction chemotherapy: the GEL/TAMO experience. Ann Oncol. 2004;15:1504–9.
60. Haioun C, Lepage E, Gisselbrecht C, et al. Survival benefit of high-dose therapy in poor-risk aggressive non-Hodgkin's lymphoma: Final analysis of the prospective LNH87-2 protocol—A Groupe d'Etude des Lymphomes de l'Adulte study. J Clin Oncol. 2000;18:3025–30.
61. Milpied N, Deconinck E, Gaillard F, et al. Initial treatment of aggressive lymphoma with high-dose chemotherapy and autologous stem-cell support. N Engl J Med. 2004;350: 1287–95.
62. Greb A, Bohlius J, Trelle S, et al. High dose chemotherapy with autologous stem cell support in first-line treatment of aggressive non-Hodgkin lymphoma—results of a comprehensive meta-analysis. Cancer Treat Rev. 2007;33:338–46.
63. Hahn T, Wolff SN, Czuczman M, et al. The role of cytotoxic therapy with hematopoietic stem cell transplantation in the treatment of diffuse large B-cell non-Hodgkin's lymphoma. Biol Blood Marrow Transplant. 2003;9:667.
64. Doocey RT, Toze CL, Connors JM, et al. Allogeneic haematopoietic stem-cell transplantation for relapsed and refractory aggressive histology non-Hodgkin lymphoma. Br J Haematol. 2005;131:223–30.
65. Kim SW, Tanimoto TE, Hirabayashi N, et al. Myeloablative allogeneic hematopoietic stem cell transplantation for non-Hodgkin's lymphoma: a nationwide survey in Japan. Blood 2006;108:382–9.
66. Peniket AJ, Ruiz de Elvira MC, Taghipour G, et al. An EBMT registry matched study of allogeneic stem cell transplants for lymphoma: allogeneic transplantation is associated with a lower relapse rate but a higher procedure-related mortality rate than autologous transplantation. Bone Marrow Transplant. 2003;31:667–78.
67. Aksentijevich I, Jones RJ, Ambinder RF, et al. Clinical outcome following autologous and allogeneic blood and marrow transplantation for relapsed diffuse large-cell non-Hodgkin's lymphoma. Biol Blood Marrow Transplant. 2006;12:965–72.
68. Robinson SP, Goldstone AH, Mackinnon S, et al. Chemoresistant or aggressive lymphoma predicts for a poor outcome following reduced-intensity allogeneic progenitor cell transplantation: an analysis from the Lymphoma Working Party of the European Group for Blood and Bone Marrow Transplantation. Blood 2002;100:4310–6.
69. Kahl C, Storer BE, Sandmaier BM, et al. Relapse risk in patients with malignant diseases given allogeneic hematopoietic cell transplantation after nonmyeloablative conditioning. Blood 2007;110:2744–8.
70. Corradini P, Dodero A, Farina L, et al. Allogeneic stem cell transplantation following reduced-intensity conditioning can induce durable clinical and molecular remissions in relapsed lymphomas: pre-transplant disease status and histotype heavily influence outcome. Leukemia 2007;21:2316–23.
71. Faulkner RD, Craddock C, Byrne JL, et al. BEAM-alemtuzumab reduced-intensity allogeneic stem cell transplantation for lymphoproliferative diseases: GVHD, toxicity, and survival in 65 patients. Blood 2004;103:428–34.
72. Rodriguez R, Nademanee A, Ruel N, et al. Comparison of reduced-intensity and conventional myeloabative regimens for allogeneic transplantation in non-Hodgkin's lymphoma. Biol Blood Marrow Transplant. 2006;12:1326–34.

73. Brice P, Simon D, Bouabdallah R, et al. High-dose therapy with autologous stem-cell transplantation (ASCT) after first progression prolonged survival of follicular lymphoma patients included in the prospective GELF 86 protocol. Ann Oncol. 2000;11:1585–90.
74. Vignot S, Mounier N, Larghero J, et al. High-dose therapy and autologous stem-cell transplantation can improve event-free survival for indolent lymphoma: a study using patients as their own controls. Cancer 2007;109:60–7.
75. Laudi N, Arora M, Burns LJ, et al. Long-term follow-up after autologous hematopoietic stem cell transplantation for low-grade non-Hodgkin lymphoma. Biol Blood Marrow Transplant. 2005;11:129–35.
76. Sabloff M, Atkins HL, Bence-Bruckler I, et al. A 15-year analysis of early and late autologous hematopoietic stem cell transplant in relapsed, aggressive, transformed, and nontransformed follicular lymphoma. Biol Blood Marrow Transplant. 2007:13;956–64.
77. Vose JM, Bierman PJ, Loberiza FR, et al. Long-term outcomes of autologous stem cell transplantation for follicular non-Hodgkin lymphoma: effect of histological grade and follicular International Prognostic Index. Biol Blood Marrow Transplant. 2008;14:36–42.
78. Rohatiner AZS, Nadler L, Davies AJ, et al. Myeloablative therapy with autologous bone marrow transplantation for follicular lymphoma at the time of second or subsequent remission: long-term follow-up. J Clin Oncol. 2007;25:2554–9.
79. Montoto S, Canals C, Rohatiner AZS, et al. Long-term follow-up of high-dose treatment with autologous haematopoietic progenitor cell support in 693 patients with follicular lymphoma: an EBMT registry study. Leukemia 2007;21:2324–31.
80. Krishnan A, Nademanee A, Fung H, et al. Does follicularity in large cell lymphoma predict outcome after autologous stem cell transplantation? Biol Blood Marrow Transplant. 2006;12:641–7.
81. Lenz G, Dreyling M, Schiegnitz E, et al. Myeloablative radiochemotherapy followed by autologous stem cell transplantation in first remission prolongs progression-free survival in follicular lymphoma: results of a prospective, randomized trial of the German Low-Grade Lymphoma Study Group. Blood 2004;104:2667–74.
82. Deconinck E, Foussard C, Milpied N, et al. High-dose therapy followed by autologous purged stem-cell transplantation and doxorubicin-based chemotherapy in patients with advanced follicular lymphoma: a randomized multicenter study by GOELAMS. Blood 2005;105:3817–23.
83. Sebban C, Mounier N, Brousse N, et al. Standard chemotherapy with interferon compared with CHOP followed by high-dose therapy with autologous stem cell transplantation in untreated patients with advanced follicular lymphoma: the GELF-94 randomized study from the Groupe d'Etude des Lymphomes de l'Adulte (GELA). Blood 2006;108:2540–4.
84. Bolwell B, Kalaycio M, Andresen S, et al. Autologous peripheral blood progenitor cell transplantation for transformed diffuse large-cell lymphoma. Clin Lymphoma. 2000;3:226–31.
85. Williams CD, Harrison CN, Lister TA, et al. High-dose therapy and autologous stem-cell support for chemosensitive transformed low-grade follicular non-Hodgkin's lymphoma: A case-matched study from the European Bone Marrow Transplant Registry. J Clin Oncol. 2001;19:727–35.
86. Rezvani AR, Storer B, Maris M, et al. Nonmyeloablative allogeneic hematopoietic cell transplantation in relapsed, refractory, and transformed indolent non-Hodgkin's lymphoma. J Clin Oncol. 2008;26:211–7.
87. van Besien K, Sobocinski KA, Rowlings PA, et al. Allogeneic bone marrow transplantation for low-grade lymphoma. Blood 1998;92:1832–6.
88. Toze CL, Barnett MJ, Connors JM, et al. Long-term disease-free survival of patients with advanced follicular lymphoma after allogeneic bone marrow transplantation. Br J Haematol. 2004;127:311–21.
89. Hosing C, Saliba RM, McLaughlin P, et al. Long-term results favor allogeneic over autologous hematopoietic stem cell transplantation in patients with refractory or recurrent indolent non-Hodgkin's lymphoma. Ann Oncol. 2003;14:737–44.

90. Vigouroux S, Michallet M, Porcher R, et al. Long-term outcomes after reduced-intensity conditioning allogeneic stem cell transplantation for low-grade lymphoma: a survey by the French Society of Bone Marrow Graft Transplantation and Cellular Therapy (SFGM-TC). Haematologica 2007;92:627–34.
91. van Besien K. The evolving role of autologous and allogeneic stem cell transplantation in follicular lymphoma. Blood Rev. 2006;20:235–44.
92. Vandenberghe E, Ruiz de Elvira C, Loberiza F, et al. Outcome of autologous transplantation for mantle cell lymphoma: a study by the European Blood and Bone Marrow Transplant and Autologous Blood and Marrow Transplant Registries. Br J Haematol. 2003;120;793–800.
93. Kasamon YL, Jones RJ, Diehl LF, et al. Outcomes of autologous and allogeneic blood or marrow transplantation for mantle cell lymphoma. Biol Blood Marrow Transplant. 2005;11:39–46.
94. Ganti AK, Bierman PJ, Lynch JC, et al. Hematopoietic stem cell transplantation in mantle cell lymphoma. Ann Oncol. 2005;16:618–24.
95. Khouri IF, Romaguera J, Kantarjian H, et al. Hyper-CVAD and high-dose methotrexate/cytarabine followed by stem-cell transplantation: an active regimen for aggressive mantle-cell lymphoma. J Clin Oncol. 1998;16:3803–9.
96. Mangel J. Leitch HA, Connors JM, et al. Intensive chemotherapy and autologous stem-cell transplantation plus rituximab is superior to conventional chemotherapy for newly diagnosed advanced stage mantle-cell lymphoma: a matched pair analysis. Ann Oncol. 2004;15:283–90.
97. Gianni AM, Magni M, Martelli M, et al. Long-term remission in mantle cell lymphoma following high-dose sequential chemotherapy and in vivo rituximab-purged stem cell autografting (R-HDS regimen). Blood 2003;102:749–55.
98. Dreyling M, Lenz G, Hoster E, et al. Early consolidation by myeloablative radiochemotherapy followed by autologous stem cell transplantation in first remission significantly prolongs progression-free survival in mantle-cell lymphoma: results of a prospective randomized trial of the European MCL Network. Blood 2005;105: 2677–84.
99. Khouri IF, Lee MS, Romaguera J, et al. Allogeneic hematopoietic transplantation for mantle-cell lymphoma: molecular remissions and evidence of graft-versus-malignancy. Ann Oncol. 1999:10:1293–9.
100. Maris MB, Sandmaier BM, Storer BE, et al. Allogeneic hematopoietic cell transplantation after fludarabine and 2 Gy total body irradiation for relapsed and refractory mantle cell lymphoma. Blood 2004;104:3535–42.
101. Khouri IF, Lee MS, Saliba RM, et al. Nonablative allogeneic stem-cell transplantation for advanced/recurrent mantle-cell lymphoma. J Clin Oncol. 2003;21:4407–12.
102. Feyler S, Prince HM, Pearce R, et al. The role of high-dose therapy and stem cell rescue in the management of T-cell malignant lymphomas: a BSBMT and ABMTRR study. Bone Marrow Transplant. 2007;40:443–50.
103. Jantunen E, Wiklund T, Juvonen E, et al. Autologous stem cell transplantation in adult patients with peripheral T-cell lymphoma: a nation-wide survey. Bone Marrow Transplant. 2004;33:405–10.
104. Rodríguez J, Caballero MD, Gutiérrez A, et al. High-dose chemotherapy and autologous stem cell transplantation in peripheral T-cell lymphoma: the GEL-TAMO experience. Ann Oncol. 2003;14:1768–75.
105. Blystad AK, Enblad G, Kvaløy S, et al. High-dose therapy with autologous stem cell transplantation in patients with peripheral T cell lymphomas. Bone Marrow Transplant. 2001;27:711–6.
106. Song KW, Mollee P, Keating A, et al. Autologous stem cell transplant for relapsed and refractory peripheral T-cell lymphoma: variable outcome according to pathological subtype. Br J Haematol. 2003;120:978–85.

107. Kewalramani T, Zelenetz AD, Teruya-Feldstein J, et al. Autologous transplantation for relapsed or primary refractory peripheral T-cell lymphoma. Br J Haematol. 2006; 134:202–7.
108. Fanin R, Ruiz de Elvira MC, Sperotto A, et al. Autologous stem cell transplantation for T and null cell CD30-positive anaplastic large cell lymphoma; analysis of 64 adult and paediatric cases reported to the European Group for Blood and Marrow Transplantation (EBMT). Bone Marrow Transplant. 1999;23:437–42.
109. Jagasia M, Morgan D, Goodman S, et al. Histology impacts the outcome of peripheral T-cell lymphomas after high dose chemotherapy and stem cell transplant. Leuk Lymphoma. 2004;45:2261–7.
110. Mounier N, Gisselbrecht C, Brière J, et al. Prognostic factors in patients with aggressive non-Hodgkin's lymphoma treated by front-line autotransplantation after complete remission: a cohort study by the Groupe d'Etude des Lymphomes de l'Adulte. J Clin Oncol. 2004;22:2826–34.
111. Mounier N, Gisselbrecht C, Brière J, et al. All aggressive lymphoma subtypes do not share similar outcome after front-line autotransplantation: a matched-control analysis from the Groupe d'Etude des lymphomas de l'Adulte (GELA). Ann Oncol. 2004; 15:1790–7.
112. Rodríguez J, Conde E, Gutiérrez A, et al. The results of consolidation with autologous stem-cell transplantation in patients with peripheral T-cell lymphoma (PTCL) in first complete remission: the Spanish Lymphoma and Autologous Transplantation Group experience. Ann Oncol. 2007;18:652–7.
113. Reimer P, Rüdiger T, Wilhelm W. The role of high-dose therapy in peripheral T-cell lymphomas. Clin Lymphoma Myeloma. 2006;6:373–9.
114. Rodríguez, J, Conde E, Gutiérrez A, et al. Frontline autologous stem cell transplantation in high-risk peripheral T-cell lymphoma: a prospective study from The Gel-Tamo Study Group. Eur J Haematol. 2007;79:32–8.
115. Kahl C, Leithäuser M, Wolff D, et al. Treatment of peripheral T-cell lymphomas (PTCL) with high-dose chemotherapy and autologous or allogeneic hematopoietic transplantation. Ann Hematol. 2002;81:646–50.
116. Corradini P, Dodero A, Zallio F, et al. Graft-versus-lymphoma effect in relapsed peripheral T-cell non-Hodgkin's lymphomas after reduced-intensity conditioning followed by allogeneic transplantation of hematopoietic cells. J Clin Oncol. 2004;22; 2172–6.
117. Wulf GG, Hasenkamp J, Jung W, et al. Reduced intensity conditioning and allogeneic stem cell transplantation after salvage therapy integrating alemtuzumab for patients with relapsed peripheral T-cell non-Hodgkin's lymphoma. Bone Marrow Transplant. 2005;36:271–3.
118. Majhail NS, Ness KK, Burns LJ, et al. Late effects in survivors of Hodgkin and non-Hodgkin lymphoma treated with autologous hematopoietic cell transplantation: a report from the bone marrow transplant survivor study. Biol Blood Marrow Transplant. 2007;13:1153–9.
119. Mielcarek M, Storer BE, Flowers ME, et al. Outcomes among patients with recurrent high-risk hematologic malignancies after allogeneic hematopoietic cell transplantation. Biol Blood Marrow Transplant. 2007;13:1160–8.
120. Jantunen E, Itälä M, Siitonen T, et al. Late non-relapse mortality among adult autologous stem cell transplant recipients: a nation-wide analysis of 1,482 patients transplanted in 1990-2003. Eur J Haematol. 2006;77:114–9.
121. Socié G, Salooja N, Cohen A, et al. Nonmalignant late effects after allogeneic stem cell transplantation. Blood 2003;101:3373–85.
122. Rizzo JD, Wingard JR, Tichelli A, et al. Recommended screening and preventive practices for long-term survivors after hematopoietic cell transplantation: joint recommendations of the European Group for Blood and Marrow Transplantation, the Center

for International Blood and Marrow Transplant Research, and the American Society of Blood and Marrow Transplantation. Biol Blood Marrow Transplant. 2006;12:138–51.

123. Armitage JO, Carbone PP, Connors JM, et al. Treatment-related myelodysplasia and acute leukemia in non-Hodgkin's lymphoma patients. J Clin Oncol. 2003;21:897–906.
124. Abruzzese E, Radford JE, Miller JS, et al. Detection of abnormal pretransplant clones in progenitor cells of patients who developed myelodysplasia after autologous transplantation. Blood 1999;94:1814–9.
125. Brown JR, Yeckes H, Friedberg JW, et al. Increasing incidence of late second malignancies after conditioning with cyclophosphamide and total-body irradiation and autologous bone marrow transplantation for non-Hodgkin's lymphoma. J Clin Oncol. 2005;23:2208–14.
126. Curtis RE, Rowlings PA, Deeg HJ, et al. Solid cancers after bone marrow transplantation. N Engl J Med. 1997;336:897–904.
127. Shimada K, Yokozawa T, Atsuta Y, et al. Solid tumors after hematopoietic stem cell transplantation in Japan: incidence, risk factors and prognosis. Bone Marrow Transplant. 2005;36:115–21.

Chapter 16
The Role of Hematopoietic Stem Cell Transplantation in Hodgkin Lymphoma

Craig Moskowitz and John Sweetenham

16.1 Introduction

Autologous hematopoietic stem cell transplantation (HSCT) has been a standard component of therapy for most patients with relapsed and refractory Hodgkin's lymphoma (HL; a.k.a. Hodgkin's disease) for many years. The emergence of new first-line therapies for HL, the application of new staging and imaging techniques and the introduction of nonmyeloablative conditioning for allogeneic HSCT have resulted in a re-evaluation of the role of stem cell transplant strategies in this disease. As first-line therapy continues to improve, the number of patients requiring salvage therapy with HSCT is likely to fall. However, it is likely that this patient population will be particularly challenging, requiring novel salvage approaches.

16.2 Autologous HSCT in Hodgkin Lymphoma

16.2.1 Relapsed Disease

The use of conventional-dose salvage therapy for patients with HL who relapse after initial chemotherapy has been disappointing. Studies in patients relapsing after MOPP (mechlorethamine, vincristine, procarbazine, and prednisone) chemotherapy showed MOPP retreatment produced second complete remission (CR) rates of approximately 50%, but that these were typically short lived with a median duration of 21 months [1]. Patients with an initial remission that lasted less than 12 months had a significantly worse progression-free (PFS) and overall survival (OS) compared with those with longer initial remissions. Long-term outcome for all patients was poor. Only 17% of the patients whose initial remission was longer than 1 year were alive at 20 years, and only 29% of those with a shorter initial remission achieved a second CR with very few surviving long term.

C. Moskowitz (✉)
Memorial Sloan-Kettering Cancer Center, New York, NY, USA
e-mail: moskowic@mskcc.org

M.R. Bishop (ed.), *Hematopoietic Stem Cell Transplantation*, Cancer Treatment and Research 144, DOI 10.1007/978-0-387-78580-6_16,

In a randomized study from the Cancer and Leukemia Group B (CALGB), patients who relapsed after initial therapy with ABVD (doxorubicin, bleomycin, vinblastine, dacarbazine) and were treated with MOPP had a 5-year failure-free survival rate of only 31%, compared with 15% for those receiving MOPP first-line and ABVD at relapse [2].

Single institution and registry studies reported superior results for patients with relapsed disease receiving high-dose therapy (HDT) and autologous HSCT, with long-term disease-free survival rates between 40% and 65% for those undergoing autologous HSCT at first relapse [3–6].

A report from Stanford University describes 60 patients with relapsed/refractory HL undergoing autologous HSCT who were compared with a matched control group treated with conventional-dose second-line therapy [4]. Four-year event-free survival (EFS) and freedom from progression (FFP) were higher in patients undergoing autologous HSCT compared with those receiving conventional-dose salvage (53% vs. 27% for EFS; 62% vs. 27% for FFP). Four-year actuarial OS was the same for both groups (54% for HDT vs. 47% for conventional dose), although the subset of patients relapsing within 1 year of first-line therapy had a higher OS when treated with autologous HSCT. The European Group for Blood and Marrow Transplantation (EBMT) reported 45% progression-free survival (PFS) at 5 years for 139 patients undergoing autologous HSCT at first relapse [7].

The first randomized trial to compare autologous HSCT with conventional-dose salvage therapy for relapsed HL was reported by the British National Lymphoma Investigation (BNLI). In this small trial 40 patients in first or subsequent relapse were randomized to receive HDT with BEAM (carmustine, etoposide, cytarabine, melphalan) or conventional-dose therapy, using the same drugs ("mini-BEAM") [8]. A significant difference in EFS was observed for patients receiving BEAM (3-year EFS = 53% for BEAM vs. 10% for mini-BEAM, $p = 0.025$). A similar difference in PFS was seen between the two arms but this did not translate into an OS difference since some patients relapsing after mini-BEAM crossed over to receive BEAM and autologous HSCT. The trial was closed early because of poor accrual.

In a subsequent study by the German Hodgkin's Lymphoma Study Group (GHSG) and EBMT, 161 patients between 16 and 60 years old with relapsed HL were randomized between two cycles of Dexa-BEAM (dexamethasone, BCNU, etoposide, cytarabine, melphalan) followed either by two further cycles of Dexa-BEAM or HDT and auto-HSCT [9]. Patients continued on the protocol only if they had chemotherapy-sensitive disease (i.e., achieved a PR or CR with the initial two cycles of Dexa-BEAM). For the 117 patients with chemotherapy-sensitive disease 3-year freedom from treatment failure (FFTF) was 55% for the HSCT arm compared with 34% in the Dexa-BEAM arm ($p = 0.019$) at a median of 39 months follow up (range, 3–78 months). This difference in FFTF was significant for patients with early (less than 1 year) or late (1 year or greater) relapses. Overall survival did not differ significantly between treatment arms (71% vs. 65%, $p = 0.331$). Again, the failure to demonstrate an OS difference is related to the "cross-over" of patients who relapsed on the Dexa-BEAM and then underwent autologous HSCT.

These results have subsequently been updated, with median follow-up now to 83 months [10] and continue to show a difference in 7-year FFTF rate was higher in the HSCT arm (32% vs. 27%). No OS difference was observed (56% vs. 57%, respectively at 7 years). Of note, no FFTF difference was observed for multiply relapsed patients.

The results of these studies have established HDT and autologous HSCT as the standard of care for patients with relapsed HL after a prior chemotherapy regimen such as MOPP or ABVD, irrespective of the duration of the initial remission or the total number of prior chemotherapy regimens.

The introduction of multi-agent dose-intensive and dose-dense regimens as initial treatment for advanced HL has raised some uncertainties regarding the role of HDT and autologous HSCT for relapsing patients. The Stanford V and escalated BEACOPP (bleomycin, etoposide, doxorubicin, cyclophosphamide, vincristine, procarbazine, prednisone) regimens both result in high rates of remission and disease-free survival, even for poor risk patients with advanced HL [11, 12]. The Stanford group initially reported 5-year actuarial PFS and OS rates of 89% and 96% for the Stanford V regimen. Of 142 patients treated, 16 relapsed, 11 of whom underwent autologous HSCT [12]. The freedom from second relapse in the entire group of 16 patients was 69% at 5 years, suggesting a high salvage rate.

Conflicting data have emerged from the GHSG with respect to the salvage rate for patients treated on their HD9 trial in advanced HL. In their original report it appeared that patients who relapsed after baseline or escalated BEACOPP were less readily salvaged by autologous HSCT than those relapsing after COPP/ABVD (cyclophosphamide, vincristine, procarbazine, prednisone/doxorubicin, bleomycin, vinblastine, dacarbazine). In a recent update, this was not confirmed although the concern still exists that patients who relapse after highly active first-line regimens may have relatively chemotherapy-resistant disease and may prove more difficult to salvage with autologous HSCT. Recent data have also emerged to suggest that ABVD can be given safely according to a dose-intensive schedule without dose delay or dose adjustment for neutropenia. This more dose-intensive ABVD regimen may prove more effective than when given according to the conventional schedule. Further follow-up will be required to clarify the ability of autologous HSCT to salvage patients who relapse after these regimens. It is unlikely that randomized trials will be conducted since the number of patients with relapsed disease will probably continue to decline as dose-dense and dose-intensive regimens are more widely accepted.

16.2.2 Refractory Disease

The prognosis for patients who do not achieve a remission with initial chemotherapy is very poor if these patients are treated with an alternative conventional-dose regimen. In a study from Milan 29 patients whose disease was refractory to treatment with MOPP/ABVD received CEP (lomustine, etoposide, prednimustine) [13]. The 5-year actuarial OS in this group was only 12%, and none of the surviving patients were disease free at the time of the report. The National Cancer Institute has reported comparable results in 51 patients with primary refractory disease after MOPP [1], in whom the median OS was 16 months. Yuen at al have reported a 4-year OS rate of 38% for 29 patients with primary refractory HL, with a 4-year PFS of 19% [4].

The role of autologous HSCT in this setting has been investigated in many registry and single institution studies. A retrospective, matched analysis from Stanford showed 4-year OS and FFP rates of 44% and 52%, respectively, for patients with primary refractory disease, which were significantly superior to those in the matched, nontransplanted group [3].

Chopra et al. reported a 6-year actuarial PFS rate of 33% for 46 patients with primary refractory disease treated with BEAM and autologous HSCT, and a similar figure was reported from Memorial Sloan-Kettering Cancer Center [6, 14]. The same group has more recently reported long-term results for 75 patients with biopsy-proven HL at the completion of primary chemotherapy or combined modality therapy [15]. All patients received standard-dose salvage therapy followed by involved field radiation therapy, and those without clinical or radiologic evidence of progression then received HDT with cyclophosphamide, etoposide and either total lymphoid irradiation or carmustine, depending upon prior radiation therapy, followed by autologous HSCT. Seven patients had progressive disease on second-line salvage therapy and did not proceed to transplant. This group had a median OS of only 4 months. For the remaining patients, subsequent outcome was related to their response to second-line salvage. Those with a reduction in disease bulk of greater than or equal to 25% had a 10-year EFS of 60% compared with 17% for those with less than 25% decrease.

Two prospective cooperative group studies in Europe have produced similar results. Ferme et al. reported results for 157 patients with induction failure or relapsed HL treated with MINE (mitoguazone, ifosfamide, vinorelbine, etoposide) followed by autologous HSCT after BEAM conditioning [16]. The 5-year OS rate in the group with primary induction failure was 30%. Constans et al. reported results for 62 patients with primary induction failure undergoing autologous HSCT with 5-year actuarial TTF and OS rates of 15% and 26%, respectively [17].

The EBMT has reported experience for patients treated with autologous HSCT after failure of induction therapy with a 5-year actuarial OS and PFS rate of 36% and 32%, respectively [18]. Similar results have been reported by the Autologous Blood and Marrow Transplant Registry of North America (ABMTR) [19].

Many of the results summarized above suggest that HDT and autologous HSCT is more effective than conventional-dose salvage therapy in the setting of primary refractory disease, but these data should be interpreted cautiously.

These retrospective studies may be subject to major selection bias. None of these studies have included an intent-to-treat analysis. Patients who have very rapidly progressive disease, poor performance status, or who fail to harvest adequate numbers of hematopoietic stem cells are excluded from these reports. In a landmark analysis from the GHSG, Josting et al. compared patients with primary induction failure who received or did not receive autologous HSCT within 6 months of progression [20]. When they excluded patients who survived less than 6 months, there was no survival advantage for autologous HSCT over conventional-dose salvage. Assessment of response in HL is difficult, especially for patients with bulky mediastinal disease and residual radiographic masses. The studies outlined above have used highly variable criteria for the definition of primary refractory disease and only two of these series have required biopsy confirmation of persistent disease. Emerging data suggest that functional imaging techniques such as [18] fluorodeoxyglucose positron emission tomography (FDG-PET) may help to identify active disease within residual masses at the completion of chemotherapy. If so, future studies of the use of autologous HSCT for primary refractory HL are likely to require positive functional imaging as a requirement for entry.

The use of "early" FDG-PET scanning in patients with advanced HL may also lead to a re-definition of refractory disease. Gallamini et al. have recently reported that the result of a PET scan performed after two cycles of ABVD in patients with advanced HL is very predictive of subsequent relapse [21]. If confirmed, it is likely that future studies will select patients for intensification of therapy based on the results of an early interim PET scan. The use of HDT and autologous HSCT may be investigated as a potential strategy for intensification of therapy in this context.

16.2.2.1 High-Dose Sequential Therapy and Tandem Autologous Transplantation

The observation that transplant outcomes are closely related to disease status and degree of cytoreduction prior to autologous HSCT has prompted some groups to explore the use of high-dose sequential therapy (HDS) or tandem autologous transplantation, using the first cycle of HDT to achieve maximal cytoreduction and the second to consolidate this response.

The GHSG has reported results from a high-dose sequential regimen in which patients received two cycles of DHAP (dexamethasone, cytarabine, cisplatin) d followed by high-dose cyclophosphamide, methotrexate, vincristine and etoposide after which they received BEAM and autologous HSCT [22]. For those patients with primary refractory disease or early relapse, the median follow-up was 40 months and the FFTF and OS rates were 62% and 78%, respectively.

Fung et al. have recently reported results for tandem autologous transplantation in 46 patients with primary refractory or high-risk relapsed HL [23]. The first high-dose regimen was single agent melphalan, and the second comprised fractionated total body irradiation or carmustine with etoposide and cyclophosphamide. Five patients did not receive the planned transplants because of inadequate stem cell collections. In an intent-to-treat analysis with a median follow-up of 5.3 years, the 5-year actuarial OS and PFS rates were 54% and 49%, respectively. Similar regimens are under investigation in several single center studies and in a prospective cooperative group study including the Southwest Oncology Group (SWOG) and the Blood and Marrow Transplant Clinical Trials Network (BMT CTN). Whether the apparently superior results from this approach represent improved efficacy or selection bias for the double-transplant procedure will require prospective evaluation.

16.2.3 Prognostic Factors for HL Patients Undergoing High-Dose Therapy and Autologous HSCT

Most early transplant studies included heavily pretreated patients, which influenced the morbidity and mortality of HDT. The introduction of granulocyte-colony-stimulating factor (G-CSF), peripheral blood progenitor cells, as opposed to bone marrow, as the stem cell graft, better transfusion practices and more effective antibiotics have decreased transplant-related mortality to less than 3% in most series. Despite this improvement in supportive care, long-term EFS has improved by at most 10% in recent autologous HSCT studies [24].

Prognostic factors that can predict for outcome are important for potential risk-adapted therapy; which has not been explored in the relapse/refractory setting. The expectation from risk-adapted therapy is a reduction in the influence of prognostic factors on outcome, by improving the results of patients in the less favorable groups. In the setting of relapsed and refractory HL, risk factors can be determined either pre or post-salvage therapy.

16.2.3.1 Presalvage Therapy Risk Factors

Many groups have reported that a number of presalvage therapy (ST) clinical parameters other than refractory disease can predict survival in patients with relapsed or refractory HL. In general, these prognostic factors can be divided into pretreatment risk factors such as (1) extent of disease (advanced stage or extranodal involvement), (2) B symptoms (or surrogate marker such as elevated ESR or IL-10), (3) remission duration of less than 1 year, (4) heavily pretreated pre-autologous HSCT as defined as receiving more than two chemotherapy regimens, or (5) a significant disease burden after ST. Evaluating outcome based upon pre-ST prognostic factors yields interesting results, and cohorts of patients are easily subdivided into favorable cohorts having 5-year EFS rates approaching 75%; not unexpectedly, unfavorable cohorts have EFS less than 30% [25–29].

A few large series are worth noting with regard to outcome based upon pre-ST prognostic factors. The Grupo Español de Linformas/Transplante Autólogo de Médula Osea (GEL/TAMO) Spanish Cooperative Group treated 375 relapsed HL patients with HDT and autologous HSCT. Patients with all three of the following risk factors—advanced stage, relapsing in a previously irradiated site, and remission duration of less than 1 year—had 5-year EFS rates of only 18% [30]. The Groupe d'Etude des Lymphomes de l'Adulte (GELA) developed a two-factor model incorporating remission duration less than 1 year and the presence of extranodal disease at relapse as adverse prognostic factors. With this model, patients with zero, one, or two risk factors had PFS rates of 93%, 59%, and 43%, respectively [31, 16]. The GHSG retrospectively analyzed risk factors at relapse in a group of 422 patients (Fig. 16.1). In multivariate analysis three factors predicted outcome: remission duration less than 1 year, advanced stage at relapse, and anemia; those patients with all three risk factors had an EFS of less than 25% [22, 20].

Lastly, the lymphoma service at Memorial Sloan–Kettering Cancer Center utilized uniform ST with ICE (ifosfamide, carboplatin and etoposide) and offered HDT and autologous HSCT only to patients with chemotherapy-sensitive disease. As analyzed by intent to treat, the 5-year EFS were 55%. Three pre-ICE risk factors were predictive of a poor outcome: extranodal sites of disease, remission duration less than 1 year, and B symptoms; 5-year EFS rates were

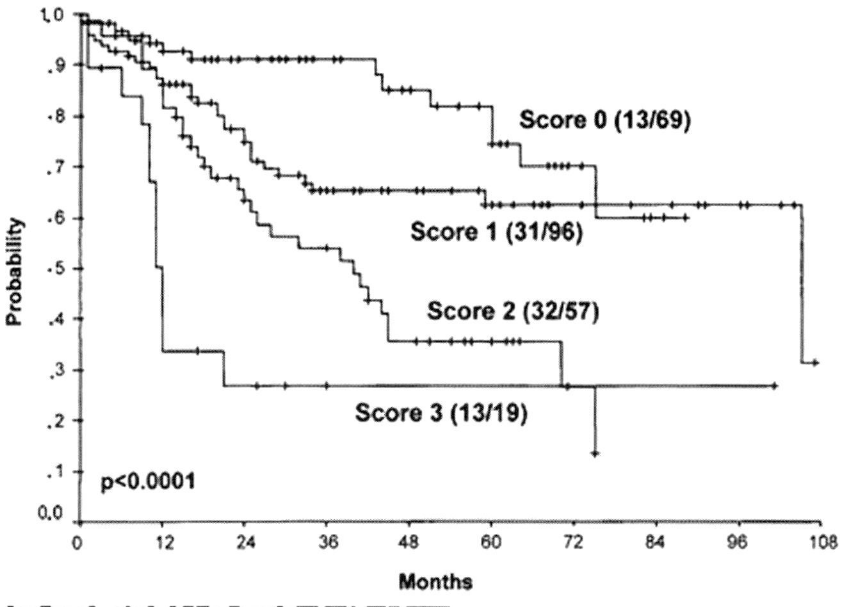

Fig. 16.1 Event-free survival based upon risk factors (remission duration less than 1 year, advanced stage at relapse, and anemia) at the time of first relapse

76%, 35% and 8% for patients with 0–1, 2, and 3 factors, respectively [32]. Other investigators have also reported that these three risk factors (RF) have an important prognostic value in the setting of relapsed/refractory HL [5].

Based upon the above information it seems very reasonable to offer patients with remission duration of <1 year with concomitant extranodal or stage IV disease at relapse investigational HDT programs.

16.2.3.2 Role of Chemotherapy-Sensitive Disease to Salvage Therapy

As with aggressive non-Hodgkin's lymphoma, chemotherapy-sensitive disease to ST is now required for transplant eligibility in the United States. There is limited information regarding the optimal ST regimen. The following requirements for an ST regimen are adequate cytoreduction in at least 75% of patients without extramedullary toxicity or severe bone marrow suppression, and with subsequent ability to collect an adequate stem cell harvest. The quality of the response to ST may be more important for outcome than originally suspected, but how this response is assessed is a matter of debate.

For two decades response to ST has been determined by Computed Tomography (CT), and transplant eligibility is based upon improvement on this imaging modality; but in the era of functional imaging, especially in HL, this dogma needs to be challenged. HL patients nearly always have residual masses after chemotherapy, and FDG-PET is more sensitive and specific than CT in determining residual disease versus fibrosis. In fact, recently, for primary therapy for the aggressive lymphomas, including HL, in order for a patient to be declared to be in CR there needs to be normalization of FDG-PET [33]. An inadequate response on CT will label a patient chemotherapy-refractory when in fact the patient may actually have had a CR on FDG-PET. Therefore three groups of patients are likely to receive an autologous HSCT for HL: those with a true CR on CT imaging and with a negative FDG-PET scan; less than CR on CT imaging with a negative FDG-PET scan and finally chemotherapy-sensitive disease on CT but with a persistently positive FDG-PET scan.

There is no doubt that chemotherapy-sensitive disease in 2007 is required for autologous HSCT eligibility; however, should a CR to ST be the goal, and how should this be determined, CT or an FDG-PET or both? Does a minimal disease state pre-autologous HSCT significantly improve outcome?

The GEL/TAMO cooperative group reported outcome based upon CT response in 357 patients undergoing autologous HSCT in their cooperative group [34]. Five-year EFS for the entire cohort was 49%; however, for those achieving a CR to ST, 68% of patients are failure-free versus 34% who had less than a CR to ST; these results are quite similar to those of our two cancer centers (Memorial Sloan-Kettering Cancer Center and Cleveland Clinic), as well as those by the group in Cologne. Unfortunately most patients do not have a true CR on CT imaging; it is unclear if the number of patients defined in a "minimal disease state" can be increased by using normalization of FDG-PET scan as a surrogate marker for CR.

The lymphoma service at M.D. Anderson Cancer Center retrospectively reviewed 211 HL patients treated with autologous HSCT and correlated the pretransplant functional imaging (FI) with FDG-PET or gallium scan with outcome [35]. A CR or unconfirmed CR (CRu) was seen in 51% of patients, a partial response (PR) in 41% of patients, and stable or progressive disease in 7% of patients. As expected FI was positive in only 6 of 110 (5%) of CR/CRu patients, but was positive in 48 of 86 (56%) of PR patients. The 3-year PFS was 69% for patients with negative FI versus 23% for patients with positive FI ($p < 0.0001$). Three groups of patients emerged with 3-year PFS of 76%, 51% and 27% for CR, FI negative less than CR and PR with positive FI ($p < 0.0001$). Data from 169 HL patients treated on consecutive Memorial Sloan-Kettering Cancer Center ST protocols for relapse and refractory HL trials have a similar outcome to that of the M.D. Anderson group (Fig. 16.2).

Current recommendations should be to do both a CT and FDG-PET scan pre- and post-ST with the goal to achieve a minimal disease state with ST. It appears that both of these imaging modalities are necessary to determine the "minimal disease state" pre-autologous HSCT.

A critical question in the FDG-PET era is how FDG-PET imaging can be used to incorporate radiation into standard salvage programs. So many medical oncologists forget that radiation therapy cures HL, yet the majority of patients transplanted for HL in the United States have not received radiation therapy as part of either initial or salvage treatment. The accuracy of radiation treatment volume can be markedly improved with the fusion of FDG-PET data and CT-

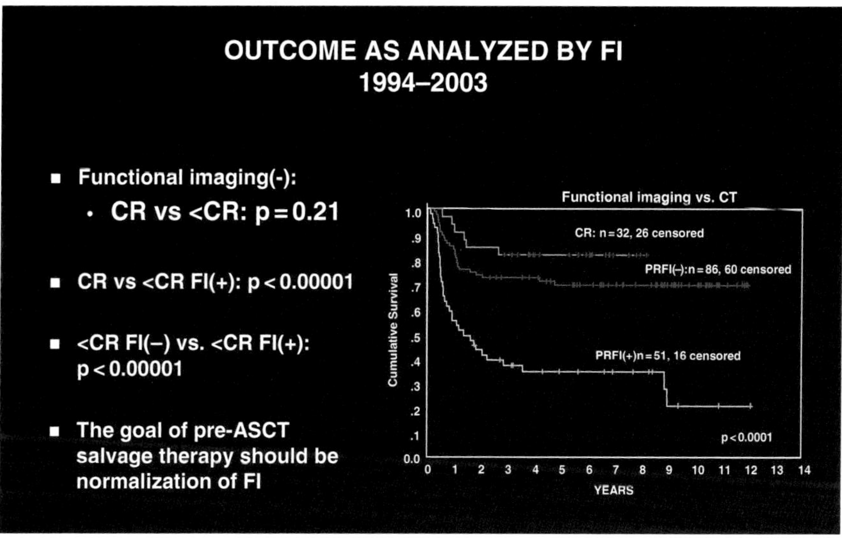

Fig. 16.2 Outcomes following HDT and autologous HSCT as determined by pretransplant response determination to computerized tomography (CT) or functional imaging (FI) with FDG-PET

simulation allowing simultaneous outlining of the treatment volumes with higher anatomic accuracy. New programs can incorporate FDG-PET information for the planning of radiotherapy pretransplant, broadening the range of radiation treatment options while minimizing the radiation dose to normal tissues. This is particularly useful for patients with bulky and/or complex mediastinal disease where the majority of HL patients fail.

16.2.4 Autologous HSCT for Hodgkin's Lymphoma in First Remission

Despite the favorable outcome for most patients with advanced HL, various investigators have identified "poor-risk" groups. The International Prognostic Factors (IPS) Project in Advanced Hodgkin's Disease identified seven adverse clinical prognostic factors [36]. Patients with no adverse factors had a 5-year FFP rate of 84% compared with only 42% for those with four or more risk factors. Some studies of autologous HSCT in first remission for patients with "poor-risk" HL have been reported, although the definition of poor risk has varied and none has used the IPS criteria. None of these studies has shown an advantage in PFS or OS for "early" autologous HSCT.

A single prospective randomized trial was conducted in 163 patients with poor risk disease (defined according to criteria reported from Memorial Sloan-Kettering Cancer Center), in CR or PR after four cycles of ABVD or similar anthracycline-based chemotherapy. These patients were randomized between high-dose therapy and autologous HSCT (83 patients) or four further cycles of chemotherapy [37]. With a median follow-up of 4 years, the 5-year FFS rates were 75% for the transplant arm, compared with 82% for the conventional therapy arm ($p = 0.4$). The corresponding OS rates were 88% vs. 88% ($p = 0.99$).

These results indicate that there is no role for HDT and autologous HSCT in first remission in this disease, largely due to the inability to identify a group of patients with a sufficiently poor prognosis to justify an intensive approach. Recently introduced dose-dense and dose-intensive regimens such as BEACOPP have been shown to be equally effective across all risk groups identified by the IPS, suggesting that this prognostic system will not have clinical utility in the future in identifying poor risk patients. New techniques such as gene expression profiling may identify poor risk patients who might benefit from early intensification of therapy, although this is likely to represent only a very small number of patients and it is unlikely that randomized trials will be possible in this group.

Recent data regarding the predictive value of "early" FI with FDG-PET suggest that this technique may identify patients with poor risk disease on conventional induction therapy who may benefit from intensification. Whether autologous HSCT will improve OS in this group will also require prospective evaluation.

16.3 Allogeneic HSCT in Hodgkin Lymphoma

The use of allogeneic HSCT in HL has been relatively limited. Early reports of the use of allogeneic transplantation using myeloablative conditioning regimens were disappointing, with high treatment-related mortality rates of 50–60% (Table 16.1). Respiratory complications were particularly common, possibly because of the prior use of extensive radiation therapy to the mediastinum. Furthermore, the presence of acute or chronic graft-versus-host diseases (GvHD) did not appear to influence the rate of relapse, suggesting that graft-versus-tumor effects may not contribute significantly to disease control in HL. A case-matched analysis of autologous and allogeneic HSCT for HL performed by the EBMT showed no difference in OS or relapse rate, but a significantly higher 4-year treatment related mortality in patients receiving allogeneic HSCT [38]. In this study, the occurrence of grade II or worse GvHD was associated with a lower relapse rate, but also with a lower survival. However, this observation suggested the possibility of a clinically exploitable graft-versus-tumor effect in HL, leading to the use of nonmyeloablative conditioning in several subsequent studies.

In a study from M.D. Anderson Cancer Center, 58 patients with relapsed or refractory HL, 48 of whom had previously undergone autologous HSCT, were treated with a reduced-intensity conditioning regimen comprising fludarabine and melphalan, with the addition of anti-thymocyte globulin for the more recent unrelated donor recipients [42]. Twenty-five patients received transplants from related donors, and 33 from matched unrelated donors. The treatment mortality rates at 100 days and 2 years were 7% and 15%, respectively. The 2-year actuarial PFS and OS were 32% and 64%, respectively. However, 24% of patients required subsequent donor lymphocyte infusions for disease progression, 35% of whom also required additional chemotherapy. The true impact of the graft-versus-tumor effect in this population is therefore difficult to assess, although in view of the very extensive prior therapy this group had received, the reported 32% PFS rate is encouraging and merits further investigation. Comparable results have been reported for several other single institution studies, summarized in Table 16.2.

A registry-based study of reduced-intensity conditioning has recently been published from the EBMT [46]. This includes 374 patients treated with a median of four prior regimens (1–8), including autologous HSCT in 288 (77%). At the

Table 16.1 Results of allogeneic HSCT with myeloablative conditioning in patients with relapsed and refractory Hodgkin's lymphoma

Reference	*n*	TRM	DFS
[39]	100	61% at 3 years	15% at 3 years
[38]	45	48% at 4 years	15% at 4 years
[40]	53	49% at 5 years	18% at 5 years
[41]	53	32% at 10 years	26% at 10 years

Table 16.2 Results of allogeneic stem cell transplantation with reduced intensity conditioning regimens in Hodgkin lymphoma

Reference	*n*	TRM	PFS
[42]	58	15% at 2 years	32% at 2 years
[43]	27	35% at 1 year	11% at 1 year for related donors and 35% at 1 year for unrelated donor
[44]	40	25% at 1 year	32% at 2 years
[45]	49	16% at 2 years	32% at 4 years

time of allogeneic HSCT, 21% of patients were in CR, 39% had a chemotherapy-sensitive relapse and 40% were in chemotherapy-resistant relapse or had not received therapy to assess chemotherapy-sensitivity prior to transplant. Matched related donors were used in 63% of patients, with 30% receiving transplant from matched unrelated donors and the remainder receiving mismatched transplants. A variety of conditioning regimens were used. The reported 100 day and 12 month treatment-related mortality was 12% and 20%, respectively. A 2-year PFS rate of 29% was reported for all patients, those with chemotherapy-resistant disease having the worse prognosis.

A recent EBMT analysis has compared outcomes after allogeneic transplantation for patients receiving myeloablative and nonmyeloablative conditioning regimens. The group receiving nonmyeloablative conditioning had a significantly lower nonrelapse mortality and significantly higher OS and PFS. The development of chronic GvHD was associated with a lower incidence of relapse and higher PFS and OS, providing some further evidence for a possible graft-versus-HL effect, which is also supported by the observed response to donor lymphocyte infusions reported for some patients with this disease.

Despite these early encouraging results for allogeneic HSCT in HL, it remains an experimental therapy that should not be used outside the context of prospective trials. Uncertainties exist regarding the optimal stem cell source, conditioning regimen and GvHD prophylaxis, all of which require prospective evaluation.

References

1. Longo DL, Duffey PL, Young RC, Hubbard SM, Idhe DC, Glatstein E, Phares JC, Jaffe ES, Urba WJ, De Vita VT Jr. Conventional-dose salvage combination chemotherapy in patients relapsing with Hodgkin's disease after combination chemotherapy: the low probability of cure. J Clin Oncol. 1992;10:210–8.
2. Canellos GP, Anderson JR, Propert KJ, Nissen N, Cooper MR, Henderson ES, Green MR, Gottlieb A, Peterson BA. Chemotherapy of advanced Hodgkin's disease with MOPP, ABVD or MOPP alternating with ABVD. New Engl J Med. 1992;327:1478–84.
3. Horning SJ, Chao NJ, Negrin RS, Hoppe RT, Long GD, Hu WW, Wong RM, Brown BW, Blume KG. High-dose therapy and autologous hematopoietic progenitor cell transplantation for recurrent or refractory Hodgkin's disease: analysis of the Stanford University results and prognostic indices. Blood 1997;89:801–13.

4. Yuen AR, Rosenberg SA, Hoppe RT, Halpern JD, Horning SJ. Comparison between conventional salvage therapy and high-dose therapy with autografting for recurrent or refractory Hodgkin's disease. Blood 1997;89:814–22.
5. Reece DE, Connors JM, Spinelli JJ, Barnett MJ, Fairey RN, Klingermann HG, Nantel SH, O'Reilly S, Shepherd JD, Sutherland HJ, Voss N, Chan K-W, Phillips GL. Intensive therapy with cyclophosphamide, carmustine, etoposide ± cisplatin, and autologous bone marrow transplantation for Hodgkin's disease in first relapse after combination chemotherapy. Blood 1994;83:1193–9.
6. Chopra R, McMillan AK, Linch DC, Yuklea S, Taghipour G, Pearce R, Patterson KG, Goldstone AH. The place of high-dose BEAM therapy and autologous bone marrow transplantation in poor-risk Hodgkin's disease. A single center eight-year study of 155 patients. Blood 1993;81:1137–45.
7. Sweetenham JW, Taghipour G, Milligan D, Blystad AK, Caballero D, Fassas A, Goldstone AH. High-dose therapy and autologous stem cell rescue for patients with Hodgkin's disease in first relapse after chemotherapy: results from the EBMT. Bone Marrow Transplant. 1997;20:745–52.
8. Linch DC, Winfield D, Goldstone AH, Moir D, Hancock B, McMillan AK, Chopra R, Milligan D, Vaughan-Hudson G. Dose intensification with autologous bone marrow transplantation in relapsed and resistant Hodgkin's disease: results of a BNLI randomized trial. Lancet 1993;341:1051–4.
9. Schmitz N, Pfistner B, Sextro M, Sieber M, Carella AM, Haenel M, Boissevain F, Zschaber R, Muller P, Kirchner H, Lohri A, Decker S, Koch B, Hasenclever D, Goldstone AH, Diehl V. Aggressive conventional chemotherapy compared with high-dose chemotherapy with autologous haemopoietic stem-cell transplantation for relapsed chemosensitive Hodgkin's disease: a randomized trial. Lancet 2002;359:2065–71.
10. Schmitz N, Haverkamp H, Josting A, Diehl V, Pfistner B, Carella AM, Haenel N, Biossvain F, Bokemeyer C, Goldstone AH. Long term follow up in relapsed Hodgkin's disease (HD): updated results of the HD-R1 study comparing conventional chemotherapy (cCT) to high-dose chemotherapy (HDCT) with autologous haemopoietic stem cell transplantation (autologous HSCT) of the German Hodgkin's Study Group (GHSG) and the Working Party Lymphoma of the European Group for Blood and Marrow Transplantation (EBMT). J Clin Oncol. 2005;23:562s (Abstract).
11. Horning SJ, Hoppe RT, Breslin S, Bartlett NL, Brown BW, Rosenberg SA. Stanford V and radiotherapy for locally extensive and advanced Hodgkin's disease: mature results of a prospective clinical trial. J Clin Oncol. 2002;20:630–7.
12. Diehl V, Franklin J, Pfreundschuh M, Lathan B, Paulus U, Hasenclever D, Tesch H, Herrmann R, Dorken B, Muller-Hermelink H-K, Duhmke E, Loeffler M. Standard and increased-dose BEACOPP chemotherapy compared with COPP-ABVD for advanced Hodgkin's disease. New Engl J Med. 2003;348:2386–95.
13. Bonfante V, Santoro A, Viviani S, Devizzi L, Balzarotti M, Soncini F, Zanini M, Valagussa P, Bonnadonna G. Outcome of patients with Hodgkin's disease failing MOPP-ABVD. J Clin Oncol. 1997;15:528–34.
14. Yahalom J, Gulati S, Toia M, Maslak P, McCarron EG, O'Brien JP, Portlock CS, Straus DJ, Phillips J, Fuks Z. Accelerated hyperfractionated total lymphoid irradiation, high-dose chemotherapy and autologous bone marrow transplantation for refractory and relapsing patients with Hodgkin's disease. J Clin Oncol. 1993;11:1062–70.
15. Moskowitz CH, Kewalramani T, Nimer SD, Gonzalez M, Zelenetz AD, Yaholom J. Effectiveness of high dose chemoradiotherapy and autologous stem cell transplantation for patients with biopsy-proven refractory Hodgkin's disease. Br J Haematol. 2004; 124:645–52.
16. Ferme C, Mounier N, Divine M, Brice P, Stamatoullas A, Reman O, Voillat L, Jaubert J, Lederlin P, Colin P, Berger F, Salles G. Intensive salvage therapy with high-dose chemoradiotherapy for patients with advanced Hodgkin's disease in relapse or failure after

initial chemotherapy: results of the Groupe D'Etudes des Lymphomes de l'adulte H89 trial. J Clin Oncol. 2002;20:467–75.
17. Constans M, Sureda A, Terol MJ, Arranz R, Caballero MD, Iriondo A, Jarque I, Carreras E, Moraleda JM, Carrera D, Leon A, Lopez A, Albo C, Diaz-Mediavilla J, Fernandez-Abellan P, Garcia-Ruiz JC, Hernandez-Navarro F, Mataix R, Petit J, Pascual MJ, Rifon J, Garcia-Conde J, Fernandez-Ranada JM, Mateos MV, Sierra J, Conde E: GEL/TAMO Cooperative Group. Autologous stem cell transplantation for primary refractory Hodgkin's disease: results and clinical variables affecting outcome. Ann Oncol. 2003;14:745–51.
18. Sweetenham JW, Carella AM, Taghipour G, Cunningham D, Marcus R, Volpe AD, Linch DC, Schmitz N, Goldstone AH. High-dose therapy and autologous stem cell transplantation for adult patients with Hodgkin's disease who do not enter complete remission after induction chemotherapy: results in 175 patients reported to the European Group for Blood and Marrow Transplantation. J Clin Oncol. 1999;17:3101–9.
19. Lazarus HM, Rowlings PA, Zhang M-J, Vose JM, Armitage JO, Bierman PJ, Gajewski JL, Gale RP, Keating A, Klein JP, Miller CB, Phillips GL, Reece DE, Sobocinski KA, van Beisen K, Horowitz MM. Autotransplants for Hodgkin's disease in patients never achieving remission: a report from the Autologous Blood and Marrow Transplant Registry. J Clin Oncol. 1999;17:534–45.
20. Josting A, Rueffer U, Franklin J, Seiber M, Diehl V, Engert A. Prognostic factors and treatment outcome in primary progressive Hodgkin lymphoma: a report from the German Hodhkin Lymphoma Study Group. Blood 2000;96:1280–6.
21. Gallamini A, Hutchings M, Rigacci L, Specht L, Merli F, Hansen M, Patti C, Loft A, Di Raimondo F, D'Amore F, Biggi A, Vitolo U, Stelitano C, Sancetta R, Trentin L, Luminari S, Iannitto E, Viviani S, Pierri I, Levis A. Early interim 2-[^{18}F] Fluoro-2-deoxy-D-glucose positron emission tomography is prognostically superior to international prognostic score in advanced Hodgkin's lymphoma: a report from a joint Italian–Danish study. J Clin Oncol. 2007;25:3746–52.
22. Josting A, Rudolph C, Mapara M, Gloosman JP, Sienawski M, Seiber M, Kirchner HH, Dorken B, Hossfiled DK, Kisro J, Metzner B, Berdel WE, Diehl V, Engert A. Cologne high-dose sequential chemotherapy in relapsed and refractory Hodgkin lymphoma: results of a large multicenter study of the German Hodgkin Lymphoma Study Group (GHSG). Ann Oncol. 2005;16:116–23.
23. Fung HC, Stiff P, Schriber J, Toor A, Smith E, Rodriguez T, Krishnan A, Molina A, Smith D, Ivers B, Kogut N, Popplewell L, Rodriguez R, Somlo G, Forman SJ, Nademanee A. Tandem autologous stem cell transplantation for patients with primary refractory or poor risk recurrent Hodgkin lymphoma. Biol Blood Marrow Transplant. 2007;13:594–600.
24. Moskowitz C. An update on the management of relapsed and primary refractory Hodgkin's disease. Semin Oncol. 2004;31:54–9.
25. Abdel Hamid TM, El Zawahry HM, Khattab NA, Mowafy TM, Awaad MM, Ali El-Din NH, Mokhtar NM. Prognostic factors of Hodgkin's lymphoma and their impact on response to chemotherapy and survival. J Egypt Natl Canc Inst. 2005;17:9–14.
26. Brice P, Bastion Y, Divine M, Nedellec G, Ferrant A, Gabarre J, Reman O, Lepage A, Ferme C. Analysis of prognostic factors after the first relapse of Hodgkin's disease in 187 patients. Cancer 1996;78:1293–9.
27. Czyz J, Dziadziuszko R, Knopinska-Postuszuy W, Hellmann A, Kachel L, Holowiecki J, Gozdzik J, Hansz J, Avigdor A, Nagler A, Osowiecki M, Walewski J, Mensah P, Jurczak W, Skotnicki A, Sedzimirska M, Lange A, Sawicki W, Sulek K, Wach M, Dmoszynska A, Kus A, Robak T, Warzocha K. Outcome and prognostic factors in advanced Hodgkin's disease treated with high-dose chemotherapy and autologous stem cell transplantation: a study of 341 patients. Ann Oncol. 2004;15:1222–30.
28. Josting A, Engert A, Diehl V, Canellos GP. Prognostic factors and treatment outcome in patients with primary progressive and relapsed Hodgkin's disease. Ann Oncol. 2002;13 Suppl 1:112–6.

29. Sarris AH. Prognostic factors in early-stage Hodgkin's disease. J Clin Oncol. 1997; 15:411–2.
30. Sureda A, Arranz R, Iriondo A, Carreras E, Lahuerta JJ, García-Conde J, Jarque I, Caballero MD, Ferrà C, López A, García-Laraña J, Cabrera R, Carrera D, Ruiz-Romero MD, León A, Rifón J, Díaz-Mediavilla J, Mataix R, Morey M, Moraleda JM, Altés A, López-Guillermo A, de la Serna J, Fernández-Rañada JM, Sierra J, Conde E. Grupo Español de Linformas/Transplante Autólogo de Médula Osea Spanish Cooperative Group. Autologous stem-cell transplantation for Hodgkin's disease: results and prognostic factors in 494 patients from the Grupo Espanol de Linfomas/Transplante Autologo de Medula Osea Spanish Cooperative Group. J Clin Oncol. 2001;19:395–404.
31. Brice P, Bouabdallah R, Moreau P, Divine M, André M, Aoudjane M, Fleury J, Anglaret B, Baruchel A, Sensebe L, Colombat P. Prognostic factors for survival after high-dose therapy and autologous stem cell transplantation for patients with relapsing Hodgkin's disease: analysis of 280 patients from the French registry. Societe Francaise de Greffe de Moelle. Bone Marrow Transplant. 1997;20:21–6.
32. Moskowitz CH, Nimer SD, Zelenetz AD, Trippett T, Hedrick EE, Filippa DA, Louie D, Gonzales M, Walits J, Coady-Lyons N, Qin J, Frank R, Bertino JR, Goy A, Noy A, O'Brien JP, Straus D, Portlock CS, Yahalom J. A 2-step comprehensive high-dose chemoradiotherapy second-line program for relapsed and refractory Hodgkin disease: analysis by intent to treat and development of a prognostic model. Blood 2001;97:616–23.
33. Cheson BD, Pfistner B, Juweid ME, Gascoyne RD, Specht L, Horning SJ, Coiffier B, Fisher RI, Hagenbeek A, Zucca E, Rosen ST, Stroobants S, Lister TA, Hoppe RT, Dreyling M, Tobinai K, Vose JM, Connors JM, Federico M, Diehl V. The international harmonization project on lymphoma. Revised response criteria for malignant lymphoma. J Clin Oncol. 2007;25:579–86.
34. Sureda A, Constans M, Iriondo A, Arranz R, Caballero MD, Vidal MJ, Petit J, López A, Lahuerta JJ, Carreras E, García-Conde J, García-Laraña J, Cabrera R, Jarque I, Carrera D, García-Ruiz JC, Pascual MJ, Rifón J, Moraleda JM, Pérez-Equiza K, Albó C, Díaz-Mediavilla J, Torres A, Torres P, Besalduch J, Marín J, Mateos MV, Fernández-Rañada JM, Sierra J, Conde E. Grupo Español de Linfomas/Trasplante Autólogo de Médula Osea Cooperative Group. Prognostic factors affecting long-term outcome after stem cell transplantation in Hodgkin's lymphoma autografted after a first relapse. Ann Oncol. 2005;16:625–33.
35. Jabbour E, Hosing C, Ayers G, Nunez R, Anderlini P, Pro B, Khouri I, Younes A, Hagemeister F, Kwak L, Fayad L. Pretransplant positive positron emission tomography/gallium scans predict poor outcome in patients with recurrent/refractory Hodgkin lymphoma. Cancer 2007;109:2481–9.
36. Hasenclever D, Diehl V, Armitage JO, Assouline D, Bjorkholm M, Brusamolino E, Canellos GP, Carde P, Crowther D, Cunningham D, Eghbali H, Ferme C, Fisher RI, Glick JH, Glimelius B, Gobbi PG, Holte H, Horning SJ, Lister TA, Longo DL, Mandelli F, Polliak A, Proctor SJ, Specht L, Sweetenham JW, Vaughan-Hudson G. A prognostic score for advanced Hodgkin's disease. New Engl J Med. 1998;339:1506–14.
37. Federico M, Bellei M, Brice P, Brugiatelli M, Nagler A, Gisselbrecht C, Moretti L, Colombat P, Luminari S, Fabbiano F, Di Renzo N, Goldstone A, Carella AM. High-dose therapy and autologous stem cell transplantation versus conventional therapy for patients with advanced Hodgkin's lymphoma responding to front-line therapy. J Clin Oncol. 2003;21:2320–5.
38. Milpied N, Fielding AK, Pearce R, Ernst P, Goldstone AH. Allogeneic bone marrow transplant is not better than autologous transplant for patients with relapsed Hodgkin's disease. J Clin Oncol. 1996;14:1291–6.
39. Gajewski JL, Phillips GL, Sobconski KA, Armitage JO, Gale RP, Champlin RE, Herzig RH, Hurd DD, Jagannath S, Lkein JP, Lazarus HM, McCarthy PL, Pavlovsky S, Peterson FB, Rowlings PA, Russell JA, Silver SM, Vose JM, Wiernik PH, Bortin MM,

Horowitz MM. Bone marrow transplants from HLA-identical siblings in advanced Hodgkin's disease. J Clin Oncol. 1996;14:572–8.
40. Anderson JE, Litzow MR, Appelbaum FR, Schoch G, Fisher LD, Buckner CD, Peterson FB, Crawford SW, Press OW, Sanders JE. Allogeneic syngeneic and autologous marrow transplantation for Hodgkin's disease: the 21-year Seattle experience. J Clin Oncol. 1993;11:2342–50.
41. Akpek G, Ambinder RF, Piantodosi S, Abrams RA, Brodsky RA, Vogelsang GB, Zahurak ML, Fuller D, Miller CB, Noga SJ, Fuchs E, Flinn IW, O'Donnell P, Seifter EJ, Mann RB, Jones RJ. Long-term results of blood and marrow transplantation for Hodgkin's lymphoma. J Clin Oncol. 2001;19:4314–21.
42. Anderlini P, Saliba R, Acholonu S, Okoroji GJ, Donato M, Giralt S, Andersson B, Ueno NT, Khouri I, De Lima M, Hosing C, Cohen A, Ippoliti C, Romaguera J, Rodriguez MA, Pro B, Fayad L, Goy A, Younes A, Champlin RE. Reduced-intensity allogeneic stem cell transplantation in relapsed and refractory Hodgkin's disease: low transplant-related mortality and impact of intensity of conditioning regimen. Bone Marrow Transplant. 2005;35:945–51.
43. Burroughs LM, Maris MB, Sandmeier BM. HLA-matched related (MRD) or unrelated donor (MUD) nonmyeloablative conditioning and hematopoietic cell transplant (HCT) for patients with advanced Hodgkin's disease (HD). Biol Blood Marrow Transplant. 2005;10 Suppl 1:73–4.
44. Alvarez I, Sureda A, Caballero MD, Urbano-Ispizua A, Ribera JM, Canales M, García-Conde J, Sanz G, Arranz R, Bernal MT, de la Serna J, Díez JL, Moraleda JM, Rubió-Félix D, Xicoy B, Martínez C, Mateos MV, Sierra J. Non-myeloablative stem cell transplantation is an effective therapy for refractory or relapsed Hodgkin's lymphoma: results of a Spanish prospective cooperative protocol. Biol Blood Marrow Transplant. 2006;12:172–83.
45. Peggs KS, Hunter A, Chopra R, Parker A, Mahendra P, Milligan D, Craddock C, Pettengell R, Dogan A, Thomson KJ, Morris EC, Hale G, Waldmann H, Goldstone AH, Linch DC, Mackinnon S. Clinical evidence of a graft-versus-Hodgkin's-lymphoma effect after reduced-intensity allogeneic transplantation. Lancet 2005;365:1934–41.
46. Sureda A, Robinson S, Canals C, Carella AM, Boogaerts MA, Caballero D, Hunter AE, Kanz L, Slavin S, Cornelissen JJ, Gramatzki M, Niederwieser D, Russell NH, Schmitz N. Reduced-intensity conditioning compared with conventional allogeneic stem-cell transplantation in relapsed or refractory Hodgkin's lymphoma: an analysis from the Lymphoma Working Party of the European Group for Blood and Marrow Transplantation. J Clin Oncol. 2008;26:455–62.

Chapter 17
Role of Hematopoietic Stem Cell Transplantation in Acute Myelogenous Leukemia and Myelodysplastic Syndrome

Martin S. Tallman, Vikram Mathews, and John F. DiPersio

17.1 Introduction

Significant advances have been made in the management of adult acute myeloid leukemia (AML—a.k.a. acute myelogenous leukemia) and myelodysplastic syndromes over the over the past several decades. However, most of these advances have been limited to young adults (<55 years) in whom the average 5-year disease-free survival (DFS) rate in AML has improved from 11% to 37% between 1970 and 2000 [1]. Over a similar period in patients who were older than 55 years at the time of diagnosis, the 5-year DFS for AML has changed marginally (6–12%) [1]. AML is a heterogeneous disease, thus options of therapy in first complete remission (CR1) depend on additional prognostic factors. With current induction regimens, 70–80% of patients with newly diagnosed AML achieve a complete remission; however, this is short-lived without consolidation therapy and most, if not all, of these patients will relapse and succumb to their illness [2, 3]. Options for post-remission induction therapy for AML in CR1 include intensive nonmyeloablative consolidative chemotherapy, autologous hematopoietic stem cell transplantation (HSCT), or allogeneic HSCT. Despite data consistently showing a significantly reduced risk of a relapse after an autologous or an allogeneic HSCT, historically this has not translated to a significantly better DFS or overall survival (OS) because of the counter effect of the treatment-related mortality (TRM) associated with these approaches.

Although the cytogenetic status of patients with AML is considered the single most important prognostic factor at diagnosis, additional markers are evolving that in conjunction with cytogenetics could help better define subsets at high risk for relapse and candidates for HSCT in CR1 [4, 5] or subsets of patients who may have a sufficiently favorable prognosis as to preclude a major benefit from HSCT in CR1. There have also been innovations and a steady

J.F. DiPersio (✉)
Division of Oncology, Campus Box 8007, Washington University Medical School, 660 South Euclid Avenue, St. Louis, MO 63110, USA
e-mail: jdipersi@im.wustl.edu

M.R. Bishop (ed.), *Hematopoietic Stem Cell Transplantation*, Cancer Treatment and Research 144, DOI 10.1007/978-0-387-78580-6_17,

improvement in the management of patients undergoing HSCT that has resulted in lower TRM and improved OS [6–10]. These improvements make it difficult to apply the data from the large prospective clinical trials, most of which were initiated more than a decade ago, to current therapeutic algorithms.

For older patients (>60 years) with newly diagnosed AML, the outcomes after any of the available modalities of therapy are poor. Recent data reporting on the use of reduced-intensity conditioning (RIC) regimens for an allogeneic HSCT in this age group are encouraging, but they remain to be validated in larger prospective clinical trials [7].

Myelodysplastic syndromes (MDS), like AML, are a heterogeneous group of clonal hematopoietic disorders characterized by ineffective hematopoiesis, marrow dysplasia and a variable rates of transformation to AML affecting predominantly the older age group (mean age = 69 years) [11]. With the aging of the population and increased awareness the incidence and prevalence of MDS has been steadily increasing over the last 20 years [12]. Consistent with the heterogeneous nature of MDS, a number of subtypes have been defined. The older FAB classification [13] of MDS has been replaced by the WHO classification [14] which divides MDS into refractory anemia (RA), refractory anemia with ringed sideroblasts (RARS), refractory cytopenia with trilineage dysplasia, deletion 5q syndrome, refractory anemia with excess blasts (RAEB) Type I (5–10% blasts), and RAEB Type II (11–20% blasts). The above diagnostic subtypes have a significant bearing both on the therapeutic intervention one might recommend and on prognosis. In addition to the subtype, the cytogenetic findings and number of cytopenias at diagnosis are important for prognosis. Despite significant progress in the understanding of the pathophysiology of MDS, which has translated into novel therapeutic interventions, allogeneic HSCT still remains the only therapy that has curative potential for MDS potential.

17.2 Hematopoietic Stem Cell Transplantation in Acute Myeloid Leukemia

The options of consolidation therapy for patients with newly diagnosed AML in CR1 include high-dose chemotherapy, autologous HSCT or an allogeneic HSCT. Risk stratification at diagnosis, age and response to induction chemotherapy are important factors that will help make the choice of the appropriate consolidation therapy. Newly diagnosed patients with AML should continue to be enrolled in clinical trials in an effort to address some of these issues. In the setting of evolving concepts and improved outcomes with different treatment modalities, treatment of newly diagnosed patients has to be individualized based not only on data from the older, large randomized prospective trials, reported a decade earlier, but also on currently available updates in the literature. In this chapter, the progress that has been made in the area of autologous and allogeneic HSCT and some of the evolving concepts are addressed.

17.2.1 *Risk Stratification of Patients with Acute Myeloid Leukemia in First Complete Remission*

Cytogenetics has been the cornerstone of risk stratification in AML [4]. The risk groups based on katyotyping as used by the cooperative groups (Cancer and Leukemia Group B, Southwest Oncology Group, and Eastern Cooperative Oncology Group) are illustrated in Table 17.1 [15]. The good, intermediate, and unfavourable risk groups have 25%, 50%, and greater than 70% probability of relapse and a 4-year probability of survival of greater than 70%, 40–50%, and less than 20%, respectively [16]. This applies to patients <60 years of age. Additional parameters, such as age, white blood cell count at diagnosis, presence of certain gene mutations, and response to induction chemotherapy can influence prognosis, while the type of consolidation therapy could potentially alter the predicted outcomes.

This risk stratification is particularly useful in making decisions regarding the type of consolidation chosen for a patient. In the good-risk group, an allogeneic HSCT with a TRM of 15–30% will not be the first option when three to four cycles of high-dose nonmyeloablative consolidation chemotherapy has been reported to achieve long-term DFS as high as 70% with a less than 5% TRM. However, a more recent analysis involving a larger number of patients than had been previously analyzed for this group, suggests that the outcome in the good risk group is likely to be lower than that was previously reported, with a 10-year overall survival of 44% [95% confidence interval (CI): 39–50%] [17, 18]. In the unfavorable group, with chemotherapy alone, only 10–20% of patients are likely to achieve long-term DFS, thus an allogeneic HSCT would be considered

Table 17.1 Risk group stratification based on cytogenetics at diagnosis

Good risk(10–15%)	t(15;17)
	t(8;21)
	inv16, t(16;16)
Standard risk (65–75%)	Normal karyotype
	del (9q)
	−y
	del 12 p
	Trisomy 8
	t(9;11)
Poor risk (15–20%)	Abnormal 5 or 7
	inv3q
	del 20q
	del 21q
	t (9;22)
	t (6;9)
	Non-t(9;11) 11q23 abnormalities with MLL rearrangements
	Complex cytogenetics (3 or more clonal abnormalities)

Modified from Slovak et al. [4]

acceptable in an effort to improve the DFS [4]. In the intermediate risk group, which constitutes close to 40–50% of all patients with AML, the options in CR1 are less clearly defined. This group is heterogeneous in its response to therapy, and most of its members have a normal karyotype. New markers could help identify subsets at a high risk of relapse and candidates for a HSCT. Some such markers, whose role in the management of AML is still evolving, are summarized in Table 17.2. Recently it was reported that using a combination of two such gene mutations (NPM1 and FLT3-ITD), a subset defined as being NPM1^{+}/FLT3-ITD^{-} among patients with a normal karyotype had a good prognosis and would probably not benefit from an allogeneic HSCT in CR1 [19]. Although the data on some of these markers are still preliminary and remain to be validated in large clinical trials, they illustrate the potential of using these markers in risk stratification at diagnosis.

Table 17.2 Newly identified prognostic markers used in the management of AML

Marker	Summary
Flt3-ITD [20, 21]	Reported in 15–35% of cases with AML. Presence associated with an adverse outcome
BAALC gene over expression [22]	Brain and acute leukemia cytoplasmic (BAALC) gene over expression has been shown to predict poor survival in patients with AML and normal cytogenetics
bcl-2 and WT1 [23]	Coexpression of apoptosis-related genes bcl-2 and WT1 has been associated with significantly inferior DFS and OS
Evi-1 mRNA [24]	Over expression of Evi-1 mRNA in patients with intermediate risk (by conventional cytogenetics), even in the absence of cytogenetic 3q26 abnormalities, identifies a subset with a worse prognosis
Partial tandem duplication of the MLL gene [25]	Partial tandem duplication of the MLL gene in one study was seen in 7.7% of patients with a normal karyotype and associated with a significantly shorter remission duration
FADD protein expression [26]	Absence of Fas-associated death domain (FADD) protein expression in AML has been associated with a worse outcome
Mutations in CCAAT/enhancer-binding protein-α [27]	Several studies, most recently by Frohling et al. [27], have demonstrated that mutations in the transcription factor CCAAT/enhancer-binding protein-α are associated with a good prognosis
VEGFR-1 levels [28]	Plasma soluble vascular endothelial growth factor receptor-1 levels have been shown to have an inverse correlation with the attainment of CR after induction chemotherapy in AML
NPM1 mutations [29]	The nucleophosmin (NPM1) gene mutations occur in 50% to 60% of adult AML with normal karyotype (AML-NK). NPM1 mutations in absence of FLT3-ITD identify a prognostically favorable subgroup in the heterogeneous AML-NK category

With the increasing use of high-throughput molecular analysis techniques, clinicians can look forward to the identification of well-defined biologic entities within the broad cytogenetically defined standard-/intermediate-risk group of patients with AML that would help in the enhanced assessment of the risk to benefit ratio of an HSCT in CR1.

17.3 Autologous Hematopoietic Stem Cell Transplantation for Acute Myeloid Leukemia

The early phase II trials of autologous bone marrow transplantation in young adults with (<60 years) with AML in CR1 showed an overall DFS ranging from 40% to 60%, relapse rates of 30–50%, and a TRM of 5–15%. Subsequent phase III trials confirmed a reduced relapse risk compared to intensive chemotherapy (summarized in Table 17.3) [15, 30–32]. In two of these trials, this reduction translated into an improved DFS; however, there was not a significant difference in OS in any of the trials [30, 32]. A recently published meta-analysis confirms these observations [33]. All these reported prospective trials had limitations, such as variable numbers of patients who actually received the assigned therapy and a high TRM (average of 12%). Most of these trials were initiated more than a decade ago, and there has been significant interval improvement in the management of patients undergoing an autologous HSCT. Most large single center data are consistent with our own experience and demonstrate no significant difference in TRM compared to high-dose consolidation chemotherapy. This reduction in TRM could potentially translate into reduced relapse risk and improved DFS and OS after an autologous HSCT. It is unlikely that a prospective trial will clarify this in the near future since to show a 10% difference in survival ($p = 0.05$, with 90% power), more than 1000 patients would need to be enrolled [34]. From the available data, some generalizations can be made. Good-risk group patients would probably not benefit significantly from an autologous HSCT in CR1 [35]. In the unfavorable group, there are no data to suggest a benefit of an autologous HSCT over chemotherapy; the outcomes after both these options appear dismal [4, 32]. Patients in the intermediate-risk group are candidates for an autologous HSCT, especially subsets with a high risk of relapse as defined by additional parameters. However, this remains to be validated in large randomized clinical trials.

Table 17.3 Relapse risk in phase III trials comparing nonmyeloablative chemotherapy, autologous HSCT and allogeneic HSCTs

Study	Allogeneic (%)	Autologous (%)	Chemotherapy (%)
GIMMEMA [30]	24	40	57
GOELAM [31]	28	45	55
MRC [32]	19	35	53
ECOG/SWOG [15]	29	48	61

The role of an autologous HSCT in the older adults (>60 years) is controversial. While it appears to be feasible, the results are inferior to that seen in young adults and in one report did not appear to improve the clinical outcome [36, 37]. Retrospective comparison of the clinical outcomes following an autologous HSCT and an RIC-regimen allogeneic HSCT from the European Group for Blood and Marrow Transplantation (EBMT) registry, which is increasingly being used in older adults, suggests that there is no difference in the overall survival, though the relapses were significantly lower in the RIC group [38].

While most of the data for the use of an autologous HSCT have been for AML in CR1, recent data suggests a role for the use of an autologous HSCT in the management of relapsed AML in second complete remission (CR2) and beyond [39]. A recently reported retrospective analysis of the Center for International Blood and Marrow Transplant Research (CIBMTR) Registry data suggests that an autologous HSCT was superior to an unrelated donor allogeneic HSCT for AML in CR2 [40].

The conventional conditioning regimen prior to an autologous HSCT has been a combination of busulphan and cyclophosphamide (BuCy) [41] or a modification of this with reduced dose of cyclophosphamide administered over 2 days (BuCy2) [42]. The role of cyclophosphamide (predominantly immunosuppressive) in this setting has been questioned, and more myeloid malignancy specific drugs in the conditioning regimen, such as a combination of idarubicin and busulfan, have been used. The preliminary data with this regimen is promising [43].

17.3.1 Role of Purging the Stem Cell Product Before Autologous Hematopoietic Stem Cell Transplantation

In an effort to reduce relapse, some investigators have purged stem cell products before infusion. The agents traditionally used in vitro for this purpose include mafosfamide and 4-hydroperoxy-cyclophosphamide (4-HC). There are retrospective data to suggest that purging is of benefit, whereas, in a large prospective trial, purging with 4-HC did not appear to be of significant benefit [15, 44, 45]. There is insufficient data to strongly recommend purging; however, the data are also inadequate to completely exclude a role for purging the stem cell product. Other experimental methods of purging the stem cell product, including exposure to hyperthermia and immunologic purging by positive selection, have potential [46, 47].

17.3.2 Role of Consolidation Therapy Before Autologous Stem Cell Transplantation

After induction of CR1, additional consolidation chemotherapy before an autologous HSCT appears to have a significant positive effect by reducing the relapse risk and improving the DFS [48, 49]. A recent retrospective analysis of the Autologous Blood and Marrow Transplant Registry(ABMTR)/International Bone Marrow Transplant Registry (IBMTR) database reached a similar conclusion [50]. The optimal consolidation regimen before an autologous HSCT remains to be defined. Extrapolating from the Cancer and Leukemia Group B studies on the optimal consolidation chemotherapy for AML, it would appear that high-dose cytosine arabinoside (3 g/m^2 every 12 h $\times$ six doses) administered for three or more courses would be ideal [2, 18]. From the published data regarding autologous HSCT in AML, two or more cycles of high-dose cytosine arabinoside-based regimen would appear to be adequate prior to the transplant [48] though the ABMTR data analysis did not show a significant difference when either standard-dose cytosine arabinoside ($<$1 g/m^2) or high-dose cytosine arabinoside (1–3 g/m^2) was used [50].

17.3.3 Source of Stem Cells for an Autologous Hematopoietic Stem Cell Transplantation: Bone Marrow Versus Peripheral Blood

Retrospective data suggest that the use of cytokine-mobilized peripheral blood stem cells (PBSC) for an autologous transplant is associated with more rapid engraftment of neutrophils and platelets [51]. However, most studies do not show an improvement in relapse risk, TRM, DFS, or OS [52].

17.3.3.1 Effect of CD34$^+$ Mobilization and Cell Dose on Outcome

Patients in CR1 after consolidation chemotherapy have a variable capacity to mobilize CD34$^+$ stem cells after cytokine administration for peripheral blood stem cell transplantation (PBSCT). Recent analysis of the European Organization for Research and Treatment of Cancer/Gruppo Italiano Malattie Ematologiche Maligne dell'Adulto data suggest that patients who have high CD34$^+$ cell yields defined as the CD34$^+$ cell dose achieved with the first apheresis have an increased risk of relapse as a continuous variable [53]. A small study from Italy also suggested that a larger cell dose in autologous bone marrow transplants is associated with a lower DFS in patients who received unpurged bone marrow cells [54]. The etiology of the association remains obscure and may represent contamination of normal CD34$^+$ progenitors with CD34$^+$ AML cells at the time of stem cell collection. Data from Brenner et al. [55] suggested that the stem cell product marked by retroviral vectors may contribute to those AML cells that relapse after an autologous HSCT. The optimal cell dose remains to be defined.

17.4 Allogeneic Hematopoietic Stem Cell Transplantation for Acute Myeloid Leukemia

Large prospective trials have consistently shown that an allogeneic HSCT with standard myeloablative conditioning regimen is the most potent antileukemia treatment for AML in CR1 with a relapse risk of 24–36% compared to 46–61% with autologous HSCT or chemotherapy (Table 17.3) [15, 30–32, 56]. However, in none of these trials did this decreased relapse risk translate to a significantly improved OS. This was due to high TRM, which ranged from 10% to 25%. An allogeneic HSCT is not an option to consider for patients in the good risk cytogenetic group in CR1 since (i) they have excellent response to therapy with high-dose chemotherapy and (ii) even if they do relapse after consolidation chemotherapy, they still respond well to an allogeneic or autologous HSCT in CR2 [57, 58]. In the intermediate and unfavorable cytogenetic groups, the TRM associated with an allogeneic HSCT may be acceptable in an effort to improve the DFS and OS. In the unfavorable group in CR1, an intergroup study showed a 5-year survival rate of 44% vs. 15% with chemotherapy or an autologous HSCT (Fig. 17.1), whereas a similar but less dramatic difference was noted in the European Organization for Research and Treatment of Cancer/Gruppo Italiano Malattie Ematologiche Maligne dell'Adulto AML-10 trial (EORTC/GIMEMA) and in the Dutch Belgian Hematolo-Oncology Cooperative Group/Swiss Group for Clinical Cancer Research (HOVON-SAKK) study [4, 59, 60]. Two other studies failed to show an advantage of an allogeneic HSCT

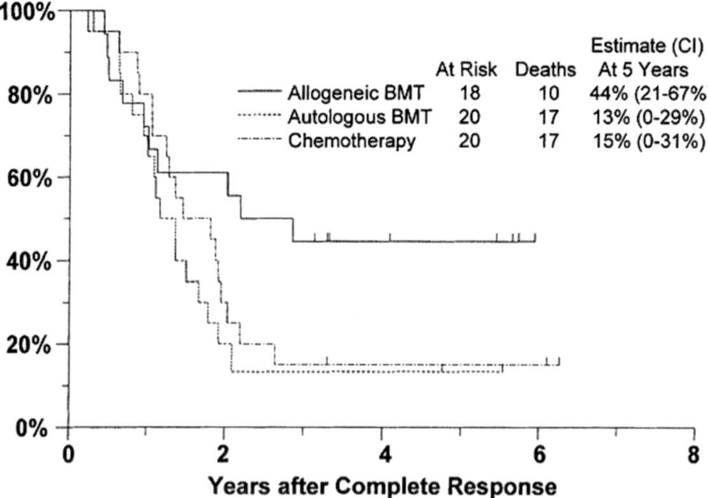

Fig. 17.1 Estimated distributions of survival by treatment arm in cases with AML in the unfavorable risk group (with permission from Slovak et al. [4])

over chemotherapy or an autologous HSCT in the unfavorable risk group [31, 56]. In all of the studies, the outcome in the unfavorable risk group with chemotherapy alone or with an autologous HSCT was dismal. Based on the available data, if a donor is available, it is reasonable to proceed with an allogeneic-related HLA-identical HSCT in CR1 with unfavourable cytogenetics. In the intermediate-risk group, the data from most large prospective clinical trials did not show an improved OS after allogeneic HSCT in CR1. However, in one study, there was a significant improvement in the DFS [15, 30–32, 56]. The optimal therapeutic strategy in this group of patients in CR1 is still evolving. If a related HLA identical donor is available, other parameters could be used to aid in the decision-making process. Some of the factors that would favor an allogeneic HSCT in CR1 include age of patient (<40 years), high white blood cell count at diagnosis (>30,000–40,000/mm^3), requirement of more than one cycle of chemotherapy to achieve CR1, and the presence of additional molecular markers (Table 17.2) that predict a high risk of relapse [20–28]. While subsets such as those with NPM1$^+$/FLT3-ITD$^-$ would probably not benefit from an allogeneic HSCT in CR1 [19]. As mentioned earlier, the data on some of these markers are still preliminary and remain to be validated in large clinical trials.

17.4.1 Role of Conditioning Regimen on Transplantation Outcomes

Two major myeloablative conditioning regimens (cyclophosphamide/total body irradiation [TBI] and cyclophosphamide/busulfan) have been used and studied in randomized trials. There are no strong data to suggest that one regimen is superior to the other; each regimen has its merits. In several retrospective studies, the use of a TBI-based regimen is associated with lower relapse rates and superior DFS [61]. In a randomized single-center study, the use of fractionated TBI to a dose of 15.75 Gy in comparison to 12 Gy was associated with a lower risk of relapse, but it did not improve survival because of increased TRM and severe acute graft-versus-host disease (GvHD) associated with the higher dose [62]. RIC regimens are increasingly being used in allogeneic HSCT in an effort to decrease regimen-related toxicity and preserve the graft-versus-leukemia effect. There are limited data on the use of RIC regimens in young patients with AML in CR1 and should probably only be considered in the setting of a clinical trial. The Medical Research Council AML-15 trial intends to allow the possibility of an RIC regimen for patients 35–45 years who have a matched donor. Even in elderly patients the use of RIC regimens that showed promise by reducing the TRM has not translated to improved event-free or OS due to the continued risk of relapse [63].

17.4.2 Role of Consolidation Chemotherapy Before an Allogeneic Hematopoietic Stem Cell Transplantation

Retrospective analysis of the IBMTR and EBMT data suggests that consolidation chemotherapy before an allogeneic HSCT does not benefit patients with AML in CR1 [64, 65]. Another retrospective analysis from a single center showed similar findings and suggested that multiple chemotherapy courses before an allogeneic HSCT had a deleterious effect [66].

17.4.3 Bone Marrow Versus Peripheral Blood Stem Cells

Retrospective analysis of the EBMT and IBMTR database showed a benefit for use of PBSC in patients with advanced AML, but no benefit was shown in patients with AML in CR1, whereas another retrospective study showed a benefit for patients with AML in CR1 who underwent a PBSCT [67, 68]. A more recent retrospective analysis of the Acute Leukemia Working Party of the EBMT suggests that there is improved outcome with the use of bone marrow versus PBSCT when the dose of bone marrow $CD34^+$ cells exceeded 2.7×10^6/kg [69]. The only prospective study addressing this issue demonstrated earlier engraftment, reduced TRM, and improved DFS with PBSCT, but there was no difference in OS [70]. A current phase III prospective Blood and Marrow Transplant-Clinical Trials Network (BMT-CTN) study is testing the outcomes of patients with hematologic malignancies (AML, acute lymphocytic leukemia, MDS, and chronic myelogenous leukemia), who are randomly assigned to receiving G-CSF mobilized PBSC versus BM after myeloablative conditioning. This study, which is expected to end in late 2008, will provide the first insight into the role of stem cells from peripheral blood versus BM on outcomes of patients undergoing matched unrelated HSCT.

17.4.4 Role of T-cell Depletion of the Allograft

Graft-versus-host disease is one of the major causes contributing to TRM after an allogeneic HSCT. T-cell depletion of the graft is one of the best ways to reduce the incidence of GvHD. Preliminary data on the use of T-cell–depleted myeloablative allogeneic HSCT for patients with AML in CR1 are exciting [6]. In this approach, the conditioning regimen would retain the benefit of intensive consolidation chemotherapy and with engraftment a graft-versus-leukemia effect could also contribute to improve the DFS, whereas the T-cell depletion would reduce the risk of severe GvHD and TRM. Ongoing clinical trials are attempting to define its role in the management of AML.

17.4.5 Role of Donor Lymphocyte Infusions for Patients Who Relapse After an Allogeneic Hematopoietic Stem Cell Transplantation

For patients with AML in CR1 who undergo an allogeneic HSCT and subsequently relapse, further options of therapy are limited. A second transplant is associated with a high TRM and cures a small minority of patients. Donor lymphocyte infusions (DLI) are an option in this situation (reviewed in Chap. 20 by Porter, Hexner, Cooley, and Miller). In retrospective analysis from two large series, the response rate varied from 15% to 30%, with durable remissions in most of the patients who responded [71, 72]. Recently retrospective data analysis of risk factor analysis and comparison of alternative strategies confirmed the benefit of DLI in this setting, though it was noted to benefit mainly a subset of patients with low tumor burden and favorable cytogenetics [73]. It would be reasonable to attempt a donor lymphocyte infusion in this setting before considering alternative strategies.

17.4.6 Matched-Unrelated Donor Hematopoietic Stem Cell Transplantation

An HLA matched-related donor may offer a survival advantage for a subset of patients with AML in CR1. Unfortunately, only 25–30% of patients are likely to have a related donor. An alternative is a matched-unrelated donor. There are limited data on the outcome of a matched-unrelated donor HSCT in comparison to other options. Preliminary retrospective analysis of the IBMTR database comparing the outcome of AML in CR1/CR2 patients treated with matched-unrelated donor versus an autologous HSCT showed a 3-year leukemia-free survival of 33% in matched-unrelated donor HSCT versus 40% with an autograft. However, there was suggestion of a selection bias with patients undergoing a matched-unrelated donor HSCT possessing more adverse features [40]. Another single center retrospective analysis of 16 patients with AML in CR1 who all had adverse prognostic features achieved a 5-year DFS of $50 \pm 12\%$ [74].

17.4.7 Haploidentical Donor Hematopoietic Stem Cell Transplantation

Haploidentical donor HSCT is an alternative source of stem cells for an allogeneic transplant in patients who do not have an HLA matched-related donor and has the advantage of being readily available. There are very limited data in the setting of AML in CR1. Recent use of T-cell–depleted grafts, mega doses of $CD34^+$ cells, and avoidance of granulocyte colony-stimulating factor after transplant to enhance NK cell recovery appear to be improving the outcome. A recent update in Perugia, Italy, suggests that, with the use of these strategies, the outcome after a haploidentical HSCT is similar to that with matched allogeneic HSCT [75]. In the setting of haploidentical HSCT for AML, killer immunoglobulin receptor ligand incompatibility in the graft-to-host direction has been shown to be associated with a decreased relapse risk, in addition to a reduced risk of graft rejection and a lower incidence of GvHD [8]. However, this benefit appears to occur only in the setting of high CD34^{+} cell doses, extensive T-cell depletion of the graft, and no post-grafting immune suppression [76]. An alternative to CD34^{+}cell selection for haploidentical HSCT is to use CD3^{+}/CD19^{+} cell-depleted grafts in an effort to retain NK cell activity; preliminary results are promising [77].

17.4.8 Cord Blood Transplantation

Umbilical cord blood is an alternative source of stem cells for an allogeneic HSCT in patients who do not have a related sibling donor (reviewed in Chap. 10 by Wagner, Brunstein, Tse, and Laughlin). Cord blood transplantation has been validated as an alternative to bone marrow transplantation in children with leukemia. In adults, cord blood transplantation is often limited by the progenitor cell dose and a high incidence of TRM [78]. A recent small series by Ooi et al. [79] reports a 2-year DFS of 76% in adults with de-novo AML in CR1. Most of the published studies of cord blood transplant in adults include subsets of patients with AML who have relapsed. There are very limited data on the outcome of cord blood transplants for patients with AML in CR1.

17.5 Hematopoietic Stem Cell Transplantation in Myelodysplastic Syndromes

Myelodysplastic syndromes (MDS) are a heterogeneous group of clonal hematopoietic disorders [11]. In addition to the previously described subtypes, the cytogenetic findings and the number of cytopenias at diagnosis are important in prognostication. Together these parameters have been used to generate a scoring system termed the International Prognostic Scoring System (IPSS) [80]. The IPSS (Table 17.4) has a bearing not only in the overall prognosis of a patient with a diagnosis of MDS but is also a useful predictor of transplantation outcomes [81, 82]. In spite of there being significant progress in the understanding of the pathophysiology of MDS, which has translated into novel therapeutic interventions, allogeneic HSCT still remains the only therapy that has curative potential in this condition, leading to the recommendations that all patients who are eligible for a transplant procedure and have an available donor should be considered for this procedure [83]. However, in reality this therapeutic option is limited to a small fraction of patients with this diagnosis since the majority of patients are over 65 years, with additional comorbidities and poor

Table 17.4 International Prognostic Scoring System (IPSS) in MDS

	Score value				
Prognostic variable	0	0.5	1.0	1.5	2.0
BM blasts (%)	<5	5–10	–	11–20	21–30
Karyotype[a]	Good	Intermediate	Poor		
Cytopenias	0/1	2/3			

With permission from Greenberg et al. [80]
Scores for risk groups are as follows: Low, 0; INT-1, 0.5–1.0; INT-2, 1.5–2.0; and High, ≥ 2.5
[a]Good, normal, –Y, del(5q), del(20q); Poor, complex (^{3}3 abnormalities) or chromosome seven anomalies; Intermediate, other abnormalities

performance status. Even when other adverse factors are not present, this group of older patients is perceived as being unable to tolerate a standard myeloablative conditioning regimen. In addition to the subtype and IPSS score at diagnosis the age and performance status of the patient are important determinants of the therapeutic options that are feasible. There is no role for an autologous HSCT in this condition.

MDS affects predominantly the older age group with significant variation in the natural history and response to therapy. No single therapeutic algorithm can be applied to this group of patients. Rather, therapy has to be tailored to the individual patient. For patients eligible to undergo an allogeneic HSCT the factors that have a bearing on the outcome following a transplant have to be weighed against the risks involved. In this chapter, some of these factors are addressed, and a broad overview of the role of an allogeneic HSCT in the management of MDS is provided.

17.5.1 Effect of Age on Transplantation Outcomes

Intuitively one could state that older MDS patients would do poorly following an allogeneic HSCT. Most studies have shown that recipient age is an important prognostic factor for nonrelapse mortality (NRM) [84] in MDS patients undergoing allogeneic HSCT. In a majority of the large trials using a myeloablative regimen with related [81, 85–87] and unrelated donor [85, 88–90] this holds true. However, in one large study by Deeg et al. [82], use of targeted busulfan levels in a myeloablative conditioning regimen showed, using a multivariate analysis, there was no significant effect of age (up to 66 years) on relapse-free survival (RFS). The data on the use of nonmyeloablative transplants for older patients are still evolving and could potentially improve the outcome of older patients undergoing an allogeneic HSCT.

17.5.1.1 Effect of International Prognostic Scoring System Score on Outcome

International Prognostic Scoring System (IPSS) scores (Table 17.4) have been clearly shown to have a bearing on the outcome following an allogeneic HSCT (Fig. 17.2) [81, 82]. In a recent publication by Deeg et al. [82] the 3-year RFS was

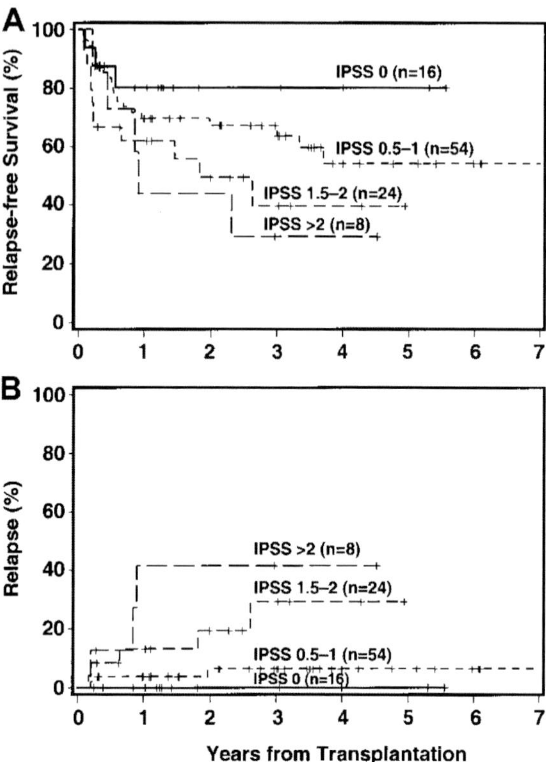

Fig. 17.2 Impact of IPSS score on clinical outcome post-allogeneic stem cell transplant (with permission from Deeg et al. [82])

80% for low-risk (IPSS score 0), which progressively decreased with increasing scores to 29% among patients with an IPSS score higher than 2 (Fig. 17.2). Earlier studies had shown a similar correlation with cytogenetic-risk groups and post-transplant outcomes in patients with MDS. Nevill et al. [91] showed a 7-year event-free survival of 51%, 40%, and 6% in the good-, intermediate- and poor-risk cytogenetic-risk groups. Since the IPSS score includes additional parameters of percentage of blasts in the bone marrow and number of cytopenias at diagnosis, which are important independent adverse factors [87], it is likely to be a more robust system to predict outcome following an allogeneic HSCT.

IPSS score also has an important bearing on decision-making with regard to proceeding with an allogeneic HSCT. In the low-risk group with a median survival of 11.8 years in patients less than 60 years of age [80], one would opt for supportive care or a reduced-intensity low-risk therapy rather than subject such an individual to the risk of TRM following an allogeneic HSCT. On the other hand, a patient with an IPSS score greater than 2 who has a median survival of a few months[80] is a candidate for an allogeneic HSCT provided a donor is available and his performance status permits the procedure to be done.

17.5.1.2 Effect of Time to Transplant from Diagnosis

While an allogeneic HSCT is the only curative therapeutic option in the management of MDS, it is also associated with the highest TRM. Nonrelapse mortality (NRM) caused by infections, GvHD and organ toxicity in large series of patients undergoing an allogeneic HSCT varies from 30% to 54% [89, 91, 92]. It would not be appropriate to expose low-risk MDS patients based on an IPSS score to these risks. However, MDS is for the most part a continuously evolving disease process with an inexorable progression to acute leukemia, and an allogeneic HSCT done in a more advanced stage of the disease process is associated with significantly worse outcomes [81, 82]. The optimal time has been a matter of controversy especially for the low- and intermediate-risk MDS. A recent publication by Cutler et al. [93] attempted to address this issue by applying a statistical technique, called a Markov model, to predict long-term outcomes under conditions of uncertainty. In patients with low or intermediate risk MDS, delayed transplantation by a fixed time interval (2–2.5 years) and prior to leukemia transformation maximized overall survival. This survival advantage was even more prominent in patients under 40 years of age in this risk group. For intermediate-2 and the high-risk group of patients an immediate transplantation improved overall survival.

17.5.1.3 Role of Induction Chemotherapy Prior to an Allogeneic HSCT

The majority of published studies has shown that patients in remission or with a lower percentage of bone marrow blasts have a lower relapse rate and improved outcome. The EBMT series on HSCT for MDS has shown that outcomes were significantly better for patients in first remission compared to patients with active disease at the time of transplant [85]. Other groups have, however, failed to demonstrate this benefit of remission induction prior to an allogeneic HSCT [82, 87, 94, 95], suggesting that it would be preferable to take patients with high-risk MDS directly to an allogeneic HSCT if they were eligible for this procedure. These studies are limited by being single-center small retrospective analyses of heterogeneous groups of patients. The study by Copeland et al. suggests that the outcome in patients receiving induction therapy is in fact worse than those taken to transplant directly, as a result of increased regimen-related toxicity (RRT) in the group receiving induction chemotherapy [95]. This issue needs to be further evaluated, especially in the setting of newer less-toxic remission induction agents, such as decitabine, clofarabine, and topotecan, preferably as a prospective study. Based on the available data it would be reasonable to recommend patients with a low percentage of bone marrow blasts proceed directly to transplant while patients with a bone marrow blast percentage closer to that of a diagnosis of AML would probably benefit from induction therapy prior to a transplant. These recommendations must also be based on the age, motivations, and comorbidities of the patient.

17.5.1.4 Conditioning Regimens for Allogeneic HSCT in MDS

Standard myeloablative conditioning regimens, both TBI-based and non-TBI-based, are associated with significant RRT and contribute to NRM. Since the majority of patients with a diagnosis of MDS are above the age of 60 years they are also a group which is less likely to tolerate these regimens. New nonmyeloablative regimens are being explored with the hope of offering an allogeneic HSCT, its graft-versus-leukemia effect, and potential for cure to this older population.

17.5.1.5 Myeloablative Conditioning Regimens

In the 1980s, studies using a cyclophosphamide plus TBI (Cy/TBI) myeloablative regimen reported DFS of 30%-40% in patients with high-risk MDS [96]. In an effort to determine if further intensification of the conditioning regimen would improve the outcome busulfan (Bu) was added to this regimen and compared with historical controls using Cy/TBI alone. The results showed that there was a decrease in relapse risk but no significant difference in survival with significantly more NRM (68% vs. 36%) [97]. From these early studies it appears that further intensification of the conditioning regimen is not a solution to improve the outcome in this disease. In the setting of unrelated matched donor transplants it has been shown that use of non-TBI-based conditioning regimens (Bu/Cy) is associated with improved outcomes both in the low- and high-risk MDS groups [89]. Overall there has been a move towards the use of non-TBI-based conditioning regimens for allogeneic HSCT in MDS. Oral busulfan with pharmacologic targeting and intravenous busulfan have been shown to reduce the incidence of RRT and NRM and improve transplant outcomes [89, 98, 99]. Recent data published by Deeg et al. using targeted busulfan levels with cyclophosphamide have shown promising results even in an older patient population with low- and high-risk MDS [82]. The data from some of the largest series using a myeloablative regimen is summarized in Table 17.5.

17.5.1.6 Nonmyeloablative Conditioning Regimens

In view of the older age group of patients with a diagnosis of MDS and the inability of a significant proportion of these patients to tolerate a standard myeloablative conditioning regimen, in the 1990s RIC and nonmyeloablative conditioning regimens for an allogeneic HSCT were actively pursued. It was hoped that this approach would reduce the RRT and NRM in this population. The most commonly used RIC regimen is a combination of fludarabine with melphalan and low-dose TBI. Results from some of the largest series published [100–105] are summarized on Table 17.6. In a majority of these studies the NRM was lower than with myeloablative regimens, but they were associated

Table 17.5 Summary of data from some large series of patients with MDS who underwent a related matched sibling allogeneic HSCT using a myeloablative conditioning regimen

Study	*n*	Age (median)	High risk MDS	Preparative regimen	NRM%	DFS% (median) %	OS% at 3 years
Sutton et al. [87]	71	37	100	TBI based	39	32	32
Appelbaum et al. [81]	251	38 (1–66)	57	TBI based 69%	42	41	NS
de Witte et al. [85]	885	NS	52	NS	43	31	46
Sierra et al. [86]	452	38 (2–64)	60	TBI based 40%	37	40	42

DFS disease-free survival, *NRM* non-relapse mortality, *NS* not stated, *OS* overall survival, *TBI* total body irradiation

with higher relapse rates, which were especially noted in the EBMT study [106]. A recent publication from the M.D. Anderson Cancer Center showed a similar correlation with an increased risk of relapse in the group receiving a less intensive conditioning regimen when comparing two reduced-intensity regimens [104]. There are a number of ongoing clinical trials addressing this issue and the optimal regimen remains to be defined.

Table 17.6 Summary of data of patients with MDS who underwent an HLA identical (related and unrelated) allogeneic HSCT using a nonmyeloablative conditioning regimen

Study	*n*	Age (median)	High Risk MDS	MUD	Preparative regimen	NRM%	DFS% (median) %	OS% at 2 years
Giralt [84]	26	57	100	33	FM or FAI	43	27	31
Parker et al. [102]	23	48	78	70	FB-Campath	26	39	48
Stuart et al. [107]	77	59	44	50	F-TBI	NS	NS	24 (high risk) 40 (low risk)
Martino et al. [106]	215	54	NS	0	Various	33		41 at 3 years 33 at 3 years
de Lima et al. [104]	26	NS	NS	NS	FM or FAI	30		Relapse risk 61% with FAI versus 30% with FM

DFS disease-free survival, *NRM* nonrelapse mortality, *NS* not stated, *OS* overall survival, *TBI* total body irradiation, *FAI* fludarabine, cytarabine and idarubicin, *FM* fludarabine and melphalan

17.5.1.7 Peripheral Blood Versus Bone Marrow as a Source of Stem Cells

Use of G-CSF mobilized peripheral blood stem cells (PBSC) has been associated with an improved outcome compared to marrow. A retrospective analysis of the EBMT data of 234 patients with a diagnosis of MDS undergoing an HLA identical sibling transplant showed an improved 2-year survival of 50% with PBSC versus 39% with bone marrow and also reduced TRM and relapses [108]. Similar reduced relapse risk and improved overall outcome was also noted in the studies published by Deeg et al. [82] and del Canizo et al. [109].

17.5.1.8 Role of Alternate Donor Sources

Alternative donor sources include a matched unrelated donor (MUD), matched or mismatched cord blood or haploidentical donor. Analysis of MUD transplants under the auspices of the National Marrow Donor Program shows comparable results to that of an HLA identical related transplant [89]. Based on the available data one would recommend a MUD transplant for a high-risk MDS. The preliminary data with cord blood transplants show their potential as a significant alternative source, especially with mismatched cord blood [110, 111]. There are insufficient data with haploidentical transplants in this condition to recommend them outside the setting of a clinical trial.

17.6 Conclusion

Significant strides have been made in the management of patients with AML. In addition to the increased understanding of the biology of the disease, ongoing developments in the field of HSCT continue to contribute to the steady improvement in the outcome of these patients. The outcomes from an HSCT have improved significantly over the past decade, thus most of the HSCT data from the large prospective trials initiated a decade ago may not be entirely consistent with the outcomes expected today. One recent publication of transplants from a single center illustrates this point with a TRM as low as 3% for patients with leukemia in CR1 undergoing an allogeneic HLA identical sibling transplant [10]. Based on very limited data, a matched unrelated HSCT could also be offered to young patients in the unfavorable risk group with AML in CR1. The optimal therapy for patients with AML in CR1 in the intermediate-risk group is evolving and several questions remain to be answered. With the available data, some guidelines can be drawn for this group, although no firm conclusions can be made. The use of new markers to identify subgroups at a high risk for relapse would help identify patients who would benefit from an HSCT. Autologous and allogeneic HSCT may have a role in this ill-defined subset of patients. There is increasing interest in RIC allogeneic HSCT especially in the elderly patient with AML. Retrospective analysis also suggests a role for autologous HSCT in patients with AML in CR2.

Unlike in AML, an allogeneic HSCT remains the only treatment with a curative potential in the management of a patient with a diagnosis of MDS. There is also no role for an autologous HSCT in this condition. However, the risks associated with an allogeneic transplant in this older population have to be weighed against the benefits. Statistical models predict that delaying an allogeneic HSCT for patients in the low-risk MDS group is associated with maximal life expectancy. Myeloablative regimens are associated with a lower risk of relapse but high TRM in patients with high-risk MDS. Recent data using myeloablative regimens with targeted busulfan levels hold promise in reducing regimen-related toxicity and reducing the risk of relapse. Preliminary data with nonmyeloablative regimens shows a definite reduction in NRM, though the high risk of relapse is of some concern, especially in patients in the high-risk group of MDS. Ongoing clinical trials may help identify an optimal nonmyeloablative regimen. Cytokine mobilized PBSC transplants appear to be superior to marrow transplants in this setting. Published data suggests that outcomes with a well HLA-matched MUD HSCT are comparable to that with a HLA identical related donor. Preliminary data with mismatched cord blood transplants are exciting but remain to be validated.

References

1. Appelbaum FR, Rowe JM, Radich J, Dick JE. Acute myeloid leukemia. Hematology Am Soc Hematol Educ Program. 2001;62–86.
2. Mayer RJ, Davis RB, Schiffer CA, et al. Intensive postremission chemotherapy in adults with acute myeloid leukemia. Cancer and Leukemia Group B. N Engl J Med. 1994;331:896–903.
3. Giles FJ, Keating A, Goldstone AH, Avivi I, Willman CL, Kantarjian HM. Acute myeloid leukemia. Hematology Am Soc Hematol Educ Program. 2002;73–110.
4. Slovak ML, Kopecky KJ, Cassileth PA, et al. Karyotypic analysis predicts outcome of preremission and postremission therapy in adult acute myeloid leukemia: a Southwest Oncology Group/Eastern Cooperative Oncology Group Study. Blood 2000;96:4075–83.
5. Mathews V, DiPersio JF. Stem cell transplantation in acute myelogenous leukemia in first remission: what are the options? Curr Hematol Rep. 2004;3:235–41.
6. Chakrabarti S, Marks DI. Should we T cell deplete sibling grafts for acute myeloid leukaemia in first remission? Bone Marrow Transplant. 2003;32:1039–50.
7. Platzbecker U, Ehninger G, Schmitz N, Bornhauser M. Reduced-intensity conditioning followed by allogeneic hematopoietic cell transplantation in myeloid diseases. Ann Hematol. 2003;82:463–68.
8. Ruggeri L, Capanni M, Urbani E, et al. Effectiveness of donor natural killer cell alloreactivity in mismatched hematopoietic transplants. Science 2002;295:2097–100.
9. Giebel S, Locatelli F, Lamparelli T, et al. Survival advantage with KIR ligand incompatibility in hematopoietic stem cell transplantation from unrelated donors. Blood 2003;102:814–9.
10. Bacigalupo A, Sormani MP, Lamparelli T, et al. Reducing transplant-related mortality after allogeneic hematopoietic stem cell transplantation. Haematologica 2004;89:1238–47.
11. Bowen D, Culligan D, Jowitt S, et al. Guidelines for the diagnosis and therapy of adult myelodysplastic syndromes. Br J Haematol. 2003;120:187–200.

12. Aul C, Germing U, Gattermann N, Minning H. Increasing incidence of myelodysplastic syndromes: real or fictitious? Leuk Res. 1998;22:93–100.
13. Bennett JM, Catovsky D, Daniel MT, et al. Proposals for the classification of the myelodysplastic syndromes. Br J Haematol. 1982;51:189–99.
14. Harris NL, Jaffe ES, Diebold J, et al. The World Health Organization classification of neoplastic diseases of the hematopoietic and lymphoid tissues. Report of the Clinical Advisory Committee meeting, Airlie House, Virginia, November, 1997. Ann Oncol. 1999;10:1419–32.
15. Cassileth PA, Harrington DP, Appelbaum FR, et al. Chemotherapy compared with autologous or allogeneic bone marrow transplantation in the management of acute myeloid leukemia in first remission. N Engl J Med. 1998;339:1649–56.
16. Lowenberg B, Griffin JD, Tallman MS. Acute myeloid leukemia and acute promyelocytic leukemia. Hematology Am Soc Hematol Educ Program. 2003;82–101.
17. Appelbaum FR, Kopecky KJ, Tallman MS, et al. The clinical spectrum of adult acute myeloid leukaemia associated with core binding factor translocations. Br J Haematol. 2006;135:165–73.
18. Byrd JC, Dodge RK, Carroll A, et al. Patients with t(8;21)(q22;q22) and acute myeloid leukemia have superior failure-free and overall survival when repetitive cycles of high-dose cytarabine are administered. J Clin Oncol. 1999;17:3767–75.
19. Schlenk RF, Corbacioglu A, Krauter J, Bullinger L, Morgan M, Spath D, et al. Gene mutations as predictive markers for post remission therapy in younger adults with normal karyotype AML. Blood 2006;108:Abstract#4.
20. Stirewalt DL, Radich JP. The role of FLT3 in haematopoietic malignancies. Nat Rev Cancer. 2003;3:650–5.
21. Kottaridis PD, Gale RE, Frew ME, et al. The presence of a FLT3 internal tandem duplication in patients with acute myeloid leukemia (AML) adds important prognostic information to cytogenetic risk group and response to the first cycle of chemotherapy: analysis of 854 patients from the United Kingdom Medical Research Council AML 10 and 12 trials. Blood 2001;98:1752–9.
22. Baldus CD, Tanner SM, Ruppert AS, et al. BAALC expression predicts clinical outcome of de novo acute myeloid leukemia patients with normal cytogenetics: a Cancer and Leukemia Group B Study. Blood 2003;102:1613–8.
23. Karakas T, Miething CC, Maurer U, et al. The coexpression of the apoptosis-related genes bcl-2 and wt1 in predicting survival in adult acute myeloid leukemia. Leukemia 2002;16:846–54.
24. Barjesteh van Waalwijk van Doorn-Khosrovani S, Erpelinck C, van Putten WLJ, et al. High EVI1 expression predicts poor survival in acute myeloid leukemia: a study of 319 de novo AML patients. Blood 2003;101:837–45.
25. Dohner K, Tobis K, Ulrich R, et al. Prognostic significance of partial tandem duplications of the MLL gene in adult patients 16 to 60 years old with acute myeloid leukemia and normal cytogenetics: a study of the Acute Myeloid Leukemia Study Group Ulm. J Clin Oncol. 2002;20:3254–61.
26. Tourneur L, Delluc S, Levy V, et al. Absence or low expression of fas-associated protein with death domain in acute myeloid leukemia cells predicts resistance to chemotherapy and poor outcome. Cancer Res. 2004;64:8101–8.
27. Frohling S, Schlenk RF, Stolze I, et al. CEBPA mutations in younger adults with acute myeloid leukemia and normal cytogenetics: prognostic relevance and analysis of cooperating mutations. J Clin Oncol. 2004;22:624–33.
28. Hu Q, Dey AL, Yang Y, et al. Soluble vascular endothelial growth factor receptor 1, and not receptor 2, is an independent prognostic factor in acute myeloid leukemia and myelodysplastic syndromes. Cancer 2004;100:1884–91.
29. Falini B, Nicoletti I, Martelli MF, Mecucci C. Acute myeloid leukemia carrying cytoplasmic/mutated nucleophosmin (NPMc + AML): biologic and clinical features. Blood 2007;109:874–85.

30. Zittoun RA, Mandelli F, Willemze R, et al. Autologous or allogeneic bone marrow transplantation compared with intensive chemotherapy in acute myelogenous leukemia. European Organization for Research and Treatment of Cancer (EORTC) and the Gruppo Italiano Malattie Ematologiche Maligne dell'Adulto (GIMEMA) Leukemia Cooperative Groups. N Engl J Med. 1995;332:217–23.
31. Harousseau JL, Cahn JY, Pignon B, et al. Comparison of autologous bone marrow transplantation and intensive chemotherapy as postremission therapy in adult acute myeloid leukemia. The Groupe Ouest Est Leucemies Aigues Myeloblastiques (GOELAM). Blood 1997;90:2978–86.
32. Burnett AK, Goldstone AH, Stevens RM, et al. Randomised comparison of addition of autologous bone-marrow transplantation to intensive chemotherapy for acute myeloid leukaemia in first remission: results of MRC AML 10 trial. UK Medical Research Council Adult and Children's Leukaemia Working Parties. Lancet 1998;351:700–8.
33. Nathan PC, Sung L, Crump M, Beyene J. Consolidation therapy with autologous bone marrow transplantation in adults with acute myeloid leukemia: a meta-analysis. J Natl Cancer Inst. 2004;96:38–45.
34. Wheatley K. Current controversies: which patients with acute myeloid leukaemia should receive a bone marrow transplantation?—a statistician's view. Br J Haematol. 2002;118:351–6.
35. Schlenk RF, Benner A, Krauter J, et al. Individual patient data-based meta-analysis of patients aged 16 to 60 years with core binding factor acute myeloid leukemia: a survey of the German Acute Myeloid Leukemia Intergroup. J Clin Oncol. 2004;22:3741–50.
36. Lashkari A, Lowe T, Collisson E, et al. Long-term outcome of autologous transplantation of peripheral blood progenitor cells as postremission management of patients > or = 60 years with acute myelogenous leukemia. Biol Blood Marrow Transplant. 2006;12:466–71.
37. Thomas X, Suciu S, Rio B, et al. Autologous stem cell transplantation after complete remission and first consolidation in acute myeloid leukemia patients aged 61-70 years: results of the prospective EORTC-GIMEMA AML-13 study. Haematologica 2007;92:389–96.
38. Herr AL, Labopin M, Blaise D, et al. HLA-identical sibling allogeneic peripheral blood stem cell transplantation with reduced intensity conditioning compared to autologous peripheral blood stem cell transplantation for elderly patients with de novo acute myeloid leukemia. Leukemia 2007;21:129–35.
39. Chantry AD, Snowden JA, Craddock C, et al. Long-term outcomes of myeloablation and autologous transplantation of relapsed acute myeloid leukemia in second remission: a British Society of Blood and Marrow Transplantation registry study. Biol Blood Marrow Transplant. 2006;12:1310–7.
40. Lazarus HM, Perez WS, Klein JP, et al. Autotransplantation versus HLA-matched unrelated donor transplantation for acute myeloid leukaemia: a retrospective analysis from the Center for International Blood and Marrow Transplant Research. Br J Haematol. 2006;132:755–69.
41. Santos GW, Tutschka PJ, Brookmeyer R, et al. Marrow transplantation for acute nonlymphocytic leukemia after treatment with busulfan and cyclophosphamide. N Engl J Med. 1983;309:1347–53.
42. Tutschka PJ, Copeland EA, Klein JP. Bone marrow transplantation for leukemia following a new busulfan and cyclophosphamide regimen. Blood 1987;70:1382–8.
43. Ferrara F, Palmieri S, De Simone M, et al. High-dose idarubicin and busulphan as conditioning to autologous stem cell transplantation in adult patients with acute myeloid leukaemia. Br J Haematol. 2005;128:234–41.
44. Gorin NC, Aegerter P, Auvert B, et al. Autologous bone marrow transplantation for acute myelocytic leukemia in first remission: a European survey of the role of marrow purging. Blood 1990;75:1606–14.

45. Miller CB, Rowlings PA, Zhang MJ, et al. The effect of graft purging with 4-hydroperoxycyclophosphamide in autologous bone marrow transplantation for acute myelogenous leukemia. Exp Hematol. 2001;29:1336–46.
46. Wierenga PK, Setroikromo R, Kamps G, Kampinga HH, Vellenga E. Differences in heat sensitivity between normal and acute myeloid leukemic stem cells: feasibility of hyperthermic purging of leukemic cells from autologous stem cell grafts. Exp Hematol. 2003;31:421–7.
47. Feller N, van der Pol MA, Waaijman T, et al. Immunologic purging of autologous peripheral blood stem cell products based on CD34 and CD133 expression can be effectively and safely applied in half of the acute myeloid leukemia patients. Clin Cancer Res. 2005;11:4793–801.
48. Sirohi B, Powles, R, Singhal S, et al. The impact of consolidation chemotherapy on the outcome of autotransplantation for acute myeloid leukemia in first remission: single center experience of 118 adult patients. Blood 2001;98:859a.
49. Cassileth P, Lee S, Litzow M, et al. Intensified induction chemotherapy in adult acute myeloid leukemia followed by high-dose chemotherapy and autologous peripheral blood stem cell transplantation: an eastern cooperative oncology group trial (E4995). Leuk Lymphoma. 2005;46:55–61.
50. Tallman MS, Perez WS, Lazarus HM, et al. Pretransplantation consolidation chemotherapy decreases leukemia relapse after autologous blood and bone marrow transplants for acute myelogenous leukemia in first remission. Biol Blood Marrow Transplant. 2006;12:204–16.
51. Korbling M, Fliedner TM, Holle R, et al. Autologous blood stem cell (ABSCT) versus purged bone marrow transplantation (pABMT) in standard risk AML: influence of source and cell composition of the autograft on hemopoietic reconstitution and disease-free survival. Bone Marrow Transplant. 1991;7:343–9.
52. de Witte T, Keating S, Suciu S, et al. A randomized comparison of the value of autologous BMT versus autologous PBSCT for patients with AML in first CR in the AML 10 trial of the EORTC, LCG and GIMEMMA. Blood 2001;98:859a.
53. Keating S, Suciu S, de Witte T, et al. The stem cell mobilizing capacity of patients with acute myeloid leukemia in complete remission correlates with relapse risk: results of the EORTC-GIMEMA AML-10 trial. Leukemia 2003;17:60–7.
54. Milone G, Indelicato F, Tornello A, et al. ABMT in CR1; Importance of infused cell dose for engraftment and LFS differs after unpurged or purged bone marrow Blood 2003;102:3681a.
55. Brenner MK, Rill DR, Moen RC, et al. Gene marking and autologous bone marrow transplantation. Ann N Y Acad Sci. 1994;716:204–14; discussion 214–205, 225–207.
56. Burnett AK, Wheatley K, Goldstone AH, et al. The value of allogeneic bone marrow transplant in patients with acute myeloid leukaemia at differing risk of relapse: results of the UK MRC AML 10 trial. Br J Haematol. 2002;118:385–400.
57. Gale RP, Horowitz MM, Rees JK, et al. Chemotherapy versus transplants for acute myelogenous leukemia in second remission. Leukemia 1996;10:13–9.
58. Linker CA, Damon LE, Ries CA, Navarro WA, Case D, Wolf JL. Autologous stem cell transplantation for advanced acute myeloid leukemia. Bone Marrow Transplant. 2002;29:297–301.
59. Suciu S, Zittoun R, Mandelli F, et al. Allogeneic versus autologous stem cell transplantation according to cytogenetic features in AML patients in first remission: results of the EORTC-GIMEMA AML-10 trial. Blood 2001;98:481a.
60. Cornelissen JJ, van Putten WL, Verdonck LF, et al. Results of a HOVON/SAKK donor versus no-donor analysis of myeloablative HLA-identical sibling stem cell transplantation in first remission acute myeloid leukemia in young and middle-aged adults: benefits for whom? Blood 2007;109:3658–66.
61. Ferry C, Socie G. Busulfan-cyclophosphamide versus total body irradiation-cyclophosphamide as preparative regimen before allogeneic hematopoietic stem cell transplantation for acute myeloid leukemia: what have we learned? Exp Hematol. 2003; 31:1182–6.

62. Clift RA, Buckner CD, Appelbaum FR, et al. Allogeneic marrow transplantation in patients with acute myeloid leukemia in first remission: a randomized trial of two irradiation regimens. Blood 1990;76:1867–71.
63. Alyea EP, Kim HT, Ho V, et al. Comparative outcome of nonmyeloablative and myeloablative allogeneic hematopoietic cell transplantation for patients older than 50 years of age. Blood 2005;105:1810–4.
64. Tallman MS, Rowlings PA, Milone G, et al. Effect of postremission chemotherapy before human leukocyte antigen-identical sibling transplantation for acute myelogenous leukemia in first complete remission. Blood 2000;96:1254–8.
65. Cahn JY, Labopin M, Sierra J, et al. No impact of high-dose cytarabine on the outcome of patients transplanted for acute myeloblastic leukaemia in first remission. Acute Leukaemia Working Party of the European Group for Blood and Marrow Transplantation (EBMT). Br J Haematol. 2000;110:308–14.
66. Robin M, Guardiola P, Dombret H, et al. Allogeneic bone marrow transplantation for acute myeloblastic leukaemia in remission: risk factors for long-term morbidity and mortality. Bone Marrow Transplant. 2003;31:877–87.
67. Champlin RE, Schmitz N, Horowitz MM, et al. Blood stem cells compared with bone marrow as a source of hematopoietic cells for allogeneic transplantation. IBMTR Histocompatibility and Stem Cell Sources Working Committee and the European Group for Blood and Marrow Transplantation (EBMT). Blood 2000;95:3702–9.
68. Russell JA, Larratt L, Brown C, et al. Allogeneic blood stem cell and bone marrow transplantation for acute myelogenous leukemia and myelodysplasia: influence of stem cell source on outcome. Bone Marrow Transplant. 1999;24:1177–83.
69. Gorin NC, Labopin M, Rocha V, et al. Marrow versus peripheral blood for geno-identical allogeneic stem cell transplantation in acute myelocytic leukemia: influence of dose and stem cell source shows better outcome with rich marrow. Blood 2003;102:3043–51.
70. Bensinger WI, Martin PJ, Storer B, et al. Transplantation of bone marrow as compared with peripheral-blood cells from HLA-identical relatives in patients with hematologic cancers. N Engl J Med. 2001;344:175–81.
71. Kolb HJ, Schattenberg A, Goldman JM, et al. Graft-versus-leukemia effect of donor lymphocyte transfusions in marrow grafted patients. Blood 1995;86:2041–50.
72. Collins RH Jr, Shpilberg O, Drobyski WR, et al. Donor leukocyte infusions in 140 patients with relapsed malignancy after allogeneic bone marrow transplantation. J Clin Oncol. 1997;15:433–44.
73. Schmid C, Labopin M, Nagler A, et al. Donor lymphocyte infusion in the treatment of first hematological relapse after allogeneic stem-cell transplantation in adults with acute myeloid leukemia: a retrospective risk factors analysis and comparison with other strategies by the EBMT Acute Leukemia Working Party. J Clin Oncol. 2007;25:4938–45.
74. Sierra J, Storer B, Hansen JA, et al. Unrelated donor marrow transplantation for acute myeloid leukemia: an update of the Seattle experience. Bone Marrow Transplant. 2000;26:397–404.
75. Aversa F, Terenzi A, Felicini R, et al. Haploidentical stem cell transplantation for acute leukemia. Int J Hematol. 2002;76 Suppl 1:165–8.
76. Davies SM, Ruggieri L, DeFor T, et al. Evaluation of KIR ligand incompatibility in mismatched unrelated donor hematopoietic transplants. Killer immunoglobulin-like receptor. Blood 2002;100:3825–7.
77. Bethge WA, Faul C, Bornhauser M, et al. Haploidentical allogeneic hematopoietic cell transplantation in adults using CD3/CD19 depletion and reduced intensity conditioning: an update. Blood Cells Mol Dis. 2008;40:13–9.
78. Barker JN, Wagner JE. Umbilical-cord blood transplantation for the treatment of cancer. Nat Rev Cancer. 2003;3:526–32.
79. Ooi J, Iseki T, Takahashi S, et al. Unrelated cord blood transplantation for adult patients with de novo acute myeloid leukemia. Blood 2004;103:489–91.

80. Greenberg P, Cox C, LeBeau MM, et al. International scoring system for evaluating prognosis in myelodysplastic syndromes. Blood 1997;89:2079–88.
81. Appelbaum FR, Anderson J. Allogeneic bone marrow transplantation for myelodysplastic syndrome: outcomes analysis according to IPSS score. Leukemia 1998;12 Suppl 1:S25–9.
82. Deeg HJ, Storer B, Slattery JT, et al. Conditioning with targeted busulfan and cyclophosphamide for hemopoietic stem cell transplantation from related and unrelated donors in patients with myelodysplastic syndrome. Blood 2002;100:1201–7.
83. Greenberg P, Bishop M, Deeg J. Practise guidelines for myelodysplastic syndromes. Oncology 1998;12:53–80.
84. Giralt S. Bone marrow transplant in myelodysplastic syndromes: new technologies, same questions. Curr Hematol Rep. 2004;3:165–72.
85. de Witte T, Hermans J, Vossen J, et al. Haematopoietic stem cell transplantation for patients with myelo-dysplastic syndromes and secondary acute myeloid leukaemias: a report on behalf of the Chronic Leukaemia Working Party of the European Group for Blood and Marrow Transplantation (EBMT). Br J Haematol. 2000; 110:620–30.
86. Sierra J, Perez WS, Rozman C, et al. Bone marrow transplantation from HLA-identical siblings as treatment for myelodysplasia. Blood 2002;100:1997–2004.
87. Sutton L, Chastang C, Ribaud P, et al. Factors influencing outcome in de novo myelodysplastic syndromes treated by allogeneic bone marrow transplantation: a long-term study of 71 patients Societe Francaise de Greffe de Moelle. Blood 1996;88:358–65.
88. Anderson JE, Anasetti C, Appelbaum FR, et al. Unrelated donor marrow transplantation for myelodysplasia (MDS) and MDS-related acute myeloid leukaemia. Br J Haematol 1996;93:59–67.
89. Castro-Malaspina H, Harris RE, Gajewski J, et al. Unrelated donor marrow transplantation for myelodysplastic syndromes: outcome analysis in 510 transplants facilitated by the National Marrow Donor Program. Blood 2002;99:1943–51.
90. de Witte T, Pikkemaat F, Hermans J, et al. Genotypically nonidentical related donors for transplantation of patients with myelodysplastic syndromes: comparison with unrelated donor transplantation and autologous stem cell transplantation. Leukemia 2001; 15:1878–84.
91. Nevill TJ, Fung HC, Shepherd JD, et al. Cytogenetic abnormalities in primary myelodysplastic syndrome are highly predictive of outcome after allogeneic bone marrow transplantation. Blood 1998;92:1910–7.
92. Runde V, de Witte T, Arnold R, et al. Bone marrow transplantation from HLA-identical siblings as first-line treatment in patients with myelodysplastic syndromes: early transplantation is associated with improved outcome. Chronic Leukemia Working Party of the European Group for Blood and Marrow Transplantation. Bone Marrow Transplant. 1998;21:255–61.
93. Cutler CS, Lee SJ, Greenberg P, et al. A decision analysis of allogeneic bone marrow transplantation for the myelodysplastic syndromes: delayed transplantation for low risk myelodysplasia is associated with improved outcome. Blood 2004;104:579–85.
94. Anderson JE, Gooley TA, Schoch G, et al. Stem cell transplantation for secondary acute myeloid leukemia: evaluation of transplantation as initial therapy or following induction chemotherapy. Blood 1997;89:2578–85.
95. Copeland EA, Penza SL, Elder PJ, et al. Analysis of prognostic factors for allogeneic marrow transplantation following busulfan and cyclophosphamide in myelodysplastic syndrome and after leukemic transformation. Bone Marrow Transplant. 2000;25:1219–22.
96. Appelbaum FR, Barrall J, Storb R, et al. Bone marrow transplantation for patients with myelodysplasia. Pretreatment variables and outcome. Ann Intern Med. 1990;112:590–7.
97. Anderson JE, Appelbaum FR, Schoch G, et al. Allogeneic marrow transplantation for myelodysplastic syndrome with advanced disease morphology: a phase II study of busulfan, cyclophosphamide, and total-body irradiation and analysis of prognostic factors. J Clin Oncol. 1996;14:220–6.

98. Slattery JT, Risler LJ. Therapeutic monitoring of busulfan in hematopoietic stem cell transplantation. Ther Drug Monit. 1998;20:543–49.
99. Andersson BS, Gajewski J, Donato M, et al. Allogeneic stem cell transplantation (BMT) for AML and MDS following i.v. busulfan and cyclophosphamide (i.v. BuCy). Bone Marrow Transplant. 2000;25 Suppl 2:S35–38.
100. Giralt S, Thall PF, Khouri I, et al. Melphalan and purine analog-containing preparative regimens: reduced-intensity conditioning for patients with hematologic malignancies undergoing allogeneic progenitor cell transplantation. Blood 2001;97:631–7.
101. Shimoni A, Giralt S, Khouri I, Champlin R. Allogeneic hematopoietic transplantation for acute and chronic myeloid leukemia: non-myeloablative preparative regimens and induction of the graft-versus-leukemia effect. Curr Oncol Rep. 2000;2:132–9.
102. Parker JE, Shafi T, Pagliuca A, et al. Allogeneic stem cell transplantation in the myelodysplastic syndromes: interim results of outcome following reduced-intensity conditioning compared with standard preparative regimens. Br J Haematol. 2002;119:144–54.
103. Martino R, van Biezen A, Iacobelli S, et al. Reduced intensity conditioning regimens for allogeneic stem cell transplants from HLA identical siblings in adults with MDS: a comparison with standard myeloablative regimens. A study of the EBMT Chronic Leukemia Working Party (EBMT-CLWP). Blood 2003;102:642 (abstract).
104. de Lima M, Anagnostopoulos A, Munsell M, et al. Non-ablative versus reduced intensity conditioning regimens in the treatment of acute myeloid leukemia and high-risk myelodysplastic syndrome. Dose is relevant for long-term disease control after allogeneic hematopoietic stem cell transplantation. Blood 2004;104:865–72.
105. Stuart JS, Cao TM, Sandmaier BM, et al. Efficacy of non-myeloablative allogeneic transplant for patients with MDS and myeloproliferative disorders. Blood 2003;102:644 (abstract).
106. Martino R, Iacobelli S, Brand R, et al. Retrospective comparison of reduced-intensity conditioning and conventional high-dose conditioning for allogeneic hematopoietic stem cell transplantation using HLA-identical sibling donors in myelodysplastic syndromes. Blood 2006;108:836–46.
107. Stuart J, Sandmeir, BM. Efficacy of non-myeloablative allogeneic transplants for patients with MDS and myeloproliferative disorders. Blood 2003;102:644ab.
108. Guardiola P, Runde V, Bacigalupo A, et al. Retrospective comparison of bone marrow and granulocyte colony-stimulating factor-mobilized peripheral blood progenitor cells for allogeneic stem cell transplantation using HLA identical sibling donors in myelodysplastic syndromes. Blood 2002;99:4370–8.
109. del Canizo MC, Martinez C, Conde E, et al. Peripheral blood is safer than bone marrow as a source of hematopoietic progenitors in patients with myelodysplastic syndromes who receive an allogeneic transplantation. Results from the Spanish registry. Bone Marrow Transplant. 2003;32:987–92.
110. Ooi J, Iseki T, Takahashi S, et al. Unrelated cord blood transplantation for adult patients with advanced myelodysplastic syndrome. Blood 2003;101:4711–3.
111. Ooi J, Iseki T, Nagayama H, et al. Unrelated cord blood transplantation for adult patients with myelodysplastic syndrome-related secondary acute myeloid leukaemia. Br J Haematol. 2001;114:834–6.

Chapter 18
Allogeneic Hematopoietic Stem Cell Transplantation for Adult Acute Lymphoblastic Leukemia

Daniel Weisdorf and Stephen Forman

18.1 Introduction

Although multidrug chemotherapy yields complete remission (CR) for nearly 90% of adults with acute lymphoblastic leukemia (ALL, a.k.a. acute lymphocytic leukemia), post-remission therapy fails to control disease recurrence for the majority [1–8]. Twenty percent of adult acute leukemia is ALL, and despite some parallels to the morphology and molecular features of pediatric ALL, where therapy is often curative [9–12], the majority of adults have high-risk phenotypes of disease, and current therapies remain inadequate. Extended leukemia-free survival (LFS) in unlikely, particularly for those with high-risk features including age greater than 35 years, elevated white blood count (WBC) at diagnosis, cytogenetically high-risk subsets and poor initial response to therapy. These further truncate the odds of extended LFS. Newer immunopathologic, molecular and monitoring techniques have improved classifications and potentially allowed risk-directed therapy. However, allogeneic hematopoietic stem cell transplantation (HSCT) remains key for many patients' survival and yet is not frequently applied. We review the biologic features of adult ALL distinguishing it from childhood ALL, highlight risk factors and techniques for identifying transplant candidates, and review the utility of allogeneic HSCT.

18.2 Epidemiology and Biology of Adult Acute Lymphoblastic Leukemia

ALL represents 20% of acute leukemia in patients over 20 years of age and occurs in two persons per 100,000; more frequently in those over 50 years of age [13]. While no defined environmental factors are closely associated with the

D. Weisdorf (✉)
University of Minnesota, Mayo Mail Code 480, Minneapolis, MN 55455, USA
e-mail: weisd001@umn.edu

M.R. Bishop (ed.), *Hematopoietic Stem Cell Transplantation*, Cancer Treatment and Research 144, DOI 10.1007/978-0-387-78580-6_18,

risks of adult ALL, prior radiation or certain chemical exposures may increase its risk, though not as much as myeloid leukemia. Neither familial clustering nor inherited syndromes increase the risk of ALL in adults, though Down's syndrome and DNA repair defects including Fanconi's anemia, Bloom syndrome, and ataxia telangiectasia yield higher risks of pediatric ALL [14, 15].

Most adults present with FAB L2 morphology, and except for those with mature B lineage L3 disease, cytochemical staining has not defined prognosis nor guided treatment planning in adult ALL [16]. Most adults have pre-B phenotype lymphoblastic ALL expressing CD 19, usually CD10, CD20, CD24, CD22, and nuclear TdT. Cytoplasmic immunoglobulin heavy chain expression confirms pre-B ALL. Only 2–3% express surface immunoglobulin, L3 morphology and thus have mature B cell ALL, which shares cytogenetic, molecular, immunologic, and prognostic features with Burkitt's lymphoma. T-cell ALL is considerably less common in adults, but frequently presents with extreme leukocytosis, male predominance, more frequent central nervous system (CNS) involvement, and sometimes a thymic mass.

As in other acute leukemias, cytogenetic and molecular classifications have dominated modern understanding of prognosis and guidance for therapy [17, 18]. The most common cytogenetic high-risk groups include t(9;22), t(4;11), t(1;19) and in mature B ALL and, t(8;14). Rearrangement of BCR/ABL in t(9;22), Philadelphia Chromosome (Ph) positive ALL is present in 25–30% and t(4;11) with 11q23 (MLL) rearrangements occur in 5% of adult ALL. These represent the dominant cytogenetic phenotypes indicating poor prognosis.

These phenotypes as well as extreme leukocytosis (>30,000/ul in pre-B and >100,000/ul in T-cell ALL) are recognized to predict poor remission induction rates and shorter remission duration, thus indicating a need for more effective therapy, usually with allogeneic HSCT. Even with recent addition of the tyrosine kinase inhibitors, imatinib or dasatinib, to multidrug intensive therapy, which has resulted in an increased rate of remission, no series indicate durable CR and thus reliably preclude the necessity of allografting in Ph-positive ALL [19–21]. Phase II trials combining imatinib with hyper-CVAD or alternative combination therapy yield encouraging 1-year survival, which might be extended when combined with follow-up allogeneic HSCT plus tyrosine kinase inhibitor supplementation [22–25]. However, prospective trials testing this approach are needed. The final indicator of poor prognosis, time to achieve CR (more than one cycle or >35 days), has predicted poor prognosis and shorter remission duration [1, 5, 6–8]. In addition, PCR or multicolor immunophenotypic flow cytometry to detect persisting minimal residual disease (MRD) after successful induction therapy indicating a high risk of early relapse may also be justification for intensified transplant therapy. Given the predictive value of MRD on subsequent relapse, transplant before overt recurrence may improve the outcome for such patients and should be tested in clinical trials [26–29].

18.3 Hematopoietic Stem Cell Transplantation for Adult Acute Lymphoblastic

18.3.1 Allogeneic HSCT for Adult Acute Lymphoblastic Leukemia in First Complete Remission

Many recent trials have described outcomes of adult ALL treated in first complete remission (CR1) with allogeneic HSCT or alternatives based upon related donor availability (biologic assignment) [3, 5, 8, 22, 30–39]. Some have analyzed outcome by the intention to treat concept of donor versus no donor, even if the transplant had not been completed. Most studies demonstrated statistically significant improvements in LFS following allogeneic HSCT (34–72%, 3-year LFS) compared to either autologous HSCT or alternative approaches (26–44%, Table 18.1). While treatment related mortality (TRM) varied between series (9–44%) and generally exceeded the TRM, with autologous HSCT (2–24%) the published analyses all demonstrated superior survival after allogeneic transplantation, particularly in patients with high-risk features of ALL.

The recent update and publication of the Medical Research Council (MRC) UK ALL XII/ECOG E2993 trial describes the largest-ever prospective assessment of optimal therapy for adult ALL [3, 8]. Following two-phased induction, 91% of patients achieved CR. Patients with HLA-compatible sibling (<age 50) were assigned to allogeneic HSCT, and others were randomly

Table 18.1 Allogeneic HLA-matched related donor HSCT in CR1

Reference	*n*	Age (median, range years)	TRM% (3 years)	LFS% (5 years)	Survival (5 years)	Relapse (%)
Thiebaut et al. [36]	116	33	44	–	46%	–
Ringden et al. [38][a]	345	34	9	61	–	33
Dombret et al. [22]	46	>15	24	–	37	50
Takeuchi et al. [5]	34	15–45	–	34	46	–
Thomas et al. [30]	100	33	18	47	51	36
Labar et al. [37]	100	15–50	23	38	41	38
Hunault et al. [31]	41	15–50	15	72	75	–
Gupta et al. [39][a]	48	34	29	40	46	–
Goldstone et al. [3]	533[b]	15–59	36[d]	–	54	24
	590[c]	–	20	–	29	37

TRM treatment related (nonrelapse) mortality, *LFS* leukemia free survival
[a]Retrospective
[b]Standard risk
[c]High risk
[d]2 years: Donor–no donor analysis

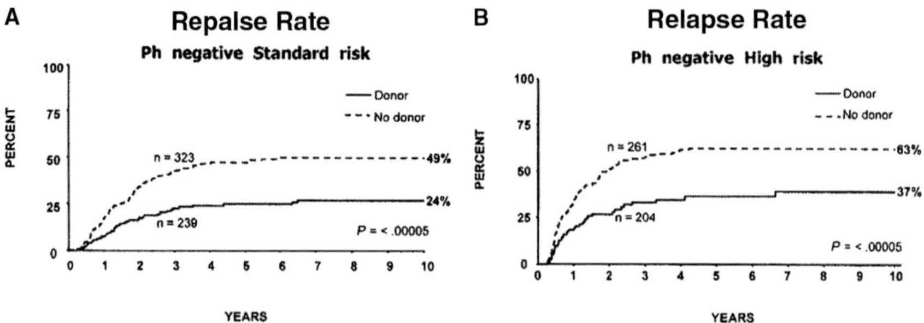

Fig. 18.1 Reduced relapse risk with available allogeneic donor for adult ALL in CR1. (**a**) Ph-negative standard risk; (**b**) Ph-negative high-risk (adapted from Goldstone et al. [3])

assigned between autologous HSCT and intensified consolidation therapy. Those with an available donor had superior survival of 5 years (53%) compared to either alternative strategy (45%), though the best protection against relapse or death was observed in standard risk patients (Ph-negative, WBC < 30,000) under age 35 due to greater TRM in the greater than 35-year-old cohort (Fig. 18.1). Allogeneic HSCT led to greater protection against relapse. Ph-positive patients, all assigned to allografting, had superior outcomes than those with no donor.

Disappointingly, survival following relapse was only 7% at 5 years, including those able to undergo allogeneic HSCT during second complete remission (CR2) (3). This emphasizes the problem for the patient who relapses, especially an early recurrence, where the chances of achieving a second remission are low. Transplants performed for patients with CR2 after early relapse often are not performed and often do not work to control disease. Outcomes were slightly better in younger adults and those with a longer duration of CR1, but importantly, the assignment of treatment during CR1 did not influence the outcome of after relapse. Outcomes were equally disappointing in patients who relapsed following either chemotherapy, autologous HSCT or allogeneic HSCT in CR1, providing a strong recommendation to seek the most effective therapy to prevent initial recurrence as the best approach to extend survival.

Several other series report extended long-term LFS (40–60%) [31, 32, 40–44] in high-risk adults with ALL. A recent multicenter analysis of 169 Ph-negative adults reported through the Center for International Blood and Marrow Transplant Research (CIBMTR) showed 39% survival at 5-year post-HSCT [45].

18.3.2 Philadelphia Chromosome-Positive Adult Acute Lymphoblastic Leukemia

For patients with Philadelphia chromosome-positive ALL, the data suggest that the use of allogeneic HSCT following induction therapy with imatinib plus chemotherapy [23] results in remarkable improvements in protection against relapse (3.5%) as compared to historical data without imatinib (47.3%, $p = 0.002$). Observed superior LFS (76% vs. 38%; $p = 0.001$) offers promise that combination tyrosine kinase inhibitor plus chemotherapy for induction and tyrosine kinase inhibitor plus allogeneic HSCT for post-remission definitive management may significantly reduce the disease burden and improve LFS for a substantive majority of patients with this common, highest risk subset of ALL in adults [24]. A prospective trial planned by the US Southwest Oncology Group (SWOG) and the Blood and Marrow Transplant Clinical Trials Network (BMT CTN) may clarify the efficacy of this approach.

18.3.3 Alternative Donor Transplantation for Adult Acute Lymphoblastic Leukemia

With no available matched sibling to allow immediate transplantation, both volunteer unrelated donor (URD; Table 18.2) or umbilical cord blood (UCB; Table 18.3) allografts are available options. Data (Fig. 18.2) from the Center for International Blood and Marrow Transplant Research (CIBMTR) reported 44% LFS in CR1 and 36% in CR2 following matched URD transplantation [33, 46–53]. Another series of high-risk URD HSCT recipients had 40% survival [33]. Longer follow-up of the adult URD recipients confirmed 5-year survival (38%) after URD HSCT with encouraging low risks of relapse (24%) [51].

Recent data, reflecting advances in higher resolution HLA typing and improvements in donor selection have reduced TRM and improved outcomes following URD allografts. National Marrow Donor Program (NMDP) data show reduction in TRM between 1999–2002 and 2003–2006 after URD HSCT. One-year TRM after myeloablative PBSC HSCT for leukemia improved from 39% to 31%. Three-year survival for adults with ALL at all stages improved

Table 18.2 Unrelated donor HSCT for adult ALL

Reference	*N*	Age (median years)	CR1 (%)	Ph+ (%)	TRM (%)	LFS% (5 years)	Survival (5 years)	Relapse (%)
Weisdorf et al. [48]	517	18	36	14	42 ± 8^a 40 ± 6^b	44 ± 8	–	14 ± 5^a 22 ± 5^b
Cornelissen et al.[47]	127	31	64	76	61 ± 9	27 (2 years)	40 ± 13^a 17^b	19 ± 7
Garderet et al.[52]	102	>14	19	–	61	21	24%	47
Kiehl et al. [33]	103	29	27	31	43	42^a 40^b	–	–
Dahlke et al. [53]	46	31	16	11	35	42	44	26
Bishop et al. [51]	76^a 83^b	27		28	45 41	37 29	38 30	15 24

[a] CR1
[b] CR2

Table 18.3 Umbilical cord blood HSCT including ALL

Reference	*n*	ALL (%)	CR1 (%)	TRM (%)	LFS (%)	Relapse (%)
Laughlin et al. [54]	150	30	20	–	23 (3 years)	–
Rocha et al. [55]	98	54	27	44	36	23
Takahashi et al. [57]	100	20	9[a,b]	9	70	17
Yanada et al. [34]	18	17	–	33	49	18
Barker et al. [49]	23	35		22	57	–
Lekakis et al. [50]	15	35	33	18	18	65
Cornetta et al. [56]	34%	9	–	65	17	16
Tomblyn et al. [58]	66%	100	20	18	50[a] 60[b]	24[a] 50[b]

[a] CR1
[b] CR2

from 19% between years 1987 and 1995 up to 29% between years 2003 and 2006 (NMDP unpublished data). For adult ALL patients in CR1, 5-year survival rates of 35–45% are expected (www.marrow.org, data 1998–2006) [46].

UCB allografts represent a new and encouraging option for patients lacking either sibling or well-matched URD sources of stem cells (reviewed in Chap. 10 by Wagner, Brunstein, Tse, and Laughlin). Adults with ALL have been included in the two largest multi-institutional analyses comparing UCB with volunteer URD transplants. A CIBMTR/New York Blood Center report [52] included 40 of 150 patients with ALL and reported similar 3-year survival [UCB 26% (19–32) vs. URD 35% (30–39)]. A second report from the European group for Blood and Marrow Transplantation (EBMT) and EuroCord included 53 ALL patients of 93 UCB grafts [33]. Two-year LFS with ALL was 34% for UCB HSCT and 33% for URD HSCT ($p = 0.021$). Encouragingly, despite

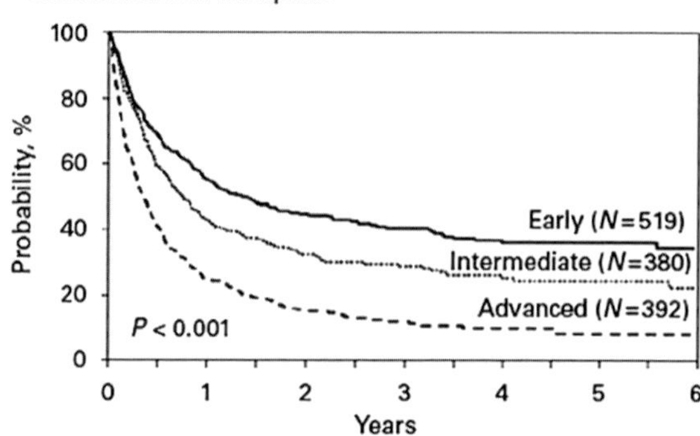

Fig. 18.2 Survival after unrelated donor HSCT for adult ALL (data from CIBMTR, 2008; www.cibmtr.org)

greater HLA disparity in the UCB grafts, graft-versus-host disease (GvHD) was significantly less frequent (26% vs. 39%) following URD transplantation [33]. Other cord blood series include ALL patients with encouraging outcomes compared to URD HSCT [49, 50, 54–57].

At the University of Minnesota, 623 HSCT patients with ALL were treated over a 25-year period [58]. They all received myeloablative, total body irradiation (TBI)-based conditioning regimen prior to HSCT, and the 5-year overall survival (OS) rate in patients receiving UCB was 46% [95% confidence interval (CI): 33–59], which was comparable to sibling donor allografts (35%; 29–41) and well-matched URD HSCT (OS = 42%; CI: 29–55). Mismatched URD grafts had inferior 5-year outcomes (OS = 21%; CI: 11–33). Multivariate analyses showed risks of LFS to be comparable between UCB and sibling transplants (relative risk for UCB = 0.8, 0.5–1.1) confirming the promise of this option for patients lacking sibling or well-matched URD for transplantation.

18.4 Graft-Versus-Leukemia in Acute Lymphoblastic Leukemia

Increased risks of relapse following T-cell depletion of an allograft or achievement of CR following donor lymphocyte infusions (DLI) for relapsed disease have documented the potency of graft-versus-leukemia (GvL) accompanying allogeneic HSCT. Unfortunately these effects have been less prominent for patients with ALL. However, both single institution and multicenter registry data [59–61] demonstrated lower risks of relapse in patients with acute and particularly chronic GvHD. Other studies documented equally potent GvL directed toward either B-cell lineage or T-cell lineage ALL and confirmed an association of chronic GvHD with better protection against relapse [62]. Though uncertainty still exists about the utility of DLI in ALL patients [62–64], this documented GvL effect has encouraged the application of reduced-intensity pre-HSCT conditioning (RIC) for patients with ALL [65–69]. Even using URD grafts, NMDP data shows improvement through reduction in 1-year TRM for 32–26% using RIC prior to HSCT for leukemia [unpublished data, NMDP, 2008]. Several recent reports suggest effective disease control, even for older patients receiving RIC HSCT for ALL, yet these favorable results are limited to those in documented complete remission. A recent report from the EBMT demonstrated 42 ± 10% 2-year LFS in adult ALL [70]. Other series using either related, unrelated, or UCB donors suggested encouraging outcomes with RIC HSCT for high-risk CR1 or CR2 ALL recipients [65–69]. Since the recent MRC/Eastern Cooperative Oncology Group (ECOG) trial demonstrated excess TRM in patients over age 35 years, further exploration of allografts using these safer, yet still potent, reduced-intensity regimens for older ALL patients will be essential and important investigations for the near future.

18.5 Opportunities for Improving Transplantation in Acute Lymphoblastic Leukemia

Superior conditioning regimens, chosen for their anti-leukemic efficacy, but also for their safety, need further study. Most series and comparisons have documented improved disease control and overall superior LFS with TBI-containing pretransplant conditioning. Investigators at the City of Hope originated substitution of etoposide plus TBI yield encouraging LFS, confirmed in multicenter trials from the Southwest Oncology Group and used in the MRC/ECOG study as well [71]. A comparative analysis of TBI combined with either cyclophosphamide or etoposide demonstrated superior disease control and outcome using TBI less than 13 Gy plus etoposide rather than cyclophosphamide, though these findings were noted only in CR2, but not CR1 HSCT recipients [72].

Radio-immunotherapy (reviewed in Chap. 13 by Gopal and Winter) using radioiodine coupled to an anti-CD45 antibody to augment marrow-targeted radiation to supplement conditioning with TBI plus cyclophosphamide suggests favorable biodistribution and tolerable toxicity [73]. This regimen only delivers 3.5–12.25 Gy to the liver yet up to 24 Gy to the marrow and spleen when combined with conventional fractionated TBI [73]. Newer approaches including helical tomotherapy to augment marrow and bone-directed radiation are being piloted in combination with chemotherapy, particularly for patients with marrow-localized resistant malignancy such as ALL [74].

Choosing the optimal donor can also augment survival, likely by reducing TRM. In the absence of a well-matched, genotypically identical sibling donor, an HLA-allele matched URD chosen by high resolution DNA based typing at HLA-A, B, C, and DRB1 yields superior survival with lowest risks of GvHD and other causes of TRM. However, closely matched donors disparate at a single HLA locus allele or antigen can still yield suitable survival and extended disease control [75]. Greater degrees of HLA mismatch are associated with more risk and poorer outcomes.

As an alternative, UCB grafts, mismatched as 0–2 HLA-A, B, DR loci with an adequate cell dose can be an excellent option to mismatched or even matched URD grafting for children and adults. Studies pioneered at the University of Minnesota indicate that two closely matched UCB grafts can augment the cell dose and assure engraftment with tolerable risks of TRM and particularly lower rates of chronic GvHD for adults in need of allografting [49, 50]. Since patients with detectable minimal residual disease or high-risk ALL phenotypes may have only brief remissions, the rapid availability of UCB grafts suggest an additional advantage, which should be elected for the proper recipient. Prompt HLA confirmation and transport to the transplant center, often achievable within 2 weeks, may permit urgent transplantation prior to another relapse and thereby reduce the ALL patients' overall risks.

18.6 Conclusions

The critical factor in improving survival in adults with ALL is identifying patients with high-risk phenotypes in order to allow planning for early-allogeneic HSCT. Initiating a donor search while initial remission induction is underway can facilitate transplantation during CR1, when long-term results are best. For patients presenting with high-risk disease t(9;22), t(4;11), mature B cell, high WBC or for those failing to promptly achieve remission, allografts in CR1 offer the most important opportunity to achieve extended LFS. Finding the right sibling match or alternatively, a well-matched URD or closely matched single or pair of UCB units can permit the curative potential of allogeneic transplantation. Monitoring of minimal residual disease, utilization of targeted therapy, tyrosine kinase inhibitors, or newer agents yet to come, might further reduce missed opportunities for disease control and improved survival. Reduced intensity conditioning for the older or sicker patient, augmented conditioning, or novel radiation delivery for those with higher risk disease also offer promise yet need to be tested in prospective, well-designed clinical trials. Based on the current data, and understanding of the benefits and limits of each approach, Fig. 18.3 shows an algorithm for the suggested management of the adult patient with ALL. The ideal management strategy

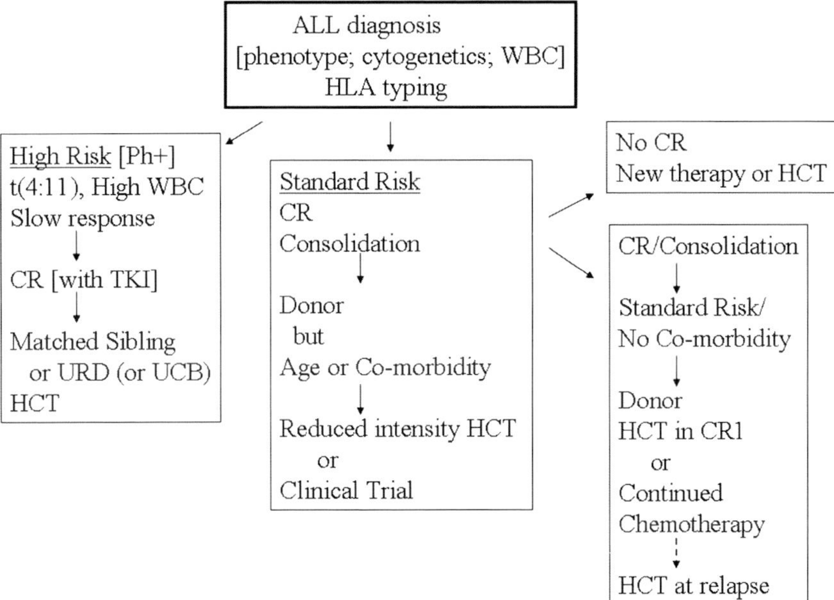

Fig. 18.3 Treatment strategy for adult ALL

for adult ALL has yet to be identified, but developing new tools and their prompt application may improve survival for all adults with ALL in the future. Scientific innovation and careful clinical translation offer both promise and great hope.

References

1. Gökbuget N, Noelzer D. Treatment of adult acute lymphoblastic leukemia. Hematology Am Soc Hematol Educ Program. 2006;133–41.
2. Annino L, Vegna ML, Camera A, et al. Treatment of adult acute lymphoblastic leukemia (ALL): long-term follow-up of the GIMEMA ALL 0288 randomized study. Blood 2002; 99:863–71.
3. Goldstone AH, Richards SH, Lazarus HM, et al. In adults with standard-risk acute lymphoblastic leukemia, the greatest benefit is achieved from a matched sibling allogeneic transplantation in first complete remission, and an autologous transplant is less effective than conventional consolidation maintenance chemotherapy in all patients: final results of the International ALL Trial (MRC UKALL XII/ECOG E2993). Blood 2008; 111:1827–33.
4. Pui CH, Evans WE. Treatment of acute lymphoblastic leukemia. N Engl J Med. 2006; 54:166–78.
5. Takeuchi J, Kyo T, Naito K, et al. Induction therapy by frequent administration of doxorubicin with four other drugs, followed by intensive consolidation and maintenance therapy for adult acute lymphoblastic leukemia: the JALSG-ALL93 study. Leukemia 2002;16:1259–66.
6. Larson RA, Dodge RK, Burns CP, et al. A five-drug remission induction regimen with intensive consolidation for adults with acute lymphoblastic leukemia: cancer and leukemia group B study 8811. Blood 1995;85:2025–37.
7. Hoelzer D, Thiel E, Loffler H, et al. Prognostic factors in a multicenter study for treatment of acute lymphoblastic leukemia in adults. Blood 1988;71:123–31.
8. Rowe JM, Buck G, Burnett AK, et al. Induction therapy for adults with acute lymphoblastic leukemia: results of more than 1500 patients from the international ALL trial: MRC UKALL XII/ECOG E2993. Blood 2005;106:3760–7.
9. Schrappe M, Reiter A, Ludwig WD, et al. Improved outcome in childhood acute lymphoblastic leukemia despite reduced use of anthracyclines and cranial radiotherapy: results of trial ALL BFM90: German-Austrian Swiss ALL BFM Study Group. Blood 2000; 95:3310–22.
10. Silverman LB, Gelber RD, Dalton VK, et al. Approved outcome for children with acute lymphoblastic leukemia: results of Dana Farber Consortium protocol 91-01. Blood 2001;97:1211–8.
11. Chessells JM, Hall E, Prentice HG, Durrant J, Bailey CC, Richards SM. The impact of age on outcome in lymphoblastic leukemia. MRC UKALL X and XA compared: a report from the MRC Paediatric and Adult Working Parties. Leukemia 1998;12:463–73.
12. Boissel N, Auclerc MF, Lhéritier V, et al. Should adolescents with acute lymphoblastic leukemia be treated as old children or young adults? Comparison of the French FRALLE-93 and LALA-94 trials. J Clin Oncol. 2003;21:774–80.
13. Sandler DP, Ross JA. Epidemiology of acute leukemia in children and adults. Semin Oncol. 1997;24:3–16.
14. Sali D, Cardis E, Sztanyik L, et al. Cancer consequences of the Chernobyl accident in Europe outside the former USSR: a review. Int J Cancer. 1996;67:343–52.
15. Hasle H, Clemmensen IH, Mikkelsen M. Risks of leukaemia and solid tumours in individuals with Down's syndrome. Lancet 2000;355:165–9.

16. Ferrando AA, Look AT. Pathobiology of acute lymphoblastic leukemia. In: Hoffman, R, Benz EJ Jr, Shattil SJ, Furie B, Cohen HJ, Silberstein LE, McGlave P, editors. Hematology. Basic principles and practices, 4th ed. Philadelphia: Elsevier Churchill Livingstone; 2005. p. 1135–54.
17. Pullarkat VA, Slovak ML, Kopecky KJ, Forman SJ, Appelbaum FR. Impact of cytogenetics on the outcome of adult acute lymphoblastic leukemia: results of Southwest Oncology Group study SWOG-9400. Blood 2008;111:2563–72.
18. Moorman AV, Harrison CJ, Buck GA, et al. Karyotype is an independent prognostic factor in adult acute lymphoblastic leukemia (ALL): analysis of cytogenetic data from patients treated on the Medical Research Council (MRC) UKALLXII/Eastern Cooperative Oncology Group (ECOG) 2993 trial. Blood 2007;109:3189–97.
19. Thomas DA, Faderl S, Cortes J, et al. Treatment of Philadelphia chromosome-positive acute lymphocytic leukemia with hyper-CVAD and imatinib mesylate. Blood 2004; 103:4396–407.
20. Wassmann B, Pfeifer H, Goekbuget N, et al. Alternating versus concurrent schedules of imatinib and chemotherapy as front-line therapy for Philadelphia-positive acute lymphoblastic leukemia (Ph+ ALL). Blood 2006;108:1469–77.
21. Ottmann OG, Wassmann B, Pfeifer H, et al. Imatinib compared with chemotherapy as front-line treatment of elderly patients with Philadelphia chromosome-positive acute lymphoblastic leukemia (Ph+ ALL). Cancer 2007;109:2068–76.
22. Dombret H, Gabert J, Boiron JM, et al. Outcome of treatment in adults with Philadelphia chromosome-positive acute lymphoblastic leukemia—results of the prospective multicenter LALA-94 trial. Blood 2002;100:2357–66.
23. Lee S, Kim YJ, Min CK, et al. The effect of first-line imatinib therapy on the outcome of allogeneic stem cell transplantation in adults with newly diagnosed Philadelphia chromosome-positive acute lymphoblastic leukemia. Blood 2005;105:3449–57.
24. Carpenter PA, Snyder DS, Flowers ME, et al. Prophylactic administration of imatinib after hematopoietic cell transplantation for high-risk Philadelphia chromosome-positive leukemia. Blood 2007;109:2791–3.
25. Kantarjian H, Thomas D, O'Brien S, et al. Long-term follow-up results of hyperfractionated cyclophosphamide, vincristine, doxorubicin, and dexamethasone (Hyper-CVAD), a dose-intensive regimen, in adult acute lymphocytic leukemia. Cancer 2004;101: 2788–801.
26. Mortuza FY, Papaioannou M, Moreira IM, et al. Minimal residual disease tests provide an independent predictor of clinical outcome in adult acute lymphoblastic leukemia. J Clin Oncol. 2002;20:1094–104.
27. Bruggemann M, Raff T, Flohr T, et al. Clinical significance of minimal residual disease quantification in adult patients with standard-risk acute lymphoblastic leukemia. Blood 2006;107:1116–23.
28. Raff T, Gokbuget N, Luschen S, et al. Molecular relapse in adult standard-risk ALL patients detected by prospective MRD monitoring during and after maintenance treatment: data from the GMALL 06/99 and 07/03 trials. Blood 2007;109:910–5.
29. Szczepanski T. Why and how to quantify minimal residual disease in acute lymphoblastic leukemia? Leukemia 2007;21:622–6.
30. Thomas X, Boiron JM, Huguet F, et al. Outcome of treatment in adults with acute lymphoblastic leukemia: analysis of the LALA-94 trial. J Clin Oncol. 2004;22:4075–86.
31. Hunault M, Harousseau JL, Delain M, et al. Better outcome of adult acute lymphoblastic leukemia after early genoidentical allogeneic bone marrow transplantation (BMT) than after late high dose therapy and autologous BMT: a GOELAMS trial. Blood 2004; 104:3028–37.
32. Thiebaut A, Vernant JP, Degos L, et al. Adult acute lymphocytic leukemia study testing chemotherapy and autologous and allogeneic transplantation: a follow-up report of the French protocol LALA87. Hematol Oncol Clin North Am. 2000;14:1353–66.

33. Kiehl MG, Kraut L, Schwerdtfeger R, et al. Outcome of allogeneic hematopoietic stem-cell transplantation in adult patients with acute lymphoblastic leukemia: no difference in relation compared with unrelated transplant in first complete remission. J Clin Oncol. 2004;22:2816–25.
34. Yanada M, Matsuo K, Suzuki T, et al. Allogeneic hematopoietic stem cell transplantation as part of postremission therapy improves survival for adult patients with high-risk acute lymphoblastic leukemia: a metaanalysis. Cancer 2006;106:2657–63.
35. Attal M, Blaise D, Marit G, et al. Consolidation treatment of adult acute lymphoblastic leukemia: a prospective, randomized trial comparing allogeneic versus autologous bone marrow transplantation and testing the impact of recombinant interleukin-2 after autologous bone marrow transplantation. Blood 1995;86:1619–28.
36. Thiebaut A, Vernanr JP, Degos L, Huguet FR, Reiffers J, Debban C, et al. Adult acute lymphocytic leukemia study testing chemotherapy and autologous and allogeneic transplantation. A follow-up report of the French protocol LALA 87. Hematol Oncol Clin North Am. 2000;14:1353–65.
37. Labar B, Suciu S, Zittoun R, Muus P, Marie JP, Fillet G, et al., EORTC Leukemia Group. Allogeneic stem cell transplantation in acute lymphoblastic leukemia and non-Hodgkin's lymphoma for patients <or = 50 years old in first complete remission: results of the EORTC ALL-3 trial. Haematologica 2004;89:809–17.
38. Ringden O, Labopin M, Bacigalupo A, Arcese W, Schaefer UW, Willemze R, et al. Transplantation of peripheral blood stem cells as compared with bone marrow from HLA-identical siblings in adult patients with acute myeloid leukemia and acute lymphoblastic leukemia. J Clin Oncol. 2002;20:4655–64.
39. Gupta V, Yi QL, Brandwein J, Minden MD, Schuh AC, Wells RA, et al. The role of allogeneic bone marrow transplantation in adult patients below the age of 55 years with acute lymphoblastic leukemia in first complete remission: a donor vs no donor comparison. Bone Marrow Transplant. 2004;33:397–404.
40. Doney K, Fisher LD, Appelbaum FR, et al. Treatment of adult acute lymphoblastic leukemia with allogeneic bone marrow transplantation: multivariate analysis of factors affecting acute graft-versus-host disease, relapse, and relapse-free survival. Bone Marrow Transplant. 1991;7:453–9.
41. Blume KG, Forman SJ, Snyder DS, et al. Allogeneic bone marrow transplantation for acute lymphoblastic leukemia during first complete remission. Transplantation. 1987; 43:389–92.
42. Vernant JP, Marit G, Maraninchi D, et al. Allogeneic bone marrow transplantation in adults with acute lymphoblastic leukemia in first complete remission. J Clin Oncol. 1988;6:227–31.
43. Sebban C, Lepage E, Vernant JP, et al. Allogeneic bone marrow transplantation in adult acute lymphoblastic leukemia in first complete remission: a comparative study. J Clin Oncol. 1994;12:2580–7.
44. Vey N, Blaise D, Stoppa AM, et al. Bone marrow transplantation in 63 adult patients with acute lymphoblastic leukemia in first complete remission. Bone Marrow Transplant. 1994;14:383–8.
45. Marks DI, Perez WS, He W, et al. Unrelated donor transplants in adults with Philadelphia-negative acute lymphoblastic leukemia in first complete remission. Blood 2008; 112:426–34.
46. Bachanova V, Weisdorf D. Unrelated donor allogeneic transplantation for adult acute lymphoblastic leukemia: a review. Bone Marrow Transplant. 2008;41:455–64
47. Cornelissen JJ, Carston M, Kollman C, et al. Unrelated marrow transplantation for adult patients with poor risk acute lymphoblastic leukemia: strong graft-versus-leukemia effect and risk factors determining outcome. Blood 2001;97:1572–7.
48. Weisdorf D, Bishop M, Dharan B, Bolwell B, Cahn JY, Cairo M, et al. Autologous versus allogeneic unrelated donor transplantation for acute lymphoblastic leukemia: comparative toxicity and outcomes. Biol Blood Marrow Transplant. 2002;8:213–20.

49. Barker JN, Weisdorf D, Wagner JE. Creation of a double chimera after the transplantation of umbilical-cord blood from two partially matched unrelated donors. N Engl J Med. 2001;24:1870–81.
50. Lekakis L, Giralt S, Couriel D, Shpall EJ, Hosing C, Khouri IF, et al. Phase II study of unrelated cord blood transplantation for adults with high-risk hematologic malignancies. Bone Marrow Transplant. 2006;38:421–6.
51. Bishop MR, Logan BR, Gandham S, et al. Long-term outcomes of adults with acute lymphoblastic leukemia after autologous or unrelated donor bone marrow transplantation: a comparative analysis by the National Marrow Donor Program and Center for International Blood and Marrow Transplant Research. Bone Marrow Transplant. 2008; 41:635–42.
52. Garderet L, Labopin M, Gorin NC, Polge E, Fouillard L, Ehringer GE, et al. Patients with acute lymphoblastic leukemia allografted with a matched unrelated donor may have a lower survival with a peripheral blood stem cell graft compared to bone marrow. Bone Marrow Transplant. 2003;31:23–9.
53. Dahlke J, Kröger N, Zabelina T, Ayuk F, Fehse N, Wolschke C, et al. Comparable results in patients with acute lymphoblastic leukemia after related and unrelated stem cell transplantation. Bone Marrow Transplant. 2006;37:155–63.
54. Laughlin MJ, Eapen M, Rubinstein P, Wagner JE, Zhang MJ, Champlin RE, et al. Outcomes after transplantation of cord blood or bone marrow from unrelated donors in adults with leukemia. N Engl J Med. 2004;351:2265–75.
55. Rocha V, Labopin M, Sanz G, Arcese W, Schwerdtfeger R, Bosi A, et al. Transplants of umbilical-cord blood or bone marrow from unrelated donors in adults with acute leukemia. N Engl J Med. 2004;351:2276–85.
56. Cornetta K, Laughlin M, Carter S, Wall D, Weinthal J, Delaney C, et al. Umbilical cord blood transplantation in adults: results of the prospective Cord Blood Transplantation (COBLT). Biol Blood Marrow Transplant. 2005;11:149–60.
57. Takahashi S, Iseki T, Ooi J, Tomonari A, Takasugi K, Shimohakamada Y, et al. Single-institute comparative analysis of unrelated bone marrow transplantation and cord blood transplantation for adult patients with hematologic malignancies. Blood 2004;104: 3813–20.
58. Tomblyn MB, DeFor TE, Tomblyn MR, MacMillan M, Higgins PD, Dusenbery KE, et al. Hematopoietic cell transplantation (HSCT) for acute lymphoblastic leukemia (ALL): 25-year experience at the University of Minnesota. J Clin Oncol. 2007;25(Suppl 185):3575.
59. Horowitz MM, Gale RP, Sondel PM, et al. Graft-versus-leukemia reactions after bone marrow transplantation. Blood 1990;75:555–62.
60. Appelbaum FR. Graft versus leukemia (GVL) in the therapy of acute lymphoblastic leukemia (ALL). Leukemia 1997;11:S15–S17.
61. Weisdorf DJ, Nesbit ME, Ramsay NKC, Woods WG, Goldman A, Kim TH, Hurd DD, McGlave PB, Kersey JH: Allogeneic bone marrow transplantation for acute lymphoblastic leukemia in remission: prolonged survival associated with acute graft vs. host disease. J Clin Oncol. 1987;5:1348–55.
62. Passweg JR, Tiberghien P, Cahn JY, et al. Graft-versus-leukemia effects in T lineage and B lineage acute lymphoblastic leukemia. Bone Marrow Transplant. 1998;21:153–8.
63. Kolb HJ, Schattenberg A, Goldman JM, et al. Graft-versus-leukemia effect of donor lymphocyte transfusions in marrow grafted patients. European Group for Blood and Marrow Transplantation Working Party Chronic Leukemia. Blood 1995;86:2041–50.
64. Collins RH, Shpilberg O, Drobyski WR, et al. Donor leukocyte infusions in 140 patients with relapsed malignancy after allogeneic bone marrow transplantation. J Clin Oncol. 1997;15:433–44.
65. Valcarcel D, Martino R, Sureda A, et al. Conventional versus reduced-intensity conditioning regimen for allogeneic stem cell transplantation in patients with hematological malignancies. Eur J Haematol. 2005;74:144–51.

66. Arnold R, Massenkeil G, Bornhäuser M, et al. Nonmyeloablative stem cell transplantation in adults with high-risk ALL may be effective in early but not in advanced disease. Leukemia 2002;16:2423–8.
67. Gutierrez-Aguirre CH, Gomez-Almaguer D, Cantu-Rodriguez OG, et al. Non-myeloablative stem cell transplantation in patients with relapsed cute lymphoblastic leukemia: results of a multicenter study. Bone Marrow Transplant. 2007;40:535–9.
68. Martino R, Giralt S, Caballero MD, Mackinnon S, Corradini P, Fernández-Avilés F, San Miguel J, Sierra J. Allogeneic hematopoietic stem cell transplantation with reduced-intensity conditioning in acute lymphoblastic leukemia: a feasibility study. Haematologica 2003;88:555–60.
69. Stein A, O'Donnell M, Snyder D, et al. Reduced-intensity stem cell transplantation for high-risk acute lymphoblastic leukemia. Biol Blood Marrow Transplant. 2007;13:134.
70. Mohty M, Labopin M, Tabrizzi R, Theorin N, Fauser AA, Rambaldi A, Maertens J, Slavin S, Majolino I, Nagler A, Blaise D, Rocha V; Acute Leukemia Working Party; European Group for Blood and Marrow Transplantation. Reduced intensity conditioning allogeneic stem cell transplantation for adult patients with acute lymphoblastic leukemia: a retrospective study from the European Group for Blood and Marrow Transplantation. Haematologica 2008;93:303–6.
71. Blume KG, Kopecky KJ, Henslee-Downey JP, et al. A prospective randomized comparison of total body irradiation-etoposide versus busulfan cyclophosphamide as preparatory regimens for bone marrow transplantation in patients with leukemia who were not in first remission: a South-West Oncology Group study. Blood 1993;81:2187–93.
72. Marks DI, Forman SJ, Blume KG, et al. A comparison of cyclophosphamide and total body irradiation with etoposide and total body irradiation as conditioning regimens for patients undergoing sibling allografting for acute lymphoblastic leukemia in first or second complete remission. Biol Blood Marrow Transplant. 2006;12:438–53.
73. Matthews DC, Appelbaum FR, Eary JF, et al. Phase I study of 131[I]-anti-CD45 antibody plus cyclophosphamide and total body irradiation for advanced acute leukemia and myelodysplastic syndrome. Blood 1999;94:1237–47.
74. Wong JY, Liu A, Schultheiss T, et al. Targeted total marrow irradiation using three-dimensional image-guided tomographic intensity-modulated radiation therapy: an alternative to standard total body irradiation. Biol Blood Marrow Transplant. 2006;12:306–15.
75. Lee SJ, Klein JP, Haagenson M, et al. High-resolution donor-recipient HLA matching contributes to the success of unrelated donor marrow transplantation. Blood 2007;110: 4576–83.

Chapter 19
Hematopoietic Stem Cell Transplantation in Children and Adolescents with Malignant Disease

Mitchell S. Cairo and Thomas G. Gross

19.1 Introduction

The origins of hematopoietic stem cell transplantation (HSCT) in children and adolescents with cancer can be traced back over 50 years ago to the original reports of Thomas et al. [1, 2]. Thomas et al. initially reported the results of syngeneic transplants in twins with leukemia who had been conditioned with superlethal doses of total body radiation (TBI) [1, 2]. Since that groundbreaking observation over 50 years ago, additional sources of stem cells have been investigated in children and adolescents with a variety of malignant conditions including human leukocyte antigen (HLA) matched sibling or related allogeneic donors, matched unrelated adult donors, sibling and unrelated cord blood donors, haploidentical donors, and autologous bone marrow or peripheral blood. Currently, there are a variety of malignant conditions that occur in children and adolescents that may benefit from HSCT during different stages of their treatment and can be subdivided into hematopoietic neoplasms and solid tumors (Table 19.1). We have summarized the state of the science of HSCT in children with cancer in the remainder of this chapter.

19.1.1 Intensity of Conditioning

Historically, myeloablation has been utilized in the conditioning regimen prior to HSCT in children and adolescents with malignant disease. This concept of myeloablative conditioning has been based on the assumption that ablative doses of cellular toxic therapy were required to circumvent potential drug resistance and were required for eradication of minimal residual malignant disease (MRD). In children and adolescents undergoing autologous HSCT,

M.S. Cairo (✉)
Morgan Stanley Children's Hospital of New York-Presbyterian, Columbia University, 3959 Broadway, CHN 10-03, New York, NY 10032, USA
e-mail: mc1310@columbia.edu

M.R. Bishop (ed.), *Hematopoietic Stem Cell Transplantation*, Cancer Treatment and Research 144, DOI 10.1007/978-0-387-78580-6_19,

Table 19.1 Malignant disease in children and adolescents successfully treated with hematopoietic stem cell transplantation (HSCT)

Hematopoietic neoplasms	Solid tumors
Acute lymphoblastic leukemia (ALL)	Neuroblastoma (NBL)
Acute myeloblastic leukemia (AML)	Wilms' tumor (WT)
Juvenile myelomonocytic leukemia (JMML)	Brain tumors (BT)
Chronic myelogenous leukemia (CML)	Ewing's sarcoma (ES)
Myelodysplastic syndrome (MDS)	Rhabdomyosarcoma (RMS)
Non-Hodgkin's lymphoma (NHL)	Germ cell tumors (GCT)
Hodgkin's lymphoma (HL)	Others

myeloablative conditioning is still required and almost exclusively utilized to eradicate post-growth and/or MRD. However, more recently the dogma that myeloablative cytotoxic therapy was required for disease eradication following allogeneic HSCT has been challenged [3]. Recent observations have suggested a potential graft-versus-tumor or graft-versus-leukemia effect following allogeneic HSCT [4]. Evidence over the past two decades has demonstrated that (1) donor lymphocyte infusions (DLI) can induce remission in patients whose disease has relapsed after allogeneic HSCT; (2) patients who develop acute or chronic graft-versus-host disease (GvHD) after allogeneic HSCT have a significantly decreased risk of leukemic relapse; and (3) that recipients of T-cell depleted allogeneic HSCT or those that are recipients of syngeneic stem cell transplantation are at a significantly higher risk of relapse compared to other recipients following unmanipulated allogeneic HSCT [5–10]. Therefore, instead of eradicating growth or MRD through ablative conditioning, alternative conditioning including non-myeloablative or reduced intensity conditioning could be utilized to suppress post-allogeneic graft rejection and that following engraftment, donor immune cells would subsequently mediate an allogeneic graft-versus-tumor effect. This

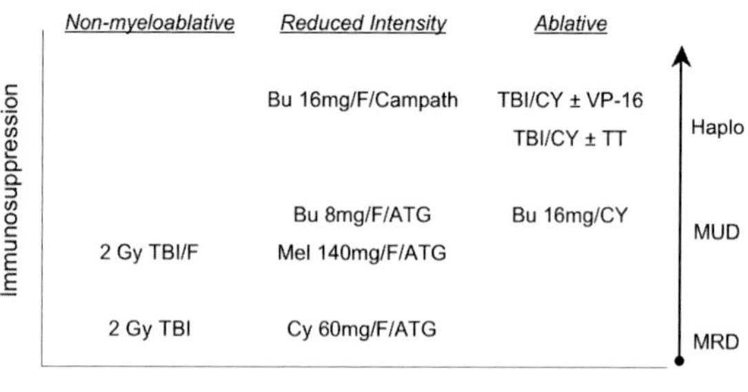

Fig. 19.1 Commonly used nonmyeloablative, reduced intensity or ablative regimens in pediatric patients. Gy, gray; TBI, total body radiation; F, fludarabine; BU, busulfan; ATG, antithymocyte globulin; MEL, melphalan; CY, cyclophosphamide; VP-16, etoposide; TT, thiotepa; Haplo, haploidentical; MUD, matched unrelated donor; MRD, matched related donor.
Source: from Satwani et al. [15]

Table 19.2 Reduced intensity AlloSCT in children and adolescents with malignant diseases

Author/Reference	*n*	Diseases	Conditioning	Donors	>90% Donor chimerism (%)	Graft failure (%)	≥Grade II GvHD (%)	Overall survival (%)
Gomez-Almaguer et al. [13]	15	AML, CML, ALL	BU (8 mg/kg)/CY (90 mg/kg)	MSD	66	NA	25	46
Del Toro et al. [11]	13	AML, CML, NBL, NHL, HL	FLU (150 mg/m^2)/ BU (6.4–8 mg/kg) or CY (60–120 mg/kg)/ ±ATG or Campath	MRD, UCB	93	7	23	78
Roman et al. [14]	8	AML	FLU (180 mg/m^2)/ BU (6.4–8 mg/ kg) ± ATG		88	12	12	63
Duerst et al. [12]	10	ALL	FLU (180 mg/m^2)/ BU (6.4 mg/kg)/ ATG ± CST	MUD,MSD	90	10	20	40

Source: From Satwani et al. [15]
AlloSCT Allogeneic stem cell transplantation, *AML* Acute myeloid leukemia, *CML* Chronic myeloid leukemia, *ALL* Acute lymphoblastic leukemia, *NBL* Neuroblastoma, *NHL* Non-Hodgkin's lymphoma, *HL* Hodgkin's disease, *BU* Busulfan, *CY* Cyclophosphamide, *FLU* Fludarabine, *ATG* Anti-thymocyte globulin, *CST* Cranio spinal radiation, *MSD* Matched sibling donor, *MRD* Matched related donor, *UCB* Umbilical cord blood, *MUD* Matched unrelated donor, *NA* Not applicable, *GvHD* Graft-versus-host disease

reduction in the intensity conditioning might then allow patients with significant comorbidities or medically infirmed patients to be treated with allogeneic HSCT for high risk malignant disease [3].

There is significant heterogeneity between the intensity of conditioning between truly nonmyeloablative regimens to moderate but reduced intensity conditioning compared to that with full myeloablative conditioning (Fig. 19.1). Figure 19.1 depicts the intensity of myelosuppression on the *x*-axis and the intensity of immunosuppression on the *y*-axis and demonstrates a variety of different conditioning regimens with varied immunosuppressive-versus-myelosuppressive intensity. We and others have piloted over the past 5 years reduced-intensity conditioning and allogeneic HSCT in a subset of children and adolescents with malignant disease [3, 11–15]. Table 19.2 summarizes the brief experience with reduced intensity conditioning and allogeneic HSCT in children and adolescents with malignant disease. While it is clear in these early studies that reduced intensity conditioning and allogeneic HSCT results in a high degree of engraftment and mixed donor chimerism in children and adolescents with previously treated malignant disease, there are many issues that still need to be addressed regarding what role and at what time in the treatment alternative intensity conditioning should be considered prior to allogeneic HSCT in children and adolescents with malignant disease. Specifically, controlled randomized perspective clinical trials will be required to determine how to best utilize this alternative conditioning strategy in selected children and adolescents with malignant disease who require allogeneic HSCT.

19.2 Hematologic Malignancies

19.2.1 Acute Lymphoblastic Leukemia (ALL)

Acute lymphoblastic leukemia (ALL, a.k.a. acute lymphocytic leukemia) is the most common pediatric malignancy and represents approximately 25% of all pediatric cancers diagnosed in children under the age of 15 years [16]. In the last 50 years there has been dramatic improvement in the outcome of treatment for childhood and adolescent ALL with expected overall survival (OS) rates to be >80% with current multiagent chemotherapy [16]. However, there are still subsets of children and adolescents with ALL who have poor prognoses and who can benefit from HSCT. These subsets of children include patients with ultra-high-risk features in first complete remission (CR), children with poor risk features in second remission, all patients in and beyond third CR, and small sets of patients in refractory relapse. Multiple donor sources have been utilized for HSCT in children and adolescents with ALL including matched family donor allogeneic HSCT as the most preferred choice; however, other allogeneic donor sources have recently been utilized including matched unrelated adult donors, unrelated cord blood donors, mismatched (haploidentical) family donors, and in select cases autologous HSCT.

A small set of children and adolescents with ALL in first CR have a less than 40% event-free survival (EFS) with standard conventional chemotherapy and may benefit from myeloablative conditioning and allogeneic HSCT in first CR. These ultra high-risk features include induction failure at day 28 of induction, subsets of children with poor cytogenetic features including t(9;22), t(4;11), and hypodiploid ($\leq$44 chromosomes), subsets of children with infant ALL and adolescents with elevated WBC at diagnosis ($\geq$200,000/mm^3). A number of studies have been performed investigating myeloablative conditioning and matched related allogeneic HSCT in children with ultra-high-risk features in first CR (Table 19.3). Three to five year EFS ranges between 50% and 84% depending on the ultra-high-risk features utilized for eligibility (Table 19.3) [17–21]. A number of studies have been single arm allogeneic HSCT trials [18, 19], and others have attempted to compare myeloablative conditioning and allogeneic HSCT vs. chemotherapy in subsets of patients with ultra-high-risk features with ALL in first CR [17, 20, 21]. We in the Children's Cancer Group (CCG) demonstrated a 56% 5-year EFS in children with ALL with ultra-high-risk features in first CR (Fig. 19.2) [19]. One of the best randomized studies reported in children with ultra-high-risk features with ALL in first CR was reported by Balduzzi et al. [17]. This report demonstrated in 77 related allogeneic HSCT recipients versus 280 children receiving standard chemotherapy with ultra-high-risk features of ALL in first CR, a significant advantage of allogeneic HSCT versus chemotherapy (5-year EFS = 57% vs. 41%; $p < 0.02$; Fig. 19.3) [17]. Additional studies in subsets of children and adolescents with ultra-high-risk features of ALL in first CR have also demonstrated that myeloablative conditioning and allogeneic HSCT have been associated with favorable results. Children and adolescents with Philadelphia chromosome positive ALL may benefit from allogeneic HSCT in first CR. We in the CCG, although with small numbers, demonstrated a 67% 5-year EFS in children with Philadelphia chromosome positive ALL in first CR following matched related donor allogeneic HSCT (Fig. 19.4) [19]. Arico et al. retrospectively reviewed the outcome of 326 children and adolescents with Philadelphia chromosome positive ALL treated with either chemotherapy or bone marrow transplantation by 10 pediatric study groups or large institutions from 1986 to 1996 [22]. Arico et al. demonstrated in this retrospective study that children and adolescents with Philadelphia chromosome positive ALL had significantly improved disease-free survival (DFS) when treated with matched related donor allogeneic HSCT versus chemotherapy alone (65% vs. 25%; $p < 0.001$; Fig. 19.5) [22]. In a subset of children and adolescents with T-cell ALL and poor response to induction prednisone therapy, allogeneic HSCT was associated with a significantly improved outcome compared to standard chemotherapy (67% vs. 42%; $p < 0.01$) [23]. However, the role of allogeneic HSCT in children with 11q23 cytogenetic abnormalities is still considered controversial. Pui et al. retrospectively reviewed the outcome in 497 children and adolescents with ALL and 11q23 abnormalities in first CR as reported by 11 study groups and single large institutions from 1983 to 1995 [24]. In this retrospective analysis there did not

Table 19.3 HSCT in children and adolescents with acute lymphoblastic leukemia

Authors	Center/Study	Allogeneic (*n*)	Chemotherapy (*n*)	Allogeneic EFS (%)	Chemotherapy EFS (%)	*p*-value
Selected studies						
First CR						
Bordigoni et al. [18]	Groupe/d'ETUDE	32	N/A	84	N/A	N/A
Uderzo et al. [20]	AIEOP/85, 87, 88, 91–93	30	130	59	47	NS
Wheeler et al. [21]	MRC UKALL[b] X & XII	101	351	45	39	NS
Balduzzi et al. [17]	EUROPE	77	280	56	41	0.02
Satwani et al. [19]	CCG/1921	29	N/A	59	N/A	N/A
Second CR						
Dopfer et al. [27]	BFM 83, 85, 87, 90 (Early relapse)	51	115	52	22	0.01
Barrett et al. [28]	IBMTR/POG	376	540	40	17	0.001
Uderzo et al. [29]	AIEOP/GITMO (Early relapse)	29	142	36	16	0.002
Wheeler et al. [30]	UKALL X	110	261	41	20	0.05
Boulad et al. [31]	MSKCC	38	37	62	26	0.03
Gaynon et al. [32]	CCG 1941	50	35	29	27	NS

HSCT hematopoietic stem cell transplantation, *CR* complete remission, *CCG* Children's Cancer Group, *BFM* Berlin-Frankfurt-Münster, *IBMTR* International Bone Marrow Transplant Registry, *POG* Pediatric Oncology Group, *GITMO* Gruppo Italiano di Trapianto di Midollo Osseo, *MSKCC* Memorial Sloan Kettering Cancer Center, *N/A* Not applicable, *EFS* event-free survival, *NS* not significant Groupe/d'ETUDE Bone marrow transplant study group (France) UKALL Medical Research Council United Kingdom Acute Lymphoblastic Leukemia AIEOP Italian Association Pediatric Oncologia Hematology

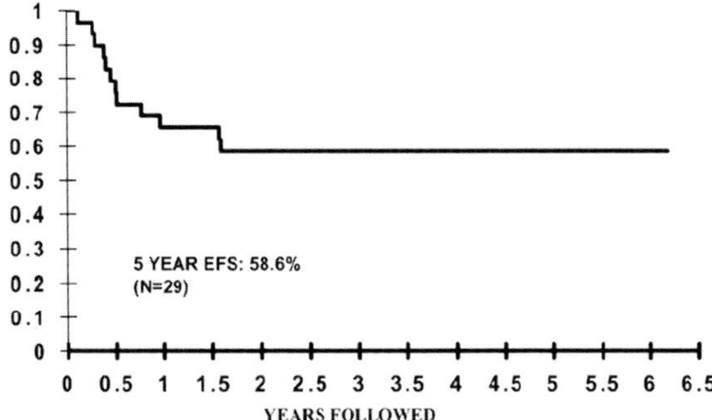

Fig. 19.2 Probability of 5-year event free survival (EFS) by Kaplan–Meier estimates in children with ultra-high-risk features of acute lymphoblastic leukemia in first complete remission treated with allogeneic bone marrow transplantation in the Children's Cancer Group 1921 study.
Source: from Satwani et al. [19], Copyright Elsevier (2007)

appear to be any benefit from allogeneic HSCT versus chemotherapy in children and adolescents with 11q23 in first CR [24]. However, in other large single institutional studies, allogeneic HSCT in children with infant ALL with 11q23 cytogenetic abnormalities have been associated with improved results compared to chemotherapy [25, 26]. Jacobsohn et al. reported a 75% OS at 5 years in 16 infants with ALL in first CR with an 11q23 cytogenetic rearrangement following HSCT from HLA matched sibling donors and from unrelated

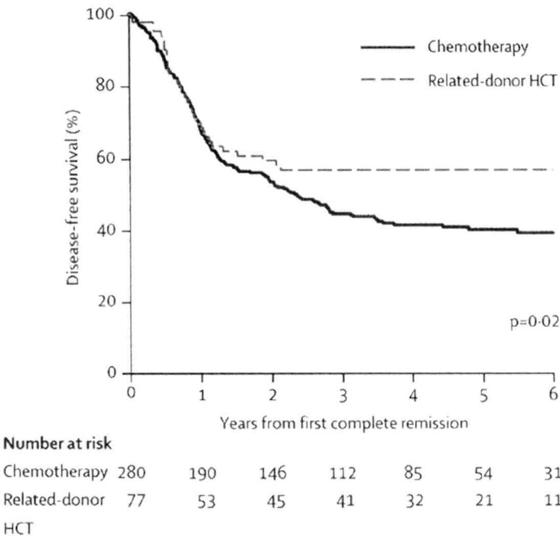

Fig. 19.3 Estimation of disease-free survival, by treatment assigned. HCT=hematopoietic cell transplantation.
Source: from Balduzzi et al. [17]. Reprinted with permission from Elsevier

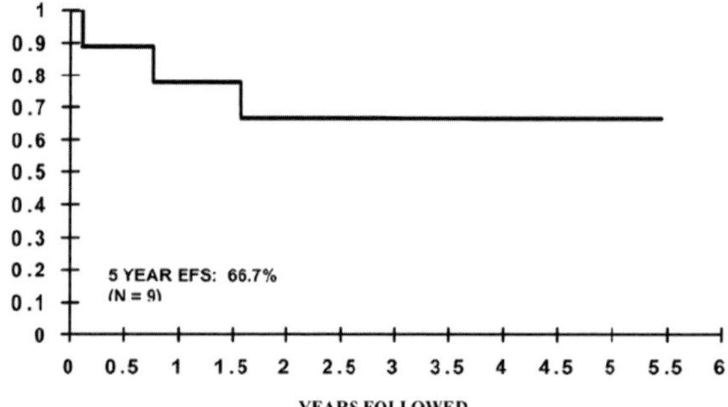

Fig. 19.4 Probability of 5-year event-free survival (EFS) by Kaplan-Meier estimates in children with Philadelphia chromosome-positive t(9,22) acute lymphoblastic leukemia in first complete remission treated with allogeneic bone marrow transplantation in the Children's Cancer Group 1921 study.
Source: from Satwani et al. [19], Copyright Elsevier (2007)

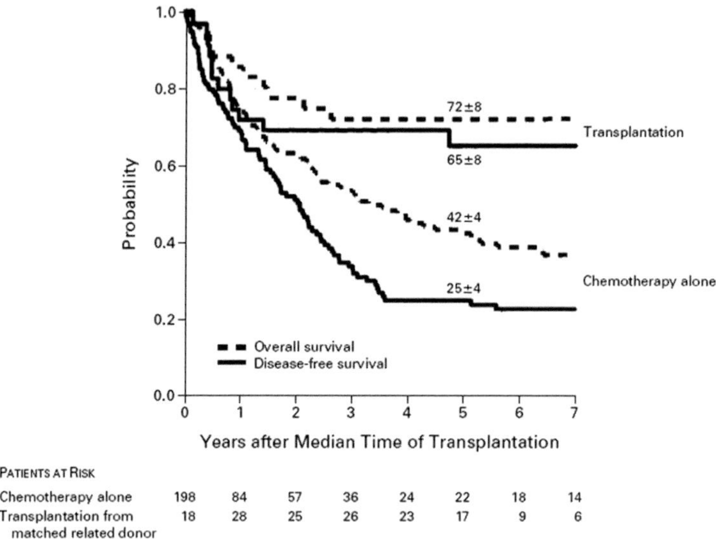

Fig. 19.5 Estimates of disease-free and overall survival (±SE) in 267 patients treated with transplantation of bone marrow from HLA-matched related donors or chemotherapy only. The curves have been adjusted for waiting time to transplantation, so that the zero on the time axis corresponds to the median time from diagnosis to transplantation (6 months); patients were assigned to this treatment group in a time-dependent fashion. Five-year estimates are shown. *P* values are from the Mantel–Byar test. $P=0.002$ for the comparison of the two treatments with respect to overall survival; $P<0.001$ for the comparison with respect to disease-free survival.
Source: from Arico et al. [22], Copyright [2000] Massachusetts Medical Society. All rights reserved

cord blood transplant donors [25]. Kosaka et al. reported a 65% 3-year EFS in 44 infants with ALL and 11q23 cytogenetic rearrangements in first CR in 29 patients who underwent HSCT in first remission [26].

The vast majority of children and adolescents with ALL who undergo HSCT do so in second remission. Although there is a high re-induction remission rate, (75–95%) in children and adolescents with HSCT in first relapse, the long-term prognosis remains dismal [33]. The prognosis for children and adolescents with ALL in second CR is dependent in large part on the duration of first CR, the site of relapse, i.e., bone marrow versus extramedullary and the immunophenotype [33–35]. A recent Berlin-Frankfurt-Münster (BFM) risk stratification for relapsed childhood ALL subdivided patients into three subgroups: high risk, intermediate, and standard risk subgroups [34]. In particular, children and adolescents with ALL who relapsed early, i.e., less than 30–36 months from diagnosis, had the poorest prognosis of all [33–35].

There have been several reported comparisons of allogeneic HSCT versus chemotherapy in children with second remission ALL, some reported by pediatric cooperative groups, some comparative studies from the International Bone Marrow Transplant Registry (IBMTR), and other large single institutional experiences (Table 19.3) [27–32]. Dopfer et al. recently reported a significantly improved EFS in children and adolescents with ALL in second CR following an early relapse with allogeneic HSCT versus chemotherapy (52% vs. 22%; $p = 0.01$; Table 19.3) [27]. In a much larger retrospective analysis Barrett et al. reported on the outcome of all children with ALL in second CR from the IBMTR following allogeneic HSCT versus a large cohort of children treated on relapsed ALL studies in the Pediatric Oncology Group (POG) [28]. Barrett et al. demonstrated significantly improved EFS in children with ALL in second CR following allogeneic HSCT versus chemotherapy (40% vs. 17%; $p = 0.001$; Table 19.3; Fig. 19.6) [28]. Similar significant improvement in survival follows allogeneic HSCT versus chemotherapy in children with ALL in second CR—especially those with early relapse—have also been demonstrated by Uderzo et al. and Wheeler et al. from the AEIOP/Gruppo Italiano di Trapianto di Midollo Osseo (GITMO) and United Kingdom ALL (UKALL) X, respectively (Table 19.3) [29, 30]. However, more recently in patients with more resistant disease, Gaynon et al. from the CCG was unable to demonstrate any significant advantage to allogeneic HSCT versus chemotherapy in children and adolescents with ALL in second CR (Table 19.3) [32]. The majority of the evidence seems to suggest that allogeneic HSCT from matched family donors versus chemotherapy provides a significant improvement in EFS in children with ALL in second CR who relapse early in their first remission or just shortly after the end of their initial therapy.

Recent advances in HSCT in children and adolescents with ALL have suggested the benefit of alternative donor sources besides matched related allogeneic HSCT donors. Other alternative donor sources have included unrelated cord blood transplant donors, matched unrelated adult donors, mismatched (haploidentical) family donors, and autologous HSCTs. We and

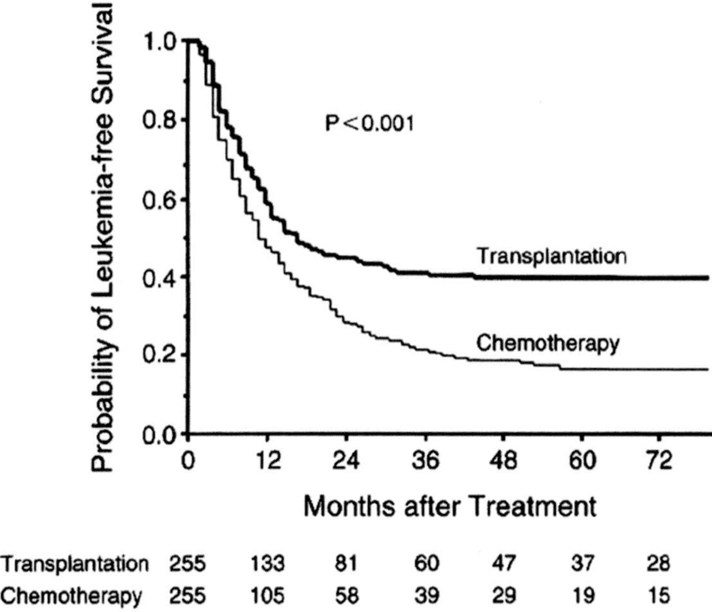

Fig. 19.6 Actuarial Probability of Leukemia-free survival in matched cohorts of children receiving chemotherapy or undergoing transplantation. The numbers below the figure indicate the numbers of children at risk.
Source: Barrett et al. [28]

others have demonstrated the success of utilizing HLA disparate (4–6 HLA matched) unrelated cord blood transplantation in children and adolescents with ALL and AML [36–40]. Matched or HLA disparate unrelated cord blood transplantation has been associated with a 30–50% EFS in children and adolescents with ALL [36–40]. Additionally, matched unrelated adult donor stem cell transplantation has also been demonstrated to be successful in children and adolescents with ALL [34, 38, 41–43]. Bunin et al. reported the outcome of 363 children with ALL in second remission who received unrelated adult donor stem cell transplantation from 1998 to 2000 and were reported to the National Marrow Donor Program (NMDP) [42]. The 5-year leukemia-free survival (LFS) was 36%. Children less than 15 years of age and those with a CR greater than 6 months had significantly improved LFS compared to their counterparts [42]. Since serious acute GvHD is a limiting factor following unrelated adult donor HSCT, Lang et al. investigated a method of $CD34^+$ cell-selection from unrelated donors prior to allogeneic HSCT [43]. In the subset analysis in children with ALL in CR following $CD34^+$ cell-selection and unrelated adult donor stem cell transplantation, the 2-year OS was 63% [43]. $CD34^+$ stem cell collection has also been utilized following haploidentical stem cell transplantation in children with ALL [44]. In children with ALL in first, second, or third CR following CD34^{+} cell-selected haploidentical stem cell transplantation, the probability of survival was 44% [44]. Autologous HSCT, especially following autologous purging, also has been demonstrated to be efficacious in children with ALL in second CR [45–47]. Ramsay et al. first demonstrated the success of autologous bone marrow transplantation in children with ALL in second and subsequent remissions following monoclonal antibody plus complement purging, and subsequently our group demonstrated the success of autologous bone marrow transplantation in childhood ALL following ex-vivo marrow purging with VP16, vincristine and verapamil, respectively [45, 46].

New advances in the use of different conditioning regimens have also been investigated prior to HSCT in children and adolescents with ALL. Original studies of conditioning therapy and allogeneic HSCT in children and adolescents with ALL utilized either TBI plus cyclophosphamide or TBI plus cytosine arabinoside [48, 49]. There have been several attempts to compare chemotherapy-only ablative conditionings versus TBI plus chemotherapy ablative conditioning in children with ALL [50, 51]. Davies et al. reported the outcome of HLA identical sibling transplants for children with ALL who received TBI plus cyclophosphamide versus busulfan plus cyclophosphamide between 1988 and 1995 and reported to the IBMTR [51]. The probability of LFS was significantly improved in children and adolescents receiving TBI and cyclophosphamide versus busulfan and cyclophosphamide and allogeneic HSCT (3-year LFS = 50% vs. 35%; $p = 0.005$) [51]. Bunin et al. reported the results of a randomized trial of busulfan and cyclophosphamide versus TBI plus chemotherapy containing conditioning regimens in children with ALL undergoing allogeneic HSCT. Again, there was a significant improvement in 3-year EFS in children with ALL receiving the TBI conditioning regimen versus busulfan and cyclophosphamide conditioning regimen [50]. These studies suggest that current TBI conditioning regimens versus chemotherapy only conditioning regimens are associated with significant improvement of EFS in children with ALL undergoing HSCT.

Most recently the American Society for Blood and Marrow Transplantation (ASBMT) reported an evidence based review of the role of cytotoxic therapy with HSCT in children with ALL [52]. Several areas of critically needed research in the future role of HSCT in children with ALL were enumerated [52]. Future studies should focus on a number of areas including the role of unrelated marrow or blood donor versus unrelated cord blood donor allogeneic transplantation, the role of haploidentical or non-family allogeneic donor versus autologous HSCT, the role of HSCT in children with ALL with 11q23 cytogenetic rearrangements, the role of reduced intensity conditioning in selected children with ALL, the role of adoptive cellular immunotherapy with or without genetic reengineering in children with ALL post-allogeneic HSCT, and the future identification of poor prognostic factors in children and adolescents with ALL in first and second CR.

19.2.2 Acute Myelogenous Leukemia

Acute myelogenous leukemia (AML) comprises approximately 20% of all childhood leukemias, and is classified using the French-American-British (FAB) system and divided into seven different subgroups (M1–M7). Over the past 20 years, there have been a number of investigations comparing allogeneic HSCT from matched sibling donors versus chemotherapy and in some studies also versus autologous HSCT in children and adolescents with AML following induction into first CR (Table 19.4) [53–58]. There are a few subtypes in children and adolescents with AML in first CR where allogeneic HSCT is not recommended, and those include children with Down's syndrome, M3 FAB sub-type (acute promyelocytic leukemia [APL]), and more recently, children with an inversion of chromosome 16.

The majority of studies have demonstrated a significant improvement in either EFS or DFS following allogeneic HSCT versus post-remission intensification chemotherapy in children with AML in first CR (Table 19.4) [53–58]. Nesbit et al. originally demonstrated a significant advantage of matched sibling allogeneic HSCT versus post-remission intensification chemotherapy in children with AML in first CR (5-year EFS = 50% vs. 36%; $p < 0.05$; Table 19.4) [54]. Ravindranath et al. demonstrated in the POG 8821 study no advantage of post-remission chemotherapy versus autologous HSCT, but an improvement in outcome following allogeneic HSCT versus either autologous HSCT or chemotherapy, in children with AML in first CR (Table 19.4) [56]. Woods et al. reported the results of CCG 2891, and it clearly demonstrated the superiority of allogeneic HSCT with matched sibling donors in children with AML in first CR versus autologous HSCT or chemotherapy (Table 19.4; Fig. 19.7) [58]. In a retrospective review of four Italian Association Pediatric Oncologia Hematology (AIEOP) AML studies in children with AML in first CR, there appeared to be a significant improvement in children receiving allogeneic HSCT versus chemotherapy (5-year EFS = 64% vs. 28%; Table 19.4) [55]. Similarly, Lie et al. reported the results of the NOPHO-AML 93 Scandinavian study in children with AML in first CR and demonstrated a significant improvement in 5-year EFS following allogeneic HSCT versus chemotherapy (64% vs. 51%; $p = 0.04$; Table 19.4) [53]. Taken together, all of these studies suggest a superiority of allogeneic HSCT versus chemotherapy following remission induction in first CR in children with AML and probably no advantage of autologous HSCT versus chemotherapy alone. However, Stevens et al. reported the results of the UKMRC10 study and demonstrated similar survival between allogeneic HSCT and post-remission intensification chemotherapy in children with AML in first CR (Table 19.4) [57]. These UKMRC10 results suggest that a small number of children may be retrieved after relapse after chemotherapy and that the high mortality rate following allogeneic HSCT may outweigh the improvement in EFS. However, despite the recent UKMRC10 results, allogeneic HSCT in children with AML in first CR is still recommended if a matched sibling

Table 19.4 HSCT for children and adolescents with acute myeloid leukemia in first complete remission

Author	Center/Group	Allogeneic (*n*)	Autologous (*n*)	Chemotherapy (*n*)	Allogeneic EFS (%)	Autologous EFS (%)	Chemotherapy EFS (%)	*p*-value
Nesbit et al. [54]	CCG 251	89	N/A	252	50	N/A	36	Allo vs. chemo 0.05
Ravindranath et al. [56]	POG 8821	89	115	117	52	38	36	Allo vs. chemo 0.06, Allo vs. Auto 0.01, Auto vs. Chemo NS
Stevens et al. [57]	UKMRC X	61	60	268	N/A	N/A	N/A	N/A
Woods et al. [58]	CCG 2891	181	179	177	55	42	47	Allo vs. chemo 0.01, Allo vs. Auto 0.001, Auto vs. Chemo NS
Pession et al. [55]	AIEOP LAME 82, 87, 87 M, 92	78	110	89	64	55	28	N/A
Lie et al. [53]	NOPHO/AML 93	53	N/A	147	64	N/A	51	Allo vs. Chemo 0.04

HSCT hematopoietic stem cell transplantation, *CCG* Children's Cancer Group, *POG* Pediatric Oncology Group, *UKMRC* United Kingdom Medical Research Council, *LAME* Leucémie Aiguë Myéloblastique Enfant, *NOPHO* Nordic Society for Pediatric Hematology and Oncology, *AML* acute myeloid leukemia, *N/A* not applicable, *EFS* event-free survival, *allo* allogeneic, *chemo* chemotherapy, *auto* autologous, *NS* not significant AIEOP Italian Association Pediatric Oncologia Hematology

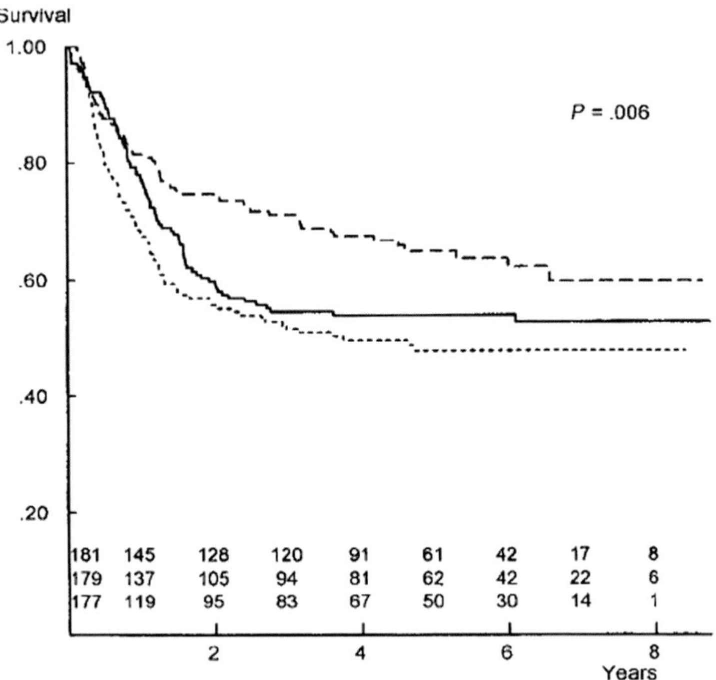

Fig. 19.7 Actuarial survival from AML remission, comparing the 3 postremission regimens from CCG-2891. Numbers are patients at risk at yearly intervals; rows are in the same order as curves. *P* value is for homogeneity. Dashed line indicates allogeneic BMT; solid line, intensive non-marrow-ablative chemotherapy; dotted line line, autologous BMT.
Source: This research was originally published in Blood. Woods et al. [58]. Copyright the American Society of Hematology

donor is available except in those patients with Down's syndrome, APL and/or inversion chromosome 16.

The role of HSCT in children and adolescents with AML outside of first remission is not as well defined. Children and adolescents relapsing or failing to achieve remission when given initial induction chemotherapy on CCG chemotherapy AML trials have only a 3-year 20% OS [59]. Nemecek et al. reported the outcome of allogeneic HSCT utilizing matched sibling donors (n = 19), mismatched related donors (n = 17), or unrelated matched donors (n = 22) in 58 children in untreated first relapse, CR2, and refractory disease [60]. The estimated 5-year DFS in patients in CR2, untreated first relapse, and refractory disease, were 58%, 36% and 9%, respectively [60]. Children and adolescents with relapsed or refractory APL who were not transplanted in first CR also may benefit from allogeneic HSCT. Bourquin et al. reported results of allogeneic HSCT from five related sibling donors and seven unrelated donors in 11 children with relapsed or refractory APL [61]. The cumulative incidence of relapse post-HSCT was only 10% with a 5-year OS rate of 73% [61]. Alternative donor sources including autologous HSCT, unrelated adult donor bone marrow transplantation, and unrelated cord blood transplantation have also been utilized in children and adolescents with AML in second CR or beyond. Godder et al. reported results from the Autologous Blood and Marrow Transplant Registry in children with AML in second CR following autologous HSCT [62]. In children with a short first CR (i.e., less than 12 months, LFS was 23% compared to children with first CR equal to or longer than 12 months; the LFS was 60% in children with AML in second CR following autologous HSCT [62]. Michel et al. reported the results of unrelated cord blood transplantation for children and adolescents with AML in second CR ($n = 47$) in patients in refractory relapse ($n = 23$) from the Euro Cord Group [63]. In children and adolescents with AML in CR2, the 2-year LFS following unrelated cord blood transplantation was 50%, and for those with refractory relapse was 21% [63]. Wall et al. reported the Cord Blood Transplantation (COBLT) study experience following unrelated donor cord blood transplantation in children less than 4 years of age with AML and ALL and demonstrated in patients in CR2 a 30% 2-year DFS [64]. Lastly, partially matched related donors and matched or mismatched unrelated adult donor stem cell transplantation is yet another option for children and adolescents with AML. Bunin et al. reported the outcomes of partial T-cell depletion of matched or mismatched unrelated or partially matched related donor bone marrow transplantation in children and adolescents with acute leukemia [65]. There were 13 patients with AML in second complete remission (CR2) following unrelated adult donor transplantation and eight patients with AML in CR2 following partially matched related donor stem cell transplantation. The 3-year EFS of all patients with AML following partial T-cell depleted unrelated or partially matched related donor stem cell transplantation in children was 34% [65].

A number of risk factors have been suggested to be important in the outcome in children and adolescents with AML in first CR including age, white blood cell count at diagnosis, unfavorable cytogenetics, intensively timed induction therapy, high WT1 expression after induction, FAB subtype, and lack of low-grade GvHD following allogeneic HSCT [66–69]. One of the major limitations of myeloablative conditioning in allogeneic HSCT has been the high degree of regimen-related mortality associated with myeloablative conditioning. Recently, Scott et al. reviewed the experience of 150 adult patients with MDS or AML conditioned with nonmyeloablative versus myeloablative conditioning treated at the Fred Hutchinson Cancer Research Center [70]. There was no significant difference in the 3-year OS or progression-free survival (PFS) between the two types of conditioning [70]. Recently we reported the preliminary results of reduced intensity conditioning with busulfan and fludarabine followed by allogeneic HSCT in children with AML who also received post-transplant targeted immunotherapy with gemtuzumab ozogamycin [14, 71]. Randomized prospective studies are needed to further address the optimal choice of transplant conditioning intensity in children and adolescents with

AML in first CR. Ruggeri et al. also has suggested that natural killer (NK) cell KIR-ligand mismatching between donor and recipient following haploidentical transplantation in adults with AML is associated with a significantly improved LFS [72]. Future studies are also warranted in determining the benefits, if any, of NK KIR-ligand mismatched unrelated donor stem cell transplantation in children with AML in CR2 or beyond.

ASBMT recently published an evidence based review on the role of cytotoxic therapy with hematopoietic stem cell transplantation in the therapy of AML in children [73]. Future areas of research for HSCT in children with AML include the role of reduced intensity conditioning, NK KIR-ligand mismatching, biologically targeted therapy, targeted immunotherapy, adoptive cellular immunotherapy, and further risk-group adapted stratification. Currently, however, allogeneic HSCT for matched sibling donor is still the preferred choice of treatment for children and adolescents in AML and CR1 except for those patients with FAB M3 subtype, Down's syndrome, and/or inversion chromosomal 16 abnormality.

19.2.3 Chronic Myelogenous Leukemia

Chronic myelogenous leukemia (CML) only accounts for approximately 5% of all childhood and adolescent leukemias. Similar to adults, allogeneic HSCT has previously been the only proven curative treatment for children with CML [74]. There are very few studies that have prospectively analyzed the outcome in children and adolescents with CML following allogeneic HSCT. Recent studies in adults following the use of imatinib have demonstrated durable responses in a high proportion of adults with CML in first chronic phase [75]. Recent studies in adults with other BCR-ABL ALL tyrosine kinase inhibitors such as dasatinib and nilotinib in imatinib-resistant CML adults have also demonstrated significant hematological and cytogenetic responses [76, 77]. The increased use and experience with BCR-ABL tyrosine kinase inhibitors in adults with CML has suggested that allogeneic HSCT for adults with CML in chronic phase is not currently the treatment of choice. However, since children and adolescents have over 70–80 years of life span following diagnosis, matched sibling allogeneic HSCT is still the preferred and only curative form of treatment in this age group with CML in chronic phase [77].

Cwynarski et al. recently reported the results of stem cell transplantation in children and adolescents for CML on behalf of the European Group for Blood and Marrow Transplantation (EBMT) Chronic Leukemia & Pediatric Working Group parties [76]. In children and adolescents in first chronic phase CML who underwent allogeneic HSCT from matched sibling donors, the LFS rate was 63% and OS rate was 75% and in 97 children in first chronic phase CML who underwent matched unrelated adult donor stem cell transplantation, the 3-year LFS rate was 56% and 3-year OS rate was 65% [76]. In children with accelerated phase CML who underwent any form of allogeneic HSCT, the 5-year OS rate was significantly less (35%) regardless of stem cell donor source ($p = 0.001$) [76]. Gamis et al. originally reported the results of unrelated adult donor bone marrow transplantation in children with CML with an estimated 5-year DFS of 45% [78]. Balduzzi et al. reported the results of unrelated adult donor marrow transplantation in 16 children with CML transplanted at the Fred Hutchinson Cancer Research Center and reported a 3-year DFS of 75% [79]. Dini et al. reported the results of 44 children and adolescents with CML following unrelated donor transplantation from eight European countries with a 3-year EFS of 50% [80].

Additional approaches to improve the efficacy of allogeneic HSCT in children and adolescents with CML have included alternative intensity conditionings, serial measurement of BCR-ABL transcripts post–transplant, and the potential role of adoptive cellular immunotherapy. Reduced-intensity conditioning offers an alternative to reduce treatment-related mortality while maintaining a significant graft-versus-CML effect following allogeneic HSCT [3, 4]. Early detection and serial measurement of BCR-ABL transcripts in the peripheral blood after allogeneic HSCT for CML is important in predicting relapse and may signal the need for alternative post-transplant treatment strategies including the use of BCR-ABL tyrosine kinase inhibitors or adoptive cellular immunotherapy [81, 82]. Furthermore, DLI in patients with CML who relapse after allogeneic HSCT has induced significant remissions and durable responses [83]. The response of DLI post-allogeneic HSCT has the highest remission induction rate and durable responses in CML compared to other forms of leukemia [83]. Further research is required to determine the optimal approach, including reduced intensity conditioning, the use of BCR-ABL tyrosine kinase inhibitors, and adoptive cellular immunotherapy in conjunction with allogeneic HSCT for children and adolescents with AML in first chronic phase for future optimization of long-term survival with a significant reduction in acute and long-term morbidity and mortality.

19.2.4 Hodgkin's Disease and Non-Hodgkin's Lymphoma

The prognosis for children and adolescents with newly diagnosed Hodgkin lymphoma (HL, a.k.a. Hodgkin's disease) is excellent with an estimated 70–90% 5-year EFS [84, 85]. However, over 25% of children with newly diagnosed HL progress and/or relapse and the outcome for this subgroup of patients is dismal. Furthermore, children and adolescents with HL treated with radiation therapy with or without chemotherapy have a significantly high risk of developing secondary malignancies and breast cancer [86, 87]. Similarly, the prognosis for children with newly diagnosed non-Hodgkin's lymphoma (NHL) is also superb with an estimated 60–95% 5-year EFS [88]. The prognosis, however, in children with recurrent NHL is also dismal with an estimated 5-year EFS of 10–30% [88–90].

In the 1980s and early 1990s when upfront chemotherapy was not intensive, the prognosis in children with HL and NHL after relapse was higher following HSCT then compared to patients today who are relapsing off of intensive upfront chemotherapy. There are a variety of NHL histologies that have been treated with HSCT in children and adolescents following induction failure, disease progression and/or relapse. Loiseau et al. first reported results in 24 children, 16 with B-NHL and eight with T-cell NHL following a busulfan conditioning regimen and autologous HSCT and reported a 33% DFS (Table 19.5) [91]. In a rather uncommon form of childhood NHL, Gordon et al. reported the results in a small number (9) of patients with peripheral T-cell lymphoma (PTCL) following TBI and thiotepa conditioning and autologous HSCT and reported a 89% DFS (Table 19.5) [92]. Philip et al. reported the results in 15 children with B-cell NHL failing upfront Lymphoma Malignancy B (LMB) therapy treated with autologous HSCT and reported only a 27% DFS (Table 19.5) [93]. Ladenstein et al. reported the results in 89 children from the EBMT registry with B-cell NHL following autologous HSCT and reported a 49% DFS in patients achieving a sensitive response after chemotherapy reinduction (Table 19.5) [94]. Kobrinsky et al. reported the results of 50 children with NHL following re-induction chemotherapy with the DECAL regimen (dexamethasone, etoposide, cisplatin, cytarabine, L-asparaginase) and who subsequently underwent autologous HSCT and reported approximately a 50% OS rate (Table 19.5) [95]. Levine et al. reported the results from IBMTR in 204 patients with lymphoblastic lymphoma with a median age of 13 years following autologous HSCT ($n = 128$) and allogeneic HSCT ($n = 76$) [96]. Although there was a significantly decreased risk of relapse following allogeneic HSCT, due to an increased risk of regimen related toxic deaths following allogeneic HSCT, there was a similar DFS between allogeneic HSCT versus autologous HSCT in patients with lymphoblastic lymphoma (36% vs. 39%) (Table 19.5) [96]. Most recently Woessmann et al. reported from the BFM Group the results in 20 children with relapsed or progressed anaplastic large cell lymphoma (ALCL) following TBI, cyclophosphamide, etoposide, and allogeneic HSCT, an impressive 75% DFS (Table 19.5) [97]. These results in children with various types of histologies of NHL suggests a DFS ranging between 25% and 75% following HSCT, and it appears that both ALCL and lymphoblastic lymphoma may respond to an allogeneic graft-versus-lymphoma effect (Table 19.5).

The results following HSCT in children with HL is similar to the results in children with NHL. Williams et al. first reported the results in 81 children with HL following a chemotherapy conditioning regimen and an autologous HSCT and reported a 40% PFS [98]. Baker et al. from the University of Minnesota reported the results in 53 children with HL following predominately a CBV (cyclophosphamide, BCNU, and etoposide) conditioning and an autologous HSCT and reported a 31% failure-free survival (Table 19.5) [99]. Further, Stoneham et al. reported the results in 51% patients with relapsed or HL who underwent autologous HSCT at the Royal Marsden following BEAM (BCNU, etoposide, cytarabine, and melphalan) conditioning and reported a 20% PFS

Table 19.5 HSCT in children with NHL and Hodgkin's lymphoma HL

Author	Center/Group	*n*	NHL histology	Donor source	Conditioning regimen	DFS/EFS
Loiseau et al. [91]	Institut Gustave Roussy	24	16 B-NHL, 8 T-NHL	Autologous	BU/CY, BU/Melphalan	33%
Gordon et al. [92]	University of Nebraska	9	PTCL	Autologous	TBI/Thiotepa	89%
Philip et al. [93]	SFOP	15	B-NHL	14 Autologous, 1 Allogeneic	BEAM/BEAC, Other	27%
Ladenstein et al. [94]	EBMT	89	B-NHL	Autologous	BACT 31, BEAM 23, BU/CY 9,Other 26	44% sensitive relapse
Kobrinsky et al. [95]	CCG	50	N/A	Autologous	N/A	50%
Levine et al. [96]	IBMTR	128, 76	LL	Autologous, Allogeneic	N/A, N/A	39%, 36%
Woessmann et al. [97]	BFM	20	ALCL	Allogeneic	TBI/CY/VP-16	75%
Williams et al. [98]	EBMT	81	HL	Autologous	76 Chemo	40% (PFS)
Baker et al. [99]	University of Minnesota	53	HL	Autologous	44 CBV, 9 Other	31% (FFS)
Stoneham et al. [100]	Royal Marsden	51	HL	Autologous	44 BEAM, 7 Other	20% (PFS)
Lieskovsky et al. [101]	Stanford	41	HL	Autologous	23 CVB, 18 Other	53% (EFS)
Harris et al. [102]	COG	38	HL	Autologous	CBV	43% (PFS)
Bradley et al. [103]	Columbia	10	HL	Autologous, Allogeneic	CBV, BU/FLU	70%

HSCT hematopoietic stem cell transplantation, *NHL* non-Hodgkin's lymphoma, *HL* Hodgkin's disease, *SFOP* Société Française di'Oncologie Pédiatrique, *EBMT* The European Group for Blood and Marrow Transplantation, *CCG* Children's Cancer Group, *IBMTR* International Bone Marrow Transplant Registry, *BFM* Berlin-Frankfurt-Münster, *COG* Children's Oncology Group, *B-NHL* B-cell non-Hodgkin's lymphoma, *T-NHL* T-cell non-Hodgkin's lymphoma, *PTCL* peripheral T-cell lymphoma, *N/A* not applicable, *LL* lymphoblastic lymphoma, *ALCL* anaplastic large cell lymphoma, *BU* busulfan, *CY* cyclophosphamide, *TBI* total body irradiation, *BACT* BCNU + cytarabine + cyclophosphamide + thioguanine, *FLU* fludarabine, *DFS* disease-free survival, *EFS* event-free survival, *PFS* progression-free survival, *FFS* failure-free survival BEAM Carmustine, etoposide, cytarabine, and melphalan BEAC Carmustine, etoposide, Ara C and cyclophosphamide VP-16 Etoposide

(Table 19.5) [100]. Lieskovsky et al. reported the results in 41 children with relapsed refractory HL from Stanford University following chemotherapy conditioning and autologous HSCT and reported a 53% EFS (Table 19.5) [101]. Lastly, Harris et al. reported the early results of 38 children with relapsed refractory HL who obtained a CR or partial response following re-induction therapy and underwent an autologous HSCT following CBV conditioning and reported a 43% PFS (Table 19.5) [102]. These results suggest that children and adolescents with relapsed refractory HL who undergo chemotherapy conditioning and an autologous HSCT have an estimated 20–50% PFS and are still at risk for long-term complications including secondary/therapy-related myelodysplastic syndromes (MDS) and AML, as well as breast cancer.

Recently, it has been identified that reduced-intensity conditioning followed by allogeneic HSCT induces a significant graft-versus-tumor effect against HL [104]. Several adult centers have piloted the use of myeloablative conditioning and autologous HSCT followed by nonmyeloablative or reduced-intensity conditioning and allogeneic HSCT for poor-risk adults with HL [105, 106]. These results of autologous HSCT following by reduced-intensity allogeneic HSCT in very poor-risk adults with HL suggests that this approach may also be beneficial in children and adolescents with resistant HL and who are at long-term risk of secondary complications. Bradley et al. has reported the initial results in 10 children and adolescents with HL treated with CBV conditioning and an autologous HSCT followed by busulfan and fludarabine conditioning and allogeneic HSCT and has reported an early 70% EFS (Table 19.5) [103]. Longer term follow up with a larger cohort and a subsequently randomized trial will need to be performed to determine whether this approach reduces the risk of HL relapse and/or reduces the risk of secondary complications compared to standard myeloablative conditioning and autologous HSCT.

19.3 Nonhematologic Malignancies

Most pediatric solid tumors are chemotherapy-sensitive. With improvements in supportive care, it has been possible to give very intense chemotherapy regimens safely to children with cancer, which has resulted in significant improvement of OS and DFS. However, there still exist some tumors, though chemotherapy-sensitive, in which the prognosis remains poor, i.e., high-risk neuroblastoma. Additionally, for patients with tumor relapse the DFS remains less than 20%. As the intensity of "standard therapy" has increased for pediatric solid tumors, the role of myeloablative chemotherapy and autologous stem cell rescue is increasingly being debated. Randomized trials are desperately needed to determine the role of autologous HSCT in pediatric solid tumors; however, due to the small number of patients, these are often not feasible without international collaboration. There is increased interest in the utility of allogeneic HSCT and the potential graft-versus-tumor effect; however, most studies are still in the pilot phase.

19.3.1 Neuroblastoma

The most common indication for autologous transplantation in pediatrics is neuroblastoma. Beginning in the mid-1980s, reports began to appear suggesting benefit of autologous HSCT for high-risk neuroblastoma. Early studies were all single arm studies with small patient numbers, differing in risk of disease and numerous conditioning regimens used, and the 3-year EFS ranged from 24% to 50%. In general, this compared favorably to the 20% expected EFS with chemotherapy alone [107]. In the late 1980s, CCG conducted a phase III study for high-risk neuroblastoma where patients were randomized following intensive induction chemotherapy to either autologous HSCT, including TBI in the conditioning, or continued intensive chemotherapy as consolidation [108]. This study enrolled 190 patients per arm and demonstrated a benefit in 3-year EFS for the transplant arm, 34% vs. 22%, but no difference in OS with late relapses, i.e., greater than 5 years, continuing to occur (Fig. 19.8). Therefore, further follow-up is required to determine the benefit of transplant on long-term EFS. Of interest, there was no difference in treatment-related deaths or hospital days between the two arms. Attempts to better overcome chemotherapy-resistance have been attempted by the use of tandem transplants as consolidation therapy. Grupp et al. reported a 58% EFS but had only a 22-month median

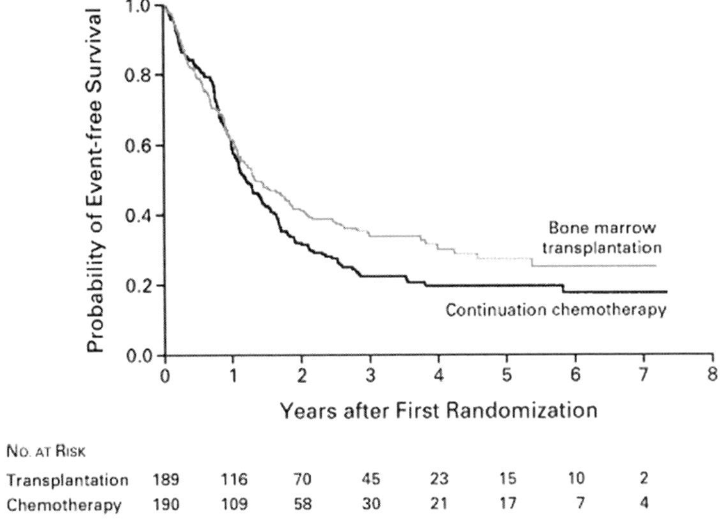

No. at Risk								
Transplantation	189	116	70	45	23	15	10	2
Chemotherapy	190	109	58	30	21	17	7	4

Fig. 19.8 Probability of event-free survival among patients assigned to bone marrow transplantation or continuation chemotherapy. Follow-up began at the time of the first randomization (8 weeks after diagnosis). The difference in survival between the two groups was significant at 3 years (P=0.034).
Source: Matthay et al. [108].

follow-up [109]. Kletzel et al. employed triple tandem myeloablative regimens each followed by autologous HSCT and reported a 3-year EFS of 57% with 38 months median follow-up [110]. However, a later report with additional patients and longer follow-up demonstrate a 38% 6-year EFS [111]. Children's Oncology Group (COG) will soon open a randomized study to test the efficacy of tandem versus standard autologous HSCT for high-risk neuroblastoma. Another strategy to gain better tumor control is to incorporate targeted therapy. A radionucleotide, metaiodobenzylguanidine (MIBG), has been shown to have specificity and activity in relapsed neuroblastoma [112], and pilot studies have been performed combining MIBG with chemotherapy followed by autologous HSCT (Table 19.6) [113].

Hematogenous dissemination is common in neuroblastoma; therefore, re-infusion of tumor contaminated stem cell products may be responsible for post-transplant relapse. A study with ex vivo genetically marked stem cells demonstrated that indeed re-infused tumor cells can contribute to post-transplant relapse [116]. Therefore, some studies have used purged stem cell products [108, 109] while others have not [110]. Though peripheral blood stem cells (PBSC) may have less tumor contamination than marrow, studies have demonstrated tumor presence in PBSC by polymerase chain reaction (PCR) [117]. COG has conducted a study to evaluate the benefit of purging autologous PBSC products for transplant of patients with neuroblastoma. The preliminary results demonstrate no advantage to patients receiving purged products versus unpurged PBSC [118].

Post-transplant treatment of MRD is another approach to decrease relapse. A CCG study demonstrated regardless to consolidation (chemotherapy vs. transplantation) there was a benefit to receiving 13-cis-retinoic acid as maintenance therapy, with the 3-year EFS being 46% vs. 29% [108]. The anti-GD2 monoclonal antibody targets neuroblastoma cells [119] and COG has an ongoing study to evaluate the toxicity and efficacy of this antibody with granulocyte-macrophage-colony-stimulating factor (GM-CSF) and interleukin-2 (IL-2) to further enhance the antibody-dependent cytotoxicity. Further research to control post-transplant MRD remains active and promising. Current approaches under investigation include cytokine therapy, adoptive cellular therapy, and tumor vaccines, as well as anti-angiogenic therapies and small molecular inhibitors of cellular proliferation pathways or to enhance tumor cell apoptosis.

Allogeneic HSCT has been performed for patients with neuroblastoma. A case control study by the European Blood and Marrow Transplant Registry (EBMTR) suggested a benefit of allogeneic transplant with the 2-year PFS being 41% compared to 35% for autologous HSCT, though due to small numbers this was not statistically significant [114]. CCG conducted a biologically randomized study comparing the outcome of patients receiving an allogeneic transplant if an HLA-identical matched sibling was available to autologous HSCT [115]. This study showed significantly more nonrelapse related mortality in the allogeneic group, and no statistical difference in relapse rate, though

Table 19.6 HSCT in children with neuroblastoma

Author	Center/Group	*n*	Donor source	Conditioning regimen	EFS (%)
Matthay et al. [108]	CCG	189, 190	Autologous Purged marrow, Chemotherapy	CEM/TBI	34 (3 years), 22 (3 years)
Grupp et al. [109]	CHOP/Dana Farber/Emory/ Primary Children's – Salt Lake	55	Autologous CD34-selected	Tandem: #1 – Carbo/VP-16/CY, #2 – Melph/TBI	59 (3 years)
Kletzel et al. [110]	Children's Memorial Hospital, Chicago	25	Autologous PBSC	Tandem: #1 – Carbo/VP-16, #2 – Carbo/VP-16, #3 – Thiotepa/CY	57 (3 years)
Ladenstein et al. [114]	EBMT (case controlled study)	34, 17	Autologous, Allogeneic	N/A	35 (2 years), 41 (2 years)
Matthay et al. [115]	CCG (biologic randomized)	36, 20	Autologous Purged marrow, Allogeneic	CEM/TBI, CEM/TBI	60 (4 years), 33 (4 years)

CCG Children's Cancer Group, *CHOP* Children's Hospital of Philadelphia, *Melph* melphalan, *PBSC* peripheral blood stem cells, *CEM* carboplatin, etoposide, melphalan, *TBI* total body irradiation, *Carbo* Carboplatin, *CY* Cyclophosphamide, *EBMT* The European Group for Blood and Marrow Transplantation, N/A not applicable vp-16 Etoposide numbers were small. With improvement in supportive care for allogeneic transplant and the use of nonmyeloablative conditioning, the role of allogeneic HSCT for high-risk neuroblastoma is being evaluated again in pilot studies by several groups [120].

19.3.2 Central Nervous System Tumors

Primary brain tumors are a diverse group of diseases that together constitute the most common solid tumor of childhood. Surgical resection remains a key element in prognosis of childhood brain tumors. Though radiation therapy is very useful in the treatment of pediatric brain tumors, it is technically more demanding, and debilitating effects on growth and neurologic development have frequently been observed following radiation therapy, especially in younger children. Many, but not all types of brain tumors seen in pediatrics have been shown to be chemotherapy-sensitive. Therapeutic strategies using high-dose chemotherapy and autologous stem cell rescue studied in children with brain tumors include (1) for chemotherapy-sensitive poor-risk tumors as consolidative therapy, (2) for chemosensitive relapsed tumors, (3) dose escalation by multiple nonmyeloablative courses of chemotherapy with stem cell rescue, and (4) an attempt to delay radiation therapy in young children. The use and utility to date of high-dose chemotherapy and stem cell rescue will be discussed for the different histologic types of brain tumors observed in children and adolescents, while the treatment of young children to delay radiation will be discussed separately (Table 19.7).

19.3.2.1 High-Grade Astrocytomas

High-grade astrocytoma, anaplastic astrocytoma, or glioblastoma multiforme are chemosensitive but have a very poor outcome even with surgery, radiation, and chemotherapy, i.e., 5-year survival of about 20% (40% for patients with total resection) [128]. Studies have suggested that some durable responses can be achieved using myeloablative chemotherapy and autologous HSCT as consolidative therapy [121, 122] for recurrent disease [123] and for hematologic support following multiple cycles of nonmyeloablative chemotherapy [129]. Though some of these results have been promising, all series have small numbers of patients, and no randomized trials have been performed to prove high-dose chemotherapy and autologous HSCT improves outcome when compared to standard therapy with surgery, radiation, and chemotherapy.

19.3.2.2 Neuroectodermal Tumors

Tumors of neuroectodermal origin, i.e., medulloblastoma and supratentorial primitive neuroectodermal tumors (Spnet), are chemosensitive, and about

Table 19.7 HSCT in children with central system tumors

Author	Center/Group	*n*	Histology	Donor source	Conditioning regimen	EFS (%)
Graham et al. [121]	Duke	6	High-grade astrocytoma or GBM	Autologous marrow	CY/Melph BU/Melph Carbo/VP-16	17 (duration not specified)
Heideman et al. [122]	St. Jude	11	High-grade astrocytoma or GBM	Autologous marrow	Thiotepa/CY	27 (2 years)
Finlay et al. [123]	CCG	18	High-grade astrocytoma or GBM	Autologous marrow	Thiotepa/VP-16	28 (3 years)
Strother et al. [124]	CCG	53, 20	Spnet (newly diagnosed)	Autologous PBSC support	Nonmyeloablative four cycles of CY/ Cisplatin/vincristine	73 (2 years)
Dunkel et al. [125]	CCG	23	Medulloblastoma	Autologous marrow or PBSC	Carbo/Thiotepa/VP-16	34 (3 years)
Broniscer et al. [126]	CCG, MSKCC	9, 8	Spnet pineoblastoma	Autologous marrow or PBSC	Carbo/Thiotepa/VP-16	62 (5 years), 0 (5 years)
Mason et al. [127]	MSKCC, Columbus Children's, Columbia, NYU, University of Wisconsin	62	Age $<$ 6 years any malignant histology	Autologous marrow	Vincristine/cisplatin/ CY/VP-16	25% (3 years)

GBM glioblastoma multiforme, *CY* cyclophosphamide, *Melph* melphalan, *BU* busulfan, *Carbo* carboplatin, *CCG* Children's Cancer Group, *Spnet* supratentorial primitive neuroectodermal tumor, *MSKCC* Memorial Sloan-Kettering Cancer Center, NYU New York University

50% of patients are long-term survivors with surgery, radiation, and chemotherapy [130, 131]. Strother et al. treated over 50 newly diagnosed patients with medulloblastoma and Spnet with multiple cycles of nonmyeloablative chemotherapy and stem cell rescue resulting in excellent short-term results (>75% 2-year PFS) [124]. Further long-term follow-up and/or a randomized trial are required to determine if this approach is beneficial as compared to standard therapy for newly diagnosed high-risk patients. However, for patients with relapsed disease long-term survival is very rare. A CCG study demonstrated 34% 3-year EFS using high-dose chemotherapy and autologous HSCT for recurrent medulloblastoma [125], and another study had 5/17 patients with recurrent Spnet alive and disease-free following myeloablative chemotherapy and autologous HSCT; however, 0/8 patients with recurrent pineoblastoma survived [126].

In general, young children with brain tumors present a particular problem. First, they have worse prognoses than older children, i.e., <40% 2-year PFS [132]. Secondly, the adverse effects on growth and neurocognitive development are significantly more profound for children less than 6 years of age. Therefore, one strategy that has been employed to delay radiation is to use myeloablative therapy with autologous stem cell rescue as consolidative therapy in these very young patients with brain tumors (Fig. 19.9) [127]. This strategy has resulted in delay in radiation and some long-term survivors. However, again longer follow-up and/or randomized trials are necessary to determine the benefit of this approach compared to standard therapy. To date, these studies have identified some types of disease in which this approach appears to provide no benefit over standard therapy, such as high-grade astrocytomas, brain stem gliomas and ependymomas [127, 133].

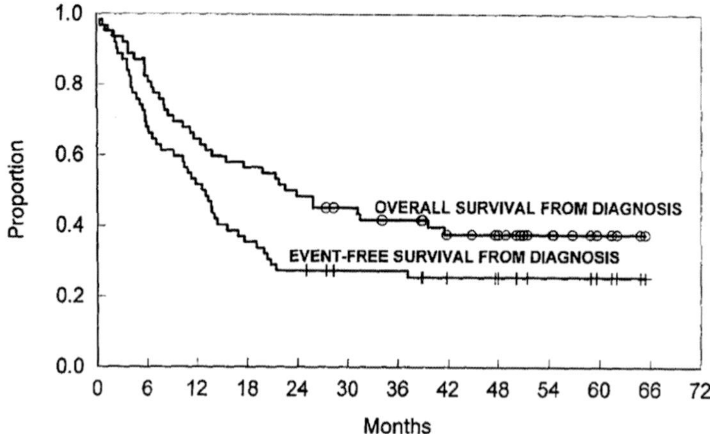

Fig. 19.9 Overall survival and event-free survival (1–3 years) from diagnosis in 62 children with primary brain tumors. (O and +) Censored times.
Source: Mason et al. [127]. Reprinted with permission from the American Society of Clinical Oncology

19.3.3 Sarcoma

Local control with surgery and/or radiation remains very important in the curative potential of sarcomas; however, outcome remains quite poor with cure rates of less than 30% for patients with metastatic disease [134, 135] and less than 10% for recurrent disease [136]. Since many sarcomas in pediatrics are chemotherapy-sensitive, myeloablative chemotherapy with autologous stem cell rescue has been used to treat metastatic or recurrent disease.

19.3.3.1 Ewing's Sarcoma

After neuroblastoma, Ewing's sarcoma is the most common nonhematologic cancer in pediatrics where SCT is employed. There have been numerous single arm studies using myeloablative chemotherapy and HSCT to treat metastatic Ewing's sarcoma, but the results have been insufficient to determine superiority versus standard therapy [137]. An EBMTR review suggested a benefit of autologous HSCT for patients with metastatic disease and suggested that melphalan-based myeloablative regimens had the most activity [138]. Results of this study have lead to the current ongoing Euro-Ewing study using myeloablative chemotherapy and autologous HSCT in nonrandomized fashion for extrapulmonary metastatic disease and with participation of select US centers addressing in a randomized fashion the role of autologous HSCT versus standard therapy, including whole lung radiation for patients with lung as the only site of metastatic disease. Tandem, myeloablative therapies followed each by autologous stem cell rescue have been shown to be feasible for high-risk Ewing's patients, but, again, the results are similar to those observed with standard therapy [139, 140]. Again, numerous single arm studies using myeloablative therapy with autologous HSCT have been performed for recurrent Ewing's sarcoma, with conclusions of efficacy of SCT being mixed. A single center retrospective multi-variate analysis demonstrated significantly improved outcome for patients who received autologous HSCT, had chemo-responsive disease at relapse, and/or had initial relapse-free interval of longer than 24 months [141]. However, there may be bias in this study as patients without chemo-responsive disease did not go on to HSCT. It has been hypothesized that the characteristic EWS-FLI fusion gene product may be a target for immune therapies [142]. Though a very interesting approach, a vaccine trial was performed in post-HSCT patients but it has been difficult to prove clinical benefit of an immune response. However, one European multi-center trial demonstrated an EFS advantage for patients who received IL-2 following autologous HSCT [143]. A single center experience of 27 Ewing's patients who received allogeneic HSCT suggested a trend toward better survival compared to the center's historical results for autologous HSCT [144]. In summary, the outcome remains poor for Ewing's sarcoma patients with metastatic or recurrent disease, and without randomized trials the role of SCT is difficult to define (Table 19.8).

Table 19.8 HSCT in children with sarcoma

Author	Center/Group	*n*	Histology	Donor source	Conditioning regimen	EFS (%)
Burdach et al. [137]	MetaEICESS	28, 26	Ewing	Autologous PBSC rescue, No PBSC	Tandem nonmyeloablative Melph/VP-16, Chemotherapy	29 (5 years), 22 (5 years)
Ladenstein et al. [138]	EBMTR	63	Ewing	Autologous marrow or PBSC	N/A	27 (5 years)
Burke et al. [139]	Children's Memorial Hospital – Chicago	8	Ewing	Autologous PBSC	Tandem: #1 – Carbo/CY/VP-16, #2 – Melph/CY or Thiotepa/CY or Melph/TBI	40 (3 years)
Hawkins et al. [140]	Seattle	16	Ewing	Autologous PBSC or marrow	BU/Melph/Thiotepa	36 (5 years)
Carli et al. [145]	European MMT	52	RMS	Autologous PBSC	High-dose Melph	30 (3 years)
Koscielniak et al. [146]	European MMT	31, 5	RMS	Autologous, Allogeneic	Melph/VP-16/carbo/TBI (26), Variable (5)	36 (2 years), 0 (2 years)
Sauerbrey et al. [147]	COSS	15	Osteosarcoma	Autologous	Variable, Single myeloablation (9), Tandem myeloablation (6)	20 (2 years)

MetaEICESS Meta European Intergroup Cooperative Ewing Sarcoma Study, *Melph* melphalan, *VP-16* etoposide, EBMTR European Bone Marrow Transplant Registry, *Carbo* carboplatin, *CY* cyclophosphamide, *TBI* total body irradiation, *BU* busulfan, *MMT* malignant mesenchymal tumor, *RMS* rhabdomyosarcoma, *COSS* Cooperative Osteosarcoma Study Group

19.3.3.2 Rhabdomyosarcoma

The outcome for patients with metastatic or recurrent rhabdomyosarcoma has not changed in decades, with survival rates being about 30% for metastatic disease [148] and less than 20% for recurrent disease [149]. Dose escalation has not demonstrated significant improvement in high-risk rhabdomyosarcoma. Myeloablative chemotherapy, including tandem cycles, followed by autologous HSCT has been attempted without much demonstrable benefit [145, 146, 150]. Long-term survival has been shown using myeloablative therapy and autologous HSCT for some patients with recurrent rhabdomyosarcoma [146]; however, a large meta-analysis demonstrated no benefit of autologous HSCT for patients with recurrent disease [151]. Therefore, outside the setting of a clinical investigation, HSCT is difficult to recommend for metastatic or recurrent rhabdomyosarcoma (Table 19.8).

19.3.3.3 Osteosarcoma

Osteosarcoma was one of the first solid tumors where dose-escalation was shown to have benefit [152, 153]. However, it has been difficult to demonstrate benefit of myeloablative therapy and autologous HSCT for high-risk or recurrent osteosarcoma [153, 147]. Currently, another approach to using stem cell support in the treatment of osteosarcoma is as rescue following radio-labeled samarium (Table 19.8) [154].

19.3.4 Wilms' Tumor

Though outcome for Wilms' tumor is excellent, for patients with relapsed disease long-term DFS is often less than 20% [155]. There have been impressive results (i.e., EFS > 50%) from single center studies using myeloablative therapy and autologous HSCT for relapsed Wilms' tumor (Fig. 19.10) [156]. A retrospective analysis of the EBMTR experience demonstrated about 50% of patients who were in CR at time of transplant were long-term disease-free survivors; however, only one of eight with measurable disease survived [157]. The French Society of Pediatric Oncology (SFOP) group conducted a prospective trial and demonstrated 50% EFS for relapsed patients [158]. However, there are now pilot studies that suggest similar results can be achieved without myeloablative chemotherapy and autologous HSCT [159, 160]. A randomized trial is needed to assess the role of autologous HSCT in relapsed Wilms' tumor; however, due to small number of patients, an international collaboration would be required.

19.3.5 Miscellaneous Tumors

Myeloablative therapy and autologous HSCT has been reported to have efficacy for many types of recurrent pediatric solid tumors. The experience consists

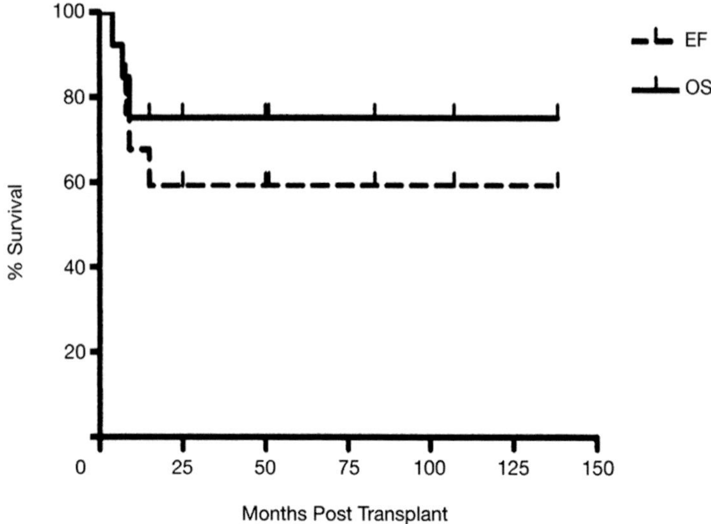

Fig. 19.10 Kaplan–Meier analysis event-free survival (EFS) and overall survival (OS) of 13 patients with relapsed Wilms' tumor from the time of high-dose chemotherapy and hematopoietic stem cell rescue.
Source: Campbell et al. [156]. Reprinted with permission from the American Society of Clinical Oncology

of only case reports in the majority of instances. Such tumors include: esthesioneuroblastoma [161], germ-cell tumors (both cranial and extracranial) [121, 162] and pulmonary blastoma [163]. A French multicenter study involving 25 patients with high-risk retinoblastoma demonstrated approximately 50% long-term DFS. Conclusion of this study was that autologous HSCT provided similar results as conventional chemotherapy for patients with residual optic disease, but superior outcome for patients with extraocular disease [164]. Autologous HSCT has been performed in patients with desmoplastic round cell tumor since the disease is usually chemotherapy-sensitive, but responses are usually very short in duration with a less than 10% 1-year survival [165]. There are reports of prolonged survival, (i.e., 3–4 years) following autologous HSCT, the vast majority of patients relapse and longer follow-up is require to determine if any patients will be cured of their disease [150].

19.4 Psychosocial Issues

As with any individual undergoing HSCT, psychosocial issues (physical, emotional, financial, etc.) for children and their families are universal and can be immense. A comprehensive discussion of such issues is beyond the scope of this review; however, a few issues that are specific or more prevalent for children and families undergoing HSCT warrant mentioning. For small children, being confined to a room can be challenging, so physical, recreational, and occupational therapy as well as child life specialists are utilized to maintain growth and development skills for small children and provide constructive distraction from the boredom of their confinement. For school-aged children educational services are often provided to afford the child opportunity to keep up academically with peers. Additionally, parents have the stress of not only caring for an ill child, but having to provide or arrange care for siblings, pressures of work and financial issues. Therefore, social workers, financial counselors and psychologists are required to provide assistance to family members as well. The psychosocial support required goes beyond the patient to the immediate and often extended family, such that for a child undergoing HSCT support often surpasses that required to support an adult through the process of HSCT.

19.5 Late Effects

Potential late sequelae of HSCT are well-described. Many of the late complications of HSCT observed in adults are also seen in children. Again, there exist some complications that are specific or more prevalent in children undergoing HSCT. The risk of long-term effects has been shown to be related to agents used in HSCT. But the cumulative affect of pre-HSCT therapy can also add to long-term deficits, e.g., hearing loss in children with neuroblastoma [166].

Complications with growth and development following high-dose chemotherapy, irradiation or complications of infections and/or GvHL continue to be a major concern for children undergoing HSCT [167]. All children who undergo HSCT require annual follow-up at a minimum to monitor growth and development. Of note, growth hormone (GH) deficiency should be monitored closely. GH deficiency has been associated not only with short stature, but obesity, hyperlipidemia, increased risk of cardiovascular disease, as well as behavioral problems which can improve after GH replacement therapy [168, 169]. Though there have been concerns about increased risk of leukemia relapse with GH replacement therapy, this has not been shown to be true with GH therapy post-HSCT [167]. Children require close monitoring to assure appropriate development through puberty, which may require hormonal replacement therapy. And bone health is very important in children, not only for increased risk of fracture but also to obtain maximal adult height. Young children are prone to develop problems as adult dentition can be significantly affected by HSCT [170]. Secondary malignancies are a concern of all patients undergoing HSCT. A study from the University of Minnesota demonstrated that cumulative risk for post-transplant lymphoproliferative disease and secondary MDS or leukemia plateaued at 1–2% at 10 years post-HSCT, while the cumulative risk of developing a solid tumor was 4% at 20 years and has not plateaued [171]. This same study showed that the younger the age at HSCT, the higher the risk of secondary malignancy—underscoring again the need for education and close surveillance for the life of the HSCT recipient.

19.6 Summary

HSCT continues to provide cures for children with malignancy. As primary therapies become more intensive and effective in curing children with cancer, patients with refractory or relapse disease have more resistant disease and are at increased risk for regimen-related toxicity. Therefore, if HSCT is to continue to benefit children with cancer, newer strategies are required to control more resistant disease while reducing toxicities. Some strategies that are very exciting and hold much promise include utilizing the graft-versus-tumor effect with the use of reduced intensity conditioning regimens; incorporation of more targeted therapies into conditioning regimens, such as radiolabeled antibodies; and improvement in early detection and therapies for prevention and treatment of regimen-related toxicities, infections, and other complications (short and long-term).

Acknowledgment The authors would like to thank Erin Morris, RN, for her expert assistance in the preparation of this manuscript.

References

1. Thomas ED, Blume KG. Historical markers in the development of allogeneic hematopoietic cell transplantation. Biol Blood Marrow Transplant. 1999;5:341–6.
2. Thomas ED, Lochte HL Jr, Lu WC, Ferrebee JW. Intravenous infusion of bone marrow in patients receiving radiation and chemotherapy. N Engl J Med. 1957;257:491–6.
3. Satwani P, Harrison L, Morris E, Del Toro G, Cairo MS. Reduced-intensity allogeneic stem cell transplantation in adults and children with malignant and nonmalignant diseases: end of the beginning and future challenges. Biol Blood Marrow Transplant. 2005;11:403–22.
4. Champlin R, Khouri I, Shimoni A, et al. Harnessing graft-versus-malignancy: non-myeloablative preparative regimens for allogeneic haematopoietic transplantation, an evolving strategy for adoptive immunotherapy. Br J Haematol. 2000;111:18–29.
5. Butturini A, Bortin MM, Gale RP. Graft-versus-leukemia following bone marrow transplantation. Bone Marrow Transplant. 1987;2:233–42.
6. Drobyski WR, Keever CA, Roth MS, et al. Salvage immunotherapy using donor leukocyte infusions as treatment for relapsed chronic myelogenous leukemia after allogeneic bone marrow transplantation: efficacy and toxicity of a defined T-cell dose. Blood 1993;82:2310–8.
7. Fefer A, Sullivan KM, Weiden P, et al. Graft versus leukemia effect in man: the relapse rate of acute leukemia is lower after allogeneic than after syngeneic marrow transplantation. Prog Clin Biol Res. 1987;244:401–8.
8. Horowitz MM, Gale RP, Sondel PM, et al. Graft-versus-leukemia reactions after bone marrow transplantation. Blood 1990;75:555–62.
9. Kolb HJ, Schattenberg A, Goldman JM, et al. Graft-versus-leukemia effect of donor lymphocyte transfusions in marrow grafted patients. Blood 1995;86:2041–50.
10. Sullivan KM, Weiden PL, Storb R, et al. Influence of acute and chronic graft-versus-host disease on relapse and survival after bone marrow transplantation from HLA-identical siblings as treatment of acute and chronic leukemia. Blood 1989;73:1720–8.
11. Del Toro G, Satwani P, Harrison L, et al. A pilot study of reduced intensity conditioning and allogeneic stem cell transplantation from unrelated cord blood and matched family donors in children and adolescent recipients. Bone Marrow Transplant. 2004;33:613–22.

12. Duerst R, Jacobsohn D, Tse W, Kletzel M. Efficacy of reduced intensity conditioning (RIC) with FLU-BU-ATG and allogeneic hematopoietic stem cell transplantation (HSCT) for pediatric ALL. Blood 2004 (abstract);104:2314.
13. Gomez-Almaguer D, Ruiz-Arguelles GJ, Tarin-Arzaga Ldel C, et al. Reduced-intensity stem cell transplantation in children and adolescents: the Mexican experience. Biol Blood Marrow Transplant. 2003;9:157–61.
14. Roman E, Cooney E, Harrison L, et al. Preliminary results of the safety of immunotherapy with gemtuzumab ozogamicin following reduced intensity allogeneic stem cell transplant in children with $CD33^+$ acute myeloid leukemia. Clin Cancer Res. 2005;11(19 Pt 2):7164s–70s.
15. Satwani P, Morris E, Bradley M, Bhatia M, van de Ven C, Cairo M. Reduced intensity and non-myeloablative allogeneic stem cell transplantation in children and adolescents with malignant and non-malignant diseases. Pediatr Blood Cancer. 2008;50(1):1–8.
16. Pui CH, Evans WE. Treatment of acute lymphoblastic leukemia. N Engl J Med. 2006;354:166–78.
17. Balduzzi A, Valsecchi MG, Uderzo C, et al. Chemotherapy versus allogeneic transplantation for very-high-risk childhood acute lymphoblastic leukaemia in first complete remission: comparison by genetic randomisation in an international prospective study. Lancet 2005;366:635–42.
18. Bordigoni P, Vernant JP, Souillet G, et al. Allogeneic bone marrow transplantation for children with acute lymphoblastic leukemia in first remission: a cooperative study of the Groupe d'Etude de la Greffe de Moelle Osseuse. J Clin Oncol. 1989;7:747–53.
19. Satwani P, Sather H, Ozkaynak F, et al. Allogeneic bone marrow transplantation in first remission for children with ultra-high-risk features of acute lymphoblastic leukemia: a children's oncology group study report. Biol Blood Marrow Transplant. 2007;13:218–27.
20. Uderzo C, Valsecchi MG, Balduzzi A, et al. Allogeneic bone marrow transplantation versus chemotherapy in high-risk childhood acute lymphoblastic leukaemia in first remission. Associazione Italiana di Ematologia ed Oncologia Pediatrica (AIEOP) and the Gruppo Italiano Trapianto di Midollo Osseo (GITMO). Br J Haematol. 1997;96:387–94.
21. Wheeler KA, Richards SM, Bailey CC, et al. Bone marrow transplantation versus chemotherapy in the treatment of very high-risk childhood acute lymphoblastic leukemia in first remission: results from Medical Research Council UKALL X and XI. Blood 2000;96:2412–8.
22. Arico M, Valsecchi MG, Camitta B, et al. Outcome of treatment in children with Philadelphia chromosome-positive acute lymphoblastic leukemia. N Engl J Med. 2000;342:998–1006.
23. Schrauder A, Reiter A, Gadner H, et al. Superiority of allogeneic hematopoietic stem-cell transplantation compared with chemotherapy alone in high-risk childhood T-cell acute lymphoblastic leukemia: results from ALL-BFM 90 and 95. J Clin Oncol. 2006;24:5742–9.
24. Pui CH, Gaynon PS, Boyett JM, et al. Outcome of treatment in childhood acute lymphoblastic leukaemia with rearrangements of the 11q23 chromosomal region. Lancet 2002;359:1909–15.
25. Jacobsohn DA, Hewlett B, Morgan E, Tse W, Duerst RE, Kletzel M. Favorable outcome for infant acute lymphoblastic leukemia after hematopoietic stem cell transplantation. Biol Blood Marrow Transplant. 2005;11:999–1005.
26. Kosaka Y, Koh K, Kinukawa N, et al. Infant acute lymphoblastic leukemia with MLL gene rearrangements: outcome following intensive chemotherapy and hematopoietic stem cell transplantation. Blood 2004;104:3527–34.
27. Dopfer R, Henze G, Bender-Gotze C, et al. Allogeneic bone marrow transplantation for childhood acute lymphoblastic leukemia in second remission after intensive primary and relapse therapy according to the BFM- and CoALL-protocols: results of the German Cooperative Study. Blood 1991;78:2780–4.

28. Barrett AJ, Horowitz MM, Pollock BH, et al. Bone marrow transplants from HLA-identical siblings as compared with chemotherapy for children with acute lymphoblastic leukemia in a second remission. N Engl J Med. 1994;331:1253–8.
29. Uderzo C, Valsecchi MG, Bacigalupo A, et al. Treatment of childhood acute lymphoblastic leukemia in second remission with allogeneic bone marrow transplantation and chemotherapy: ten-year experience of the Italian Bone Marrow Transplantation Group and the Italian Pediatric Hematology Oncology Association. J Clin Oncol. 1995;13:352–8.
30. Wheeler K, Richards S, Bailey C, Chessells J. Comparison of bone marrow transplant and chemotherapy for relapsed childhood acute lymphoblastic leukaemia: the MRC UKALL X experience. Medical Research Council Working Party on Childhood Leukaemia. Br J Haematol. 1998;101:94–103.
31. Boulad F, Steinherz P, Reyes B, et al. Allogeneic bone marrow transplantation versus chemotherapy for the treatment of childhood acute lymphoblastic leukemia in second remission: a single-institution study. J Clin Oncol. 1999;17:197–207.
32. Gaynon PS, Harris RE, Altman AJ, et al. Bone marrow transplantation versus prolonged intensive chemotherapy for children with acute lymphoblastic leukemia and an initial bone marrow relapse within 12 months of the completion of primary therapy: Children's Oncology Group study CCG-1941. J Clin Oncol. 2006;24:3150–6.
33. Gaynon PS. Childhood acute lymphoblastic leukaemia and relapse. Br J Haematol. 2005;131:579–87.
34. Borgmann A, von Stackelberg A, Hartmann R, et al. Unrelated donor stem cell transplantation compared with chemotherapy for children with acute lymphoblastic leukemia in a second remission: a matched-pair analysis. Blood 2003;101:3835–9.
35. Roy A, Cargill A, Love S, et al. Outcome after first relapse in childhood acute lymphoblastic leukaemia—lessons from the United Kingdom R2 trial. Br J Haematol. 2005;130:67–75.
36. Bradley MB, Cairo MS. Cord blood immunology and stem cell transplantation. Hum immunol. 2005;66:431–46.
37. Cairo MS, Wagner JE. Placental and/or umbilical cord blood: an alternative source of hematopoietic stem cells for transplantation. Blood 1997;90:4665–78.
38. Eapen M, Rubinstein P, Zhang MJ, et al. Comparable long-term survival after unrelated and HLA-matched sibling donor hematopoietic stem cell transplantations for acute leukemia in children younger than 18 months. J Clin Oncol. 2006;24:145–51.
39. Rocha V, Cornish J, Sievers EL, et al. Comparison of outcomes of unrelated bone marrow and umbilical cord blood transplants in children with acute leukemia. Blood 2001;97:2962–71.
40. Styczynski J, Cheung YK, Garvin J, et al. Outcomes of unrelated cord blood transplantation in pediatric recipients. Bone Marrow Transplant. 2004;34:129–36.
41. Afify Z, Hunt L, Green A, Guttridge M, Cornish J, Oakhill A. Factors affecting the outcome of stem cell transplantation from unrelated donors for childhood acute lymphoblastic leukemia in third remission. Bone Marrow Transplant. 2005;35:1041–7.
42. Bunin N, Carston M, Wall D, et al. Unrelated marrow transplantation for children with acute lymphoblastic leukemia in second remission. Blood 2002;99:3151–7.
43. Lang P, Handgretinger R, Niethammer D, et al. Transplantation of highly purified $CD34^+$ progenitor cells from unrelated donors in pediatric leukemia. Blood 2003;101:1630–6.
44. Klingebiel T, Handgretinger R, Lang P, Bader P, Niethammer D. Haploidentical transplantation for acute lymphoblastic leukemia in childhood. Blood Rev. 2004;18:181–92.
45. Houtenbos I, Bracho F, Davenport V, et al. Autologous bone marrow transplantation for childhood acute lymphoblastic leukemia: a novel combined approach consisting of ex vivo marrow purging, modulation of multi-drug resistance, induction of autograft vs leukemia effect, and post-transplant immuno- and chemotherapy (PTIC). Bone Marrow Transplant. 2001;27:145–53.

46. Ramsay N, LeBien T, Nesbit M, et al. Autologous bone marrow transplantation for patients with acute lymphoblastic leukemia in second or subsequent remission: results of bone marrow treated with monoclonal antibodies BA-1, BA-2, and BA-3 plus complement. Blood 1985;66:508–13.
47. Ribera JM, Ortega JJ, Oriol A, et al. Comparison of intensive chemotherapy, allogeneic, or autologous stem-cell transplantation as postremission treatment for children with very high risk acute lymphoblastic leukemia: PETHEMA ALL-93 Trial. J Clin Oncol. 2007;25:16–24.
48. Brochstein JA, Kernan NA, Groshen S, et al. Allogeneic bone marrow transplantation after hyperfractionated total-body irradiation and cyclophosphamide in children with acute leukemia. N Engl J Med. 1987;317:1618–24.
49. Coccia PF, Strandjord SE, Warkentin PI, et al. High-dose cytosine arabinoside and fractionated total-body irradiation: an improved preparative regimen for bone marrow transplantation of children with acute lymphoblastic leukemia in remission. Blood 1988;71:888–93.
50. Bunin N, Aplenc R, Kamani N, Shaw K, Cnaan A, Simms S. Randomized trial of busulfan vs total body irradiation containing conditioning regimens for children with acute lymphoblastic leukemia: a Pediatric Blood and Marrow Transplant Consortium study. Bone Marrow Transplant. 2003;32:543–8.
51. Davies SM, Ramsay NK, Klein JP, et al. Comparison of preparative regimens in transplants for children with acute lymphoblastic leukemia. J Clin Oncol. 2000;18:340–7.
52. Hahn T, Wall D, Camitta B, et al. The role of cytotoxic therapy with hematopoietic stem cell transplantation in the therapy of acute lymphoblastic leukemia in children: an evidence-based review. Biol Blood Marrow Transplant. 2005;11:823–61.
53. Lie SO, Abrahamsson J, Clausen N, et al. Treatment stratification based on initial in vivo response in acute myeloid leukaemia in children without Down's syndrome: results of NOPHO-AML trials. Br J Haematol. 2003;122:217–25.
54. Nesbit ME Jr, Buckley JD, Feig SA, et al. Chemotherapy for induction of remission of childhood acute myeloid leukemia followed by marrow transplantation or multiagent chemotherapy: a report from the Children's Cancer Group. J Clin Oncol. 1994;12:127–35.
55. Pession A, Rondelli R, Basso G, et al. Treatment and long-term results in children with acute myeloid leukaemia treated according to the AIEOP AML protocols. Leukemia 2005;19:2043–53.
56. Ravindranath Y, Yeager AM, Chang MN, et al. Autologous bone marrow transplantation versus intensive consolidation chemotherapy for acute myeloid leukemia in childhood. Pediatric Oncology Group. N Engl J Med. 1996;334:1428–34.
57. Stevens RF, Hann IM, Wheatley K, Gray RG. Marked improvements in outcome with chemotherapy alone in paediatric acute myeloid leukemia: results of the United Kingdom Medical Research Council's 10th AML trial. MRC Childhood Leukaemia Working Party. Br J Haematol. 1998;101:130–40.
58. Woods WG, Neudorf S, Gold S, et al. A comparison of allogeneic bone marrow transplantation, autologous bone marrow transplantation, and aggressive chemotherapy in children with acute myeloid leukemia in remission. Blood 2001;97:56–62.
59. Wells RJ, Adams MT, Alonzo TA, et al. Mitoxantrone and cytarabine induction, high-dose cytarabine, and etoposide intensification for pediatric patients with relapsed or refractory acute myeloid leukemia: Children's Cancer Group Study 2951. J Clin Oncol. 2003;21:2940–7.
60. Nemecek ER, Gooley TA, Woolfrey AE, Carpenter PA, Matthews DC, Sanders JE. Outcome of allogeneic bone marrow transplantation for children with advanced acute myeloid leukemia. Bone Marrow Transplant. 2004;34:799–806.
61. Bourquin JP, Thornley I, Neuberg D, et al. Favorable outcome of allogeneic hematopoietic stem cell transplantation for relapsed or refractory acute promyelocytic leukemia in childhood. Bone Marrow Transplant. 2004;34:795–8.

62. Godder K, Eapen M, Laver JH, et al. Autologous hematopoietic stem-cell transplantation for children with acute myeloid leukemia in first or second complete remission: a prognostic factor analysis. J Clin Oncol. 2004;22:3798–804.
63. Michel G, Rocha V, Chevret S, et al. Unrelated cord blood transplantation for childhood acute myeloid leukemia: a Eurocord Group analysis. Blood 2003;102:4290–7.
64. Wall DA, Carter SL, Kernan NA, et al. Busulfan/melphalan/antithymocyte globulin followed by unrelated donor cord blood transplantation for treatment of infant leukemia and leukemia in young children: the Cord Blood Transplantation study (COBLT) experience. Biol Blood Marrow Transplant. 2005;11:637–46.
65. Bunin N, Aplenc R, Leahey A, et al. Outcomes of transplantation with partial T-cell depletion of matched or mismatched unrelated or partially matched related donor bone marrow in children and adolescents with leukemias. Bone Marrow Transplant. 2005;35:151–8.
66. Alonzo TA, Wells RJ, Woods WG, et al. Postremission therapy for children with acute myeloid leukemia: the children's cancer group experience in the transplant era. Leukemia 2005;19:965–70.
67. Lapillonne H, Renneville A, Auvrignon A, et al. High WT1 expression after induction therapy predicts high risk of relapse and death in pediatric acute myeloid leukemia. J Clin Oncol. 2006;24:1507–15.
68. Neudorf S, Sanders J, Kobrinsky N, et al. Allogeneic bone marrow transplantation for children with acute myelocytic leukemia in first remission demonstrates a role for graft versus leukemia in the maintenance of disease-free survival. Blood 2004; 103:3655–61.
69. Woods WG, Kobrinsky N, Buckley J, et al. Intensively timed induction therapy followed by autologous or allogeneic bone marrow transplantation for children with acute myeloid leukemia or myelodysplastic syndrome: a Children's Cancer Group pilot study. J Clin Oncol. 1993;11:1448–57.
70. Scott BL, Sandmaier BM, Storer B, et al. Myeloablative vs nonmyeloablative allogeneic transplantation for patients with myelodysplastic syndrome or acute myelogenous leukemia with multilineage dysplasia: a retrospective analysis. Leukemia 2006;20:128–35.
71. Roman E, Cooney E, Militano O, et al. Reduced intensity allogeneic stem cell transplantation followed by targeted consolidation immunotherapy with gemtuzumab ozogamicin in children and adolescents with $CD33^+$ acute myeloid leukemia. Biol Blood Marrow Transplant. 2007 (abstract);13:30–1.
72. Ruggeri L, Capanni M, Urbani E, et al. Effectiveness of donor natural killer cell alloreactivity in mismatched hematopoietic transplants. Science 2002;295:2097–100.
73. Oliansky DM, Rizzo JD, Aplan PD, et al. The role of cytotoxic therapy with hematopoietic stem cell transplantation in the therapy of acute myeloid leukemia in children: an evidence-based review. Biol Blood Marrow Transplant. 2007;13:1–25.
74. Goldman JM, Apperley JF, Jones L, et al. Bone marrow transplant for patients with chronic myeloid leukemia. N Engl J Med. 1986;314:202–7.
75. Druker BJ, Guilhot F, O'Brien SG, et al. Five-year follow-up of patients receiving imatinib for chronic myeloid leukemia. N Engl J Med. 2006;355:2408–17.
76. Cwynarski K, Roberts IA, Iacobelli S, et al. Stem cell transplantation for chronic myeloid leukemia in children. Blood 2003;102:1224–31.
77. Goldman JM, Druker BJ. Chronic myeloid leukemia: current treatment options. Blood 2001;98:2039–42.
78. Gamis AS, Haake R, McGlave P, Ramsay NK. Unrelated-donor bone marrow transplantation for Philadelphia chromosome-positive chronic myelogenous leukemia in children. J Clin Oncol. 1993;11:834–8.
79. Balduzzi A, Gooley T, Anasetti C, et al. Unrelated donor marrow transplantation in children. Blood 1995;86:3247–56.
80. Dini G, Rondelli R, Miano M, et al. Unrelated-donor bone marrow transplantation for Philadelphia chromosome-positive chronic myelogenous leukemia in children: experience

of eight European Countries. The EBMT Paediatric Diseases Working Party. Bone Marrow Transplant. 1996;18 Suppl 2:80–5.
81. Kaeda J, O'Shea D, Szydlo RM, et al. Serial measurement of BCR-ABL transcripts in the peripheral blood after allogeneic stem cell transplantation for chronic myeloid leukemia: an attempt to define patients who may not require further therapy. Blood 2006;107:4171–6.
82. Olavarria E, Kanfer E, Szydlo R, et al. Early detection of BCR-ABL transcripts by quantitative reverse transcriptase-polymerase chain reaction predicts outcome after allogeneic stem cell transplantation for chronic myeloid leukemia. Blood 2001;97:1560–5.
83. Dazzi F, Szydlo RM, Cross NC, et al. Durability of responses following donor lymphocyte infusions for patients who relapse after allogeneic stem cell transplantation for chronic myeloid leukemia. Blood 2000;96:2712–6.
84. Cairo MS, Bradley MB. Lymphoma. In: Kliegman RM, Behrman RE, Jenson HB, Stanton BF, editors. Nelson textbook of pediatrics. Philadelphia: Elsevier; 2007. p. 2123–6.
85. Hudson MM, Donaldson SS. Treatment of pediatric Hodgkin's lymphoma. Semin Hematol. 1999;36:313–23.
86. Bhatia S, Robison LL, Oberlin O, et al. Breast cancer and other second neoplasms after childhood Hodgkin's disease. N Engl J Med. 1996;334:745–51.
87. Ng AK, Bernardo MV, Weller E, et al. Second malignancy after Hodgkin disease treated with radiation therapy with or without chemotherapy: long-term risks and risk factors. Blood 2002;100:1989–96.
88. Cairo MS, Raetz E, Perkins SL. Non-Hodgkin's lymphoma in children. In: Kufe DW, Bast RC, Hait WN, et al., editors. Cancer medicine, 7th ed. Ontario: BC Decker Inc.; 2005. p. 1962–76.
89. Cairo MS, Sposto R, Hoover-Regan M, et al. Childhood and adolescent large-cell lymphoma (LCL): a review of the Children's Cancer Group experience. Am J Hematol. 2003;72:53–63.
90. Cairo MS, Sposto R, Perkins SL, et al. Burkitt's and Burkitt-like lymphoma in children and adolescents: a review of the Children's Cancer Group experience. Br J Haematol. 2003;120:660–70.
91. Loiseau HA, Hartmann O, Valteau D, et al. High-dose chemotherapy containing busulfan followed by bone marrow transplantation in 24 children with refractory or relapsed non-Hodgkin's lymphoma. Bone Marrow Transplant. 1991;8:465–72.
92. Gordon BG, Warkentin PI, Weisenburger DD, et al. Bone marrow transplantation for peripheral T-cell lymphoma in children and adolescents. Blood 1992;80:2938–42.
93. Philip T, Hartmann O, Pinkerton R, et al. Curability of relapsed childhood B-cell non-Hodgkin's lymphoma after intensive first line therapy: a report from the Societe Francaise d'Oncologie Pediatrique. Blood 1993;81:2003–6.
94. Ladenstein R, Pearce R, Hartmann O, Patte C, Goldstone T, Philip T. High-dose chemotherapy with autologous bone marrow rescue in children with poor-risk Burkitt's lymphoma: a report from the European Lymphoma Bone Marrow Transplantation Registry. Blood 1997;90:2921–30.
95. Kobrinsky NL, Sposto R, Shah NR, et al. Outcomes of treatment of children and adolescents with recurrent non-Hodgkin's lymphoma and Hodgkin's disease with dexamethasone, etoposide, cisplatin, cytarabine, and l-asparaginase, maintenance chemotherapy, and transplantation: Children's Cancer Group Study CCG-5912. J Clin Oncol. 2001;19:2390–6.
96. Levine JE, Harris RE, Loberiza FR Jr, et al. A comparison of allogeneic and autologous bone marrow transplantation for lymphoblastic lymphoma. Blood 2003;101:2476–82.
97. Woessmann W, Peters C, Lenhard M, et al. Allogeneic haematopoietic stem cell transplantation in relapsed or refractory anaplastic large cell lymphoma of children and

adolescents—a Berlin-Frankfurt-Munster group report. Br J Haematol. 2006;133:176–82.
98. Williams CD, Goldstone AH, Pearce R, et al. Autologous bone marrow transplantation for pediatric Hodgkin's disease: a case-matched comparison with adult patients by the European Bone Marrow Transplant Group Lymphoma Registry. J Clin Oncol. 1993; 11:2243–9.
99. Baker KS, Gordon BG, Gross TG, et al. Autologous hematopoietic stem-cell transplantation for relapsed or refractory Hodgkin's disease in children and adolescents. J Clin Oncol. 1999;17:825–31.
100. Stoneham S, Ashley S, Pinkerton CR, Wallace WH, Shankar AG. Outcome after autologous hemopoietic stem cell transplantation in relapsed or refractory childhood Hodgkin disease. J Pediatr Hematol Oncol. 2004;26:740–5.
101. Lieskovsky YE, Donaldson SS, Torres MA, et al. High-dose therapy and autologous hematopoietic stem-cell transplantation for recurrent or refractory pediatric Hodgkin's disease: results and prognostic indices. J Clin Oncol. 2004;22:4532–40.
102. Harris RE, Termuelin A, Cairo MS, et al. Safety and efficacy of CBV followed by autologous PBSC transplant in children with lymphoma after failed induction or first relapse—a Children's Oncology Group Study. Pediatr Blood Cancer. 2006 (abstract);46:843.
103. Bradley B, Cooney E, George D, et al. A pilot study of myeloalative (MA) autologous stem cell (AutoSCT) followed by reduced intensity (RI) allogeneic transplantation (AlloSCT) in children and adolescents with relapsed/refractory Hodkin disease (HD) and non-Hodgkin lymphoma (NL). Pediatr Blood Cancer. 2006 (abstract);46:852.
104. Peggs KS, Hunter A, Chopra R, et al. Clinical evidence of a graft-versus-Hodgkin's-lymphoma effect after reduced-intensity allogeneic transplantation. Lancet 2005; 365:1934–41.
105. Carella AM, Cavaliere M, Lerma E, et al. Autografting followed by nonmyeloablative immunosuppressive chemotherapy and allogeneic peripheral-blood hematopoietic stem-cell transplantation as treatment of resistant Hodgkin's disease and non-Hodgkin's lymphoma. J Clin Oncol. 2000;18:3918–24.
106. Gutman JA, Bearman SI, Nieto Y, et al. Autologous transplantation followed closely by reduced-intensity allogeneic transplantation as consolidative immunotherapy in advanced lymphoma patients: a feasibility study. Bone Marrow Transplant. 2005;36:443–51.
107. Matthay K. Hematopoietic cell transplantation for neuroblastoma. In: Blume K, Forman S, Appelbaum F, editors. Thomas' hematopoietic cell transplantation, 3rd ed. Oxford: Blackwell Publishing Ltd; 2004. p. 1333–44.
108. Matthay KK, Villablanca JG, Seeger RC, et al. Treatment of high-risk neuroblastoma with intensive chemotherapy, radiotherapy, autologous bone marrow transplantation, and 13-cis-retinoic acid. Children's Cancer Group. N Engl J Med. 1999;341:1165–73.
109. Grupp SA, Stern JW, Bunin N, et al. Rapid-sequence tandem transplant for children with high-risk neuroblastoma. Med Pediatr Oncol. 2000;35:696–700.
110. Kletzel M, Katzenstein HM, Haut PR, et al. Treatment of high-risk neuroblastoma with triple-tandem high-dose therapy and stem-cell rescue: results of the Chicago Pilot II Study. J Clin Oncol. 2002;20:2284–92.
111. Kletzel M, Cohn S, Morgan E, Kalapurakal J, Jacobsohn D, Duerst R. The Chicago pilot #2 for high risk (HR) neuroblastoma (NBL) patients (pts): a 4-year update. Pediatr Blood Cancer. 2006 (abstract);47:462.
112. Matthay KK, DeSantes K, Hasegawa B, et al. Phase I dose escalation of 131I-metaiodobenzylguanidine with autologous bone marrow support in refractory neuroblastoma. J Clin Oncol. 1998;16:229–36.
113. Yanik GA, Levine JE, Matthay KK, et al. Pilot study of iodine-131-metaiodobenzylguanidine in combination with myeloablative chemotherapy and autologous stem-cell support for the treatment of neuroblastoma. J Clin Oncol. 2002;20:2142–9.

114. Ladenstein R, Lasset C, Hartmann O, et al. Comparison of auto versus allografting as consolidation of primary treatments in advanced neuroblastoma over one year of age at diagnosis: report from the European Group for Bone Marrow Transplantation. Bone Marrow Transplant. 1994;14:37–46.
115. Matthay KK, Seeger RC, Reynolds CP, et al. Allogeneic versus autologous purged bone marrow transplantation for neuroblastoma: a report from the Children's Cancer Group. J Clin Oncol. 1994;12:2382–9.
116. Rill DR, Santana VM, Roberts WM, et al. Direct demonstration that autologous bone marrow transplantation for solid tumors can return a multiplicity of tumorigenic cells. Blood 1994;84:380–3.
117. Mattano LA Jr, Moss TJ, Emerson SG. Sensitive detection of rare circulating neuroblastoma cells by the reverse transcriptase-polymerase chain reaction. Cancer Res 1992;52:4701–5.
118. Kreissman SG, Villablanca JG, Diller L, et al. Response and toxicity to a dose-intensive multi-agent chemotherapy induction regimen for high risk neuroblastoma (HR-NB): a Children's Oncology Group (COG A3973) study. J Clin Oncol. 2007 (abstract);25:9505.
119. Cheung NK, Kushner BH, Cheung IY, et al. Anti-G(D2) antibody treatment of minimal residual stage 4 neuroblastoma diagnosed at more than 1 year of age. J Clin Oncol. 1998;16:3053–60.
120. Yamashiro DJ, Lee A, Bhatia M, et al. Feasibility of autologous stem cell transplant followed by reduced intensity allogeneic stem cell transplantation for high risk neuroblastoma: a single institution pilot study. Biol Blood Marrow Transplant. 2007 (abstract);13:68.
121. Graham ML, Herndon JE II, Casey JR, et al. High-dose chemotherapy with autologous stem-cell rescue in patients with recurrent and high-risk pediatric brain tumors. J Clin Oncol. 1997;15:1814–23.
122. Heideman RL, Douglass EC, Krance RA, et al. High-dose chemotherapy and autologous bone marrow rescue followed by interstitial and external-beam radiotherapy in newly diagnosed pediatric malignant gliomas. J Clin Oncol. 1993;11:1458–65.
123. Finlay JL, Goldman S, Wong MC, et al. Pilot study of high-dose thiotepa and etoposide with autologous bone marrow rescue in children and young adults with recurrent CNS tumors. The Children's Cancer Group. J Clin Oncol. 1996;14:2495–503.
124. Strother D, Ashley D, Kellie SJ, et al. Feasibility of four consecutive high-dose chemotherapy cycles with stem-cell rescue for patients with newly diagnosed medulloblastoma or supratentorial primitive neuroectodermal tumor after craniospinal radiotherapy: results of a collaborative study. J Clin Oncol. 2001;19:2696–704.
125. Dunkel IJ, Boyett JM, Yates A, et al. High-dose carboplatin, thiotepa, and etoposide with autologous stem-cell rescue for patients with recurrent medulloblastoma. Children's Cancer Group. J Clin Oncol. 1998;16:222–8.
126. Broniscer A, Nicolaides TP, Dunkel IJ, et al. High-dose chemotherapy with autologous stem-cell rescue in the treatment of patients with recurrent non-cerebellar primitive neuroectodermal tumors. Pediatr Blood Cancer. 2004;42:261–7.
127. Mason WP, Grovas A, Halpern S, et al. Intensive chemotherapy and bone marrow rescue for young children with newly diagnosed malignant brain tumors. J Clin Oncol. 1998;16:210–21.
128. Fouladi M, Hunt DL, Pollack IF, et al. Outcome of children with centrally reviewed low-grade gliomas treated with chemotherapy with or without radiotherapy on Children's Cancer Group high-grade glioma study CCG-945. Cancer 2003;98:1243–52.
129. Jakacki RI, Siffert J, Jamison C, Velasquez L, Allen JC. Dose-intensive, time-compressed procarbazine, CCNU, vincristine (PCV) with peripheral blood stem cell support and concurrent radiation in patients with newly diagnosed high-grade gliomas. J Neurooncol. 1999;44:77–83.
130. Cohen BH, Zeltzer PM, Boyett JM, et al. Prognostic factors and treatment results for supratentorial primitive neuroectodermal tumors in children using radiation

and chemotherapy: a Children's Cancer Group randomized trial. J Clin Oncol. 1995;13:1687–96.

131. Evans AE, Jenkin RD, Sposto R, et al. The treatment of medulloblastoma. Results of a prospective randomized trial of radiation therapy with and without CCNU, vincristine, and prednisone. J Neurosurg. 1990;72:572–82.
132. Duffner PK, Horowitz ME, Krischer JP, et al. Postoperative chemotherapy and delayed radiation in children less than three years of age with malignant brain tumors. N Engl J Med. 1993;328:1725–31.
133. Zacharoulis S, Levy A, Chi SN, et al. Outcome for young children newly diagnosed with ependymoma, treated with intensive induction chemotherapy followed by myeloablative chemotherapy and autologous stem cell rescue. Pediatr Blood Cancer. 2007;49:34–40.
134. Miser JS, Krailo MD, Tarbell NJ, et al. Treatment of metastatic Ewing's sarcoma or primitive neuroectodermal tumor of bone: evaluation of combination ifosfamide and etoposide—a Children's Cancer Group and Pediatric Oncology Group study. J Clin Oncol. 2004;22:2873–6.
135. Paulussen M, Ahrens S, Burdach S, et al. Primary metastatic (stage IV) Ewing tumor: survival analysis of 171 patients from the EICESS studies. European Intergroup Cooperative Ewing Sarcoma Studies. Ann Oncol. 1998;9:275–81.
136. Bacci G, Longhi A, Ferrari S, Mercuri M, Versari M, Bertoni F. Prognostic factors in non-metastatic Ewing's sarcoma tumor of bone: an analysis of 579 patients treated at a single institution with adjuvant or neoadjuvant chemotherapy between 1972 and 1998. Acta Oncol. 2006;45:469–75.
137. Burdach S, Meyer-Bahlburg A, Laws HJ, et al. High-dose therapy for patients with primary multifocal and early relapsed Ewing's tumors: results of two consecutive regimens assessing the role of total-body irradiation. J Clin Oncol. 2003;21:3072–8.
138. Ladenstein R, Lasset C, Pinkerton R, et al. Impact of megatherapy in children with high-risk Ewing's tumours in complete remission: a report from the EBMT Solid Tumour Registry. Bone Marrow Transplant. 1995;15:697–705.
139. Burke MJ, Walterhouse DO, Jacobsohn DA, Duerst RE, Kletzel M. Tandem high-dose chemotherapy with autologous peripheral hematopoietic progenitor cell rescue as consolidation therapy for patients with high-risk Ewing family tumors. Pediatr Blood Cancer. 2007;49:196–8.
140. Hawkins D, Barnett T, Bensinger W, Gooley T, Sanders J. Busulfan, melphalan, and thiotepa with or without total marrow irradiation with hematopoietic stem cell rescue for poor-risk Ewing-Sarcoma-Family tumors. Med Pediatr Oncol. 2000;34:328–37.
141. Barker LM, Pendergrass TW, Sanders JE, Hawkins DS. Survival after recurrence of Ewing's sarcoma family of tumors. J Clin Oncol. 2005;23:4354–62.
142. Dagher R, Long LM, Read EJ, et al. Pilot trial of tumor-specific peptide vaccination and continuous infusion interleukin-2 in patients with recurrent Ewing sarcoma and alveolar rhabdomyosarcoma: an inter-institute NIH study. Med Pediatr Oncol. 2002;38:158–64.
143. Burdach S, Nurnberger W, Laws HJ, et al. Myeloablative therapy, stem cell rescue and gene transfer in advanced Ewing tumors. Bone Marrow Transplant. 1996;18 Suppl 1:S67–8.
144. Landenstein R, Peters C, Zoubek A, et al. The role of megatherapy (MGT) followed by stem cell rescue (SCR) in high risk Ewing's tumors (ET): 11 years single center experience. Med Pediatr Oncol. 1996 (abstract);24:237.
145. Carli M, Colombatti R, Oberlin O, et al. High-dose melphalan with autologous stem-cell rescue in metastatic rhabdomyosarcoma. J Clin Oncol. 1999;17:2796–803.
146. Koscielniak E, Klingebiel TH, Peters C, et al. Do patients with metastatic and recurrent rhabdomyosarcoma benefit from high-dose therapy with hematopoietic rescue? Report of the German/Austrian Pediatric Bone Marrow Transplantation Group. Bone Marrow Transplant. 1997;19:227–31.

147. Sauerbrey A, Bielack S, Kempf-Bielack B, Zoubek A, Paulussen M, Zintl F. High-dose chemotherapy (HDC) and autologous hematopoietic stem cell transplantation (ASCT) as salvage therapy for relapsed osteosarcoma. Bone Marrow Transplant. 2001;27:933–7.
148. Breitfeld PP, Lyden E, Raney RB, et al. Ifosfamide and etoposide are superior to vincristine and melphalan for pediatric metastatic rhabdomyosarcoma when administered with irradiation and combination chemotherapy: a report from the Intergroup Rhabdomyosarcoma Study Group. J Pediatr Hematol Oncol. 2001;23:225–33.
149. Pappo AS, Anderson JR, Crist WM, et al. Survival after relapse in children and adolescents with rhabdomyosarcoma: a report from the Intergroup Rhabdomyosarcoma Study Group. J Clin Oncol. 1999;17:3487–93.
150. Boulad F, Kernan NA, LaQuaglia MP, et al. High-dose induction chemoradiotherapy followed by autologous bone marrow transplantation as consolidation therapy in rhabdomyosarcoma, extraosseous Ewing's sarcoma, and undifferentiated sarcoma. J Clin Oncol. 1998;16:1697–706.
151. Weigel BJ, Breitfeld PP, Hawkins D, Crist WM, Baker KS. Role of high-dose chemotherapy with hematopoietic stem cell rescue in the treatment of metastatic or recurrent rhabdomyosarcoma. J Pediatr Hematol Oncol. 2001;23:272–6.
152. Schabel FM Jr, Griswold DP Jr, Corbett TH, Laster WR Jr. Increasing the therapeutic response rates to anticancer drugs by applying the basic principles of pharmacology. Cancer 1984;54 Suppl 6:1160–7.
153. Valteau-Couanet D, Kalifa C, Benhamou E, et al. Phase II study of high-dose thiotepa (HDT) and hematopoietic stem cell transplantation (SCT) support in children with metastatic osteosarcoma. Med Pediatr Oncol. 1996 (abstract);24:239.
154. Anderson PM, Wiseman GA, Dispenzieri A, et al. High-dose samarium-153 ethylene diamine tetramethylene phosphonate: low toxicity of skeletal irradiation in patients with osteosarcoma and bone metastases. J Clin Oncol. 2002;20:189–96.
155. Grundy P, Breslow N, Green DM, Sharples K, Evans A, D'Angio GJ. Prognostic factors for children with recurrent Wilms' tumor: results from the Second and Third National Wilms' Tumor Study. J Clin Oncol. 1989;7:638–47.
156. Campbell AD, Cohn SL, Reynolds M, et al. Treatment of relapsed Wilms' tumor with high-dose therapy and autologous hematopoietic stem-cell rescue: the experience at Children's Memorial Hospital. J Clin Oncol. 2004;22:2885–90.
157. Garaventa A, Hartmann O, Bernard JL, et al. Autologous bone marrow transplantation for pediatric Wilms' tumor: the experience of the European Bone Marrow Transplantation Solid Tumor Registry. Med Pediatr Oncol. 1994;22:11–4.
158. Pein F, Michon J, Valteau-Couanet D, et al. High-dose melphalan, etoposide, and carboplatin followed by autologous stem-cell rescue in pediatric high-risk recurrent Wilms' tumor: a French Society of Pediatric Oncology study. J Clin Oncol. 1998;16:3295–301.
159. Abu-Ghosh AM, Krailo MD, Goldman SC, et al. Ifosfamide, carboplatin and etoposide in children with poor-risk relapsed Wilms' tumor: a Children's Cancer Group report. Ann Oncol. 2002;13:460–9.
160. Dome JS, Liu T, Krasin M, et al. Improved survival for patients with recurrent Wilms tumor: the experience at St. Jude Children's Research Hospital. J Pediatr Hematol Oncol. 2002;24:192–8.
161. Nguyen QA, Villablanca JG, Siegel SE, Crockett DM. Esthesioneuroblastoma in the pediatric age-group: the role of chemotherapy and autologous bone marrow transplantation. Int J Pediatr Otorhinolaryngol. 1996;37:45–52.
162. Devalck C, Tempels D, Ferster A, et al. Long-term disease-free survival in a child with refractory metastatic malignant germ cell tumor treated by high-dose chemotherapy with autologous bone marrow rescues. Med Pediatr Oncol. 1994;22:208–10.
163. Schmaltz C, Sauter S, Opitz O, et al. Pleuro-pulmonary blastoma: a case report and review of the literature. Med Pediatr Oncol. 1995;25:479–84.

164. Namouni F, Doz F, Tanguy ML, et al. High-dose chemotherapy with carboplatin, etoposide and cyclophosphamide followed by a haematopoietic stem cell rescue in patients with high-risk retinoblastoma: a SFOP and SFGM study. Eur J Cancer 1997;33:2368–75.
165. Kretschmar CS, Colbach C, Bhan I, Crombleholme TM. Desmoplastic small cell tumor: a report of three cases and a review of the literature. J Pediatr Hematol Oncol. 1996;18:293–8.
166. Trahair TN, Vowels MR, Johnston K, et al. Long-term outcomes in children with high-risk neuroblastoma treated with autologous stem cell transplantation. Bone Marrow Transplant. 2007;40:741–6.
167. Sanders JE. Growth and development after hematopoietic cell transplantation. In: Blume KG, Forman S, Appelbaum FR, editors. Thomas' hematopoietic cell transplantation, 3rd ed. Oxford: Blackwell Publishing Ltd.; 2004. p. 929–43.
168. Stabler B, Siegel PT, Clopper RR, Stoppani CE, Compton PG, Underwood LE. Behavior change after growth hormone treatment of children with short stature. J Pediatr. 1998;133:366–73.
169. Vance ML, Mauras N. Growth hormone therapy in adults and children. N Engl J Med 1999;341:1206–16.
170. Dahllof G, Rozell B, Forsberg CM, Borgstrom B. Histologic changes in dental morphology induced by high dose chemotherapy and total body irradiation. Oral Surg Oral Med Oral Pathol. 1994;77:56–60.
171. Baker KS, DeFor TE, Burns LJ, Ramsay NK, Neglia JP, Robison LL. New malignancies after blood or marrow stem-cell transplantation in children and adults: incidence and risk factors. J Clin Oncol. 2003;21:1352–8.

Chapter 20
Cellular Adoptive Immunotherapy After Autologous and Allogeneic Hematopoietic Stem Cell Transplantation

David L. Porter, Elizabeth O. Hexner, Sarah Cooley, and Jeffrey S. Miller

20.1 Introduction

HSCT remains the best if not only curative therapy for many patients with hematologic malignancies. The success of HSCT is related not just to the high dose conditioning therapy, but at least in the setting of allogeneic HSCT, the donor graft itself can provide powerful "graft-versus-leukemia" (GvL) activity critically important for the cure of many patients. The relevant cellular immune components of the donor graft include at least T cells, natural killer (NK) cells and B cells, all recognized in various settings as potential effectors of the GvL (or graft-versus-tumor, GvT) effect. Although GvL activity was identified in some of the earliest murine models of HSCT [1], it took many years to unequivocally prove GvL activity was critical in clinical transplantation. Numerous observations implicated mature donor T cells as primarily mediators of GvL, and a tight association of GvL activity and graft-versus-host disease (GvHD) was repeatedly observed [2]. Ultimately, the use of donor leukocyte infusions (DLI) to treat relapsed leukemia provided the first direct evidence for a GvL reaction in the clinical setting. More recently, accumulating evidence shows that in the proper setting, natural killer (NK) cells also possess potent anti-tumor activity and hold great promise for cellular immunotherapy without the risk of graft-versus-host disease. Defining the precise cellular effectors and the target antigens for the GvL response will be necessary to maximize the anticancer effects of cellular therapy while minimizing the risk of GvHD. Ultimately adoptive immunotherapy after HSCT offers a powerful approach for immunologic control of cancer and infections, and has far reaching implications for the immunological control of human disease.

D.L. Porter (✉)
Division of Hematology-Oncology, University of Pennsylvania Medical Center, 16 Penn Tower, 3400 Spruce St, Philadelphia, PA, USA
e-mail: david.porter@uphs.upenn.edu

M.R. Bishop (ed.), *Hematopoietic Stem Cell Transplantation*, Cancer Treatment and Research 144, DOI 10.1007/978-0-387-78580-6_20,

20.1.1 DLI for Chronic Myelogenous Leukemia

The classic and most potent example of successful allogeneic cellular therapy is the use of DLI for chronic myelogenous leukemia (CML). Kolb et al. first reported that three patients with relapsed CML after allogeneic HSCT all achieved a complete cytogenetic remission after buffy coat infusions from the original transplant donor [3]. This report was quickly followed by a number of studies confirming that DLI could induce complete remissions for the majority of similar patients with relapse of chronic phase CML [4, 5]. Furthermore, several studies also showed that the majority of patients achieved a complete molecular response when assayed by high sensitivity polymerase chain reaction (PCR) techniques. Two large retrospective registry analyses have better quantitated the GvL activity of DLI as shown in Table 20.1. These data are remarkably consistent with single institution trials and

Table 20.1 Response rates to donor leukocyte infusions to treat relapse after allogeneic bone marrow transplantation[a]

Disease	Response rate
CML chronic phase	76% (28/37) [7]
	79% (53/67) [6]
CML advanced phase	28% (5/18) [7]
	12% (1/8) [6]
AML	15% (6/39) [7]
	29% (5/17) [6]
	36% (16/44) [8][b]
	34% (54/159) [9]
	62% (10/16) [10][c]
ALL	18% (2/11) [7]
	0% (0/12) [6]
	13% (2/15) [11]
MDS	40% (2/5) [7]
	25% (1/4) [6]
	21% (3/14) [12][d]
NHL	0/6 (0%) [7]
Multiple myeloma	50% (2/4) [7]
	31% (4/13) [13]
	22% (6/27) [14]
	9% (2/22) [15][e]

AML acute myelogenous leukemia, *ALL* acute lymphocyte leukemia, MDS myelodysplasia, *NHL* non-Hodgkin's lymphoma, *CML* chronic myelogenous leukemia, *EBMT* European Group for Blood and Marrow Transplantation

[a]Representative response rates are illustrated from either registry data or in some cases, larger series of *DLI* for a specific indication

[b]All patients were pretreated with chemotherapy by design of the protocol

[c]Only 25% long-term survivors without disease

[d]No long-term disease-free survivors due to toxicity or relapse in three responders

[e]A total of 25 patients were treated. An additional three patients achieved a complete response after treatment with chemotherapy before DLI.

show that 76–79% of patients treated with DLI for relapsed chronic phase CML achieve complete cytogenetic and molecular remission [6, 7].

DLI is most effective for patients with chronic phase relapse but disappointing for patients with accelerated phase or blast crisis; remissions were observed in only 12–28% of these patients. Even those patients with advanced phase CML who respond to DLI are less likely to enjoy prolonged remissions [16, 17] and have relapses rates of over 40% [16]. On the contrary, the majority of remissions are durable in patients treated for early phase relapse of CML. A review of long-term follow-up data from the North American registry showed that only 5 of 39 (13%) DLI recipients for CML relapsed; this included 2 of 32 (6%) recipients of DLI for early phase relapse and three of seven (43%) recipients of DLI for advanced phase relapse of CML [18]. The probability of both event free and overall survival was 73% at 3 years (Fig. 20.1). In another report on long-term outcomes after DLI for CML, the Hammersmith group reported that only 4 of 44 (9%) patients had a recurrence of CML 15–87 weeks after remission [17] with a 3-year probability of molecular remission of 68%. Their data confirmed that advanced phase CML and a short duration of remission after transplant were poor prognostic factors after DLI. In a subsequent report from Sweden, 3-year leukemia-free survival was similar at 85% after DLI for cytogenetic or molecular relapse of CML but 0% for patients treated at hematologic relapse [19]. Late relapses in these long-term follow-up studies raise the concern that the GvL effects provided by donor T cells might have a limited life span.

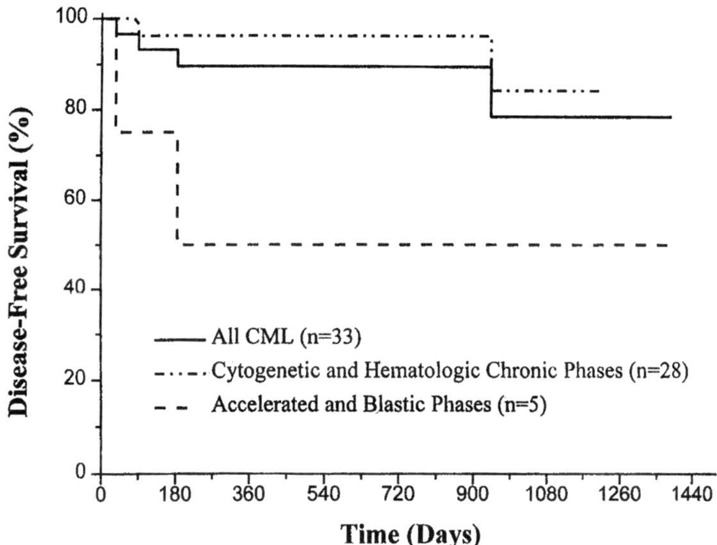

Fig. 20.1 Disease-free survival after DLI for CML, reprinted with permission from Collins et al. [7]

20.1.2 DLI for Acute Myelogenous Leukemia

The activity of DLI for relapsed acute myelogenous leukemia (AML) has been disappointing. This is not surprising since early data suggested that GvL activity against AML was relatively weak [2, 20]. Several initial case series described remissions after DLI for relapsed AML [21, 22], but all reports included only small numbers of heterogeneous patients with few responses. Three large retrospective analyses have been performed to estimate the anticipated outcomes after DLI for AML [6, 7, 9] (Table 20.1). Overall, response rates vary between 15% and 34% and 2-year overall survival between 9% and 20%.

One of the limitations to successful DLI for relapsed AML has been the rapid progression of leukemia before a GvL effect can be manifested. After DLI for CML, the median time to response may be over 40 days [4]. Given the latency of GvL activity it is logical to consider treatment prior to DLI with cytoreductive chemotherapy. DLI can then be given either as consolidation after achieving a remission, or during a chemotherapy-induced nadir.

Three important and illustrative studies using DLI for relapsed advanced myeloid malignancies illustrate the controversies using pre-DLI chemotherapy. Two prospective trials included patients treated with induction chemotherapy, followed 7–14 days later by a defined dose of G-CSF mobilized peripheral blood mononuclear cells as the source of DLI [8, 10]. Complete remissions were achieved in 47% (27/57) and 63% (10/16) of patients respectively. Overall survival was 19% and 31% at 2 years. Several important findings can be highlighted. For patients who achieved complete remission after chemotherapy and DLI, 1- and 2-year survival rates were approximately 50% and 40% respectively, compared to a 1-year survival of 0–5% in nonresponders. Therefore, for patients whose disease can be controlled, there does appear to be a potent antileukemic effect of DLI. The most important predictor of survival was time from transplant to relapse; 1-year survival for patients relapsing more than 6 months after HSCT was about 50% compared to 0–10% for patients relapsing less than 6 months from transplant (Fig. 20.2) [8, 10]. Thus, for the group of patients who relapse within 6 months after HSCT, novel manipulations of DLI or other therapy should be considered.

A more recent retrospective analysis was conducted by the European Group for Blood and Marrow Transplantation (EBMT). This study was particularly informative and clarified a number of prognostic factors associated with outcomes after DLI [9]. The study was designed to compare outcomes after AML relapse ($n = 399$) between patients that did ($n = 171$) and did not ($n = 228$) receive DLI. After adjusting for differences between groups, the 2-year overall survival was 21% for DLI recipients compared to 9% for patients who did not receive DLI. Factors associated with better outcome was relapse greater than 5 months from HSCT, age less than 37 years, and use of DLI. For DLI recipients specifically, remission at the time of DLI or <35% marrow blasts were both associated with better survival as was female sex and favorable cytogenetics. In

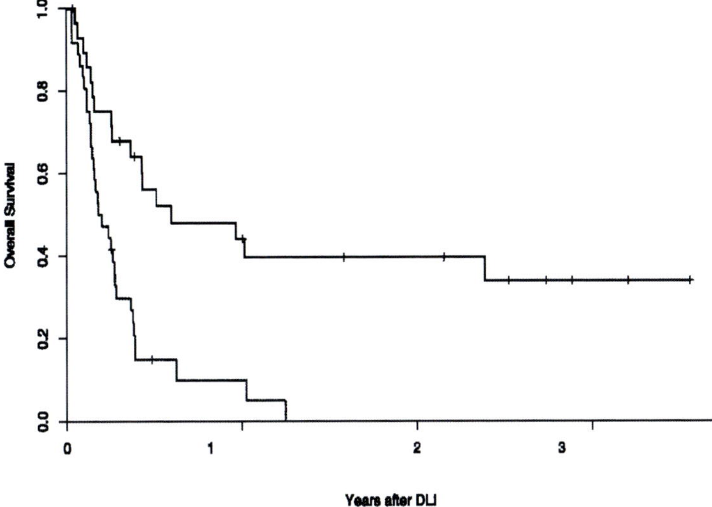

Fig. 20.2 Survival after chemotherapy followed by DLI for AML; post-transplant remission >6 months (*solid line*), post-transplant remission <6 months (*dashed line*), reprinted with permission from Levine et al. [8]

the best risk patients in remission or with favorable cytogenetics, 2-year overall survival (OS) was estimated to be 56% (Fig. 20.3). Though it is possible that remission induction prior to DLI is simply preselecting the best risk patients, it may also imply that DLI is likely to be most effective when given for a minimal disease burden. In this study, two other nonoverlapping prognostic groups were identified: Female recipients not in remission with a low tumor burden had a 2-year OS of 21% while all other patients had an estimated 9% 2-year OS. Two-year OS was 15% for patients given DLI during aplasia or with active disease. Clearly there remains an important role for DLI. Newer methods to

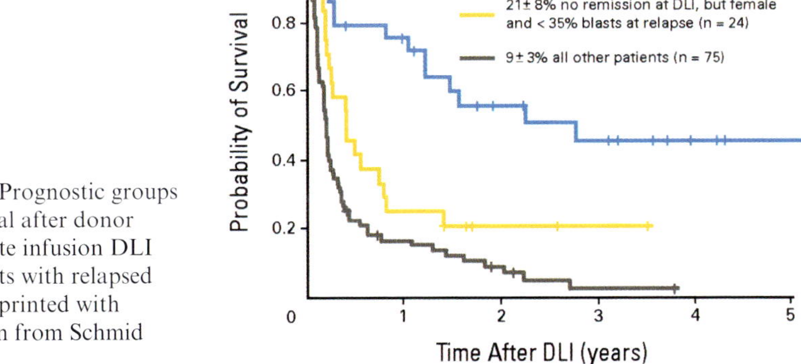

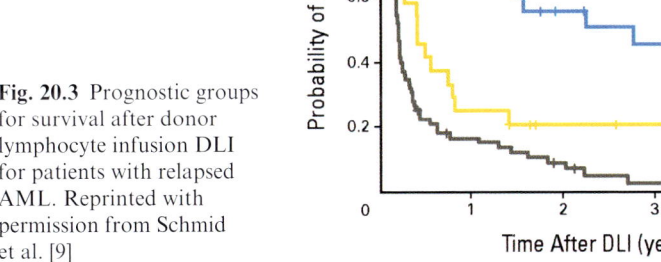

Fig. 20.3 Prognostic groups for survival after donor lymphocyte infusion DLI for patients with relapsed AML. Reprinted with permission from Schmid et al. [9]

enhance anti-leukemic effects of allogeneic cellular therapy should be aggressively investigated, particularly in the high risk group of patients.

There is little long-term follow-up information after DLI for AML, but most data suggest that many of the DLI-induced remissions are not durable. In one report of long-term follow-up, event-free survival after achieving CR for relapsed AML was only 31% at 3 years [18]. Interestingly, there are a surprisingly large number of patients whose relapses after DLI are characterized by extramedullary disease in the absence of marrow involvement [23]. This observation suggests that AML can recur either in a sanctuary site or in a subset of cells with specific properties that escape immunologic recognition [10, 24]. More effective and/or other site specific therapy should be considered when treating extramedullary relapse.

20.1.3 DLI for Myelodysplasia

There are only limited data on the role of DLI in relapsed MDS. Some trials of DLI have included patients with MDS, but response rates are not reported separately from patients with AML [8]. In general, response rates have been low and long-term survival disappointing. It is important to note however that myelodysplastic syndromes are quite heterogeneous and can vary from very indolent to very aggressive diseases. In those patients with an indolent course, the response to DLI may be higher than in patients with AML or more aggressive subtypes of MDS.

Overall response rates to DLI for MDS are between 14% and 45%, and it can be anticipated than a number of patients will ultimately relapse, thus limiting DFS [6, 7, 12, 25, 26]. In a recent and sobering report, for 16 recipients of DLI for relapsed MDS treated between 1993 and 2004, all 13 patients who did not respond died of their disease 3–20 months after DLI. Only 3 of 14 evaluable patients (21%) responded; one died of subsequent relapse less than 6 months from DLI, and two long-term responders died of toxicity 65 and 68 months after DLI. Nevertheless, there is compelling evidence that a meaningful GvL reaction will occur in some patients with MDS.

20.1.4 DLI for Acute Lymphocytic Leukemia

Although GvL activity against acute lymphocytic leukemia (ALL, a.k.a. acute lymphoblastic leukemia) is weak [2], the potential for DLI to induce remissions for relapsed ALL is well established. In fact, one of the first known cases of successful DLI was a child with relapsed ALL, who was in remission at least 15 years following the infusion [27].

Unfortunately, many subsequent reports using DLI for relapsed ALL have been disappointing. The EBMT reported that no patient with relapsed ALL achieved remission from DLI alone, and the median survival was less than 6 months after DLI; in addition, all patients who received chemotherapy or were in CR relapsed a median of 15 months after treatment [6]. Collins et al. described 44 patients treated in various ways at different centers for relapsed ALL [11]. Fifteen patients received no pre-DLI chemotherapy while the remainder were treated with chemotherapy and received DLI at their nadir. Regardless of pre-treatment, patients had uniformly poor outcomes. Of 15 patients who received no pre-DLI chemotherapy, only two (13%) responded. Response rates were 20% for the 25 recipients of DLI given at a chemotherapy-induced nadir. Five of these seven responders relapsed 42–1112 days after remission; overall survival was 13% at 3 years and only three patients remained alive and disease-free.

A more recent prospective trial included 10 relapsed ALL patients treated with standard chemotherapy and granulocyte-colony-stimulating factor (G-CSF)-stimulated DLI at nadir [28]. Although seven patients were in remission following treatment, two died of complications related to GvHD, four relapsed 120–991 days after CR, and only one remained alive in CR though over 3 years from DLI. Therefore, taken together, these data support an important GvL effect against ALL, but only in a minority of patients.

20.1.5 DLI in Myeloma, Non-Hodgkin's Lymphoma, and Hodgkin's Lymphoma

There is compelling data for a meaningful graft-versus-myeloma (GvM) effect after both conventional [29] and nonmyeloablative allogeneic HSCT [30, 31]. It is also clear that DLI can induce remissions in some patients who relapse after allogeneic HSCT [32]. However, while response rates of up to 60% have been reported, complete responses have occurred in only 25–30% of patients, and are sustained in 0–18% of patients [14, 15]. The North American multicenter analysis reported complete remissions in two of 22 patients who received DLI alone but both patients relapsed 10 and 26 weeks after CR [15]. Interestingly, Kroger et al. administered DLI in combination with low dose thalidomide to 18 patients with relapsed MM after allogeneic HSCT [33]. There were 12 responses, four complete remissions, and 100% estimated 2-year survival. The contribution of thalidomide versus DLI could not be separated but data suggest that other therapies may enhance response rates to DLI. These data highlight that DLI can generate a meaningful GvM effect for a minority of patients, but significant toxicity and relapse limit the success for myeloma.

While indirect evidence also suggests that non-Hodgkin's lymphoma (NHL) and Hodgkin's lymphoma (HL, a.k.a. Hodgkin's disease) are susceptible to graft-versus-lymphoma induction [34, 35], outcome data after DLI for relapse of NHL or HL are also quite limited. While no responses in six patients with NHL were reported to the North American DLI registry [7], a number of small reports do show that DLI can induce a meaningful graft-versus-lymphoma reaction [36, 37].

There is remarkably little data on the use of DLI for relapsed HL, though there is compelling evidence that a graft-versus-lymphoma reaction can be generated [38]. DLI has been used most frequently for relapse or persistent disease after nonmyeloablative allogeneic HSCT. Response rates of 56% (50% complete remissions) [39] and 54% [40] have been noted for recipients of DLI for relapsed HL. The M.D. Anderson Cancer Center Group reported four of nine (44%) DLI recipients responded for a median of 7 months but had only one ongoing response [41]. Therefore, cellular therapy for HL holds significant promise, but new methods to enhance and sustain graft-versus-lymphoma responses are clearly needed.

20.1.6 Unrelated Donor Lymphocyte Infusions

Donor lymphocyte infusions are being used with increasing frequency after unrelated donor HSCT (reviewed in [42]). A number of studies described above have included recipients of unrelated DLI (UDLI) [6, 7, 17], but in most cases specific outcomes compared to sibling DLI have not been provided. The two large retrospective studies suggested that UDLI and related DLI result in similar outcomes but included small numbers of patients [6, 7]. Two other studies have focused primarily on the role of unrelated DLI for relapsed disease. In one study for relapsed CML, outcomes after related DLI in 18 patients were compared directly to outcomes for 12 recipients of UDLI [43]. A cytogenetic remission was achieved in 73% of related DLI recipients compared to 64% of UDLI recipients ($p = 0.71$). There was a trend toward more grade II–IV acute GvHD after UDLI (58% vs. 39%) that did not reach statistical significance ($p = 0.09$) possibly due to the small numbers of patients studied. The incidence of chronic GvHD was 49% for all patients and was not dependent on the donor source. The only factor associated with response was disease stage at the time of DLI, similar to other reports [6, 7, 44]; patients treated in cytogenetic or molecular relapse were seven times more likely to respond when compared to patients treated in hematologic relapse.

In a larger retrospective analysis, 58 recipients of UDLI were identified through the National Marrow Donor Program database [44]. Patients received UDLI for relapse of CML ($n = 25$), AML ($n = 23$), ALL ($n = 7$) or other diseases ($n = 3$). The donor and recipient were HLA-mismatched in at least 21% of cases and the median cell dose administered was 1.0×10^8 mononuclear cells (MNC)/kg. For patients with active disease at the time of DLI, complete remissions were achieved in 46% of patients with CML, 42% of patients with AML, and two of four patients with ALL. The incidence of grade II–IV acute GvHD was 25% and chronic GvHD occurred in 41% of patients, both in keeping with data from large series of related DLI. The estimated disease-free survival (DFS) for all recipients at 1 year after complete remission was 65% for patients with CML, 23% for AML, and 30% for ALL. As anticipated, overall survival appeared superior for patients with early-phase relapse of CML compared with patients with advanced-phase relapse. There was no association of cell dose with GvHD, response, survival, or DFS. Only a longer time interval from transplant to relapse and transplant to UDLI was associated with improved survival and DFS respectively. There was also no obvious association between acute and chronic GvHD and disease response, in contrast to several [6, 7, 45], though not all [46] related DLI studies.

It should be noted that comparisons of UDLI to related DLI are difficult, largely because of the small numbers of patients studied, the relatively short follow-up in most studies, and the retrospective nature of the data. Nevertheless, the complete remission rates for recipients of UDLI appear at least similar to rates reported in related DLI studies [6, 7]. Given these data and the generally accepted poor outcome after relapse from unrelated donor HSCT, cellular therapy is clearly feasible and appears to be an appropriate approach for patients who relapse with leukemia after unrelated donor marrow grafting.

20.1.7 Complications of DLI

20.1.7.1 Graft-Versus-Host Disease

Acute and chronic GvHD are the major direct complications from DLI and develop in 40–60% of patients (for a review of GvHD after DLI see [47]). Severe acute GvHD (grade III–IV) develops in approximately 20–35% of conventional DLI recipients and has been associated with treatment related mortality rates of 10–20% [48]. It can take many weeks after infusion before manifestations of acute GvHD are noted. Chronic GvHD occurs in 30–60% of recipients of DLI. In most studies, GvHD correlates with GvL activity and response [6, 7]. In the North America analysis, over 90% of complete responders developed acute GvHD and 88% of responders developed chronic GvHD. Of 23 patients who did not experience GvHD, only three achieved a complete remission. In 92 patients who had no response, only 35% had acute GvHD and only 13% had chronic GvHD [7]. In the EBMT analysis, 41% of DLI recipients developed grade II–IV acute GvHD [6]. Interestingly, DLI from an unrelated donor carries a similar risk of GvHD as related donors [44]. However, it is also important to emphasize numerous complete responses are seen in patients without any sign of GvHD providing important evidence for GvL activity separate from GvHD.

20.1.7.2 Marrow Aplasia

Pancytopenia has been reported in 18–50% of recipients of DLI [6, 7], but sustained marrow aplasia occurs in only 2–5% of patients. Typically pancytopenia resolves without therapy, though in some cases, sustained marrow aplasia has been reversed successfully with infusion of additional donor stem cells [4, 49]. The cause of aplasia after DLI is not completely understood. It is likely in part a manifestation of GvHD, analogous to transfusion-associated GvHD. It may be most pronounced when there is little donor hematopoiesis to support hematologic recovery, since lack of residual donor chimerism can predict for marrow aplasia after DLI [49, 50]. However, the use of $CD34^+$ cell-enriched donor cells as the source of DLI does not seem to prevent pancytopenia in many cases [51] suggesting that other mechanisms may lead to pancytopenia.

20.2 Cellular Therapy After Allogeneic Stem Cell Transplantation for Nonrelapse Complications

The limited immune reconstitution after allogeneic HSCT can result in several major and potentially life-threatening infectious and malignant complications, and donor T cell infusions have been remarkable effective at restoring cell-mediated immunity and treating or preventing a number of nonrelapse complications after HSCT [52]. For instance, DLI has been dramatically effective treating Epstein–Barr Virus (EBV) associated post-transplant lymphoproliferative disorders (PTLD). PTLD is typically of donor origin, develops due to uncontrolled proliferation of EBV-infected B-cells in the absence of appropriate viral-specific immunity and T-cell regulation [53] and historically has been associated with a high mortality rate [54]. After allogeneic HSCT, T cells from a donor who has had prior EBV exposure will induce complete remission in the majority of patients with PTLD [55, 56]. More recently, EBV-specific T cells have been generated and expanded ex-vivo and used effectively to both treat and prevent EBV-related complications after allogeneic HSCT. Since these cells have EBV-specificity, there is minimal risk for GvHD or other complications [52, 57].

Donor leukocyte infusions have been effective for prevention of other viral complications after allogeneic HSCT. For instance, adoptive immunotherapy with cytomegalovirus (CMV)-specific T cells can restore CMV-specific immunity and prevent viral reactivation. In one example, $CD8^+$ T cells from CMV seropositive marrow donors were cloned and infused into transplant recipients [58, 59]. Transient survival of the T cell clones was documented, and an increase in the circulating CMV-specific cytotoxic T cells was noted in most cases. Although these cells did not persist in patients with poor $CD4^+$ helper function, no patient in this small cohort developed CMV viremia.

DLI have also been used to reverse acute life threatening infections after allogeneic HSCT caused by adenovirus [60] and respiratory syncytial virus [61]. These examples further emphasize the broad potential application of this therapy to treat infections after allogeneic HSCT. In the future, it is likely that allogeneic adoptive immunotherapy will have a wide range of clinical applications to both treat and prevent malignant and infectious complications after allogeneic cell transplantation.

20.2.1 Novel Approaches for Cellular Therapy After Allogeneic HSCT

The success of DLI remains limited both by lack of efficacy in all diseases but CML, and by toxicity largely related to GvHD. A number of innovative and novel approaches are being tested to both minimize GvHD and to improve responses to allogeneic cellular therapy (Table 20.2).

20.2.1.1 Low Dose DLI and Dose Escalation

In patients with relapse of early phase CML, a schedule of low dose DLI followed by dose escalation seems to minimize the risk of GvHD [46]. This strategy resulted in complete remissions in 86% of patients and only one patient developed acute GvHD. A retrospective analysis of 298 recipients of DLI similarly found that an initial low T cell dose ($\leq 2 \times 10^7$/kg) was associated with less GvHD and improved survival compared to recipients of who received higher initial T cell doses [62]. The treatment related mortality at 3 years was 5% with the low initial dose compared to 20% with the higher initial doses; the overall response rate was similar regardless of the initial T cell dose. This escalating dose strategy may not be practical for patients with relapse of more aggressive diseases such as acute leukemia, since rapid disease progression will occur before an effective GvL response can be generated in many cases.

It is not completely clear why dose escalation of DLI minimizes GvHD. In some cases, there is likely an important effector to target cell ratio responsible for GvL induction. However, protection from GvHD using dose escalation of DLI may not simply be due to infusion of lower cell doses over time. It is possible that the delayed administration of higher doses of DLI minimizes GvHD; for instance, T cell infusions given soon after transplant are more likely to induce severe GvHD than when delayed from the initial transplant [63, 64]. Homeostatic proliferation—the extensive expansion of T cells that happens in

Table 20.2 Newer approaches to donor leukocyte infusions

- Low dose DLI followed by dose escalation
- Depletion of GVHD reactive cells
- Graft-manipulation and infusion of selected T cell subsets (i.e. after $CD8^+$ cell depletion or $CD4^+$ cell selection)
- Inactivate alloreactive T cells (i.e., through engineering with suicide genes; photochemical inactivation; chemotherapy inactivation, irradiation)
- Tumor or antigen-specific T cells
- Minor histocompatibility antigen-specific T cells
- Lymphodepletion of host prior to DLI
- Ex-vivo activation and expansion of donor T cells through costimulation
- Generation and infusion of Th2 type T cells
- Infusion of T-regulatory cells

the setting of lymphopenia—could explain, at least in part, this early, more exuberant graft-versus-host reaction. Another intriguing explanation is that low doses of donor T cells (and/or delayed administration of additional DLI) may not induce an initial GvL reaction, but may result in generation of regulatory cells (or induction of anergy) that inhibit GvHD; only subsequent higher doses of DLI would be sufficient to overcome this effect and induce a GVH reaction. This possibility is supported by animal experiments showing that graft-versus-host tolerance could not be abrogated by the transfusion of lymphocytes from the marrow donor unless the donor was immunized against the recipient [65].

20.2.1.2 Depletion of GvHD Effector Cells

Data from preclinical models and after allogeneic HSCT implicate $CD8^+$ T cells as primary mediators of GvHD while $CD4^+$ cells seem most important for effective GvL induction. $CD8^+$-depleted DLI have been used to treat relapsed CML after allogeneic HSCT [66, 67], and outcomes suggest that GvL activity can be retained with minimal GvHD; in small numbers of patients, the majority of responses have been sustained [68], though the overall clinical impact of this approach will require direct comparison to unmanipulated DLI.

20.2.1.3 Inactivation of GvHD Effector Cells

Irradiated donor T cells have been given as DLI based on the hypothesis that they would induce GvL effects at the time of infusion but could not proliferate in response to allo-antigens; preliminary data suggest these cells do retain GvL activity and result in minimal GvHD [69]. Amotosalen-treated donor T cells can result in photochemical inactivation and have been tested as DLI in mice. These cells enhanced immune reconstitution, provided antiviral immunity, and were protective against a leukemia challenge without causing GvHD, suggesting that this novel clinical approach could separate GvHD and GvL activity [70].

20.2.1.4 Genetic Modification of Donor T Cells to Contain a Suicide Gene

A more specific approach designed to both limit and modulate GvHD without altering GvL reactivity has been the use of genetically modified donor cells engineered to contain a suicide-gene. The best example has been the development of donor lymphocytes transduced with the herpes simplex thymidine kinase (HSV-TK) gene, rendering these cells sensitive to treatment with ganciclovir [71]. HSV-TK modified T cells successfully induced complete remissions in patients with PTLD, and acute GvHD was effectively treated with ganciclovir; drug treatment resulted in a decrease in the number and activity of allo-reactive cells as well as a decrease in the number of cells containing the HSV-TK gene [72].

20.2.1.5 Tumor-Specific DLI

The most effective and efficient method of inducing GvL without GvHD would be to use tumor-specific T cells. Leukemia-specific donor T cells have been isolated and expanded in-vitro. Preliminary data in small numbers of patients demonstrate that this strategy is feasible and can induce complete remission for relapsed CML with minimal toxicity [73]. Unfortunately, this approach is not only quite complicated and time consuming, tumor reactive T cell clones cannot be isolated in the majority of cases. Furthermore, in most circumstances, the target antigens for GvL induction are not known. Reasons for this relative resistance to immunotherapy may include inadequate cell surface presentation of molecules that can be recognized by the donor T cells, failure to express costimulatory molecules [74], sanctuary sites, a rapid proliferative rate of the malignancy, or other mechanisms [75]. It is also possible that malignant stem cells may be more resistant to immunologic control than more mature leukemia cells.

In some cases GvL reactive targets may be leukemia specific [76, 77], a hypothesis supported by the fact that in some cases GvL occurs in the absence of clinical GvHD. In other cases the targets may be minor histocompatibility antigens differentially expressed on hematopoietic cells [78]. This would explain why in most (though not all) studies, GvHD is strongly associated with GvL. Cytotoxic T lymphocytes (CTL) have been generated against mismatched mHag that demonstrate leukemia-specific cell lysis in vitro [79, 80]. In three recipients of DLI for relapsed CML, an increase in mHag HA-1 and HA-2 specific $CD8^+$ T cells was noted [80]. Unfortunately, only a small minority of patients will have polymorphic differences with their HLA-matched donor for HA-1 and HA-2 mHags, restricting the potential use of these targets to limited numbers of patients.

Other minor histocompatibility antigens may be critical and may be the same antigens that are the targets of GvHD. For example this effect may be important when female donors are used for male recipients. Y chromosome encoded proteins are some of the best-studied mHags; they are unique to the recipient and can function as potent mediators of both GvL and GvHD [81, 82].

Proteinase 3 (P3) is another potential target antigen. It is over-expressed in myeloid leukemias and cytotoxic T cells specific for P3 and the HLA-A2 restricted P3 peptide PR1 have been found to lyse selectively CML cells in vitro [83]. A strong correlation between PR1-specific CTLs and clinical response after both interferon treatment and allogeneic BMT has been noted [84]. These findings support the use of P3 vaccination strategies [85] but also raise the possibility of using PR1-specific T cells for selective adoptive immunotherapy.

Wilm's tumor protein, WT1, is another endogenous host protein that is overexpressed in myeloid malignancies [86] that could serve as a tumor specific target for cellular therapy. Vaccine strategies using WT1 have been explored in animal models (reviewed in [86]), and it is logical to begin testing WT1 specific T cells generated and expanded in vitro as tumor-specific DLI. Other potential tumor-associated antigens that may serve as targets for immunotherapy include

NY-ESO-1, a cancer-testis antigen found also preferentially on myeloma cells [87], and the melanoma-associate antigen PRAME, an HLA-24 restricted antigen on AML cells [88].

Another attractive and obvious target for donor T cells would be the BCR/ABL protein, and in fact, CTLs reactive to BCR/ABL have been identified in CML patients [77]. Unfortunately, vaccination with a BCR/ABL fusion peptide did not induce cytotoxic T cells in CML patients [89]. It remains unknown if BCR/ABL is an important target antigen for GvL induction.

Generation of tumor-specific DLI can be quite laborious, and at least presently, this technology is confined to a limited number of research laboratories. Nevertheless, as the target antigens and effector cells for GvL induction become better characterized, new techniques for cell selection and expansion will allow tumor-specific adoptive immunotherapy to become reality.

20.2.1.6 Lymphodepletion Prior to DLI

A number of other methods are actively being tested to try and maximize GvL reactivity of allogeneic cellular therapy. Miller and colleagues used chemotherapy prior to DLI, hypothesizing that host lymphodepletion would result in donor T cell expansion and activation [90]. Fifteen patients were pretreated with fludarabine and high dose cyclophosphamide and received DLI 48 h after chemotherapy. This regimen resulted in significant lymphopenia and with evidence of T cell proliferation 14 days after chemotherapy, but the trial was stopped early because 47% of patients developed grade III–IV acute GvHD (accounting for 5 of 11 deaths). It is unclear whether the high rate of GvHD was due to lymphodepletion and lymphocyte expansion or possibly to the close proximity of DLI to chemotherapy and organ toxicity to the donor cell infusion. Regardless, this study raises additional concern about the routine use and timing of pre-DLI chemotherapy.

20.2.1.7 Ex-Vivo Costimulation and Expansion for Activated DLI

A different strategy to enhance GvL after DLI uses ex-vivo activated donor T cells for GvL induction. In vivo, inadequate T cell activation could occur for many reasons, including lack of costimulatory ligands on tumor cells, failure to present antigens to T cells, direct suppression of cytotoxic effector cells by suppressor T cells or cytokines, failure to stimulate $CD4^+$ cells, or quantitative lack of sufficient cytotoxic effector cells. Nonspecific activation and ex-vivo expansion could enhance the anti-tumor potential of donor T cells and overcome possible in-vivo suppression of T cell activation [91]; these cells could overcome disease-induced anergy, preserve and augment CD4 function, and enhance GvT activity. Activated donor T cells have been produced by costimulation and expansion through exposure to magnetic beads coated with anti-CD3 (OKT3) and anti-CD28 [92].

A phase I trial of ex-vivo costimulated and expanded cells, referred to as activated DLI, has been performed at the University of Pennsylvania. Conventional DLI was administered to all patients followed by escalating doses of ex-vivo costimulated donor T cells for relapse of diseases other than chronic phase CML after allogeneic HSCT [93]. Eight of 17 evaluable patients achieved a complete remission, including two of four patients with AML, four of seven patients with ALL, one patient with CLL, and one of two patients with NHL (mantle cell lymphoma). Although four complete responders subsequently relapsed, four were alive in remission a median 23 months after activated DLI. Activated DLI was well tolerated without excessive toxicity; only two patients developed grade III acute GvHD and four patients developed chronic GvHD. No patient died of complication related to GvHD. Overall, the response rates were impressive in diseases that historically do not respond well to DLI, suggesting that activated DLI may offer an advantage for GvL induction.

Ex-vivo expanded donor T cells have also been used in a slightly different strategy. Fowler et al. selectively expanded Th2 cells after nonmyeloablative allogeneic HSCT and found that these cells enhanced lymphocyte recovery without an apparent increase in GvHD [94]. It is not known if these cells possess GvT activity or might function only to limit GvHD without inhibiting GvT effects of other effector cells.

20.2.2 Activated T Cell Therapy After Autologous HSCT

There is significant rationale for considering autologous T cell therapy after autologous HSCT. It is well known that autologous HSCT results in significant and prolonged T cell deficiency, particularly when $CD34^+$-selected cells are used [95]. Furthermore, absolute lymphocyte counts after autologous HSCT have been associated with improved DFS and OS [96, 97]. Early lymphoid recovery therefore can be important to limit infectious complications, provide potential anti-tumor activity, and perhaps permit other effective immune modulation such as vaccine therapies.

However, there are a number of limitations to T cell therapy after autologous HSCT. Heavily pretreated patients may already be lymphopenic, and techniques for lymphoid expansion, until recently, have been limited. Techniques have now been developed to grow and expand $CD4^+$ T cells for adoptive transfer in clinical trials. One approach is based on the use of artificial antigen presenting cells composed of antibodies to CD3 (OKT-3) and CD28 immobilized on magnetic beads. T cells can therefore be activated and costimulated and can be expanded logarithmically [92].

An initial trial was performed in 16 patients with high risk NHL undergoing $CD34^+$-selected autologous HSCT [98]. Prior to HSCT, autologous T cells were collected and expanded ex-vivo and infused on day 14 after HSCT. The CD3/

CD28 culture procedure at least partially reversed impaired cytokine responsiveness in T cells in both in vitro and in vivo assays. Lymphocyte recovery was rapid and several patients developed delayed lymphocytosis. While 3 patients were alive and disease free, it was not possible to determine the contribution of the ex-vivo costimulated T cells to disease control in the pilot trial.

More recently, ex-vivo costimulated autologous T cells and pneumococcal vaccine were given as combined immunotherapy to patients with multiple myeloma after autologous HSCT [99]. Four groups of subjects were randomized to receive a T cell dependent pneumococcal vaccine (or not) prior to T cell apheresis and HSCT, and all subjects were vaccinated 30 and 90 days following HSCT. Groups then received either early infusion (day 12 following HSCT) or delayed infusion (day 100) of expanded T cells. The randomized design was able to show that a single infusion of costimulated T cells could accelerate T cell reconstitution. Importantly, this approach led to improved T cell proliferation in response to vaccine and nonvaccine antigens compared to patients who did not receive autologous T cells. Furthermore, the combined immunotherapy approach of early post-transplant infusion of in-vivo vaccine primed, ex-vivo expanded costimulated T cells and post-transplant immunizations improved severe immune defects found in control patients within 1 month after transplant. The group who received a pretransplant vaccine in addition to a booster had significantly higher pneumococcal titers on day 42, which were sustained; this marker of B cell function confirmed clinically significant, antigen specific, functional T cell help. This approach will clearly enhance the ability to perform effective post-transplant immunization against infectious organisms and now presents the promise of developing effective tumor-specific immunization strategies in the early post-transplant period.

20.3 Natural Killer Cell Therapy

It is clear that cells other than T cells also can effect potent anti-tumor responses both in vitro and in the setting of clinical HSCT. Natural killer (NK) cells are perhaps the most potent and best studied cellular component, other than T cells, with a great deal of potential for immunotherapy (reviewed also in Chap. 3 by Ruggeri, Zhang, and Farag). NK cells are innate immune effectors that mediate the nonspecific lysis of targets and produce inflammatory cytokines important in the innate immune response to tumors and viruses. NK cells can kill tumors without requiring prior sensitization, and they do not have memory. Their functions are regulated by a complex balance of activating and inhibitory signals transferred via several classes of receptors. Some receptors, including those in the killer immunoglobulin-like receptors (KIR) family, recognize "self" MHC class I antigens [100]. Self-tolerance is mediated by inhibitory KIR, which transmit signals that interrupt the cytolytic pathway after they bind their cognate class I HLA ligands. The loss of KIR-ligand expression by an infected or malignant target thus renders it susceptible to NK cell lysis. In addition, a number of activating receptors must be ligated to determine whether a target will be killed by NK cells. NK cells can be easily isolated in high quantity from donor lymphopheresis products and do not cause GvHD when infused. These characteristics make NK cells an attractive cell population to exploit for anti-tumor immunotherapy. Several clinical strategies have been developed using alloreactive NK cells for therapeutic benefit.

20.3.1 Biologic Basis of Cellular Therapy with NK Cells: Immunologic Principles

20.3.1.1 Definition of NK Cells

NK cells are large granular lymphocytes that were first described in 1975 for their ability to lyse virally infected and tumor targets without MHC-restriction or prior sensitization [101, 102]. In 1987 they were further characterized for their ability to mediate the rejection of allogeneic or parental-strain hematopoietic grafts in lethally irradiated mice [103], a function that was first noted in 1971 when the phenomenon of "hybrid resistance" was defined [104]. As effector cells of the innate immune system they play an important role in immune surveillance. Human NK cells are found in the bone marrow, spleen, lymph nodes, and peripheral blood (PB), where they compose approximately 10–15% of the lymphocyte pool. NK cells are defined phenotypically by their expression of CD56 and by their lack of T cell markers (CD3, CD4 and T cell receptors) and are distinct from $CD3^+/CD56^+$ lymphocytes, which are not NK cells. Blood NK cells are further categorized by their level of CD56 expression, which correlates with their effector functions. Approximately 10% of NK cells are $CD56^{bright}$, a subset that is more proliferative and produces more cytokines (especially IFN-γ), whereas the $CD56^{dim}$ subset is more cytotoxic and bears Fc receptors to mediate antibody dependent cellular cytotoxicity (ADCC) [105]. Cytokine-activated cells, sometimes referred to as lymphokine-activated killer (LAK) cells, show more proliferation, increased cytokine production, and higher cytotoxicity to kill targets than do resting NK cells [106]. NK cells respond to IL-2, IL-15 and IL-21, all of which signal via the IL-2 receptor β chain [107–109], as well as the combination of IL-12 and IL-18, which is an especially strong stimulant to increase IFN-γ production [110].

20.3.2 NK Cell Functions

20.3.2.1 Cytokine Production

NK cells are major producers of several cytokines such as granulocyte colony-stimulatory factor (G-CSF), granulocyte-macrophage colony-stimulatory factor (GM-CSF), IL-5, tumor necrosis factor (TNF), interferon gamma

(IFN-γ), and transforming growth factor beta (TGF-β). These, in turn, can stimulate or inhibit hematopoiesis and the effects of other immune cells. These cytokines and cell–cell interactions may stimulate dendritic cells (DC) to activate both NK cells and T cells, providing a link between the innate and adaptive immune systems [111]. The interaction between DC and NK cells leads to mutual co-activation of each cell type.

20.3.2.2 Cytotoxicity

NK cells have demonstrated in vivo anti-tumor cytotoxicity against both hematologic malignancies and a wide variety of solid tumors, including breast, ovarian, hepatocellular and colon cancer [112, 113], as well as against virally-infected cells. Most NK cells kill directly using perforin and granzyme, but they can also use Fas ligand (FasL) and tumor necrosis factor related apoptosis inducing ligand (TRAIL) pathways [114]. In addition, NK cells mediate antibody-dependent cellular cytotoxicity via CD16 (FcR(III), the Fc receptor that recognizes Ig coated targets [115]. The recognition and response to a wide array of foreign, damaged, malignant, and virally infected cells is regulated through a complex network of cell–cell interactions. NK cells express (β2 integrins and CD2, which bind to target adhesion molecules such as ICAM-1 and LFA-3. In addition, NK cells express several classes of activating and inhibitory receptors, which are both MHC class I-specific and nonspecific. The net balance of signals, dependent on both the target phenotype and the NK cell receptor repertoire, determines whether or not a target is lysed.

20.3.2.3 Class I Recognizing NK Cell Receptors

Human NK cells express killer immunoglobulin-like receptors (KIR), type I transmembrane molecules belonging to the Ig superfamily, which are all are encoded on chromosome 19. KIR are named by the number of extracellular immunoglobulin domains (2D or 3D) and the length of the intracellular tail, which determines whether they are stimulatory (short) or inhibitory (long). A nomenclature committee has assigned a cluster of designation (CD) number of CD158 for the KIR genes with individual loci designated by a small letter ± a number (e.g., KIR3DL1 = CD158e1) [116]. All individuals contain the framework genes KIR3DL3, KIR2DL4, and KIR3DL2. In addition, a variable number of activating and inhibitory genes are inherited, and population studies show different evolutionary patterns [117]. Individuals with only one activating receptor (2DS4) are referred to as having an A KIR haplotype. Individuals with more than one activating receptor are referred to as having a B KIR haplotype. These genes are highly polymorphic, and new alleles continue to be reported. Some of these polymorphisms are functionally important. For example, KIR3DL1*004 is not expressed on the surface, so it cannot function to recognize ligand [118]. Murine NK cells do not express KIR but do express Ly49 receptors of the same class [119]. While the ligands for many KIR are unknown, the inhibitory receptors KIR2DL1, KIR2DL2/KIR2DL3, and KIR3DL1 bind HLA class I C2, C1, and Bw4 alleles, respectively. The KIR repertoire is determined primarily by KIR genotype and at steady state is only minimally affected by class I HLA (KIR-ligand) genes, which segregate independently (chromosome 6). The recognition of self-class I HLA by the higher affinity inhibitory receptors suppresses NK cell effector responses, including cell mediated lysis and cytokine release [120]. Both human and murine NK cells express CD94, which heterodimerizes with the NKG2 family of C-type lectin receptors. They are either inhibitory (NKG2A) or activating (NKG2C/E) and recognize nonclassical HLA-E [121]. NKG2D is unique in that it does not heterodimerize with CD94, and it recognizes stress-induced molecules such as MHC class I polypeptide-related sequence A/B (MICA and MICB) and the class I like CMV homologous ULBP proteins, which are often upregulated on tumor or virally infected cells [122, 123] NK cells also express Ig-like transcript (ILT) receptors, some of which bind classic HLA or HLA-G, expressed in the placenta and on fetal tissue. Several other receptors have been identified that regulate killing of MHC class I-negative targets, including but not limited to the natural cytotoxicity receptors (NCR) NKp30, NKp46, and NKp44; 2B4, which binds CD48; and leukocyte-associated immunoglobulin-like receptor-1 (LAIR-1).

20.3.2.4 NK Cell Alloreactivity

In 1985 Ljunggren and Karre described the phenomenon of "missing self," by which the loss of MHC class I expression renders autologous targets more sensitive to NK-mediated killing, providing a mechanism by which these innate killer cells can recognize tumor or virally-infected cells [124]. The discovery of class I-specific inhibitory KIR and the observation that cloned NK cells all express self-inhibitory receptors [125] led to the belief that mature peripheral blood NK cells must express "at least one" inhibitory NKR for self-MHC class I to prevent autoreactivity [126]. Although recent reports of murine [127] and human [128, 129] NK cells lacking self-inhibitory receptors challenge this model of autoreactivity, the concept remains important for clinical applications involving alloreactive NK cell clones that may be generated by using donor NK cells expressing inhibitory KIR for which the recipient lacks the appropriate ligand (Fig. 20.4).

20.3.2.5 Understanding the Role of Activating NK Cell Receptors

The stepwise evolution of the innate and adaptive immune systems in response to viral pathogens is well illustrated by the example of murine cytomegalovirus (MCMV). Although the downregulation of MHC class I expression in infected cells allows them to evade recognition by T cells, it makes them good NK cell targets. MCMV also upregulates the expression of the m144 gene, a

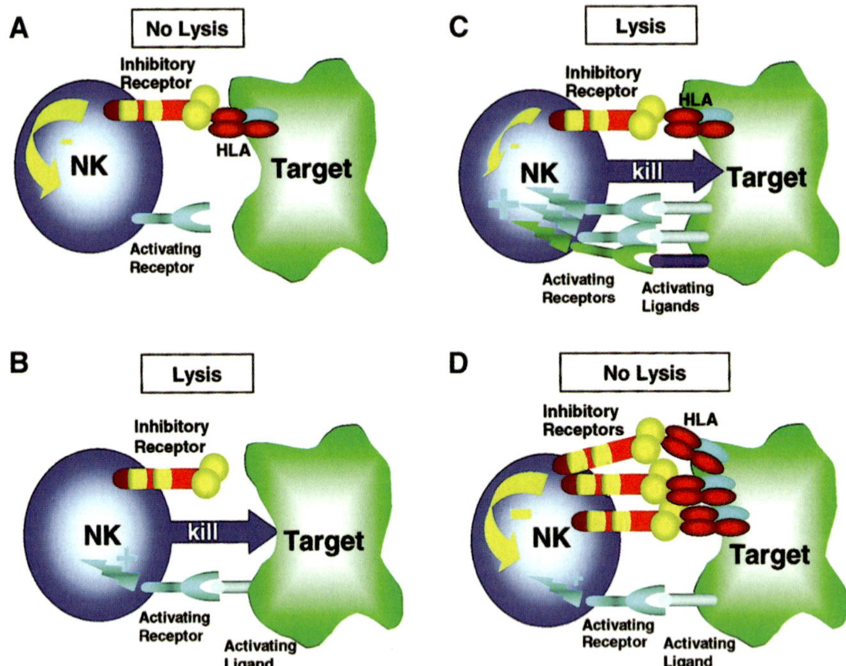

Fig. 20.4 Regulation of NK cell response by activating and inhibitory receptors. Inhibitory receptors (e.g., inhibitory KIR, CD94/NKG2A) recognize and engage their ligands, MHC class I molecules (HLA) on the surface of the target tumor cell, thereby initiating an inhibitory signal. Activating receptors (e.g., activating KIR, CD94/NKG2C, NKG2D) bind ligands on the target cell surface and trigger NK cell activation and target cell lysis. (**a**) When inhibitory receptors engage HLA in the absence of an activating receptor/ligand interaction, a net negative signal is generated, resulting in no target cell lysis. (**b**) Conversely, when activating receptors engage their ligands on target cells in the absence of inhibitory receptor/ligand interaction, a net activation signal is generated, resulting in target cell lysis. This scenario is likely operative in NK alloreactivity in the setting of KIR epitope mismatch. More complex physiologic scenarios are shown in **c** and **d** with both inhibitory and activating receptor/ligand signals being generated when an NK cell interacts with a target cell. (**c**) Here, the activating receptor/ligand interactions predominate over weaker inhibitory receptor/ligand signals with the net result of NK cell activation and target cell lysis. This net result may occur when activation receptors and ligands are upregulated, thereby amplifying the net activation signal to exceed the inhibitory signal. For example, the activating ligands MICA/B and ULBPs are expressed highly in stressed or transformed cells, thereby activating NKG2D/PI3K pathways that are not susceptible to inhibitory signals (see text for details). Alternatively, when expression of self-MHC class I ligands is decreased in the setting of viral infection or transformation, the net signal may be positive, also resulting in target cell lysis. (**d**) Here, inhibitory receptor/ligand interactions result in a net negative signal that prevents NK cell lysis of the target cell. This process may occur constantly as NK cells survey normal host tissues. Not shown is the scenario of absence of both inhibitory and activating signals that results in no NK cell activation. Reprinted with permission from Farag et al. [185]

mimic of MHC class I, which is recognized by NK cell inhibitory receptors, protecting the cell. In response, murine NK cells express Ly49H, an activating receptor, which recognizes the MCMV glycoprotein m157 [130, 131]. This case in point provides "proof of principle" that activating receptors may recognize viral proteins. A similar role for human activating receptors is supported by studies of patients with HIV, showing an association between AIDS progression and the activating receptor KIR3DS1 [132]. It has recently been shown that this activating KIR does not directly recognize Bw4 as its cognate ligand. It is presumed that infectious natural ligands for activating KIR will be discovered, somewhat analogous to the role of conserved pathogen associated microbial proteins (PAMPs) and toll-like receptors [133].

20.3.2.6 NK Cell Development

Human NK cells are derived from $CD34^+$, $CD38^-$, HLA DR^-, lin-1^- marrow-derived progenitors. Their maturation is induced by IL-15, fms-like tyrosine kinase 3 (flt3) ligand, c-kit ligand or stem cell factor (SCF), IL-7, and IL-3 [134-136]. Discrete stages of NK cell development in lymphoid tissues are defined by the acquisition of IL-15-responsiveness [137]. The $CD56^{bright}$ subset, which is more proliferative, may be more primitive than $CD56^{dim}$ NK cells. The $CD56^{dim}$ subset expresses high frequency of KIR, the variegated expression of which is controlled by transcriptional regulation of several homologous promoters under epigenetic control [138, 139]. In healthy subjects the KIR repertoire is predicted mainly by the KIR genotype, although it is influenced by HLA class I KIR ligand status [140]. The wide allelic variation in KIR genes includes several common alleles exhibiting poor or no surface expression [118, 141-143]. Interestingly, while NKG2A is increased, KIR expression is decreased on NK cells reconstituting in patients after allogeneic HSCT. This may be partially explained by a significantly higher frequency of $CD56^{bright}$ cells present after transplant, suggesting that there is a developmental delay in this lineage similar to that seen in T cells [129]. Developing strategies to manipulate KIR repertoire formation may be important since the frequency of KIR expression correlates with clinical outcomes [116, 144].

20.3.2.7 Development of Self-tolerance

The developmental mechanism by which NK cells acquire function yet remain self-tolerant has been referred to as NK cell education. Several models have been proposed to explain the integration of inhibitory receptor expression with the acquisition of effector functions. "Disarming" refers to the suppression of effector function in maturing NK cells that receive stimulatory signals unopposed by inhibitory signals via self-MHC receptors, analogous to the development of T cell anergy [145]. "Licensing" describes a terminal differentiation step by which NK cells only acquire mature function when they receive an appropriate signal via an inhibitory receptor ligating with self-MHC

[146, 147]. Alternatively, self-tolerance may be the result of a coordinated genetic developmental sequence during which mature NK function is synchronized with the acquisition of adequate expression of self-inhibitory molecules [129, 148].

20.3.3 NK Cell Clinical Applications

20.3.3.1 Early Autologous NK Cell-Based Therapy

The first therapeutic trials using adoptive immunotherapy were performed in the 1980s when several groups tested autologous lymphokine-activated killer (LAK) cells to treat a variety of malignancies. Peripheral blood mononuclear cells were stimulated ex vivo with IL-2 and then re-infused with high-dose IL-2 to treat immune-sensitive malignancies including melanoma, lymphoma, and renal cell cancer. Although it was shown that the cytotoxicity was mainly mediated by NK cells, limited clinical benefit was seen [149]. The significant toxicity of the capillary leak syndrome induced by high-dose IL-2 led to trials using low-dose subcutaneous IL-2, either alone or in combination with LAK cells, to activate patient NK cells in vivo. These strategies failed to show efficacy in patients with CML, lymphoma, and breast cancer [150].

Subsequent discoveries explained the failure of autologous LAK and NK-cell based therapies. Many groups demonstrated that because host lymphocytes compete with infused cells for access to cytokines and other growth factors, successful expansion of adoptively transferred lymphocytes requires adequate lymphodepletion or "clearing of space" [151]. Rosenberg's group at the NIH developed a successful therapy for melanoma using cyclophosphamide (60 mg/kg/day $\times$ 2) followed by fludarabine (25 mg/m^2/day $\times$ 5 days) to induce T cell lymphopenia prior to the infusion of cytotoxic T cells [152]. While the induction of lymphopenia prior to the adoptive transfer of NK cells may enhance their expansion, investigators abandoned autologous strategies after the discovery of inhibitory KIR and their role in preventing NK cell killing of "self" MHC-expressing tumor cells. The inherent self-tolerance of autologous NK cells prompted researchers to explore the use of allogeneic donor sources.

20.3.4 Allogeneic NK Cell Therapy

20.3.4.1 Rationale

The current generation of therapeutic trials uses allogeneic NK cells and is based on a better understanding of the signaling pathways that regulate the anti-tumor activity of NK cells. Tumors that express ligands for activating NK receptors have proven to be more responsive targets to NK cell-based strategies, but it is difficult to alter tumor phenotype in vivo. Therefore, more interest has been focused on ways to manipulate the interactions between inhibitory KIR and their ligands. The selection of NK cell or stem cell donors based on their KIR ligand status in relation to the patient would, in theory, increase the potential for NK cell alloreactivity. Enthusiasm for this strategy was generated by the 2002 report from Perugia in which Ruggeri et al. published that KIR ligand mismatch between patients and their donors was associated with improved outcomes in myeloid leukemia after T cell deplete haploidentical HSCT [153].

20.3.4.2 Allogeneic NK Cell Strategies

The two main strategies to harness the therapeutic power of alloreactive NK cells are (1) HSCT (see Chap. 3 by Ruggeri, Zhang, and Farag) and (2) adoptive transfer of NK cells. Each approach has its own advantages and disadvantages. Adoptively transferred NK cells, obtained either from donor lymphopheresis products or from umbilical cord blood units, can be expanded either in vitro or in vivo. As ex vivo expansion techniques have not been perfected, currently most clinical protocols include a preparative regimen of lymphodepleting chemotherapy [154] to facilitate in vivo expansion of the adoptively transferred NK cells. Treatment-related toxicity is minimal because NK cells do not induce GvHD. However, the efficacy of adoptive transfer protocols is limited by the transient nature of the NK anti-tumor effect. Alternatively, the beneficial effects of alloreactive NK cells can be incorporated into allogeneic HSCT protocols by selecting donors based on one of several KIR mismatch algorithms. While these strategies assume the risks of HSCT (higher treatment-related mortality, GvHD, etc.) they provide a permanently engrafted potentially alloreactive NK cell pool which can provide ongoing anti-tumor activity. A third option, to include adoptively transferred NK cells in standard HSCT protocols, may incorporate advantages of both strategies while lessening the cumulative toxicity associated with two separate therapeutic procedures.

20.3.4.3 Determination of NK Cell Alloreactivity

Regardless of the treatment strategy, the first step is to select a suitable allogeneic donor. The subtleties between the various methods by which the potential for KIR alloreactivity between donor and recipient has been defined have caused confusion. The Perugia group used the KIR-ligand mismatch or KIR-ligand incompatibility model, which predicts that donor-derived NK cells will be alloreactive in the GvH direction when recipients lack C2, C1 or Bw4 alleles that are present in the donor. This model assumes that donors express inhibitory KIR for their HLA class I KIR ligands, and does not predict NK alloreactivity using HLA compatible transplants or for the approximately 1/3 of recipients who express all three KIR ligands. A KIR ligand match calculator based on this model, which requires knowledge of both the donor and recipient HLA types, is available on the Immuno Polymorphism Database (IPD) http://www.ebi.ac .uk/ipd/kir/ligand.html. Alternatively, the KIR-ligand absence model categorizes recipients based on their C2, C1, and Bw4 allele status with no regard to the donor status. As most human populations have high frequencies of inhibitory KIR specific for C2, C1, and Bw4 alleles, it is assumed that most donor-derived NK cells will express inhibitory KIR, and that alloreactive potential is based on the number of KIR ligands a recipient lacks. The receptor-ligand model is based on a comparison of the donor inhibitory KIR genotype with the recipient KIR ligand status, where it is not assumed that donor class I HLA type can be used as predictor of inhibitory KIR expression. As KIR genes have multiple alleles with variable functional activity and expression levels, this model may be more precise if based not just on donor KIR genotype but on functional measures of KIR phenotype. This model allows for NK alloreactivity in HLA identical transplants where recipients lack KIR ligands for inhibitory KIR expressed on self-tolerant clones in the donor that may be alloreactive in the post-transplant setting.

20.3.4.4 Adoptive NK Cell Transfer with In Vivo Expansion

Adoptive cellular transfer allows for short-term anti-tumor activity using alloreactive NK cells. While many investigators are developing techniques for ex vivo NK cell expansion there are several potential limitations. Most importantly, NK cells stimulated by supraphysiologic concentrations of cytokines tend to undergo apoptosis when removed from ongoing stimulation and may not persist or expand in vivo. In addition marked size changes occur with activation which may alter homing characteristics in vivo. Consequently, it seems appropriate to develop strategies for in vivo NK cell expansion. The safety and success of this approach was established in a trial using in vivo expanded haploidentical, related-donor NK cell infusions to treat 43 patients with metastasis melanoma, metastatic renal cell carcinoma, refractory HL, and refractory AML [155]. The trial, which tested three preparative chemotherapy regimens of differing intensity, confirmed that successful NK cell expansion was only seen in the AML cohort who received the fully lymphodepleting cyclophosphamide and fludarabine regimen used by Rosenberg. Patients received NK cell infusions on day 0 following one or two doses of intravenous cyclophosphamide (60 mg/kg) days 4 and 5 and daily intravenous fludarabine (25 mg/m^2) days 5 to 1, followed by 10 million units of subcutaneous IL-2 administered over 2 weeks. Successful expansion was only seen in higher-dose cyclophosphamide and fludarabine, which was the only regimen to induce pancytopenia. Additionally, it was the only one to induce a surge of endogenous IL-15 after chemotherapy. A significant inverse correlation was seen between the IL-15 levels and the absolute lymphocyte count, and high levels correlated with successful NK cell expansion, supporting the importance of IL-15 for NK cell homeostasis.

In vivo expansion of NK cells was assessed using a PCR-based chimerism assay, with successful expansion defined by the presence of measurable donor NK cells at 2 weeks, following the IL-2 therapy. Eight of 15 evaluable patients had successful in vivo NK cell expansion, and the circulating donor-derived NK cells were functional in standard cytotoxicity assays. Clinical efficacy correlated with in vivo NK expansion and KIR ligand mismatch. Of the 19 patients with poor prognosis AML, five achieved complete remissions. The remission patients had significantly higher proportions of circulating NK cells, which were significantly more cytotoxic against K562 targets, suggesting that the observed clinical efficacy was mediated in part by the in vivo-expanded allogeneic donor NK cells. Furthermore, in this small cohort four of the 19 NK donors were predicted to exhibit alloreactivity based on KIR ligand mismatch in the GvH direction. CR was achieved in three of the four (75%) KIR ligand mismatch and only two of 15 (13%) KIR ligand match patients, supporting a role for KIR ligand mismatching in the treatment of AML.

Adoptive transfer of allogeneic NK cells is being studied in several other disease settings. Currently testing of NK cell expansion and anti-tumor activity is ongoing using the same protocol to treat metastatic breast cancer, which is sensitive to NK cell lysis in vitro [156]. There are also plans to treat NHL, chronic lymphocytic leukemia, and ovarian cancer, and other investigators are beginning to explore adoptively transferred NK cells for the treatment of multiple myeloma, hepatocellular carcinoma, melanoma, and renal cell carcinoma [157, 158].

Another approach to achieve the aforementioned benefits of NK alloreactivity has been to incorporate adoptive transfer of allogeneic NK cells into standard HSCT protocols. NK cell products are infused either prior to or during the early recovery phase. To test the potential NK-mediated effects protocols have been developed for patients with poor prognosis AML that combine the infusion of allogeneic haploidentical or umbilical cord blood (UCB)-derived NK cell products with standard haploidentical or UCB HSCT after nonmyeloablative vs. fully ablative preparative regimens, respectively. Other groups are using NK cell DLI after haploidentical HSCT to consolidate engraftment in adults with AML [159] or children with leukemia and solid tumors [160].

20.3.4.5 Therapeutic Limitations and Future Directions for NK Cell Therapy

There are several potential limitations to the therapeutic potential of adoptively transferred allogeneic NK cells. The NK cell yield from lymphopheresis collections is limited. Although NK cells can be successfully expanded in vivo, the success is unpredictable, and the expanded cell population circulates for a limited period. Additionally, the homing signals required to direct NK cells to tumor sites are not fully understood. Furthermore, the alloreactivity of in vivo expanded NK cell populations may be heterogeneous due to variable KIR repertoire expression or to differences in NK cell or accessory cell subsets. The use of monoclonal antibodies that block NK cell inhibitory receptors may increase anti-tumor killing [161], and more sophisticated techniques for subset selection in NK cell products may affect the interaction between the innate and adaptive immune responses; for example, removing any regulatory T cells that can suppress NK cell proliferation and killing may also improve the immune effector functions of the expanding NK cells [162]. NK cell expansion may be improved by refining the use of lymphodepleting chemotherapy or the use of concurrent exogenous cytokine therapy. Irradiated cell lines such as NK92 and KHYG-1 may provide an inexhaustible supply of highly cytotoxic NK cells, but their in vivo survival is not well known [163, 164]. Alternatively, large numbers of NK cells may be derived from umbilical cord blood sources [134]. Ex vivo expanded cells from any source can be genetically modified to express tumor-specific receptors. For example the NK92 cell line has been transfected with a chimeric antigen receptor for HER2/neu, which conferred superior cytotoxicity against HER2/neu positive targets [165]. Lastly, the anti-tumor activity of NK cells depends not only on the KIR ligand mismatch status, but also on tumor expression of appropriate activating ligands. For example, the lack of efficacy of KIR mismatched transplants in lymphoid leukemias may be due to their low expression of LFA-1 or NKG2D-ligands. Future strategies to enhance activating ligand expression on tumor cells are needed to increase their susceptibility to NK cell mediated lysis. Other avenues of research for NK cell immunotherapy include engineering NK cells with transferred genes, incorporating NK cells into dendritic cell vaccine therapies, and combination therapy with immunomodulatory drugs such as thalidomide, toll-like receptor agonists, and monoclonal antibodies to target ADCC.

20.4 Regulation of Immune Function with Cellular Therapy After Stem Cell Transplantation

In addition to the potential for direct anti-tumor activity, there is a great deal of interest in, and rationale behind, using cellular therapy for immune modulation. A great deal of evidence now supports the role of a specific population of T cells capable of regulating immune reactivity. In addition, some nonhematopoietic cells, such as mesenchymal stromal cells (MSC), appear to be important mediators of immune function. It is now possible to isolate and manipulate these cell populations and a number of clinical trials are underway to test the potential of cellular therapy for immune regulation after HSCT.

20.4.1 Regulatory T Cell Therapy

Adoptive immunotherapy with regulatory T cells (Treg) after transplant holds promise as a different and exciting means of controlling GvHD while maintaining anti-tumor efficacy. Tregs are distinguished by a $CD4^{+}CD25^{+}Foxp3^{+}$ phenotype; low/absent expression of the IL-7 receptor (CD127) may further improve the specificity for defining Tregs [166, 167]. In animal models, eradication of tumor with concomitant suppression of lethal GvHD was observed when nonphysiologic ratios of Tregs to conventional T cells were transferred [168]. Isolation and ex vivo expansion of Treg for clinical use has been shown to be feasible [169]. Culture conditions generally require high concentrations of IL-2; expansion in the presence of rapamycin appears to favor Treg proliferation [170, 171]. A clinical trial using prophylactic DLI with isolated naturally occurring Treg is ongoing in Europe; a clinical trial using expanded Treg (via CD3/CD28 costimulation) is expected to open soon in the United States [172]. However, since Tregs are in part defined by CD25 expression, it is important to determine if these products are contaminated with activated T cells, and careful safety analyses will be needed for any adoptive immunotherapy trial.

In addition to naturally occurring Tregs, which develop in the thymus, there is another, inducible T cell population with regulatory/suppressive activity that has been described as T regulatory type 1 (Tr1) cells [173]. These antigen specific cells arise in the periphery in the presence of IL-10, and have a unique suppressive cytokine profile that regulates T cells, APCs, and B cells. As of yet, these cells cannot be distinguished by cell surface markers but can be generated ex vivo in the presence of recipient cells and IL-10 with the goal of culturing cells with GvHD suppressive properties; Tr1 cells are currently in clinical trials of haploidentical HSCT [172]. Together, these clinical studies of T cells with regulatory function will lead to further studies of adoptive immunotherapy for both GvHD and disease relapse.

20.4.2 Mesenchymal Stromal Cells

Nonhematopoietic stem cells (embryonic and adult tissue derived), capable of giving rise to a variety of somatic tissues, have been of great interest in regenerative medicine. Among the first adult derived cells described from bone marrow and other tissues are MSC, which are fibroblast-like plastic adherent cells of nonhematopoietic cell origin [174]. Although they are termed mesenchymal stem cells by several investigators, the International Society for Cellular Therapy position paper encouraged a name change to mesenchymal stromal cells (MSC) to accurately reflect the fact that many reports do not qualify these cells as stem cells and because not all MSC are alike [175]. Part of the difficulty in comparing MSC between labs are differences in culture techniques and the lack of distinct surface antigens that accurately distinguish developmental maturity or differentiating capacity. The major interest in MSC in HSCT is their potential immunomodulatory effects.

MSC have been described to produce a number of cytokines [176] or to suppress allogeneic T cells stimuli in mixed lymphocyte reaction assays or by other nonspecific stimuli [177]. More detailed in vitro studies show that MSC can alter the cytokine secretion profile of dendritic cells (DC), T cell, and NK cells to induce a tolerant phenotype [178]. Specifically, MSC can mature type 1 DC to decrease TNF-a secretion, mature type 2 DC to increase the suppressive factor IL-10, and can cause an increase in regulatory T cells. These changes lead to a shift from TH1 to TH2 responses in T cells and a decrease in interferon-g production by NK cells. Taken together, these reports and studies transplanting human cells into immunodeficient mice [179, 180] suggest that MSC may play a role in facilitating engraftment and modulating GvHD much like the Treg discussed above. One concern about these reports is whether all the in vitro findings will be important in vivo. This concern is highlighted by a study evaluating the effects of mouse MSC. Although these murine MSC have potent suppressive effects on T cells in vitro, they had no clinical benefit on the incidence or severity in a bone marrow transplant model. Clinical trials using human MSC are under study in several centers.

The first report of clinical use of human MSC was by Koc et al. in which autologous MSC were infused in women with breast cancer [181]. Conclusions from this study were MSC infusions were safe, and hematopoietic recovery was rapid, but this phase I-II study could not definitively compare effects on engraftment. In 2004, LeBlanc and colleagues first reported clinical benefit in treating grade IV GvHD of the gut and liver after two infusions of $1\text{–}2 \times 10^6$ haploidentical MSC [182]. A follow-up study by this group in eight patients showed six responses demonstrating the potential promise of this therapy [183]. MSC have been safely coinfused with HSCT after sibling transplant [184], and other trials are in progress. In summary, MSC remain a promising cellular therapy to enhance the safety of or to treat complications of HSCT.

20.5 Conclusions and Future Directions

It is clear that adoptive immunotherapy can provide powerful anti-tumor activity in hematologic malignancies, and the challenge is now to enhance its efficacy while limiting toxicity. Better insight into factors promoting isolated GvT activity without GvHD is needed to improve the safety of cellular therapy; NK cell therapies have the advantage of providing anti-tumor effects without GvHD, and the optimal role of NK cells is being actively investigated. Common to all cellular therapeutic approaches is that disease type and stage and time to relapse are highly predictive of response, highlighting the need for more effective therapies and earlier interventions. Novel combinations of immunomodulatory drugs and cytokines may enhance tumor responses, especially in those diseases for which responses to conventional DLI are disappointing.

Strategies aimed at the problem of waning immunity following allogeneic HSCT or successful DLI are being developed. New approaches using prophylaxis, repeated dosing, and dose escalation of DLI, are now feasible with modern ex vivo expansion techniques. For both NK and T cell therapies—both allogeneic and autologous—it is being increasingly recognized that lymphodepletion significantly alters both response to immunization and toxicity. More insight into the basic mechanisms of both tumor immune escape and the role of lymphodepletion/homeostatic proliferation of T cells is needed, and should translate into safer and more effective therapeutic strategies. Regulatory T cell expansion (ex vivo or in vivo) may be able to modulate graft-versus-host reactions, and may prove useful both for active treatment of GvHD and for improving the therapeutic window of cellular therapy in general. Ultimately, new insights into the identity of important target antigens and the biologic mechanisms of GvT activity will allow optimization of cellular therapy after HSCT and will dramatically alter the ability to harness and transfer these powerful immune cells to cure human disease.

Acknowledgments This work was supported in part by grants from The Leukemia & Lymphoma Society (7000-02) and NIH (K24 CA11787901) (DLP) and P01 CA111412 and P01 CA65493 (JM).

References

1. Barnes D, Loutit J. Treatment of murine leukaemia with x-rays and homologous bone marrow. Br J Haematol. 1957;3:241–52.
2. Horowitz M, Gale R, Sondel P, Goldman J, Dersey J, Kolb H, Rimm A, Ringden O, Rozman C, Speck B, Truitt R, Zwaan F, Bortin M. Graft-versus-leukemia reactions after bone marrow transplantation. Blood 1990;75:555–62.
3. Kolb H, Mittermuller J, Clemm C, Holler E, Ledderose G, Brehm G, Heim M, Wilmanns W. Donor leukocyte transfusions for treatment of recurrent chronic myelogenous leukemia in marrow transplant patients. Blood 1990;76:2462–5.
4. Porter D, Roth M, McGarigle C, Ferrara J, Antin J. Induction of graft-versus-host disease as immunotherapy for relapsed chronic myeloid leukemia. N Engl J Med. 1994;330:100–6.
5. Bacigalupo A, Soracco M, Vassallo F, Abate M, Van Lint MT, Gualandi F, Lamparelli T, Occhini D, Mordini N, Bregante S, Figari O, Benvenuto F, Sessarego M, Fugazza G, Carlier P, Valbonesi M. Donor lymphocyte infusions (DLI) in patients with chronic myeloid leukemia following allogeneic bone marrow transplantation. Bone Marrow Transplant. 1997;19:927–32.
6. Kolb H, Schattenberg A, Goldman J, Hertenstein B, Jacobsen N, Arcese W, Ljungman P, Ferrant A, Verdonck L, Niederwieser D, van Rhee F, Mittermueller J, de Witte T, Holler E, Ansari H. Graft-versus-leukemia effect of donor lymphocyte transfusions in marrow grafted patients. Blood 1995;86:2041–50.
7. Collins R, Shpilberg O, Drobyski W, Porter D, Giralt S, Champlin R, Goodman S, Wolff S, Hu W, Verfaillie C, List A, Dalton W, Ognoskie N, Chetrit A, Antin J, Nemunaitis J. Donor leukocyte infusions in 140 patients with relapsed malignancy after allogeneic bone marrow transplantation. J Clin Oncol. 1997;15:433–44.
8. Levine J, Braun T, Penza S, Beatty P, Cornetta K, Martino R, Drobyski W, Barrett A, Porter D, Giralt S, Horowitz M, Leis J, Johnson M, Collins R. Prospective trial of chemotherapy and donor leukocyte infusions for relapse of advanced myeloid malignancies after allogeneic stem cell transplantation. J Clin Oncol. 2002;20:405–12.
9. Schmid C, Labopin M, Nagler A, Bornhauser M, Finke J, Fassas A, Volin L, Gurman G, Maertens J, Bordigoni P, Holler E, Ehninger G, Polge E, Gorin NC, Kolb HJ, Rocha V. Donor lymphocyte infusion in the treatment of first hematological relapse after allogeneic stem-cell transplantation in adults with acute myeloid leukemia: a retrospective risk

factors analysis and comparison with other strategies by the EBMT Acute Leukemia Working Party. J Clin Oncol. 2007;25:4938–45.
10. Choi SJ, Lee JH, Kim S, Seol M, Lee YS, Lee JS, Kim WK, Chi HS, Lee KH. Treatment of relapsed acute myeloid leukemia after allogeneic bone marrow transplantation with chemotherapy followed by G-CSF-primed donor leukocyte infusion: a high incidence of isolated extramedullary relapse. Leukemia 2004;18:1789–97.
11. Collins RH Jr, Goldstein S, Giralt S, Levine J, Porter D, Drobyski W, Barrett J, Johnson M, Kirk A, Horowitz M, Parker P. Donor leukocyte infusions in acute lymphocytic leukemia. Bone Marrow Transplant. 2000;26:511–16.
12. Campregher PV, Gooley T, Scott BL, Moravec C, Sandmaier B, Martin PJ, Deeg HJ, Warren EH, Flowers ME. Results of donor lymphocyte infusions for relapsed myelodysplastic syndrome after hematopoietic cell transplantation. Bone Marrow Transplant. 2007;40:965–71.
13. Lokhorst HM, Schattenberg A, Cornelissen JJ, Thomas LL, Verdonck LF. Donor leukocyte infusions are effective in relapsed multiple myeloma after allogeneic bone marrow transplantation. Blood 1997;90:4206–11.
14. Lokhorst HM, Schattenberg A, Cornelissen JJ, van Oers MH, Fibbe W, Russell I, Donk NW, Verdonck LF. Donor lymphocyte infusions for relapsed multiple myeloma after allogeneic stem-cell transplantation: predictive factors for response and long-term outcome. J Clin Oncol. 2000;18:3031–7.
15. Salama M, Nevill T, Marcellus D, Parker P, Johnson M, Kirk A, Porter D, Giralt S, Levine J, Drobyski W, Barrett A, Horowitz M, Collins R. Donor leukocyte infusions for multiple myeloma. Bone Marrow Transplant. 2000;26:1179–84.
16. Porter D, Collins R, Drobyski W, Connors J, Van Hoef M, Antin J. Long-term follow-up of 55 patients who achieved complete remission (CR) after donor leukocyte infusions (DLI) for relapse after allogeneic bone marrow transplantation (BMT). Blood 1997; 90:549a.
17. Dazzi F, Szydlo RM, Cross NC, Craddock C, Kaeda J, Kanfer E, Cwynarski K, Olavarria E, Yong A, Apperley JF, Goldman JM. Durability of responses following donor lymphocyte infusions for patients who relapse after allogeneic stem cell transplantation for chronic myeloid leukemia. Blood 2000;96:2712–6.
18. Porter D, Collins R, Shpilberg O, Drobyski W, Connors J, Sproles A, Antin J. Long-term follow-up of patients who achieved complete remission after donor leukocyte infusions. Biol Blood Marrow Transplant. 1999;5:253–61.
19. Carlens S, Remberger M, Aschan J, Ringden O. The role of disease stage in the response to donor lymphocyte infusions as treatment for leukemic relapse. Biol Blood Marrow Transplant. 2001;7:31–8.
20. Gale R, Horowitz M, Ash R, Champlin R, Goldman J, Rimm A, Ringden O, Veum Stone J, Bortin M. Identical-twin bone marrow transplants for leukemia. Ann Intern Med. 1994;120:646–52.
21. Porter D, Roth M, Lee S, McGarigle C, Ferrara J, Antin J. Adoptive immunotherapy with donor mononuclear cell infusions to treat relapse of acute leukemia or myelodysplasia after allogeneic bone marrow transplantation. Bone Marrow Transplant. 1996;18:975–80.
22. Szer J, Grigg A, Phillipos G, Sheridan W. Donor leucocyte infusions after chemotherapy for patients relapsing with acute leukaemia following allogeneic BMT. Bone Marrow Transplant. 1993;11:109–11.
23. Cunningham I. Extramedullary sites of leukemia relapse after transplant. Leuk Lymphoma. 2007;47:1754–67.
24. Chong G, Byrnes G, Szer J, Grigg A. Extramedullary relapse after allogeneic bone marrow transplantation for haematological malignancy. Bone Marrow Transplant. 1011;26:1011–5.
25. Porter D, Antin J. Adoptive immunotherapy for relapsed leukemia following allogeneic bone marrow transplantation. Leuk Lymphoma. 1995;17:191–7.

26. Depil S, Deconinck E, Milpied N, Sutton L, Witz F, Jouet JP, Damaj G, Yakoub-Agha I, Societe Francaise de Greffe de Moelle et Therapie c. Donor lymphocyte infusion to treat relapse after allogeneic bone marrow transplantation for myelodysplastic syndrome. Bone Marrow Transplant. 2004;33:531–4.
27. Slavin S, Morecki S, Weiss L, Or R. Donor lymphocyte infusion: the use of alloreactive and tumor-reactive lymphocytes for immunotherapy of malignant and nonmalignant diseases in conjunction with allogeneic stem cell transplantation. J Hematother Stem Cell Res. 2002;11:265–76.
28. Choi SJ, Lee JH, Kim S, Lee YS, Seol M, Ryu SG, Lee JS, Kim WK, Jang S, Park CJ, Chi HS, Lee KH. Treatment of relapsed acute lymphoblastic leukemia after allogeneic bone marrow transplantation with chemotherapy followed by G-CSF-primed donor leukocyte infusion: a prospective study. Bone Marrow Transplant. 2005;36:163–9.
29. Bjorkstrand BB, Ljungman P, Svensson H, Hermans J, Alegre A, Apperley J, Blade J, Carlson K, Cavo M, Ferrant A, Goldstone AH, de Laurenzi A, Majolino I, Marcus R, Prentice HG, Remes K, Samson D, Sureda A, Verdonck LF, Volin L, Gahrton G. Allogeneic bone marrow transplantation versus autologous stem cell transplantation in multiple myeloma: a retrospective case-matched study from the European Group for Blood and Marrow Transplantation. Blood 1996;88:4711–8.
30. Badros A, Barlogie B, Morris C, Desikan R, Martin SR, Munshi N, Zangari M, Mehta J, Toor A, Cottler-Fox M, Fassas A, Anaissie E, Schichman S, Tricot G, Aniassie E. High response rate in refractory and poor-risk multiple myeloma after allotransplantation using a nonmyeloablative conditioning regimen and donor lymphocyte infusions. Blood 2001;97:2574–9.
31. Bruno B, Rotta M, Patriarca F, Mordini N, Allione B, Carnevale-Schianca F, Giaccone L, Sorasio R, Omede P, Baldi I, Bringhen S, Massaia M, Aglietta M, Levis A, Gallamini A, Fanin R, Palumbo A, Storb R, Ciccone G, Boccadoro M. A comparison of allografting with autografting for newly diagnosed myeloma. N Engl J Med. 2007;356:1110–20.
32. Tricot G, Vesole D, Jagannath S, Hilton J, Munshi N, Barlogie B. Graft-versus-myeloma effect: proof of principle. Blood 1996;87:1196–8.
33. Kroger N, Shimoni A, Zagrivnaja M, Ayuk F, Lioznov M, Schieder H, Renges H, Fehse B, Zabelina T, Nagler A, Zander AR. Low-dose thalidomide and donor lymphocyte infusion as adoptive immunotherapy after allogeneic stem cell transplantation in patients with multiple myeloma. Blood 2004;104:3361–3.
34. Ratanatharathorn V, Uberti J, Karanes C, Abella E, Lum LG, Momin F, Cummings G, Sensenbrenner LL. Prospective comparative trial of autologous versus allogeneic bone marrow transplantation in patients with non-Hodgkin's lymphoma. Blood 1994;84:1050–5.
35. Jones R, Ambinder R, Piantadosi S, Santos G. Evidence of a graft-versus-lymphoma effect associated with allogeneic bone marrow transplantation. Blood 1991;77:649–53.
36. Bernard M, Dauriac C, Drenou B, Leberre C, Branger B, Fauchet R, Le Prise PY, Lamy T. Long-term follow-up of allogeneic bone marrow transplantation in patients with poor prognosis non-Hodgkin's lymphoma. Bone Marrow Transplant. 1999;23:329–33.
37. Robinson S, Goldstone AH, Mackinnon S, Carella A, Russell N, DeElvira R, Taghipour G, Schmitz N. Chemoresistant or aggressive lymphoma predicts for a poor outcome following reduced intensity allogeneic progenitor cell transplantation: an analysis from the Lymphoma Working Party of the European Group for Blood and Bone Marrow Transplantation. Blood 2002;100:4310–6.
38. Porter D, Stadtmauer EA, Lazarus H. "GVHD": graft-versus host disease or graft-versus Hodgkin's disease? An old acronym with new meaning. Bone Marrow Transplant. 2003;31:739–46.
39. Peggs KS, Hunter A, Chopra R, Parker A, Mahendra P, Milligan D, Craddock C, Pettengell R, Dogan A, Thomson KJ, Morris EC, Hale G, Waldmann H, Goldstone AH, Linch DC, Mackinnon S. Clinical evidence of a graft-versus-Hodgkin's-lymphoma effect after reduced-intensity allogeneic transplantation. Lancet 2005;365:1934–41.

40. Alvarez I, Sureda A, Caballero MD, Urbano-Ispizua A, Ribera JM, Canales M, Garcia-Conde J, Sanz G, Arranz R, Bernal MT, de la Serna J, Diez JL, Moraleda JM, Rubio-Felix D, Xicoy B, Martinez C, Mateos MV, Sierra J. Nonmyeloablative stem cell transplantation is an effective therapy for refractory or relapsed Hodgkin lymphoma: results of a Spanish prospective cooperative protocol. Biol Blood Marrow Transplant. 2006; 12:172–83.
41. Anderlini P, Champlin RE. Reduced intensity conditioning for allogeneic stem cell transplantation in relapsed and refractory Hodgkin lymphoma: where do we stand? Biol Blood Marrow Transplant. 2006;12:599–602.
42. Loren A, Porter D. Donor leukocyte infusions after unrelated donor hematopoietic stem cell transplantation. Curr Opin Oncol. 2006;18:107–14.
43. van Rhee R, Savage D, Blackwell J, Orchard K, Dazzi F, Lin F, Chase A, Bungey J, Cross N, Apperley J, Szydlo R, Goldman J. Adoptive immunotherapy for relapse of chronic myeloid leukemia after allogeneic bone marrow transplant: equal efficacy of lymphocytes from sibling and matched unrelated donors. Bone Marrow Transplant. 1998;21:1055–61.
44. Porter D, Collins R, Hardy C, Kernan N, Drobyski W, Giralt S, Flowers M, Casper J, Leahey A, Parker P, Mick R, Bate-Boyle B, King R, Antin J. Treatment of relapsed leukemia after unrelated donor marrow transplantation with unrelated donor leukocyte infusions. Blood 2000;95:1214–21.
45. Porter D, Antin J. Adoptive immunotherapy in bone marrow transplantation. In: Burakoff S, Deeg H, Ferrara J, editors. Graft-versus-host disease. New York: Marcel Dekker; 1997. p. 733–54.
46. Mackinnon S, Papadopoulos E, Carabasi M, Reich L, Collins N, Boulad F, Castro-Malaspina H, Childs B, Gillio A, Kernan N, Small T, Young J, O'Reilly R. Adoptive immunotherapy evaluating escalating doses of donor leukocytes for relapse of chronic myeloid leukemia after bone marrow transplantation: separation of graft-versus-leukemia responses from graft-versus-host disease. Blood 1995;86:1261–8.
47. Porter D, Levine J. GVHD and GVL after donor leukocyte infusion. Semin Hematol. 2007;43:53–61.
48. Porter D, Antin J. Graft-versus-leukemia effect of allogeneic bone marrow transplantation and donor mononuclear cell infusions. In: Winter J, editor. Blood stem cell transplantation. Norwell: Kluwer Academic Publishers; 1997. p. 57–86.
49. Chiorean EG, DeFor TE, Weisdorf DJ, Blazar BR, McGlave PB, Burns LJ, Brown C, Miller JS. Donor chimerism does not predict response to donor lymphocyte infusion for relapsed chronic myelogenous leukemia after allogeneic hematopoietic cell transplantation. Biol Blood Marrow Transplant. 2004;10:171–7.
50. Keil F, Haas OA, Fritsch G, Kalhs P, Lechner K, Mannhalter C, Reiter E, Niederwieser D, Hoecker P, Greinix HT. Donor leukocyte infusion for leukemic relapse after allogeneic marrow transplantation: lack of residual donor hematopoiesis predicts aplasia. Blood 1997;89:3113–7.
51. Flowers M, Leisenring W, Beach K, Riddell S, Radich J, Higano C, Rowley S, Chauncey T, Bensinger W, Sanders J, Anasetti C, Storb R, Wade J, Appelbaum F, Martin P. Granulocyte colony-stimulating factor given to donors before apheresis does not prevent aplasia in patients treated with donor leukocyte infusion for recurrent chronic myeloid leukemia after bone marrow transplantation. Biol Blood Marrow Transplant. 2000; 6:321–6.
52. Gustafsson A, Levitsky V, Zou JZ, Frisan T, Dalianis T, Ljungman P, Ringden O, Winiarski J, Ernberg I, Masucci MG. Epstein-Barr virus (EBV) load in bone marrow transplant recipients at risk to develop posttransplant lymphoproliferative disease: prophylactic infusion of EBV-specific cytotoxic T cells. Blood 2000;95:807–14.
53. Loren AW, Porter DL, Stadtmauer EA, Tsai DE. Post-transplant lymphoproliferative disorder: a review. Bone Marrow Transplant. 2003;31:145–55.

54. Shapiro R, McClain K, Frizzera G, Gajl-Peczalska K, Kersey J, Blazar B, Arthur D, Patton D, Greenberg J, Burke B, Ramsay N, McGlave P, Filipovich A. Epstein-Barr virus associated B cell lymphoproliferative disorders following bone marrow transplantation. Blood 1988;71:1234–43.
55. Porter D, Orloff G, Antin J. Donor mononuclear cell infusions as therapy for B-cell lymphoproliferative disorder following allogeneic bone marrow transplant. Transplant Sci. 1994;4:11–15.
56. Papadopoulos E, Ladanyi M, Emanuel D, Mackinnon S, Boulad F, Carabasi M, Castro-Malaspina J, Childs B, Gillio A, Small T, Young J, Kernan N, O'Reilly R. Infusions of donor leukocytes to treat Epstein-Barr virus-associated lymphoproliferative disorders after allogeneic bone marrow transplantation. N Engl J Med. 1994;330:1185–91.
57. Rooney C, Smith C, Ng C, Loftin S, Sixbey J, Gan Y, Srivastava DK, Bowman L, Krance R, Brenner M, Heslop H. Infusion of cytoxic T cells for the prevention and treatment of Epstein-Barr virus-induced lymphoma in allogeneic transplant recipients. Blood 1998; 92:1549–55.
58. Riddell S, Watanabe K, Goodrich J, Li C, Agha M, Greenberg P. Restoration of viral immunity in immunodeficient humans by adoptive transfer of T cell clones. Science 1992;257:238–41.
59. Walter E, Greenberg P, Gilbert M, Finch R, Watanabe K, Thomas E, Riddell S. Reconstitution of cellular immunity against cytomegalovirus in recipients of allogeneic bone marrow by transfer of T-cell clones from the donor. N Engl J Med. 1995; 333:1038–44.
60. Hromas R, Cornetta K, Srour E. Donor leukocyte infusion as therapy of life-threatening adenoviral infections after T-cell-depleted bone marrow transplantation. Blood 1994;84(5):1689–90.
61. Kishi Y, Kami M, Oki Y, Kazuyama Y, Kawabata M, Miyakoshi S, Morinaga S, Suzuki R, Mori S, Muto Y. Donor lymphocyte infusion for treatment of life-threatening respiratory syncytial virus infection following bone marrow transplantation. Bone Marrow Transplant. 2000;26:573–6.
62. Guglielmi C, Arcese W, Dazzi F, Brand R, Bunjes D, Verdonck LF, Schattenberg A, Kolb HJ, Ljungman P, Devergie A, Bacigalupo A, Gomez M, Michallet M, Elmaagacli A, Gratwohl A, Apperley J, Niederwieser D. Donor lymphocyte infusion for relapsed chronic myelogenous leukemia: prognostic relevance of the initial cell dose. Blood 2002;100:397–405.
63. Sullivan K, Weiden P, Storb R, Witherspoon R, Fefer A, Fisher L, Buckner C, Anasetti C, Appelbaum F, Badger C, Beatty P, Bensinger W, Berenson R, Bigelow C, Cheever M, Clift R, Deeg H, Doney K, Greenberg P, Hansen J, Hill R, Loughran T, Martin P, Neiman P, Peterson F, Sanders J, Singer J, Stewart P, Thomas E. Influence of acute and chronic graft-versus-host disease on relapse and survival after bone marrow transplantation from HLA-identical siblings as treatment of acute and chronic leukemia. Blood 1989;73:1720–8.
64. Johnson B, Drobyski W, Truitt R. Delayed infusion of normal donor cells after MHC-matched bone marrow transplantation provides an antileukemia reaction without graft-versus-host disease. Bone Marrow Transplant. 1993;11:329–36.
65. Weiden P, Storb R, Tsoi M, Graham T, Lerner K, Thomas E. Infusion of donor lymphocytes into stable canine radiation chimeras: implications for mechanism of transplantation tolerance. J Immunol. 1978;116:1212–9.
66. Alyea E, Soiffer R, Canning C, Neuberg D, Schlossman R, Pickett C, Collins H, Wang Y, Anderson K, Ritz J. Toxicity and efficacy of defined doses of $CD4^+$ donor lymphocytes for treatment of relapse after allogeneic bone marrow transplant. Blood 1998;91:3671–80.
67. Giralt S, Hester J, Huh Y, Hirsch-Ginsberg C, Rondon G, Seong D, Lee M, Gajewski J, Van Besien K, Khouri I, Mehra R, Przepiorka D, Korbling M, Talpaz M, Kantarjian H, Fischer H, Deisseroth A, Champlin R. CD8-depleted donor lymphocyte infusion as

treatment for relapsed chronic myelogenous leukemia after allogeneic bone marrow transplantation. Blood 1995;86:4337–43.
68. Shimoni A, Gajewski J, Donato M, Martin T, O'Brien S, Talpaz M, Cohen A, Korbling M, Champlin R, Giralt S. Long-term follow-up of recipients of CD8 depleted donor lymphocyte infusions for the treatment of chronic myelogenous leukemia relapsing after allogeneic progenitor cell transplantation. Biol Blood Marrow Transplant. 2001; 7:568–75.
69. Waller EK, Ship AM, Mittelstaedt S, Murray TW, Carter R, Kakhniashvili I, Lonial S, Holden JT, Boyer MW. Irradiated donor leukocytes promote engraftment of allogeneic bone marrow in major histocompatibility complex mismatched recipients without causing graft-versus-host disease. Blood 1999;94:3222–33.
70. Truitt RL, Johnson BD, Hanke C, Talib S, Hearst JE. Photochemical treatment with S-59 psoralen and ultraviolet: a light to control the fate of naive or primed T lymphocytes in vivo after allogeneic bone marrow transplantation. J Immunol. 1999;163:5145–56.
71. Servida P, Rossini S, Traversari C, Ferrari G, Bonini C, Nobili N, Vago L, Faravelli A, Vanzulli A, Mavillio F, Bordignon C. Gene transfer into peripheral blood lymphocytes for in vivo immunomodulation of donor anti-tumor immunity in a patient affected by EBV-induced lymphoma. Blood 1993;82:214a.
72. Bonini C, Ferrari G, Verzeletti S, Servida P, Zappone E, Ruggieri L, Ponzoni M, Rossini S, Mavilio F, Traversari C, Bordignon C. HSV-TK gene transfer into donor lymphocytes for control of allogeneic graft-versus-leukemia. Science 1997;276:1719–24.
73. Falkenburg JH, Wafelman AR, Joosten P, Smit WM, van Bergen CA, Bongaerts R, Lurvink E, van der Hoorn M, Kluck P, Landegent JE, Kluin-Nelemans HC, Fibbe WE, Willemze R. Complete remission of accelerated phase chronic myeloid leukemia by treatment with leukemia-reactive cytotoxic T lymphocytes. Blood 1999;94:1201–8.
74. Cardoso AA, Seamon MJ, Afonso HM, Ghia P, Boussiotis VA, Freeman GJ, Gribben JG, Sallan SE, Nadler LM. Ex vivo generation of human anti-pre-B leukemia-specific autologous cytolytic T cells. Blood 1997;90:549–61.
75. Kolb HJ, Schmid C, Barrett AJ, Schendel DJ. Graft-versus-leukemia reactions in allogeneic chimeras. Blood 2004;103:767–76.
76. Bocchia M, Korontsvit T, Xu Q, Mackinnon S, Yang SY, Sette A, Scheinberg DA. Specific human cellular immunity to bcr-abl oncogene-derived peptides. Blood 1996;87:3587–92.
77. Clark RE, Dodi IA, Hill SC, Lill JR, Aubert G, Macintyre AR, Rojas J, Bourdon A, Bonner PL, Wang L, Christmas SE, Travers PJ, Creaser CS, Rees RC, Madrigal JA. Direct evidence that leukemic cells present HLA-associated immunogenic peptides derived from the BCR-ABL b3a2 fusion protein. Blood 2001;98:2887–93.
78. Voogt PJ, Goulmy E, Veenhof WF, Hamilton M, Fibbe WE, Van Rood JJ, Falkenburg JH. Cellularly defined minor histocompatibility antigens are differentially expressed on human hematopoietic progenitor cells. J Exp Med. 1988;168:2337–47.
79. Mutis T, Verdijk R, Schrama E, Esendam B, Brand A, Goulmy E. Feasibility of immunotherapy of relapsed leukemia with ex vivo-generated cytotoxic T lymphocytes specific for hematopoietic system-restricted minor histocompatibility antigens. Blood 1999;93: 2336–41.
80. Marijt WA, Heemskerk MH, Kloosterboer FM, Goulmy E, Kester MG, van der Hoorn MA, van Luxemburg-Heys SA, Hoogeboom M, Mutis T, Drijfhout JW, van Rood JJ, Willemze R, Falkenburg JH. Hematopoiesis-restricted minor histocompatibility antigens HA-1- or HA-2-specific T cells can induce complete remissions of relapsed leukemia. Proc Natl Acad Sci USA. 2003;100:2742–7.
81. Miklos DB, Kim HT, Zorn E, Hochberg EP, Guo L, Mattes-Ritz A, Viatte S, Soiffer RJ, Antin JH, Ritz J. Antibody response to DBY minor histocompatibility antigen is induced after allogeneic stem cell transplantation and in healthy female donors. Blood 2004;103:353–9.
82. Randolph SS, Gooley TA, Warren EH, Appelbaum FR, Riddell SR. Female donors contribute to a selective graft-versus-leukemia effect in male recipients of HLA-matched, related hematopoietic stem cell transplants. Blood 2004;103:347–52.

83. Molldrem J, Dermime S, Parker K, Jiang YZ, Mavroudis D, Hensel N, Fukushima P, Barrett AJ. Targeted T-cell therapy for human leukemia: cytotoxic T lymphocytes specific for a peptide derived from proteinase 3 preferentially lyse human myeloid leukemia cells. Blood 1996;88:2450–7.
84. Molldrem JJ, Lee PP, Wang C, Felio K, Kantarjian HM, Champlin RE, Davis MM. Evidence that specific T lymphocytes may participate in the elimination of chronic myelogenous leukemia. Nat Med. 2000;6:1018–23.
85. Heslop HE, Stevenson FK, Molldrem JJ. Immunotherapy of hematologic malignancy. Hematology Am Soc Hematol Educ Program. 2003: 331–49.
86. Rosenfeld C, Cheever MA, Gaiger A. WT1 in acute leukemia, chronic myelogenous leukemia and myelodysplastic syndrome: therapeutic potential of WT1 targeted therapies. Leukemia 2003;17:1301–12.
87. Atanackovic D, Arfsten J, Cao Y, Gnjatic S, Schnieders F, Bartels K, Schilling G, Faltz C, Wolschke C, Dierlamm J, Ritter G, Eiermann T, Hossfeld DK, Zander AR, Jungbluth AA, Old LJ, Bokemeyer C, Kroger N. Cancer-testis antigens are commonly expressed in multiple myeloma and induce systemic immunity following allogeneic stem cell transplantation. Blood 1103;109:1103–12.
88. Greiner J, Schmitt M, Li L, Giannopoulos K, Bosch K, Schmitt A, Dohner K, Schlenk RF, Pollack JR, Dohner H, Bullinger L. Expression of tumor-associated antigens in acute myeloid leukemia: implications for specific immunotherapeutic approaches. Blood 2006;108:4109–17.
89. Pinilla-Ibarz J, Cathcart K, Korontsvit T, Soignet S, Bocchia M, Caggiano J, Lai L, Jimenez J, Kolitz J, Scheinberg DA. Vaccination of patients with chronic myelogenous leukemia with bcr-abl oncogene breakpoint fusion peptides generates specific immune responses. Blood 2000;95:1781–7.
90. Miller JS, Weisdorf DJ, Burns LJ, Slungaard A, Wagner JE, Verneris MR, Cooley S, Wangen R, Fautsch SK, Nicklow R, Defor T, Blazar BR. Lymphodepletion followed by donor lymphocyte infusion (DLI) causes significantly more acute graft-versus-host disease than DLI alone. Blood 2007;110:2761–3.
91. Liebowitz D, Lee K, CH J. Costimulatory approaches to adoptive immunotherapy. Curr Opin Oncol. 1998;10:533–41.
92. Levine BL, Bernstein WB, Connors M, Craighead N, Lindsten T, Thompson CB, June CH. Effects of CD28 costimulation on long-term proliferation of $CD4^{+}$ T cells in the absence of exogenous feeder cells. J Immunol. 1997;159:5921–30.
93. Porter DL, Levin BL, Bunin N, Stadtmauer EA, Luger SM, Goldstein S, Loren A, Phillips J, Nasta S, Perl A, Schuster S, Tsai D, Sohal A, Veloso E, Emerson S, June CH. A Phase I trial of donor lymphocyte infusions expanded and activated ex-vivo via CD3/CD28 co-stimulation. Blood 2006;107(4):1325–31.
94. Fowler DH, Odom J, Steinberg SM, Chow CK, Foley J, Kogan Y, Hou J, Gea-Banacloche J, Sportes C, Pavletic S, Leitman S, Read EJ, Carter C, Kolstad A, Fox R, Beatty GL, Vonderheide RH, Levine BL, June CH, Gress RE, Bishop MR. Phase I clinical trial of costimulated, IL-4 polarized donor $CD4^{+}$ T cells as augmentation of allogeneic hematopoietic cell transplantation. Biol Blood Marrow Transplant. 2006;12:1150–60.
95. Guillaume T, Rubinstein DB, Symann M. Immune reconstitution and immunotherapy after autologous hematopoietic stem cell transplantation. Blood 1998;92:1471–90.
96. Porrata LF, Gertz MA, Litzow MR, Lacy MQ, Dispenzieri A, Inwards DJ, Ansell SM, Micallef IN, Gastineau DA, Elliott M, Hogan WJ, Hayman SR, Tefferi A, Markovic SN. Early lymphocyte recovery predicts superior survival after autologous hematopoietic stem cell transplantation for patients with primary systemic amyloidosis. Clin Cancer Res. 2005;11:1210–8.
97. Boulassel MR, Herr AL, de BEMD, Galal A, Lachance S, Laneuville P, Routy JP. Early lymphocyte recovery following autologous peripheral stem cell transplantation is associated with better survival in younger patients with lymphoproliferative disorders. Hematology 2006;11:165–70.

98. Laport GG, Levine BL, Stadtmauer EA, Schuster SJ, Luger SM, Grupp S, Bunin N, Strobl FJ, Cotte J, Zheng Z, Gregson B, Rivers P, Vonderheide RH, Liebowitz DN, Porter DL, June CH. Adoptive transfer of costimulated T cells induces lymphocytosis in patients with relapsed/refractory non-Hodgkin lymphoma following CD34^{+}-selected hematopoietic cell transplantation. Blood 2003;102:2004–13.
99. Rapoport A, Stadtmauer E, Aqui N, Badros A, Cotte J, Chrisley L, Velosa E, Zheng Z, Westphal S, Mair R, Chi N, Ratterree B, Pochran M, Natt S, Hinkle J, Sickles C, Sohal A, Ruehle K, Lynch C, Zhang L, Porter D, Luger S, Guo C, Fang H, Blackwelder W, Hankey M, Mann D, Edelman R, Frasch C, Levine B, Cross A, June C. Restoration of immunity in lymphopenic individuals with cancer by vaccination and adoptive T-cell transfer. Nat Med. 2005;11:1230–7.
100. Lanier LL. NK cell recognition. Annu Rev Immunol. 2005;23:225–74.
101. Herberman RB, Ortaldo JR. Natural killer cells: their roles in defenses against disease. Science 1981;214:24–30.
102. Kiessling R, Petranyi G, Klein G, Wigzel H. Genetic variation of in vitro cytolytic activity and in vivo rejection potential of non-immunized semi-syngeneic mice against a mouse lymphoma line. Int J Cancer. 1975;15:933–40.
103. Murphy WJ, Kumar V, Bennett M. Acute rejection of murine bone marrow allografts by natural killer cells and T cells. Differences in kinetics and target antigens recognized. J Exp Med. 1987;166:1499–509.
104. Cudkowicz G, Bennett M. Peculiar immunobiology of bone marrow allografts. II. Rejection of parental grafts by resistant F1 hybrid mice. J Exp Med. 1971;134: 1513–28.
105. Cooper MA, Fehniger TA, Caligiuri MA. The biology of human natural killer-cell subsets. Trends Immunol. 2001;22:633–40.
106. Rayner AA, Grimm EA, Lotze MT, Chu EW, Rosenberg SA. Lymphokine-activated killer (LAK) cells. Analysis of factors relevant to the immunotherapy of human cancer. Cancer 1985;55:1327–33.
107. Carson WE, Giri JG, Lindemann MJ, Linett ML, Ahdieh M, Paxton R, Anderson D, Eisenmann J, Grabstein K, Caligiuri MA. Interleukin (IL) 15 is a novel cytokine that activates human natural killer cells via components of the IL-2 receptor. J Exp Med. 1994;180:1395–403.
108. Trinchieri G. Interleukin-12 and the regulation of innate resistance and adaptive immunity. Nat Rev Immunol. 2003;3:133–46.
109. Young HA, Ortaldo J. Cytokines as critical co-stimulatory molecules in modulating the immune response of natural killer cells. Cell Res. 2006;16:20–24.
110. Singh SM, Yanagawa H, Hanibuchi M, Miki T, Okamura H, Sone S. Augmentation by interleukin-18 of MHC-nonrestricted killer activity of human peripheral blood mononuclear cells in response to interleukin-12. Int J Immunopharmacol. 2000;22:35–43.
111. Walzer T, Dalod M, Robbins SH, Zitvogel L, Vivier E. Natural-killer cells and dendritic cells: "l'union fait la force". Blood 2005;106:2252–8.
112. Re F, Staudacher C, Zamai L, Vecchio V, Bregni M. Killer cell Ig-like receptors ligand-mismatched, alloreactive natural killer cells lyse primary solid tumors. Cancer 2006;107:640–8.
113. Armeanu S, Bitzer M, Lauer UM, Venturelli S, Pathil A, Krusch M, Kaiser S, Jobst J, Smirnow I, Wagner A, Steinle A, Salih HR. Natural killer cell-mediated lysis of hepatoma cells via specific induction of NKG2D ligands by the histone deacetylase inhibitor sodium valproate. Cancer Res. 2005;65:6321–9.
114. Russell JH, Ley TJ. Lymphocyte-mediated cytotoxicity. Annu Rev Immunol. 2002; 20:323–70.
115. Lanier LL, Ruitenberg JJ, Phillips JH. Functional and biochemical analysis of CD16 antigen on natural killer cells and granulocytes. J Immunol. 1988;141:3478–85.
116. Marsh SG, Parham P, Dupont B, Geraghty DE, Trowsdale J, Middleton D, Vilches C, Carrington M, Witt C, Guethlein LA, Shilling H, Garcia CA, Hsu KC, Wain H.

Killer-cell immunoglobulin-like receptor (KIR) nomenclature report, 2002. Tissue Antigens 2003;62:79–86.
117. Yawata M, Yawata N, Abi-Rached L, Parham P. Variation within the human killer cell immunoglobulin-like receptor (KIR) gene family. Crit Rev Immunol. 2002;22:463–82.
118. Pando MJ, Gardiner CM, Gleimer M, McQueen KL, Parham P. The protein made from a common allele of KIR3DL1 (3DL1*004) is poorly expressed at cell surfaces due to substitution at positions 86 in Ig domain 0 and 182 in Ig domain 1. J Immunol. 2003;171:6640–9.
119. Yokoyama WM, Daniels BF, Seaman WE, Hunziker R, Margulies DH, Smith HR. A family of murine NK cell receptors specific for target cell MHC class I molecules. Semin Immunol. 1995;7:89–101.
120. Vales-Gomez M, Reyburn HT, Mandelboim M, Strominger JL. Kinetics of interaction of HLA-C ligands with natural killer cell inhibitory receptors. Immunity 1998;9:337–44.
121. Houchins JP, Yabe T, McSherry C, Bach FH. DNA sequence analysis of NKG2, a family of related cDNA clones encoding type II integral membrane proteins on human natural killer cells. J Exp Med. 1991;173:1017–20.
122. Lopez-Botet M, Angulo A, Guma M. Natural killer cell receptors for major histocompatibility complex class I and related molecules in cytomegalovirus infection. Tissue Antigens. 2004;63:195–203.
123. Cao W, Xi X, Hao Z, Li W, Kong Y, Cui L, Ma C, Ba D, He W. RAET1E2, a soluble isoform of the UL16 binding protein RAET1E produced by tumor cells, inhibits NKG2D-mediated NK cytotoxicity. J Biol Chem. 2007;282:18922–8.
124. Ljunggren HG, Karre K. In search of the "missing self": MHC molecules and NK cell recognition. Immunol Today. 1990;11:237–44.
125. Valiante NM, Uhrberg M, Shilling HG, Lienert-Weidenbach K, Arnett KL, D'Andrea A, Phillips JH, Lanier LL, Parham P. Functionally and structurally distinct NK cell receptor repertoires in the peripheral blood of two human donors. Immunity 1997; 7:739–51.
126. Raulet DH, Vance RE, McMahon CW. Regulation of the natural killer cell receptor repertoire. Annu Rev Immunol. 2001;19:291–330.
127. Fernandez NC, Treiner E, Vance RE, Jamieson AM, Lemieux S, Raulet DH. A subset of natural killer cells achieves self-tolerance without expressing inhibitory receptors specific for self-MHC molecules. Blood 2005;105:4416–23.
128. Anfossi N, Andre P, Guia S, Falk CS, Roetynck S, Stewart CA, Breso V, Frassati C, Reviron D, Middleton D, Romagne F, Ugolini S, Vivier E. Human NK cell education by inhibitory receptors for MHC class I. Immunity 2006;25:331–42.
129. Cooley S, Xiao F, Pitt M, Gleason M, McCullar V, Bergemann T, McQueen KL, Guethlein LA, Parham P, Miller JS. A subpopulation of human peripheral blood NK cells that lacks inhibitory receptors for self MHC is developmentally immature. Blood 2007;110:578–86.
130. Farrell HE, Vally H, Lynch DM, Fleming P, Shellam GR, Scalzo AA, Davis-Poynter NJ. Inhibition of natural killer cells by a cytomegalovirus MHC class I homologue in vivo. Nature 1997;386:510–4.
131. Voigt V, Forbes CA, Tonkin JN, Degli-Esposti MA, Smith HR, Yokoyama WM, Scalzo AA. Murine cytomegalovirus m157 mutation and variation leads to immune evasion of natural killer cells. Proc Natl Acad Sci USA. 2003;100:13483–8.
132. Martin MP, Qi Y, Gao X, Yamada E, Martin JN, Pereyra F, Colombo S, Brown EE, Shupert WL, Phair J, Goedert JJ, Buchbinder S, Kirk GD, Telenti A, Connors M, O'Brien SJ, Walker BD, Parham P, Deeks SG, McVicar DW, Carrington M. Innate partnership of HLA-B and KIR3DL1 subtypes against HIV-1. Nat Genet. 2007;39:733–40.
133. Trinchieri G, Sher A. Cooperation of toll-like receptor signals in innate immune defence. Nat Rev Immunol. 2007;7:179–90.
134. Miller JS, McCullar V. Human natural killer cells with polyclonal lectin and immunoglobulinlike receptors develop from single hematopoietic stem cells with preferential expression of NKG2A and KIR2DL2/L3/S2. Blood 2001;98:705–13.

135. Yu H, Fehniger TA, Fuchshuber P, Thiel KS, Vivier E, Carson WE, Caligiuri MA. Flt3 ligand promotes the generation of a distinct CD34(+) human natural killer cell progenitor that responds to interleukin-15. Blood 1998;92:3647–57.
136. Muench MO, Humeau L, Paek B, Ohkubo T, Lanier LL, Albanese CT, Barcena A. Differential effects of interleukin-3, interleukin-7, interleukin 15, and granulocyte-macrophage colony-stimulating factor in the generation of natural killer and B cells from primitive human fetal liver progenitors. Exp Hematol. 2000;28:961–73.
137. Freud AG, Yokohama A, Becknell B, Lee MT, Mao HC, Ferketich AK, Caligiuri MA. Evidence for discrete stages of human natural killer cell differentiation in vivo. J Exp Med. 2006;203:1033–43.
138. Antony PA, Piccirillo CA, Akpinarli A, Finkelstein SE, Speiss PJ, Surman DR, Palmer DC, Chan CC, Klebanoff CA, Overwijk WW, Rosenberg SA, Restifo NP. $CD8^+$ T cell immunity against a tumor/self-antigen is augmented by $CD4^+$ T helper cells and hindered by naturally occurring T regulatory cells. J Immunol. 2005;174:2591–601.
139. Trompeter HI, Gomez-Lozano N, Santourlidis S, Eisermann B, Wernet P, Vilches C, Uhrberg M. Three structurally and functionally divergent kinds of promoters regulate expression of clonally distributed killer cell Ig-like receptors (KIR), of KIR2DL4, and of KIR3DL3. J Immunol. 2005;174:4135–43.
140. Uhrberg M, Valiante NM, Shum BP, Shilling HG, Lienert-Weidenbach K, Corliss B, Tyan D, Lanier LL, Parham P. Human diversity in killer cell inhibitory receptor genes. Immunity 1997;7:753–63.
141. Kikuchi-Maki A, Yusa S, Catina TL, Campbell KS. KIR2DL4 is an IL-2-regulated NK cell receptor that exhibits limited expression in humans but triggers strong IFN-gamma production. J Immunol. 2003;171:3415–25.
142. Maxwell LD, Wallace A, Middleton D, Curran MD. A common KIR2DS4 deletion variant in the human that predicts a soluble KIR molecule analogous to the KIR1D molecule observed in the rhesus monkey. Tissue Antigens 2002;60:254–8.
143. Leung W, Iyengar R, Triplett B, Turner V, Behm FG, Holladay MS, Houston J, Handgretinger R. Comparison of killer Ig-like receptor genotyping and phenotyping for selection of allogeneic blood stem cell donors. J Immunol. 2005;174: 6540–5.
144. Cooley S, McCullar V, Wangen R, Bergemann TL, Spellman S, Weisdorf DJ, Miller JS. KIR reconstitution is altered by T cells in the graft and correlates with clinical outcomes after unrelated donor transplantation. Blood 2005;106:4370–6.
145. Gasser S, Raulet DH. Activation and self-tolerance of natural killer cells. Immunol Rev. 2006;214:130–42.
146. Alyea EP, Kim HT, Ho V, Cutler C, Gribben J, DeAngelo DJ, Lee SJ, Windawi S, Ritz J, Stone RM, Antin JH, Soiffer RJ. Comparative outcome of nonmyeloablative and myeloablative allogeneic hematopoietic cell transplantation for patients older than 50 years of age. Blood 2005;105:1810–4.
147. Yokoyama WM, Kim S. Licensing of natural killer cells by self-major histocompatibility complex class I. Immunol Rev. 2006;214:143–54.
148. Parham P. Taking license with natural killer cell maturation and repertoire development. Immunol Rev. 2006;214:155–60.
149. Rosenberg SA, Lotze MT, Muul LM, Chang AE, Avis FP, Leitman S, Linehan WM, Robertson CN, Lee RE, Rubin JT, et al. A progress report on the treatment of 157 patients with advanced cancer using lymphokine-activated killer cells and interleukin-2 or high-dose interleukin-2 alone. N Engl J Med. 1987;316:889–97.
150. Burns LJ, Weisdorf DJ, DeFor TE, Vesole DH, Repka TL, Blazar BR, Burger SR, Panoskaltsis-Mortari A, Keever-Taylor CA, Zhang MJ, Miller JS. IL-2-based immunotherapy after autologous transplantation for lymphoma and breast cancer induces immune activation and cytokine release: a phase I/II trial. Bone Marrow Transplant. 2003;32:177–86.

151. Dummer W, Niethammer AG, Baccala R, Lawson BR, Wagner N, Reisfeld RA, Theofilopoulos AN. T cell homeostatic proliferation elicits effective antitumor autoimmunity. J Clin Invest. 2002;110:185–92.
152. Dudley ME, Wunderlich JR, Robbins PF, Yang JC, Hwu P, Schwartzentruber DJ, Topalian SL, Sherry R, Restifo NP, Hubicki AM, Robinson MR, Raffeld M, Duray P, Seipp CA, Rogers-Freezer L, Morton KE, Mavroukakis SA, White DE, Rosenberg SA. Cancer regression and autoimmunity in patients after clonal repopulation with antitumor lymphocytes. Science 2002;298:850–4.
153. Ruggeri L, Capanni M, Urbani E, Perruccio K, Shlomchik WD, Tosti A, Posati S, Rogaia D, Frassoni F, Aversa F, Martelli MF, Velardi A. Effectiveness of donor natural killer cell alloreactivity in mismatched hematopoietic transplants. Science 2002;295:2097–100.
154. Muranski P, Boni A, Wrzesinski C, Citrin DE, Rosenberg SA, Childs R, Restifo NP. Increased intensity lymphodepletion and adoptive immunotherapy – how far can we go? Nat Clin Pract Oncol. 2006;3:668–81.
155. Miller JS, Soignier Y, Panoskaltsis-Mortari A, McNearney SA, Yun GH, Fautsch SK, McKenna D, Le C, Defor TE, Burns LJ, Orchard PJ, Blazar BR, Wagner JE, Slungaard A, Weisdorf DJ, Okazaki IJ, McGlave PB. Successful adoptive transfer and in vivo expansion of human haploidentical NK cells in patients with cancer. Blood 2005; 105:3051–7.
156. Cooley S, Burns LJ, Repka T, Miller JS. Natural killer cell cytotoxicity of breast cancer targets is enhanced by two distinct mechanisms of antibody-dependent cellular cytotoxicity against LFA-3 and HER2/neu. Exp Hematol. 1999;27:1533–41.
157. Igarashi T, Wynberg J, Srinivasan R, Becknell B, McCoy JP Jr, Takahashi Y, Suffredini DA, Linehan WM, Caligiuri MA, Childs RW. Enhanced cytotoxicity of allogeneic NK cells with killer immunoglobulin-like receptor ligand incompatibility against melanoma and renal cell carcinoma cells. Blood 2004;104:170–7.
158. Ohira M, Ohdan H, Mitsuta H, Ishiyama K, Tanaka Y, Igarashi Y, Asahara T. Adoptive transfer of TRAIL-expressing natural killer cells prevents recurrence of hepatocellular carcinoma after partial hepatectomy. Transplantation 2006;82: 1712–9.
159. Passweg JR, Tichelli A, Meyer-Monard S, Heim D, Stern M, Kuhne T, Favre G, Gratwohl A. Purified donor NK-lymphocyte infusion to consolidate engraftment after haploidentical stem cell transplantation. Leukemia 2004;18:1835–8.
160. Koehl U, Esser R, Zimmermann S, Tonn T, Kotchetkov R, Bartling T, Sorensen J, Gruttner HP, Bader P, Seifried E, Martin H, Lang P, Passweg JR, Klingebiel T, Schwabe D. Ex vivo expansion of highly purified NK cells for immunotherapy after haploidentical stem cell transplantation in children. Klin Padiatr. 2005;217:345–50.
161. Koh CY, Blazar BR, George T, Welniak LA, Capitini CM, Raziuddin A, Murphy WJ, Bennett M. Augmentation of antitumor effects by NK cell inhibitory receptor blockade in vitro and in vivo. Blood 2001;97:3132–7.
162. Barao I, Hanash AM, Hallett W, Welniak LA, Sun K, Redelman D, Blazar BR, Levy RB, Murphy WJ. Suppression of natural killer cell-mediated bone marrow cell rejection by $CD4^+$ $CD25^+$ regulatory T cells. Proc Natl Acad Sci USA. 2006;103:5460–5.
163. Suck G, Branch DR, Smyth MJ, Miller RG, Vergidis J, Fahim S, Keating A. KHYG-1, a model for the study of enhanced natural killer cell cytotoxicity. Exp Hematol. 2005;33:1160–71.
164. Suck G. Novel approaches using natural killer cells in cancer therapy. Semin Cancer Biol. 2006;16:412–8.
165. Uherek C, Tonn T, Uherek B, Becker S, Schnierle B, Klingemann HG, Wels W. Retargeting of natural killer-cell cytolytic activity to ErbB2-expressing cancer cells results in efficient and selective tumor cell destruction. Blood 2002;100:1265–73.
166. Jiang S, Camara N, Lombardi G, Lechler RI. Induction of allopeptide-specific human $CD4^+$ $CD25^+$ regulatory T cells ex vivo. Blood 2003;102:2180–6.

167. Seddiki N, Santner-Nanan B, Martinson J, Zaunders J, Sasson S, Landay A, Solomon M, Selby W, Alexander SI, Nanan R, Kelleher A, Fazekas de St Groth B. Expression of interleukin (IL)-2 and IL-7 receptors discriminates between human regulatory and activated T cells. J Exp Med. 2006;203:1693–1700.
168. Edinger M, Hoffmann P, Ermann J, Drago K, Fathman CG, Strober S, Negrin RS. $CD4^+$ $CD25^+$ regulatory T cells preserve graft-versus-tumor activity while inhibiting graft-versus-host disease after bone marrow transplantation. [see comment]. Nat Med. 2003;9:1144–50.
169. Hoffmann P, Boeld TJ, Eder R, Albrecht J, Doser K, Piseshka B, Dada A, Niemand C, Assenmacher M, Orso E, Andreesen R, Holler E, Edinger M. Isolation of $CD4^+$ $CD25^+$ regulatory T cells for clinical trials. Biol Blood Marrow Transplant. 2006;12: 267–74.
170. Battaglia M, Stabilini A, Roncarolo MG. Rapamycin selectively expands $CD4^+$ $CD25^+$ $FoxP3^+$ regulatory T cells. Blood 2005;105:4743–8.
171. Keever-Taylor CA, Browning MB, Johnson BD, Truitt RL, Bredeson CN, Behn B, Tsao A. Rapamycin enriches for CD4(+) CD25(+) CD27(+) Foxp3(+) regulatory T cells in ex vivo-expanded CD25-enriched products from healthy donors and patients with multiple sclerosis. Cytotherapy 2007;9:144–57.
172. Roncarolo MG, Battaglia M. Regulatory T-cell immunotherapy for tolerance to self antigens and alloantigens in humans. Nat Rev Immunol. 2007;7:585–98.
173. Groux H, O'Garra A, Bigler M, Rouleau M, Antonenko S, de Vries JE, Roncarolo MG. A $CD4^+$ T-cell subset inhibits antigen-specific T-cell responses and prevents colitis. Nature 1997;389:737–42.
174. Pittenger MF, Mackay AM, Beck SC, Jaiswal RK, Douglas R, Mosca JD, Moorman MA, Simonetti DW, Craig S, Marshak DR. Multilineage potential of adult human mesenchymal stem cells. Science 1999;284:143–7.
175. Horwitz EM, Le Blanc K, Dominici M, Mueller I, Slaper-Cortenbach I, Marini FC, Deans RJ, Krause DS, Keating A. Clarification of the nomenclature for MSC: the International Society for Cellular Therapy position statement. Cytotherapy 2005;7:393–5.
176. Majumdar MK, Thiede MA, Mosca JD, Moorman M, Gerson SL. Phenotypic and functional comparison of cultures of marrow-derived mesenchymal stem cells (MSCs) and stromal cells. J Cell Physiol. 1998;176:57–66.
177. Le Blanc K, Tammik L, Sundberg B, Haynesworth SE, Ringden O. Mesenchymal stem cells inhibit and stimulate mixed lymphocyte cultures and mitogenic responses independently of the major histocompatibility complex. Scand J Immunol. 2003;57:11–20.
178. Aggarwal S, Pittenger MF. Human mesenchymal stem cells modulate allogeneic immune cell responses. Blood 2005;105:1815–22.
179. Maitra B, Szekely E, Gjini K, Laughlin MJ, Dennis J, Haynesworth SE, Koc ON. Human mesenchymal stem cells support unrelated donor hematopoietic stem cells and suppress T-cell activation. Bone Marrow Transplant. 2004;33:597–604.
180. Noort WA, Kruisselbrink AB, in't Anker PS, Kruger M, van Bezooijen RL, de Paus RA, Heemskerk MH, Lowik CW, Falkenburg JH, Willemze R, Fibbe WE. Mesenchymal stem cells promote engraftment of human umbilical cord blood-derived CD34(+) cells in NOD/SCID mice. Exp Hematol. 2002;30:870–8.
181. Koc ON, Gerson SL, Cooper BW, Dyhouse SM, Haynesworth SE, Caplan AI, Lazarus HM. Rapid hematopoietic recovery after coinfusion of autologous-blood stem cells and culture-expanded marrow mesenchymal stem cells in advanced breast cancer patients receiving high-dose chemotherapy. J Clin Oncol. 2000;18:307–16.
182. Le Blanc K, Rasmusson I, Sundberg B, Gotherstrom C, Hassan M, Uzunel M, Ringden O. Treatment of severe acute graft-versus-host disease with third party haploidentical mesenchymal stem cells. Lancet 2004;363:1439–41.
183. Ringden O, Uzunel M, Rasmusson I, Remberger M, Sundberg B, Lonnies H, Marschall HU, Dlugosz A, Szakos A, Hassan Z, Omazic B, Aschan J, Barkholt L, Le Blanc K.

Mesenchymal stem cells for treatment of therapy-resistant graft-versus-host disease. Transplantation 2006;81:1390–7.

184. Lazarus HM, Koc ON, Devine SM, Curtin P, Maziarz RT, Holland HK, Shpall EJ, McCarthy P, Atkinson K, Cooper BW, Gerson SL, Laughlin MJ, Loberiza FR Jr, Moseley AB, Bacigalupo A. Cotransplantation of HLA-identical sibling culture-expanded mesenchymal stem cells and hematopoietic stem cells in hematologic malignancy patients. Biol Blood Marrow Transplant. 2005;11:389–98.

185. Farag SS, Fehniger TA, Ruggeri L, Velardi A, Caligiuri MA. Natural killer cell receptors: new biology and insights into the graft-versus-leukemia effect. Blood 2002; 100:1935–47.

Chapter 21
Improvements in the Prevention and Management of Infectious Complications After Hematopoietic Stem Cell Transplantation

Juan C. Gea-Banacloche and James C. Wade

21.1 Introduction

Infections continue to play an important role in the management of transplant recipients and remain the primary cause of post-transplant, nonrelapse mortality. Several advances in the diagnosis and treatment of infections have taken place over the last few decades. It is still too early to be certain how these new approaches will impact the outcome for patients undergoing hematopoietic stem cell transplantation (HSCT), but there is no question they have impacted clinical practice. Antibiotic prophylaxis during neutropenia, new antifungal and antiviral agents, serological tests for aspergillosis and other fungal infections, the development of molecular techniques for the diagnosis of viral and parasitic infections, and the continued emergence of new pathogens are topics that are relevant and will be reviewed in this chapter.

21.2 Advances in Prevention and Treatment of Bacterial Infections After Transplantation

21.2.1 Prevention of Bacterial Infections

21.2.1.1 Antibacterial Prophylaxis During Neutropenia

The use of antibacterial prophylaxis during neutropenia has received considerable attention after the publication of several meta-analyses [1, 2] and a randomized controlled trial by Bucaneve and colleagues [3]. The meta-analyses suggested the use of prophylactic antibiotics to prevent fever during neutropenia was associated with improved survival, particularly in high-risk patients.

J.C. Gea-Banacloche (✉)
Experimental Transplantation and Immunology Branch, National Cancer Institute, National Institutes of Health, Bethesda, Maryland, USA
e-mail: banacloj@mail.nih.gov

M.R. Bishop (ed.), *Hematopoietic Stem Cell Transplantation*,
Cancer Treatment and Research 144, DOI 10.1007/978-0-387-78580-6_21,

The randomized controlled trial showed a decrease in the episodes of fever and neutropenia, a decrease in episodes of bacteremia, and a decrease in cost, but infection-related mortality was not significantly decreased [3]. These and other studies have contributed to recent clinical practice guidelines endorsing the use of antibacterial prophylaxis for patients who are going to develop profound neutropenia [absolute neutrophil count (ANC) < 100] that is expected to persist for longer than 7 days [4]. A variety of different antibiotics have been studied for this type of prophylaxis, but the largest study used levofloxacin at a dose of 500 mg once daily starting with the initiation of myelosuppressive chemotherapy.

Potential complications of antibacterial prophylaxis include colonization with resistant organisms, shifts in antibacterial susceptibility patterns and increased risk of developing *C. difficile* colitis and other antibiotic-associated toxicities [5]. There is a paucity of data to fully understand the actual incidence of these problems, but interestingly, some trials have reported a reduction in antibiotic treatment costs for the group who received antibacterial prophylaxis [6].

An additional concern is what constitutes the best management of patients who despite antibacterial prophylaxis develop fever during their period of neutropenia. To date there is a paucity of data to help the transplant physician decide on the appropriate antimicrobial modification for such patients, but coverage with broad-spectrum antimicrobial activity that takes into account the risk of antibiotic-resistant organisms or fungal pathogens is recommended.

21.2.1.2 Prophylaxis of Pneumococcal Disease

Streptococcus pneumoniae infections are documented in 2–8.6/1000 patients transplanted [7, 8]. Late infections (4 months to 10 years after transplant) are most common in patients with active chronic graft-versus-host disease (GvHD) and poor immune reconstitution and have been attributed to inadequate antibody production and functional hyposplenism [7, 9]. Vaccination and antibiotic prophylaxis should be considered. Vaccination with the 23-valent polysaccharide vaccine is recommended for all transplant recipients at their 1 year after transplant anniversary [10, 11]. The current European Guidelines of the Infectious Diseases Working Party of the EBMT also recommend the heptavalent conjugate vaccine for adults with chronic GvHD (who typically do not respond to the polysaccharide vaccine) [11]. *S. pneumoniae* prophylaxis with penicillin for adults following transplant has been recommended by the Centers for Disease Control (CDC)/American Society of Blood And Marrow Transplantation/Infectious Diseases Society of America (IDSA) guidelines for all patients with chronic GvHD who are being actively treated [10]. Other transplant experts suggest beginning universal penicillin prophylaxis at 6 months after transplant for all allogeneic transplant recipients. The local patterns of penicillin resistance place these universal recommendations into question, and we advise antibiotic prophylaxis (i.e., penicillin, trimethoprim-sulfamethoxazole, azithromycin or levofloxacin) for patients with active chronic GvHD. We vaccinate all transplant recipients with the conjugated vaccine at 12 months and transplant recipients at the National Institutes of Health (NIH) receive an additional vaccination at 6 months after transplantation. This approach has been shown to be effective in a small randomized, double blind trial among allogeneic transplant recipients whose donors also were vaccinated [12]. Given that the responses to immunization are not universal and compliance with long-term oral antibiotics is uncertain, we believe that it is critical that all transplant recipients be promptly seen by a physician when they develop fever. We typically recommend, for such patients, the use of empirical antibiotics that contain excellent activity against *Streptococcus pneumoniae*.

21.2.2 Management of Fever During Neutropenia

The latest versions of the IDSA and National Cancer Center Networks (NCCN) Guidelines on this topic remain current [4, 13], but several studies have been completed since these guidelines were published. The mainstay of therapy continues to be the use of broad-spectrum beta-lactam antibiotics that incorporate excellent activity against *Pseudomonas aeruginosa*. The different agents seem to have similar overall efficacy, and local antibiotic susceptibility patterns are the most important factor in the decision to use ceftazidime, cefepime, imipenem, meropenem, or piperacillin/tazobactam. A recent meta-analysis suggested that carbapenems may be associated with more pseudomembranous colitis, and that cefepime may be associated with increased overall mortality [14]. The importance of this later finding still needs to be confirmed, but is disconcerting. The use of aminoglycosides combined with a beta-lactam antibiotic is effective but is generally associated with increased toxicity [15, 16], and we reserve such combinations for cases of infections associated with shock, when the broadest coverage is mandatory. Glycopeptide antibiotics like vancomycin are not usually needed before a Gram-positive infection has been documented [17]. However, there are some transplant experts who believe that in the presence of fluoroquinolone prophylaxis such empiric Gram-positive specific antibiotic therapy is justified. The common practice of adding vancomycin empirically after 48 h of fever was compared to placebo in a randomized controlled trial and was found to be ineffective and thus is not routinely recommended [18]. A recent randomized trial suggested that linezolid could be safely substituted for vancomycin when required during treatment of fever and neutropenia [19], but there are no data to answer the question if linezolid should be part of the initial empirical regimen during fever and neutropenia in patients who are colonized with vancomycin-resistant enterococci (VRE).

21.2.3 Bacterial Infections Caused by Specific Pathogens

21.2.3.1 Clostridium difficile

Clostridium difficile colitis presents special challenges in the transplant setting, especially when it presents during periods of neutropenia or at times in which the patient is at high risk for the development of GvHD. The presence of abdominal pain and diarrhea during periods of neutropenia may suggest neutropenic enterocolitis, but it is important to rule out *C. difficile*, as it can be the cause of or a contributing factor to this syndrome and requires specific treatment.

The diagnosis of *C. difficile* colitis relies on the detection of its toxins in the stool. Practical considerations now preclude many centers from performing the cell culture cytoxicity assay, which is still considered the "gold standard" diagnostic test. Currently available EIA tests that detect toxins A and B seem to offer reasonable sensitivity (80–90% range) and specificity (approximately 95%) [20]. The practice of repeating the stool test several times before accepting a negative result is commonly used but unsupported by clinical evidence [21]. We believe that HSCT recipients who develop diarrhea should have stools tested for the presence of *C. difficile* toxin, and if negative should undergo sigmoidoscopy or colonoscopy and biopsy to evaluate the patient for the cause of diarrhea and to exclude other illnesses including GvHD and cytomegalovirus (CMV) enteritis. *C. difficile* colitis has also been reported to result in an increased incidence and severity of GvHD, [22], and this association underscores the necessity to establish a correct diagnosis in HSCT recipients.

The treatment of *C. difficile* is still controversial. The available randomized controlled trials have been repeatedly reviewed systematically, and meta-analyses and practice guidelines have been published [23–26]. In summary, treatment should incorporate the discontinuation of the offending agents (most commonly antibiotics) where possible, and while mild cases may not benefit from specific antibiotic treatment, most transplant recipients with *C. difficile* colitis require treatment [23, 24]. It is unknown which antibiotic is best for a severe case of *C. difficile*, but several guidelines recommend using metronidazole (250–500 mg p.o. q8h) as a first-line agent and reserving vancomycin (125–250 mg p.o. q6h) for metronidazole failures [26, 27]. Some experts believe that oral vancomycin is more effective than metronidazole in patients with cancer, but this perception seems to be based more on poor efficacy of metronidazole in recent case series than to older comparative studies [28], although the most recent clinical trial did show that vancomycin was better in cases of severe disease [29]. The antiparasitic agent nitazoxanide has efficacy that may be comparable to metronidazole and could be used as a possible second-line treatment [30]. The expected response to treatment is rapid defervescence (if fever is present) and resolution of the diarrhea over 4–6 days [31]. Relapses following completion of treatment are quite common (10–45%), but most respond to standard retreatment. A variety of approaches (based on expert opinion) have been attempted for patients with persistently relapsing infection including tapered metronidazole or vancomycin, "pulsed" dose vancomycin, probiotics (of unproven efficacy and potentially dangerous for patients with suppressed immune systems), steroids, intravenous immunoglobulin, and stool implants [27, 31, 32].

21.2.3.2 Vancomycin-Resistant Enterococcus

The frequency of vancomycin-resistant enterococcus (VRE) colonization and infections has increased among transplant recipients. The mortality of transplant recipients who develop VRE bacteremia is high, and is reported to be associated with attributable-mortality. There continues to be controversy regarding the actual role of VRE infection in patient death, and some experts have suggested that VRE colonization and infection are really just a marker of the "overall severity of illness," A case-control study from the Mayo Clinic found that transplant patients colonized with VRE were twice as likely to die by day 100 compared with noncolonized transplant recipients [33]. A study from Memorial Sloan-Kettering followed 92 patients who were screened for stool colonization with VRE. Thirty-seven (40.2%) of the 92 were colonized, and more than one third of those colonized developed VRE bacteremia before day 35. The authors determined that the attributable/contributory mortality of the infection was 35.7% (5 of 14), and suggest empirical coverage of VRE be considered for patients who are known to be colonized with VRE when they develop fever and neutropenia [34]. Until this question is more fully addressed in a prospective controlled trial, we recommend that transplant physicians have a low threshold for instituting treatment for pathogens like VRE that are resistant to multiple antibiotics.

The treatment of established VRE bacteremia is difficult, but removal of indwelling venous access devices appears to be an important part of the treatment approach. Linezolid, daptomycin, and quinupristin/dalfopristin are typically considered first-line agents. Linezolid and quinupristin/dalfopristin for VRE bacteremia were compared in a controlled trial in cancer patients, and both exhibited only modest efficacy (58% and 43%, respectively) [35]. Antibiotic-associated side effects were different for both: Linezolid is associated with marrow suppression while quinupristin/dalfopristin can cause severe debilitating myalgias. Daptomycin, which has the theoretical advantage of being bactericidal against enterococci, was used on nine neutropenic patients with fever and VRE bacteremia and resulted in four cures [36]. Tigecycline exhibits in vitro activity and there are anecdotal reports of its successful use when other alternatives are unavailable. However, its real clinical efficacy is unknown.

21.2.3.3 Resistant Gram-Negative Bacilli

The incidence of infections caused by Gram-negative bacilli resistant to multiple antibiotics is increasing. These infections tend to occur among severely ill immunocompromised patients with indwelling catheters who have received multiple courses of antibiotics. Multi-resistant *Pseudomonas aeruginosa* and *Acinetobacter baumannii*, carbapenem-resistant *Klebsiella*, and *Stenotrophomonas maltophilia* are examples of these pathogens that can be difficult to treat and constitute a significant infection problem in some hospitals. A detailed overview of each one of these pathogens is beyond the scope of this review, but some general points can be made. The general strategies to treat these infections include one or more of the following [37]: (1) infection source control including the removal of the indwelling venous access catheter and/or drainage of abscesses; (2) continuous infusion of beta-lactam antibiotics to achieve concentrations well above the measured MIC; and (3) use of antibiotic combinations in an attempt to achieve an additive or synergistic effect. In some cases of Acinetobacter infection the use of colistin or polymyxin B, tigecycline or high-dose ampicillin-sulbactam has been reported to be helpful. Inhaled colistin has also been reported as adjuvant therapy for pneumonia caused by Acinetobacter and Pseudomonas species [38].

21.3 Infectious Complications of Venous Access Devices in Patients Who Undergo HSCT

Reliable vascular access is an essential feature of HSCT care, but clinical management of catheter-related infections, infection risks associated with different catheter types, and strategies for prevention of catheter-related infections remain important clinical issues that transplant physicians must continue to address. Several of these important clinical questions are discussed below.

21.3.1 Catheter-Associated Infections, Microbiology and Clinical Management

The organisms that most commonly cause catheter-associated bloodstream infections mirror the microbial spectrum of pathogens that cause present day hospital acquired infections. Pooled data from the late 1990s and early 2000s indicate that coagulase-negative staphylococci are still most common (37%), but enterococci have become much more prevalent at 13% [39]. Antimicrobial susceptibility patterns continue to evolve with more than 50% of hospital acquired *S. aureus* being methicillin (oxacillin) resistant, and these pathogens have more frequently been isolated from community-acquired infections. The number of enterococcal isolates resistant to vancomycin (VRE) continues to increase, and in several studies this incidence has been reported to approach 26%. *Candida* spp. cause 8% of hospital acquired infections, and antimicrobial resistance has also increased for these isolates. SCOPE data suggests that 10% of *C. albicans* will be resistant to fluconazole, and that more than 50% of all *Candida* spp. infections will be caused by nonalbicans species including *C. glabrata* and *C. krusei*. Gram-negative infections are increasingly caused by Enterobacteriaceae that produce extended spectrum beta-lactamases (ESBLs), and are often resistant to many other antibiotics.

Catheter-associated infections are routinely categorized either as an entrance or exit site infection (henceforth "exit site infection"), a tunnel or port-pocket infection, and/or a catheter-associated bloodstream infection. Importantly, the first two infection groups are usually defined based on clinical characteristics and may not have a specific pathogen identified. Entrance or exit site infections represent infection localized to the skin and soft tissue that surrounds the catheter entrance but is distal to the first catheter cuff. Entrance or exit site infections are usually not associated with a bloodstream infection. Tunnel or port-pocket infections involve the catheter tunnel track from the catheter cuff or subcutaneous port pocket to the catheter entrance into the vein. Tunnel and port pocket infections are frequently accompanied by positive blood cultures (30–40%). The clinical manifestations of a tunnel or port pocket infection can be variable and range from minimal inflammation if the patient is neutropenic, to a painful cellulitis that rapidly progresses to soft tissue necrosis and ulceration. Port pocket infections pose a significant clinical challenge because the local site may be asymptomatic.

The largest prospective, single center trial of cuffed catheters (Hickman catheters) like those frequently used for patients who undergo HSCT was conducted more than two decades ago in non-transplant patients with cancer [40]. Over the course of 10 years (1978–1987), all cuffed catheters [single (n = 312) or double lumen (n = 378) Hickman catheters] that were placed in adult patients with cancer were prospectively assessed. The report chronicles the outcome of 134,273 catheter days (IVD). Infectious complications included 160 exit site infections (1.19/1000 IVD days), 46 tunnel infections (0.34/1000 IVD days) and 397 bloodstream infections (2.96/1000 IVD days). Two hundred thirty-one of 690 catheters were free of all infection complications. Multivariate analysis revealed that the risk of developing a catheter-associated infectious complication was increased when a double lumen rather than a single lumen catheter was placed, when the patient's weight exceeded 125% of his or her ideal body weight, or when the catheter was placed during a period of neutropenia. Catheter insertion by dedicated surgeons decreased the risk of noninfectious complications but was not an important factor in the development of infectious complications.

21.3.2 Infectious Complications of Venous Access Devices

21.3.2.1 Exit Site Infections

In the above mentioned trial, exit site infections occurred a median of 80 days (range from 1 to 1210 days) from catheter placement. The most commonly identified pathogens were *S. aureus* (35). Bloodstream infections occurred rarely (13/160 infections). Almost all (150/160) infections were successfully treated without catheter removal, suggesting that catheter removal is usually not necessary for the successful management of an exit site infection

21.3.2.2 Tunnel infections

Tunnel infections in this report occurred a median of 70 days (range 2–727 days) after placement, and their incidence was similar for double and single lumen catheters (0.35 vs. 0.26/1000 IVD). Twelve of the 46 infections were associated with a bloodstream infection, and 12 infections were caused by *S. aureus*. Gram-negative bacilli, other Gram-positive cocci, atypical mycobacteria, and fungi also were reported to cause tunnel infections. Only 22 of 46 infections were successfully managed without catheter removal, and five of the remaining 24 infections had slow or poor infection control with just antibiotic therapy. This experience suggests that a serious tunnel or port pocket infection should be managed with immediate or early catheter removal and broad-spectrum antibiotics that include activity against *S. aureus*.

21.3.2.3 Catheter-Associated Bloodstream Infections

The above study from the University of Maryland Cancer Center made no attempt to determine if the catheter was the primary cause of the bloodstream infection. Rather they reported on the clinical outcome of all bloodstream infections that occurred in these patients during the time that the catheter was in place. Three hundred ninety-seven bloodstream infections occurred during the 134,000 catheter days. Only 25 of these bloodstream infections were clearly associated with exit site or tunnel infections. Gram-positive cocci were the most frequent pathogens (138/397), with coagulase-negative staphylococci recovered from blood cultures in 62 patients. Fifty-four of 62 coagulase-negative staphylococcal bloodstream infections and 26 of 28 *S. aureus* bloodstream infections were successfully treated without catheter removal. This report describes no episodes of bloodstream infection with vancomycin-resistant enterococci, but only 1 of 14 vancomycin-sensitive enterococcal bloodstream infections required catheter removal for infection control. Enterobacteraciae were recovered from 111 of 397 bloodstream infections, and 107 were successfully treated without catheter removal. *Pseudomonas aeruginosa* was recovered from 29 bloodstream infections, and 27 were successfully treated without catheter removal. Eight episodes of *Bacillus* spp. bacteremia and five episodes of *Corynebacterium jeikeium* occurred in this patient cohort, and five and four episodes, respectively, required catheter removal. Of 46 episodes of yeast or mold bloodstream infection, 21 required catheter removal. Nineteen of the remaining 25 fungal infections had persistent fungemia, but the catheter was left in place because the infected patient had terminal cancer. Several other reports, literature reviews, and clinical care guidelines have suggested that bloodstream infections caused by organisms such as yeast and fungi, atypical mycobacteria, *Bacillus* spp, *S. aureus*, *P. aeruginosa*, *Stenotrophomonas maltophilia*, *Corynebacterium jeikeium*, and vancomycin-resistant enterococci may be particularly difficult to manage with antimicrobial therapy alone, and thus for these pathogens it is recommended that catheter removal occur immediately once these pathogens are identified.

21.3.3 Specific Questions Regarding Catheter-Related Infections

21.3.3.1 Is a PICC Line Safer than a Tunneled, Cuffed and Surgically Placed Central Venous Catheter?

Reliable data on catheter type and risk of infection are now available from a meta-analysis published by Maki and colleagues, who reviewed 200 prospective studies in adult patients [41]. In the meta-analysis PICC lines were associated with a slightly lower risk of catheter-associated infection when compared to central venous catheters that are both tunneled and cuffed (1.1 vs. 1.6/1000 IVD days). The placement of a PICC line is usually less traumatic to the patient and is associated with a decrease in placement costs; thus, it may have a role in the management of patients undergoing HSCT.

21.3.3.2 Do Antimicrobial Impregnated Catheters Decrease the Risk of Catheter-Related Infections Associated with Long-Term Indwelling Venous Access Devices?

In the largest prospective randomized trial in patients with cancer, Hanna et al. reported the rate of catheter-related bloodstream infections was lower for the antimicrobial impregnated PICC lines than the nontunneled, noncuffed subclavian central venous catheters (0.25 infections vs. 1.28 infections per 1000 IVD days) [42]. Antimicrobial-impregnated catheters are in general more expensive, but the increased cost may be offset by the substantially lower costs to insert a PICC line than a surgical placed tunneled catheter [43]

21.3.3.3 Is a Surgically Implanted Central or Peripheral Venous Port Safer than a Cuffed and Tunneled Central Venous Catheter?

Apparently, yes (0.1 vs. 1.6 BSI/1000 IVD days) [41, 44]. However, most subcutaneous ports provide limited venous access, and thus a subcutaneous port for patients undergoing HSCT may limit the health care team's ability to adequately deliver care.

21.3.3.4 Which Approaches are Important for the Prevention or Reduction of Catheter-Related Infections?

Measures to minimize the risk of infections associated with venous access devices must strike a balance between patient safety and cost. Methods and approaches to meet these goals have been clearly outlined in the Center for Disease Control and Prevention Recommendations [45]. The CDC report acknowledges that prevention approaches must adjust to a changing knowledge base and technology. Several of the more important recommendations include:

- *Hand Hygiene and Aseptic Technique*: Good hand hygiene before catheter insertion and during catheter maintenance and manipulation are critical infection prevention techniques. Good hand hygiene can be achieved through the use of waterless alcohol-based products, or antibacterial soap and water combined with adequate rinsing. The level of barrier protection during catheter insertion should include maximal sterile barrier techniques that consist of caps, masks, sterile gowns, sterile gloves and large sterile drapes. Such sterile barrier techniques are also appropriate for PICC line placement.
- *Skin Antisepsis*: Povidone iodine has been the most widely used antiseptic for cleansing insertion sites, but in one study, site preparation with 2% aqueous chlorhexidine-gluconate significantly lowered the bloodstream infection rates when compared to 10% povidone-iodine or 70% alcohol [46].
- *Catheter Site Dressing Regimens*: A meta-analysis has assessed studies that compared the risk of catheter-associated bloodstream infections and the different types of catheter dressings [47]. The risk of infection appears to be similar regardless of whether the catheter is dressed with a transparent, semipermeable polyurethane dressing, or qauze and tape.
- *Systemic Antibiotic Prophylaxis*: Prophylactic oral or parenteral antibiotics or antifungal drugs do not appear to reduce the incidence of catheter-associated bloodstream infections in adults.
- *Antibiotic Lock Prophylaxis*: Antibiotic lock prophylaxis using antibiotic solutions that contain vancomycin and/or ciprofloxacin have been tested as an approach to decrease the risk of catheter-associated bloodstream infections. A meta-analysis suggested the usefulness of such prophylaxis and reported a decrease in the rate of bloodstream infections by vancomycin-susceptible organisms [48] (53). However, because the use of vancomycin is an independent predictor for the acquisition or development of VRE, the practice of vancomycin locks is not recommended.

Pronovost and colleagues employed five of the most important CDC recommendations in a multi-hospital (108 hospitals) ICU setting (54). They implemented (1) hand hygiene, (2) full-barrier precautions during insertion, (3) skin cleansing with chlorhexidine, (4) avoiding the femoral insertion site, and (5) removal of unnecessary catheters. They analyzed more than 375,000 catheter days, and reported almost complete elimination of catheter-related infections among patients who had a catheter placed [49]. It is unclear what the impact of such an approach would have on HSCT patients with indwelling venous access devices, but a transplant center catheter management approach is strongly encouraged.

21.3.3.5 What is the Appropriate Approach for Obtaining Blood Cultures from Patients with Suspected Infection Who Have a Long-Term Indwelling Venous Access Device?

The volume of cultured blood (20–40 cc) is clearly the most important factor in maximizing the recovery of organisms [50]. However, if the goal of the blood culture technique is to also define the role of the catheter in the bloodstream infection, several different techniques have been studied and could be considered [51–55]. These are commonly based on the premise that a higher bacterial load is present in the blood cultured from the contaminated catheter than in the blood drawn from a peripheral site or a different catheter, and it will result in a quantitative difference in the amount of bacterial colonies recovered or the time needed for the culture to become positive. The first method is the concordance between the recovery of blood culture isolates from cultures drawn through the vascular access device and a peripheral vein. Second is the identification of at least a fivefold or greater quantitative difference in the number of organisms recovered in paired blood cultures drawn from the venous device and a peripheral vein. Third is the identification of a difference of more than 1000 colony forming units/ml of blood between quantitative blood cultures drawn from the venous access device and peripheral vein, and fourth is the differential in time to positive results from blood cultures drawn from the venous access device and a peripheral vein. All of these methods have potential value but all have major limitations. The method that relies on the differential in time to positive results may be the method best suited for clinical use since it has the advantage of not requiring expensive and time-consuming quantitative methodologies, and these time determinations are automatically provided by modern blood-culture bottle automated readers. Using this method, a catheter infection is deemed to be present when the blood culture drawn through the catheter is positive at least 120 min earlier than the blood culture drawn from a peripheral vein. This technique provides a pooled sensitivity of 0.9 and pooled specificity of 0.72 [54].

These approaches may help to decide if an episode of bacteremia is related to the catheter or not [56]. However, most transplant clinicians do not rely on such laboratory information to determine if the IV catheter should be immediately removed as part of the infection management approach, but rather rely on clinical response and the recovered pathogen to define the role for removing the vascular access device.

21.4 Advances in the Prevention and Treatment of Fungal Infections After Hematopoietic Stem Cell Transplantation

Invasive fungal infections (IFIs) are now the most common cause of infectious mortality after transplant, but the prognosis of some of these infections appears to have improved during the past decade. The attributable mortality of invasive aspergillosis following transplant has been reported in a retrospective study performed at the Fred Hutchinson Cancer Research Center to have decreased from 40% in 1990–1992 to 20% in the period 2002–2004 [57]. This improvement in outcome is likely multifactorial, but new therapies have likely had a major impact.

21.4.1 Prevention of Invasive Fungal Infections

Transplant recipients are at risk for invasive fungal infections during three well-defined periods: The first is the period of neutropenia (<40 days after transplant); the second is the period of greatest risk of developing graft-versus-host disease (day 40–180); and the third, which applies only to allogeneic HSCT recipients, occurs late (>6 months after transplant) and is likely a marker for poor post-transplant immune reconstitution. Tailored prophylaxis taking into consideration the conditioning regimen, the specific active immunosuppression, and other risk factors may be an approach that has greatest value, and we recommend it over the classic universal recommendations of the past.

21.4.1.1 Prevention of Fungal Infections During Neutropenia

The incidence of invasive aspergillosis and other mold infections early after transplant is directly proportional to the patient's duration of profound neutropenia and history of previously treated fungal disease. Trials that compare antifungal agents may fail to show significant differences among them if the period of neutropenia is too short or if its degree is too limited for patients to be at risk for the development of aspergillosis or other mold infections.

Fluconazole prophylaxis has been the standard of care since randomized trials were first published in the 1990s and reported a decrease in the incidence of IFI [58] and an improvement in overall survival [59]. The survival advantage of fluconazole was maintained when the antifungal agent was continued until day 75 after transplant. [59, 60]. The transplant conditioning regimen used for the patients included in these fluconazole trials differs from many of today's reduced-intensity regimens and must be considered when recommendations of antifungal prophylaxis are developed and updated. Fluconazole is only effective prophylaxis against *Candida albicans*, and if other pathogens are thought to be a priority a different agent should be considered. Itraconazole has been compared to fluconazole in several trials [61–63]. Although itraconazole has activity against *Aspergillus* and fluconazole does not, the outcomes associated with itraconazole usage have not consistently been better than when fluconazole is prescribed. This seems related mainly to intolerance, bioavailability, and side effects of itraconazole [64]. Micafungin, an echinocandin, was found in a large trial to be equivalent to fluconazole [65] and resulted in fewer episodes of invasive aspergillosis, although this latter difference was not statistically significant ($p = 0.07$). Posaconazole has been tested in a randomized controlled trial of nontransplant patients with prolonged neutropenia and been found to provide better protection against fungal infections than either fluconazole or itraconazole [66]. This experience has led some authorities to recommend posaconazole prophylaxis as the standard of care for HSCT recipients [4].

21.4.1.2 Empirical Addition of Antifungal Therapy During Neutropenia

The addition of empirical antifungal coverage after 4–7 days of persistent fever has become the accepted standard of care. Empirical antifungal coverage continues because of the difficulty with the early diagnosis of fungal disease and also the availability of new antifungal agents that are less toxic than amphotericin B. The fact remains, however, than even in the largest trials of persistent fever during neutropenia, only a small minority of patients are ever documented to have a fungal infection [67, 68]. A new strategy based on serial patient surveillance using CT scans and the galactomannan antigen assay has been proposed [69], and a proof-of-principle study suggests it may be possible for transplant clinicians to be more selective with their use of empiric antifungal therapy [70]. We recommend a thorough search (including meticulous physical exam, CT of chest and sinuses, and galactomannan and beta-D-glucan antigen) for invasive fungal infections in transplant recipients with persistent fever during a period of neutropenia. Such a search can result in classification of patients as being either at low or high likelihood of having an active IFI thus allowing for a risk-based intervention. If patients have no evidence of fungal infection other than the persistent fever, watchful waiting and serial galactomannan antigen assays may be a reasonable approach, although many transplant physicians will error on the side of initiating empirical treatment with caspofungin [68], voriconazole [67], or liposomal amphotericin B [71]. Alternatively, if a pulmonary nodule or sinusitis is discovered, the likelihood of invasive mold infection is very high, and we recommend more aggressive diagnostic measures plus the immediate initiation of broad-spectrum antifungal therapy with either voriconazole or amphotericin B. For patients who appear to be more ill we recommend combining either of these agents with an echinocandin like caspofungin with the hope of improving the antifungal activity with the most profound immunosuppression.

21.4.1.3 Prevention of Fungal Infections During Treatment of Graft-Versus-Host Disease

Patients with severe acute GvHD receiving corticosteroids are the group at highest risk for invasive fungal infections after transplant. One randomized controlled trial has specifically targeted this population and compared fluconazole with posaconazole, a newer azole with no intravenous formulation, limited oral bioavailability but a very broad spectrum of antifungal activity including *Aspergillus* and many zygomycetes [72]. This prophylaxis trial confirmed the important principle that an agent active against aspergillosis is superior to fluconazole when patients are at high-risk of aspergillosis. The reported success of posaconazole is remarkable considering the fact that some patients experience decreased oral absorption because of gut GvHD. It is not known if a different broad-spectrum antifungal agent that could be administered intravenously like voriconazole or an echinocandin would perform as well as posaconazole in this clinical setting, but certainly such trials need to be conducted.

The Blood and Transplant-Clinical Trials Network (BMT-CTN) in the United States has recently reported in abstract a comparison of oral voriconazole to fluconazole as prophylaxis for aspergillosis among patients undergoing a myeloablative allogeneic transplant [73]. This study failed to show an improvement in overall patient survival between patient groups, but the incidence of *Aspergillus* infection was lower among patients randomized to receive voriconazole. The results from this well designed, randomized, double-blind trial are a bit surprising and again raise questions of the oral bioavailability of these agents in patients who may experience malabsorption from either cytotoxic conditioning regimens or GvHD.

We routinely prescribe fluconazole 400 mg/day as our preferred post-transplant antifungal prophylaxis. This decision is based on the fact that our average time from transplant to neutrophil recovery is relatively short (<10 days of profound neutropenia), and the risk of mold infection is low. We do not routinely use posaconazole during neutropenia in our transplant population, but if enhanced antifungal prophylaxis directed against aspergillosis is needed (i.e., expected prolonged neutropenia, concomitant risk factors, prior history of aspergillosis) we recommend voriconazole. Voriconazole is chosen over posaconazole because it does not require a concomitant fatty meal to enhance absorption and can be administered parenterally if oral therapy is not feasible. We also routinely switch from fluconazole to voriconazole in patients who develop GvHD and receive a daily cumulative dose of corticosteroids that is equal to or higher than 1 mg/kg/day of prednisone. Posaconazole has shown to be effective in this latter setting, and is an excellent alternative [4].

For patients where fluconazole or other azoles cannot be used (e.g., because drug interactions or suspicion of liver toxicity), we substitute an echinocandin such as caspofungin [65]. Of note, caspofungin may alter cyclosporine pharmacokinetics and increase the area under the curve (AUC) and peak levels. While the manufacturer does not recommend the use of caspofungin in patients receiving cyclosporine, it can be safely employed if careful blood level monitoring is performed.

21.4.2 Diagnosis and Management of Invasive Fungal Infections

21.4.2.1 The Empirical Management of Positive Blood Cultures with Yeast

The development of blood cultures for yeast demands that the clinician question whether the blood culture isolate is most likely to be *Candida* (by far the most common yeast) or another yeast (e.g., *Cryptococcus, Trichosporon, Rhodotorula, Histoplasma, Blastoschizomyces*). This decision is important because treatment options will differ. Most transplant patients receive prophylaxis with fluconazole or another azole antifungal agent. Consequently, when fungemia develops it is most frequently caused by a nonalbicans *Candida* species (*C. glabrata*, *C. krusei*). Such infection may originate from the gastrointestinal tract or may be catheter-related. The catheter-associated infections are believed to occur when there is introduction of yeast into the soft tissues surrounding the catheter from the adjacent colonized skin or through the introduction of contaminated infusates. The formation of catheter-associated biofilm allows the yeast to grow and thrive despite the administration of the antifungal therapy.

Several studies have compared amphotericin B, fluconazole and echinocandins for treatment of invasive candidiasis (mainly candidemia in nonneutropenic patients) [74–77]. Although some published guidelines and experts still recommend a lipid formulation of amphotericin B in patients who are clinically unstable, most transplant and infectious disease physicians now consider an echinocandin (caspofungin, anidulafungin or micafungin) the treatment of choice for invasive or disseminated *Candida* spp. infections. All echinocandins are available only in an intravenous form, and the differences between them in antimicrobial spectrum (e.g., caspofungin has limited activity against *C. parapsilosis*) and toxicity are of unknown clinical significance. As a general rule, we recommend that the intravenous catheter be removed from all infected patients once the blood culture isolate is reported to be a yeast or mold.

21.4.2.2 Management of Invasive Fungal Infections

The management of fungal infections after transplant raises several critical clinical issues including:

1. What is the optimal empirical antifungal treatment of choice and what is the role for combinations of antifungal antibiotics?
2. What is the optimal approach for diagnosing an invasive fungal infection, and what are the roles of bronchoscopy, biopsy and noninvasive assays (galactomannan and beta-D-glucan antigen) in establishing a diagnosis?
3. Is it appropriate clinical management to consider the concomitant use of voriconazole and sirolimus?
4. What is the optimal dose of lipid formulation amphotericin B?
5. Is amphotericin B still the treatment of choice for zygomycetes infections after transplant, and if a lipid-formulation of amphotericin B is used, what is the optimal dose?

A new fever with a pulmonary nodule during broad-spectrum antibiotic treatment of fever and neutropenia or for the patient who is receiving immunosuppression for GvHD is very suggestive of a mold infection. *Aspergillus* is by far the most common mold, but other pathogens including zygomycetes (*Mucor*, *Rhizopus* and others, all resistant to voriconazole), Fusarium and Scedosporium must be considered. Thus the first question the clinician must consider is the need for empiric coverage of zygomycosis versus treatment with therapy targeted primarily against aspergillosis. The primary clinical feature that has been identified as a risk factor for zygomycosis is voriconazole prophylaxis, and thus specific empiric therapy for zygomycoses is most important in patients who have previously received voriconazole. The decision to prescribe treatment that is active against zygomycosis has in the past relied exclusively on a lipid formulation of amphotericin B, but posaconazole may also be effective treatment for such infections. Treatment that is directed primarily against aspergillosis would employ the empiric use of voriconazole. Voriconazole was found to be superior to amphotericin in a randomized controlled trial [78], has the advantages of a much lower toxicity profile than amphotericin B products, and unlike posaconazole is available in both an oral and IV formulation. However, voriconazole lacks antimicrobial activity against zygomycosis and thus the risk of a zygomycoses infection makes the decision of greater importance.

The diagnostic use of galactomannan antigen (in serum or bronchoalveolar lavage) in this setting has been recommended, but considerable uncertainty remains. Serum galactomannan antigen assay has shown more value when used as a screening test repeated serially over time rather than as a one-time test [79, 80]. A positive result is specific for aspergillosis, but the incidence of false negative results in serum is common and leaves the clinician faced with the questions of whether the patient truly does not have invasive aspergillosis, the patient has invasive aspergillosis but the test is a false negative, or the infection is caused by a non-*Aspergillus* mold. False positives are much less common but have been described, on occasion, when the patient was receiving concomitant piperacillin-tazobactam [81]. The BMT-CTN in their recently completed fungal prophylaxis trial attempted to answer the question about the relative value of serial glactomannan antigen assay as an early indicator of aspergillosis among recipients of a myeloablative, related donor, allogeneic transplant. Analysis is not yet complete but preliminary results suggest little clinical utility for such testing.

It is not known which empirical antifungal regimen results in the best patient outcomes. When tested in a randomized controlled trial both single agent voriconazole and amphotericin B resulted in low overall response rates for the subgroups of allogeneic transplant recipients and neutropenic patients with invasive aspergillosis [78]. Invasive mold infections may progress quickly during periods of neutropenia or severe T-cell immune suppression, and thus despite the lack of definitive prospective data the concept of empiric combination antifungal therapy for patients who are very ill or have more significant immune suppression remains controversial but attractive. Evidence from animal studies suggests that the combination of an azole and echinocandin is superior to an azole alone for invasive aspergillosis [82], and a retrospective clinical study in humans provides some additional support for such combination therapy [83]. The primary arguments against combination therapy rest on concerns about toxicity and cost. Despite these issues we frequently will prescribe initial treatment with either voriconazole plus caspofungin or liposomal amphotericin B and caspofungin and then adjust therapy as permitted based on the results of the patient's diagnostic workup and clinical response. We do not recommend that agents from all three classes (an azole with amphotericin and echinocandin) of antifungal therapy be combined. While there is animal and laboratory data that suggests potential antagonism when such an approach is utilized [84], there is no clinical data that either supports or refutes the value of such combination treatment.

Not all patients with invasive aspergillosis will respond to treatment with azole antibiotics like voriconazole or posaconazole. It is possible that some of the failures that have been reported with voriconazole are secondary to inadequate serum levels [85]. There is ample evidence that shows the inter-individual variability when oral voriconazole dosing is utilized, and this has resulted in the NIH transplant team recommending that voriconazole levels be monitored in patients whose infections appear to be failing to respond. The Milwaukee transplant team rarely performs voriconazole serum monitoring primarily because of the difficulty in obtaining such clinical results, but they do have a standard policy to increase the administered daily dose or to switch to IV therapy if there is concern about a patient's clinical response or the adequacy of a patient's oral absorption.

Empiric treatment does not replace the need for implementation of aggressive methods to identify a specific etiologic diagnosis, and thus many of these patients must undergo additional diagnostic procedures if a specific pathogen is to be identified. The diagnosis of pulmonary or sinus infections with molds continues to rely first on CT scanning of these body sites for initial detection. Unfortunately, radiographic identification of an active or progressive infection does not establish the specific etiologic pathogen. Invasive procedures including bronchoscopy, bronchoalveolar lavage and biopsy have relatively low sensitivities (50–60%), but a positive result is diagnostic [86, 87]. Additional tissue biopsies including endoscopic sinus biopsy and thoracoscopic lung biopsy should be considered early in a patient's course when a diagnosis is critical and the patient's clinical status allows him or her to more easily tolerate such invasive procedures. Transplant physicians continue to search for diagnostic approaches that result in a high level of specificity and sensitivity but decrease procedure-associated morbidity. The use of serum or BAL fluid galactomannan antigen assays continues to be studied and recommended by some experts, but most transplant physicians have cared for patients with biopsy proven aspergillosis who have had repetitively negative serum galactomannan antigen assays. The reasons for these false negative cases is unclear but perhaps reflect a limited amount of disease at the time the infection is first identified or is caused by molds other than *Aspergillus* that have a similar histological appearance. This latter possibility is significant since it has been reported that at least 10–20% of histologically proven invasive mold infections will be culture negative [86].

A question that is now more frequently being asked is what is the appropriate therapy for infections caused by zygomycetes? Is it a lipid-formulation of amphotericin B, and if so what is the appropriate dose, or is treatment with an agent like posaconazole an appropriate alternative? Amphotericin B has been the gold standard, but clinical results in HSCT recipients have been disappointing.

Some experts believe that the poor clinical response to amphotericin B therapy is a reflection of insufficient dosage, but a randomized trial reported that 10 mg/kg/day of liposomal amphotericin B was no more effective than 3 mg/kg/day in the treatment of confirmed mold infection [88], although most of these patients were infected with *Aspergillus* and not zygomycetes. It is unknown what the best dose of amphotericin B for zygomycosis is, but we recommend a dose of 5 mg/kg/day. It is also important to recall that posaconazole has activity against many of the zygomycetes (not all), and we and others have had anecdotal experience suggesting that posaconazole therapy may be effective treatment for such infections when they occur in an HSCT recipient. Posaconazole is associated with significantly less toxicity than the amphotericin B products, but its lack of an IV formulation can make drug tolerance and absorption a significant concern.

The final question relates to the concomitant use of azole antifungal agents and immunosuppressive agents like cyclosporine, tacrolimus or sirolimus. Schemes for dose adjustment have been developed but frequent monitoring of the serum levels in patients receiving voriconazole and one of the calcineurin inhibitors is critical. An even more difficult question is the appropriate management of patients who may be receiving concomitant voriconazole and sirolimus. There is a "black box" warning emphasizing the interaction between these two drugs, and it is well known that voriconazole therapy significantly increases the serum levels of sirolimus (AUC increases up to 10-fold). Yet, the need to prescribe voriconazole for some patients receiving sirolimus is real. Thus it is suggested that by reducing the sirolimus dose by 90% and carefully monitoring sirolimus levels, these agents can be successfully co-administrated [89].

21.5 Pneumocystis Infection After Stem Cell Transplantation

Pneumocystis is now classified as a "nonmold" fungus. Although some controversy persists regarding nomenclature. We have chosen to follow current recommendations by which the name *Pneumocystis carinii* applies to the rat pathogen and *Pneumocystis jiroveci* to the organism that is isolated in humans [90]. The acronym "PCP" to signify Pneumocystis pneumonia has been maintained, and is still frequently used. Prophylaxis against Pneumocystis pneumonia (PCP) is universally recommended after HSCT [10], and if compliance is maintained it results in relatively low incidence of disease (23 cases in 14 years at the M.D. Anderson, for an incidence of 386 cases per 100,000 [91], or 1.3–2.4% of patients transplanted at Brigham and Women's Hospital or the University of Minnesota. Most cases seem to occur after discontinuing prophylaxis or during periods of intensive immunosuppression for the treatment of GvHD [91, 92]. PCP infections commonly present with a combination of fever, hypoxemia and interstitial pulmonary infiltrates. However, many PCP cases have co-infections, and the radiological manifestation of these infections can vary and include pleural effusion, alveolar infiltrates, pneumothorax, but with little or no fever. The preferred

PCP prophylaxis is trimethoprim/sulfamethoxazole (TMP/SMX), and several dosing regimens are effective (one single-strength tablet daily, one double-strength tablet daily or one double-strength tablet three times/week). Unfortunately, some patients tolerate TMP/SMX poorly with the development of hematologic, gastrointestinal and cutaneous toxicity. Leucovorin, which has been used to minimize the myelotoxicity of TMP/SMX, was reported in patients with HIV/AIDS to be associated with an increased rate of treatment failure and death and thus should be used with caution [93].

Although potentially convenient, inhaled pentamidine is a prophylaxis approach that is expensive and clearly inferior to TMP/SMX. Pentamidine prophylaxis has been reported to be associated with an incidence of breakthrough infection that approaches 10% [94]. The preferred second-line prophylaxis is dapsone at a dose of 50 mg BID or 100 mg/day. Dapsone appears to be highly effective but does have a small incidence of breakthrough infection of approximately 3%. Dapsone is well tolerated by most patients, including those who previously developed a rash to TMP/SMX. The presence of G-6 PD deficiency should be excluded before starting dapsone prophylaxis, so to minimize the risk of dapsone-induced hemolytic anemia. Atovaquone suspension 1500 mg/day may be used, but published experience in HSCT recipients is limited. Atovaquone is expensive and poor oral tolerance has made compliance for some patients difficult. PCP prophylaxis is recommended for at least 3 months following an autologous HSCT and for 6–12 months or until all immunosuppression has been discontinued for allogeneic transplant recipients.

Treatment of PCP infections after HSCT at both the NIH and Medical College of Wisconsin follows the guidelines developed by the CDC, the NIH, and the IDSA for HIV-infected patients [95]. TMP/SMX (15–20 mg/kg based on the trimethoprim dose) is the treatment of choice, even for the rare patient who develops disease as a breakthrough of TMP/SMX prophylaxis. Intravenous pentamidine 4 mg/kg/day is the second choice for severe disease. All patients with an arterial $PO_2 < 70$ mmHg should receive concomitant corticosteroids (prednisone 40 mg by mouth twice a day for days 1–5, 40 mg daily for days 6–10, and 20 mg daily for days 11–21). For mild to moderate disease, other options that can be considered include atovaquone suspension (750 mg PO bid with food); dapsone (50 mg PO twice daily or 100 mg PO once a day); dapsone and trimethoprim (dapsone 100 mg PO daily and TMP 15 mg/kg/day PO in three divided doses); or primaquine and clindamycin (primaquine 15–30 mg (base) PO daily and clindamycin 600–900 mg/6–8 h IV or 300–450 mg/6–8 h PO).

21.6 Viral Infections Associated with Hematopoietic Stem Cell Transplantation

Differences in incidence and outcome of viral infections after stem cell transplantation are based on the intensity and duration of T-cell mediated immune suppression, and even among allogeneic transplant recipients the immune dysfunction may vary based on the stem cell product, donor-recipient matching, composition of the conditioning regimen, and the occurrence and severity of GvHD [10].

Infections caused by herpes simplex virus (HSV), varicella-zoster virus (VZV), CMV, Respiratory Syncytial Virus (RSV), Parainfluenza viruses, and Influenza viruses are well recognized. Newly recognized aspects of these infections, the emergence of new viral pathogens (human herpesvirus-6, BK virus, adenovirus, and human metapneumovirus) [96–98], and the development of new diagnostic techniques and therapy are addressed in this section.

21.6.1 Herpesviruses

The group of herpesviruses consists of eight members. Primary and reactivation infections are characteristic of these pathogens. Viral latency can be predicted by pretransplant serological screening, and is useful for disease management. Antiviral therapy is now routinely used for prevention and therapy [10, 97, 98]. Currently available drugs include acyclovir and its prodrug valacyclovir, penciclovir and its prodrug famciclovir, ganciclovir and its prodrug valganciclovir, foscarnet, and cidofovir. Maribavir is a new agent being tested. Viral immunization remains investigational, except for the varicella-virus vaccination.

21.6.1.1 Herpes Simplex Virus

Herpes simplex virus (HSV) infections in patients undergoing HSCT are almost exclusively reactivation infections. They are very common approaching 90% of stem cell transplant recipients [10, 97, 98]. HSV infection and disease occur early after transplant and frequently recur if immunosuppression persists. Mucocutaneous HSV disease will frequently present with an atypical appearance, and can mimic other pathogens (i.e., *Candida*), treatment-induced mucositis, or mucosal (oral and labial) GvHD. HSV infections among HSCT recipients are characteristically more invasive, heal more slowly, are associated with prolonged viral shedding, and may disseminate. Treatment and prophylaxis of HSV infections can be administered either orally or intravenously, and acyclovir resistance has remained relatively infrequent [99]. Treatment for infections caused by acyclovir-resistant isolates is foscarnet, but resistance to foscarnet also occurs. Cidofovir is the only available treatment for double-resistant HSV isolates, but HSV reactivation may occur despite cidofovir treatment. HSV prophylaxis with acyclovir is highly efficacious, and the duration of HSV prophylaxis must be individualized. We recommend that antiviral prophylaxis be continued during the first 100 days after transplant but more prolonged prophylaxis usually occurs because these same antiviral agents are used as prophylaxis for varicella-zoster virus. Longer durations of HSV prophylaxis maybe needed for patients with severe immunosuppression, active GvHD, or a history of frequent HSV reactivations.

21.6.1.2 Varicella-Zoster Virus

The clinical manifestations of varicella-zoster virus (VZV) infections include chickenpox and herpes zoster (shingles). Chickenpox results from a primary VZV infection, and herpes zoster is due to viral reactivation of latent VZV. The incidence of VZV infection ranges from 25% of patients who receive an autologous HSCT, to 55–60% among allogeneic HSCT recipients [10, 100]. Infection risk is greatest during the first 12 months after transplant, but late onset disease occurs because of persistent immunosuppression or age-associated immune senescence. The majority of VZV infections in adult patients after transplant are reactivation infections, and 80% present with localized dermatomal disease [100]. Patients who are VZV naïve are at risk for primary infection with either wild type or vaccine strains, and should be counseled about the risk of developing such an infection. Primary VZV infection can be severe, and measures to prevent exposure and intervene early after exposure are recommended [101].

VZV syndromes of importance include trigeminal zoster with keratitis and retinal necrosis, encephalitis, Ramsey–Hunt syndrome, secondary bacterial and yeast infections, and post-zoster pain [100]. Hepatic or gastrointestinal VZV disease is an important entity, and may present with few or no skin lesions. This presentation may result in delayed diagnosis and has been associated with a high case-fatality rate [102]. PCR testing may be useful diagnostically in such cases where available, as the virus may be found in peripheral blood [103]. Treatment of VZV disease should include the early institution of antiviral therapy (valacyclovir, acyclovir or famciclovir) [97, 98, 100]. There is no evidence that intravenous immunoglobulin or corticosteroids add benefit in the treatment of VZV disease in transplant recipients. Prevention of VZV reactivation among patients who undergo stem cell transplantation remains controversial. Acyclovir and valacyclovir are highly effective, yet, despite its efficacy in preventing VZV disease, antiviral prophylaxis is not routinely recommended by many of the clinical care guidelines [10, 98]. The reluctance to recommend routine prophylaxis appears based on observations that VZV disease may still occur after the discontinuation of VZV prophylaxis. A recently published study of HSCT recipients using oral acyclovir showed that late VZV infection is likely to be caused by persistent immunosuppression, and that acyclovir prophylaxis does not predispose to late VZV disease [104]. We routinely prescribe antiviral prophylaxis (valacyclovir 500 mg daily or acyclovir 800 mg BID) for at least the first year after stem cell transplantation.

21.6.1.3 Cytomegalovirus

Cytomegalovirus (CMV) disease manifestations include pneumonia, enteritis, encephalitis, retinitis, hepatitis, cholangitis, cystitis, nephritis, sinusitis, and marrow suppression [105, 106]. T-cell function is paramount in the control of CMV, and inclusion of T-cell depleting agents (i.e., alemtuzumab) as part of the conditioning regimen, or T-cell depleted stem cell grafts appears to increase the risk of CMV infection and disease. In the absence of effective antiviral prophylaxis, the incidence of CMV infection among patients who undergo hematopoietic stem cell transplantation ranges from 5% to 75%. [107]. Non-myeloablative transplant conditioning regimens do not appear to significantly decrease the cumulative incidence of CMV infection [108]. Patients undergoing an autologous stem transplant have a low risk of CMV infection, but CD 34 selection of the autologous stem product increases the risk of CMV disease and CMV-associated death [109].

Diagnosis of CMV infection and disease has improved with the development of techniques for rapid culture, CMV antigen assays, and PCR-based molecular tests [110]. Treatment consists of ganciclovir and/or foscarnet [10, 97, 111]. Cidofovir has also been used, but the response rate seems to be lower [112]. Concomitant IVIG appears helpful only when patients suffer from CMV interstitial pneumonia [10].

CMV negative or leukocyte-depleted blood products are effective CMV prevention for CMV seronegative patients. Prophylaxis of infection or early preemptive intervention remains the foundation of effective CMV infection management for patients who are seropositive for CMV pretransplant [107]. Both of these approaches have significantly lowered the risk of early mortality from CMV disease, but the occurrence of "late cytomegalovirus infection and disease," inadequate options for safe and effective CMV prophylaxis for patients with latent CMV infection and poor immune reconstitution allow CMV disease to continue to impact patient survival.

"Late CMV infection" after stem cell transplant is common (3–17% of allogeneic transplant recipients) and is associated with a 13-fold increase in post-transplant mortality [113]. The primary risk factor for late CMV infection is CMV specific T-cell dysfunction [114]. Surrogate markers for this immunosuppression include active GvHD, high-dose steroid therapy, low CD4 cell count, early post-transplant treatment for CMV infection or the need for donor lymphocyte infusions [113]. Late CMV disease has many presentations, but retinitis, sinusitis, encephalitis and marrow failure appear more common than in early CMV disease. Treatment of late CMV infection relies on CMV surveillance (3–12 months after transplant or longer in patients with chronic GvHD), and preemptive therapy with ganciclovir or other effective anti-CMV therapy. The role of oral valganciclovir as preemptive therapy remains to be defined, but some transplant groups have reported success [115]. We remain concerned with the documented increased exposure to ganciclovir levels by using the oral route and the resultant increase in hematologic toxicity [116, 117]. In general we prefer the flexibility of weight- and renal-adjusted dosing of IV ganciclovir.

"CMV infection prophylaxis" remains an attractive option for both early and late CMV infection, but early prophylaxis approaches were associated with increased treatment associated toxicity [118, 119]. Preliminary results from a randomized, phase II trial of Maribavir, suggests that infection and disease prophylaxis may be possible with this agent. Maribavir is a selective UL 97 viral protein-kinase inhibitor, and unlike other currently available anti-CMV agents does not inhibit CMV DNA polymerase [120]. The early analysis of 111 patients treated after engraftment with Maribavir or placebo showed that Maribavir decreased the incidence of CMV infection and disease. Maribavir toxicity was mild and appeared to not adversely affect marrow function [121]. Additional studies are now ongoing and are critical to clarify the utility of this new anti-CMV agent.

21.6.1.4 Human Herpesvirus-6

Human herpesvirus-6 (HHV-6) is a ubiquitous herpesvirus that infects most persons early in life. Two major viral variants have been identified (A and B), but the B variant is most frequently associated with disease among transplant recipients [122]. Longitudinal studies in HSCT recipients found that HHV-6 reactivation occurred a median of 20 days after transplantation, and viral shedding for some patients was prolonged and did not always correlate with viral disease [122]. A clinical syndrome of CNS dysfunction, impaired memory, secondary (hypothalamic) hypothyroidism, and delayed platelet engraftment are common disease manifestations [122-124]. HHV-6 viremia among allogeneic transplant recipients has been associated with an increase in all-cause mortality, and appears to be increased when patients are transplanted for disease other than first remission, when donor and recipient are sex mismatched, and when transplant patients are younger [122]. We have recently diagnosed and treated four transplant patients for HHV-6 viremia who developed CNS dysfunction and delayed platelet recovery. All four of these patients had undergone an autologous transplant for multiple myeloma following melphalan conditioning. Fortunately, all patients responded to a prolonged courses of antiviral therapy.

Foscarnet, ganciclovir, and cidofovir have been used as treatment for HHV-6 infections. Prospective studies are needed to better understand the importance of HHV-6 infection among transplant recipients, to define disease spectrum, and to define therapy options.

21.6.1.5 Adenovirus

Adenovirus is a DNA virus categorized by 51 human serotypes. Primary infection is acquired from either a respiratory droplet or the oral-fecal route. Most infections among adult stem cell transplant recipients seem to be viral reactivation [125]. Clinical manifestations vary with serotype and range from viremia to pneumonia, hepatitis, gastrointestinal disease, cystitis, nephritis, and conjunctivitis [126]. Control of adenovirus appears to be T-cell mediated, and allogeneic stem cell transplant recipients appear to be at greatest risk of infection and disease [127]. Risk factors for infection and disease include unrelated donor transplantation, GvHD, T-cell depleted stem cell product, younger patient age, total body irradiation, and adenovirus viremia [127]. The incidence of infection in stem cell recipients has been reported to range from 5% to 29%, with viral disease occurring in 5–8% of patients. Adenovirus disease may be severe, with viral-associated death reported to range from 30% to 50% [127].

Standard detection methods for adenovirus include cell culture, shell vial assays, and direct antigen detection. Quantitative PCR assays are now suitable for detection of adenovirus in blood [128]. There are no controlled treatment trials for adenovirus infection, but cidofovir is active in vitro and has shown promise for the management of clinical disease [129]. The availability of techniques for molecular monitoring of adenovirus in the blood suggests that preemptive treatment of early adenovirus disease is potentially possible. In a study of 62 HSCT recipients who received a T-cell replete stem cell product, Erard and colleagues detected adenovirus by PCR in the plasma of 88% of patients who developed adenovirus disease [130]. All patients with proven and possible adenovirus disease had at least 103 viral copies/ml, and the adenoviremia preceded the development of disease by 1–7 weeks [130].

21.6.1.6 BK Virus

BK virus is a ubiquitous, DNA polyoma virus that is believed to cause nephropathy and graft loss among renal transplant recipients. This virus has been reported to also cause pneumonia [131]. There is increasing evidence that BK virus plays an important role in some cases of hemorrhagic cystitis and renal impairment in patients who undergo HSCT, but viral tissue invasion has only recently been demonstrated [132–134]. BK viruria is reported to occur in up to 95% of stem cell transplantation recipients, with the onset of viral shedding occurring a median of 41 days after transplant. BK viruria may be prolonged and severe. Symptoms of some patients can persist for more than 1 month. Diagnostic tests have been developed, and a highly sensitive quantitative PCR assay for BK virus detection in blood and urine is now available. In a case–control study of hemorrhagic cystitis among HSCT recipients, BK plasma DNA levels greater than 10,000 copies/ml were highly associated with post-engraftment BK virus-associated hemorrhagic cystitis [133]. Treatment of hemorrhagic cystitis at the present time remains supportive and should be supplemented with hydration and platelet support for patients who are thrombocytopenic. Refractory hemorrhagic cystitis is rare but can be catastrophic. Anti-viral therapy for BK virus remains inadequate, but cidofovir has in vitro BK virus activity and leflunomide, an immunosuppressive agent used to treat rheumatoid arthritis, has been reported to be active against BK virus infection [135].

Table 21.1 Respiratory viruses (including PSV)/management approach (respiratory virus treatment flow chart)

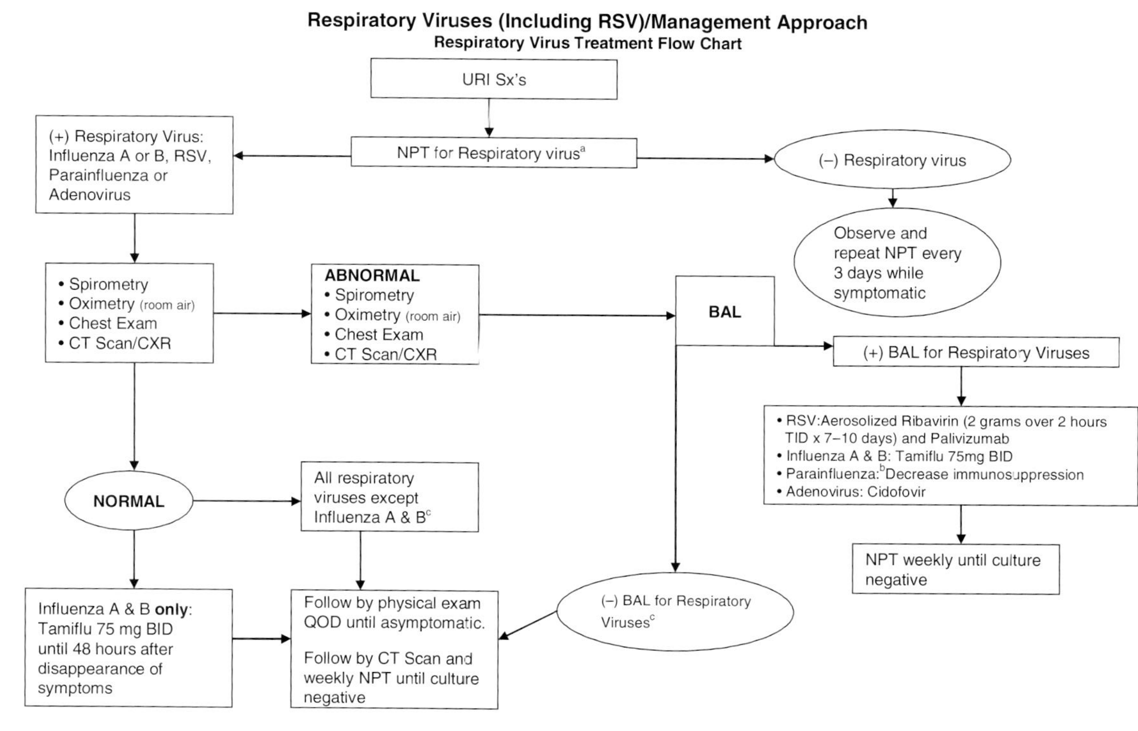

NPT nasopharyngeal wash or swab, *CXR* chest radiograph, *BAL* bronchial alveolar lavage
[a]Molecular detection or shell viral culture
[b]Tamiflu or aerosolized ribavirin + IVIg may be beneficial
[c]Aeroslized ribavirin (2g over 2 h, TID x 7 days) may be indicated if NPT(+) for RSV

21.6.1.7 Respiratory Viruses

Respiratory viruses including (RSV), parainfluenza virus and influenza virus A and B are widespread in the community and easily transmitted to patients who have undergone HSCT [136, 137]. Infections are spread by airborne droplets and contact with the hands of infected persons. Infection control measures are critical and should consist of meticulous hand washing, annual influenza vaccination, early infection detection, and both respiratory and contact isolation of infected health care workers and patients. Patients who develop respiratory virus infections prior to the initiation of treatment or transplantation should when possible have their transplant delayed [138]. RSV and influenza are primarily winter viruses, but parainfluenza virus infections that are most prevalent during the summer months can occur at anytime during the year. The clinical syndromes of these viruses range from the common cold to sinusitis, pharyngitis, tracheobronchitis, bronchiolitis and pneumonia. Respiratory virus infections among transplant recipients are associated with a more prolonged infection (i.e., RSV shedding may exceed 100 days vs. 21 days for immunocompetent children); a higher frequency of nosocomial acquisition (55–83% of exposed immunocompromised patients will become infected), and a higher rate of pneumonia, polymicrobial infection, and death. The risk of death from a respiratory viral pneumonia may be significant and has ranged from 9% to 82% [136, 137].

Rapid diagnosis is made by viral antigen or nuclei acid detection. An RT-PCR assay that detects RNA from RSV, influenza A and B, and parainfluenza viruses from nasal wash and nasopharyngeal specimens is highly sensitive and readily available. However, because of the incidence of false negative tests the study should be repeated if the patient's symptoms persist. A scheme for the management of patients who undergo hematopoietic stem cell transplantation and are suspected to have a respiratory virus infection is outlined in Figure 21.1. Neuraminidase inhibitors like tamiflu (oseltamivir) appear helpful for both influenza A and B, but more prolonged treatment may be needed for stem cell transplant recipients and patients who develop pneumonia. RSV pneumonia is treated with aerosolized ribavirin with or without palivizumab [137]. Management of patients with nonpneumonic RSV infections is unclear, but we routinely recommend that such patients who are severely immunocompromised be treated with 7–10 days of aerosolized ribavirin 2 g TID [139]. While there continues to be debate regarding the utility of the influenza vaccination in transplant recipients, our approach is to annually vaccinate all such patients and their household contacts.

21.6.1.8 Human Metapneumovirus

Human metapneumovirus (hMPV) is a newly discovered RNA paramyxovirus. Most children by 5 years of age are seropositive. This virus infection occurs primarily during winter months and can manifest as both upper and lower respiratory tract disease [140]. Results from a retrospective study suggested that hMPV infection can be a significant cause of idiopathic pneumonia syndrome after hematopoietic stem cell transplantation [141]. Five patients among 200 tested had hMPV detected in archived bronchial alveolar lavage specimens. All five positive patients had an upper respiratory tract infection that preceded their pneumonia, and four of five patients died of respiratory failure. Lung tissue obtained at autopsy from the four patients who died had pathologic changes consistent with idiopathic pneumonia syndrome. Prospective studies of the role of hMPV as a cause of infection for transplant recipients are needed. There is no established treatment for hMPV infections although ribavirin appears to have in vitro antiviral activity.

21.7 Summary

Management of infections in HSCT recipients as reviewed in this chapter illustrates the dynamic nature of the challenges that patients and their health care team will face as long as transplantation is associated with periods of profound immune dysfunction. The past decade has seen a significant increase in overall survival of HSCT recipients. Two of the major factors responsible for this improved outcome have been early diagnosis and preemptive therapy of CMV infection and the ability to prevent some fungal pathogens with fluconazole prophylaxis. Despite these significant successes, natural selection keeps providing the transplant team and HSCT recipient new infectious disease challenges.

Transplant approaches must be developed that can provide improved primary disease control and at the same time preserve immune function. Until that time comes, transplant teams must remain vigilant about infection risks, implement all reasonable prevention measures, and remain aware of both the commonly recognized infectious pathogens and the new pathogens or antimicrobial-resistant organisms that may evolve as a consequence of the use of antimicrobial agents. We would like to emphasize the importance of basic infectious principles that have been lumped in the past under the umbrella of "standard infection control measures." These include but are not limited to hand washing, providing clean air and water to our patients, and isolation of patients known to be colonized with pathogens that are unusually virulent, resistant to antimicrobial therapy, and/or easily spread among patients and health care workers. Basic infection control practices coupled with advancing measures for infection prevention and early infection diagnosis and management are likely to provide not only the best transplant outcomes but also the highest health care value. These time-honored aspects of care for the HSCT recipient will likely never go out of style, but at the same time, frame the challenge summarized by the statement, "Where there is immune dysfunction there will continue to be increased risk of infectious complications that will need to be addressed."

References

1. Gafter-Gvili A, Fraser A, Paul M, Leibovici L. Meta-analysis: antibiotic prophylaxis reduces mortality in neutropenic patients. Ann Intern Med. 2005;142(12 Pt 1):979–95.
2. van de Wetering MD, de Witte MA, Kremer LC, Offringa M, Scholten RJ, Caron HN. Efficacy of oral prophylactic antibiotics in neutropenic afebrile oncology patients: a systematic review of randomised controlled trials. Eur J Cancer. 2005;41:1372–82.
3. Bucaneve G, Micozzi A, Menichetti F, et al. Levofloxacin to prevent bacterial infection in patients with cancer and neutropenia. N Engl J Med. 2005;353:977–87.
4. Freifeld AG, Segal BH, Baden LR, et al. Prevention and treatment of cancer-related infections. Presented at 12th Annual NCCN Conference, Hollywood. 2007. http://www.nccn.org Accessed March 2007.
5. Baden LR. Prophylactic antimicrobial agents and the importance of fitness. N Engl J Med. 2005;353:1052–4.
6. Leibovici L, Paul M, Cullen M, et al. Antibiotic prophylaxis in neutropenic patients: new evidence, practical decisions. Cancer 2006;107:1743–51.
7. Engelhard D, Cordonnier C, Shaw PJ, et al. Early and late invasive pneumococcal infection following stem cell transplantation: a European Bone Marrow Transplantation survey. Br J Haematol. 2002;117:444–50.
8. Youssef S, Rodriguez G, Rolston KV, Champlin RE, Raad II, Safdar A. *Streptococcus pneumoniae* infections in 47 hematopoietic stem cell transplantation recipients: clinical characteristics of infections and vaccine-breakthrough infections, 1989–2005. Medicine 2007;86:69–77.
9. Kulkarni S, Powles R, Treleaven J, et al. Chronic graft versus host disease is associated with long-term risk for pneumococcal infections in recipients of bone marrow transplants. Blood 2000;95:3683–6.
10. Guidelines for preventing opportunistic infections among hematopoietic stem cell transplant recipients. MMWR Recomm Rep. 2000;49(RR-10):1–125,CE1–7.
11. Ljungman P, Engelhard D, de la Camara R, et al. Vaccination of stem cell transplant recipients: recommendations of the Infectious Diseases Working Party of the EBMT. Bone Marrow Transplant. 2005;35:737–46.
12. Kumar D, Chen MH, Welsh B, et al. A randomized, double-blind trial of pneumococcal vaccination in adult allogeneic stem cell transplant donors and recipients. Clin Infect Dis. 2007;45:1576–82.
13. Hughes WT, Armstrong D, Bodey GP, et al. 2002 guidelines for the use of antimicrobial agents in neutropenic patients with cancer. Clin Infect Dis. 2002;34:730–51.
14. Paul M, Yahav D, Fraser A, Leibovici L. Empirical antibiotic monotherapy for febrile neutropenia: systematic review and meta-analysis of randomized controlled trials. J Antimicrob Chemother. 2006;57:176–89.
15. Paul M, Soares-Weiser K, Leibovici L. Beta lactam monotherapy versus beta lactam-aminoglycoside combination therapy for fever with neutropenia: systematic review and meta-analysis. BMJ 2003;326:1111.
16. Furno P, Bucaneve G, Del Favero A. Monotherapy or aminoglycoside-containing combinations for empirical antibiotic treatment of febrile neutropenic patients: a meta-analysis. Lancet Infect Dis. 2002;2:231–42.
17. Paul M, Borok S, Fraser A, Vidal L, Cohen M, Leibovici L. Additional anti-Gram-positive antibiotic treatment for febrile neutropenic cancer patients. Cochrane Database Syst Rev (Online) 2005;:CD003914.
18. Cometta A, Kern WV, De Bock R, et al. Vancomycin versus placebo for treating persistent fever in patients with neutropenic cancer receiving piperacillin-tazobactam monotherapy. Clin Infect Dis. 2003;37:382–9.
19. Jaksic B, Martinelli G, Perez-Oteyza J, Hartman CS, Leonard LB, Tack KJ. Efficacy and safety of linezolid compared with vancomycin in a randomized, double-blind study of febrile neutropenic patients with cancer. Clin Infect Dis. 2006;42:597–607.

20. Russmann H, Panthel K, Bader RC, Schmitt C, Schaumann R. Evaluation of three rapid assays for detection of *Clostridium difficile* toxin A and toxin B in stool specimens. Eur J Clin Microbiol Infect Dis. 2007;26:115–9.
21. Mohan SS, McDermott BP, Parchuri S, Cunha BA. Lack of value of repeat stool testing for *Clostridium difficile* toxin. Am J Med. 2006;119:356 e7–8.
22. Chakrabarti S, Lees A, Jones SG, Milligan DW. *Clostridium difficile* infection in allogeneic stem cell transplant recipients is associated with severe graft-versus-host disease and nonrelapse mortality. Bone Marrow Transplant. 2000;26:871–6.
23. Nelson R. Antibiotic treatment for *Clostridium difficile*-associated diarrhea in adults. Cochrane Database Syst Rev. (Online) 2007;:CD004610.
24. Bricker E, Garg R, Nelson R, Loza A, Novak T, Hansen J. Antibiotic treatment for *Clostridium difficile*-associated diarrhea in adults. Cochrane Database Syst Rev. (Online) 2005;:CD004610.
25. Fekety R. Guidelines for the diagnosis and management of *Clostridium difficile*-associated diarrhea and colitis. American College of Gastroenterology, Practice Parameters Committee. Am J Gastroenterol. 1997;92:739–50.
26. Gerding DN. Treatment of *Clostridium difficile*-associated diarrhea and colitis. Curr Top Microbiol Immunol. 2000;250:127–39.
27. Aslam S, Hamill RJ, Musher DM. Treatment of *Clostridium difficile*-associated disease: old therapies and new strategies. Lancet Infect Dis. 2005;5:549–57.
28. Teasley DG, Gerding DN, Olson MM, et al. Prospective randomised trial of metronidazole versus vancomycin for *Clostridium difficile*-associated diarrhoea and colitis. Lancet 1983;2:1043–6.
29. Zar FA, Bakkanagari SR, Moorthi KM, Davis MB. A comparison of vancomycin and metronidazole for the treatment of *Clostridium difficile*-associated diarrhea, stratified by disease severity. Clin Infect Dis. 2007;45:302–7.
30. Musher DM, Logan N, Hamill RJ, et al. Nitazoxanide for the treatment of *Clostridium difficile* colitis. Clin Infect Dis. 2006;43:421–7.
31. Bartlett JG. Narrative review: the new epidemic of *Clostridium difficile*-associated enteric disease. Ann Intern Med. 2006;145:758–64.
32. Aas J, Gessert CE, Bakken JS. Recurrent *Clostridium difficile* colitis: case series involving 18 patients treated with donor stool administered via a nasogastric tube. Clin Infect Dis. 2003;36:580–5.
33. Zirakzadeh A, Gastineau DA, Mandrekar JN, Burke JP, Johnston PB, Patel R. Vancomycin-resistant enterococcal colonization appears associated with increased mortality among allogeneic hematopoietic stem cell transplant recipients. Bone Marrow Transplant. 2007.
34. Weinstock DM, Conlon M, Iovino C, et al. Colonization, bloodstream infection, and mortality caused by vancomycin-resistant enterococcus early after allogeneic hematopoietic stem cell transplant. Biol Blood Marrow Transplant. 2007;13:615–21.
35. Raad I, Hachem R, Hanna H, et al. Prospective, randomized study comparing quinupristin-dalfopristin with linezolid in the treatment of vancomycin-resistant *Enterococcus faecium* infections. J Antimicrob Chemother. 2004;53:646–9.
36. Poutsiaka DD, Skiffington S, Miller KB, Hadley S, Snydman DR. Daptomycin in the treatment of vancomycin-resistant *Enterococcus faecium* bacteremia in neutropenic patients. J Infect. 2007;54:567–71.
37. Giamarellou H. Treatment options for multidrug-resistant bacteria. Expert Rev Anti Infect Ther. 2006;4:601–18.
38. Kwa AL, Loh C, Low JG, Kurup A, Tam VH. Nebulized colistin in the treatment of pneumonia due to multidrug-resistant *Acinetobacter baumannii* and *Pseudomonas aeruginosa*. Clin Infect Dis. 2005;41:754–7.
39. Wisplinghoff H, Bischoff T, Tallent SM, Seifert H, Wenzel RP, Edmond MB. Nosocomial bloodstream infections in US hospitals: analysis of 24,179 cases from a prospective nationwide surveillance study. Clin Infect Dis. 2004;39:309–17.

40. Newman KA, Reed WP, Bustamante CI, Schimpff SC, Wade JC. Venous access devices utilized in association with intensive cancer chemotherapy. Eur J Cancer Clin Oncol. 1989;25:1375–8.
41. Maki DG, Kluger DM, Crnich CJ. The risk of bloodstream infection in adults with different intravascular devices: a systematic review of 200 published prospective studies. Mayo Clin Proc. 2006;81:1159–71.
42. Hanna H, Benjamin R, Chatzinikolaou I, et al. Long-term silicone central venous catheters impregnated with minocycline and rifampin decrease rates of catheter-related bloodstream infection in cancer patients: a prospective randomized clinical trial. J Clin Oncol. 2004;22:3163–71.
43. Darouiche RO, Berger DH, Khardori N, et al. Comparison of antimicrobial impregnation with tunneling of long-term central venous catheters: a randomized controlled trial. Ann Surg. 2005;242:193–200.
44. Groeger JS, Lucas AB, Thaler HT, et al. Infectious morbidity associated with long-term use of venous access devices in patients with cancer. Ann Intern Med. 1993;119:1168–74.
45. O'Grady NP, Alexander M, Dellinger EP, et al. Guidelines for the prevention of intravascular catheter-related infections. The Hospital Infection Control Practices Advisory Committee, Center for Disease Control and Prevention, U.S. Pediatrics 2002;110:e51.
46. Maki DG, Ringer M, Alvarado CJ. Prospective randomised trial of povidone-iodine, alcohol, and chlorhexidine for prevention of infection associated with central venous and arterial catheters. Lancet 1991;338:339–43.
47. Gillies D, O'Riordan L, Carr D, Frost J, Gunning R, O'Brien I. Gauze and tape and transparent polyurethane dressings for central venous catheters. Cochrane Database Syst Rev (Online). 2003;:CD003827.
48. Safdar N, Maki DG. Use of vancomycin-containing lock or flush solutions for prevention of bloodstream infection associated with central venous access devices: a meta-analysis of prospective, randomized trials. Clin Infect Dis. 2006;43:474–84.
49. Pronovost P, Needham D, Berenholtz S, et al. An intervention to decrease catheter-related bloodstream infections in the ICU. N Engl J Med. 2006;355:2725–32.
50. Weinstein MP. Current blood culture methods and systems: clinical concepts, technology, and interpretation of results. Clin Infect Dis. 1996;23:40–6.
51. Raad I, Hanna H, Maki D. Intravascular catheter-related infections: advances in diagnosis, prevention, and management. Lancet Infect. Dis. 2007;7:645–57.
52. Safdar N, Fine JP, Maki DG. Meta-analysis: methods for diagnosing intravascular device-related bloodstream infection. Ann Intern Med. 2005;142:451–66.
53. Siegman-Igra Y, Anglim AM, Shapiro DE, Adal KA, Strain BA, Farr BM. Diagnosis of vascular catheter-related bloodstream infection: a meta-analysis. J Clin Microbiol. 1997;35:928–36.
54. Raad I, Hanna HA, Alakech B, Chatzinikolaou I, Johnson MM, Tarrand J. Differential time to positivity: a useful method for diagnosing catheter-related bloodstream infections. Ann Intern Med. 2004;140:18–25.
55. Hanna R, Raad II. Diagnosis of catheter-related bloodstream infection. Curr Infect Dis Rep. 2005;7:413–9.
56. Mermel LA, Farr BM, Sherertz RJ, et al. Guidelines for the management of intravascular catheter-related infections. Clin Infect Dis. 2001;32:1249–72.
57. Upton A, Kirby KA, Carpenter P, Boeckh M, Marr KA. Invasive aspergillosis following hematopoietic cell transplantation: outcomes and prognostic factors associated with mortality. Clin Infect Dis. 2007;44:531–40.
58. Goodman JL, Winston DJ, Greenfield RA, et al. A controlled trial of fluconazole to prevent fungal infections in patients undergoing bone marrow transplantation [see comments]. N Engl J Med. 1992;326:845–51.
59. Slavin MA, Osborne B, Adams R, et al. Efficacy and safety of fluconazole prophylaxis for fungal infections after marrow transplantation—a prospective, randomized, double-blind study. J Infect Dis. 1995;171:1545–52.

60. Marr KA, Seidel K, Slavin MA, et al. Prolonged fluconazole prophylaxis is associated with persistent protection against candidiasis-related death in allogeneic marrow transplant recipients: long-term follow-up of a randomized, placebo-controlled trial. Blood 2000;96:2055–61.
61. Oren I, Rowe JM, Sprecher H, et al. A prospective randomized trial of itraconazole vs fluconazole for the prevention of fungal infections in patients with acute leukemia and hematopoietic stem cell transplant recipients. Bone Marrow Transplant. 2006;38:127–34.
62. Marr KA, Crippa F, Leisenring W, et al. Itraconazole versus fluconazole for prevention of fungal infections in patients receiving allogeneic stem cell transplants. Blood 2004;103:1527–33.
63. Winston DJ, Maziarz RT, Chandrasekar PH, et al. Intravenous and oral itraconazole versus intravenous and oral fluconazole for long-term antifungal prophylaxis in allogeneic hematopoietic stem-cell transplant recipients. A multicenter, randomized trial. Ann Intern Med. 2003;138:705–13.
64. Vardakas KZ, Michalopoulos A, Falagas ME. Fluconazole versus itraconazole for antifungal prophylaxis in neutropenic patients with haematological malignancies: a meta-analysis of randomised-controlled trials. Br J Haematol. 2005;131(1):22–8.
65. van Burik JA, Ratanatharathorn V, Stepan DE, et al. Micafungin versus fluconazole for prophylaxis against invasive fungal infections during neutropenia in patients undergoing hematopoietic stem cell transplantation. Clin Infect Dis. 2004;39:1407–16.
66. Cornely OA, Maertens J, Winston DJ, et al. Posaconazole vs. fluconazole or itraconazole prophylaxis in patients with neutropenia. N Engl J Med. 2007;356:348–59.
67. Walsh TJ, Pappas P, Winston DJ, et al. Voriconazole compared with liposomal amphotericin B for empirical antifungal therapy in patients with neutropenia and persistent fever. N Engl J Med. 2002;346:225–34.
68. Walsh TJ, Teppler H, Donowitz GR, et al. Caspofungin versus liposomal amphotericin B for empirical antifungal therapy in patients with persistent fever and neutropenia. N Engl J Med. 2004;351:1391–402.
69. Maertens J, Deeren D, Dierickx D, Theunissen K. Preemptive antifungal therapy: still a way to go. Current opinion in infectious diseases 2006;19:551–6.
70. Maertens J, Theunissen K, Verhoef G, et al. Galactomannan and computed tomography-based preemptive antifungal therapy in neutropenic patients at high risk for invasive fungal infection: a prospective feasibility study. Clin Infect Dis. 2005;41:1242–50.
71. Walsh TJ, Finberg RW, Arndt C, et al. Liposomal amphotericin B for empirical therapy in patients with persistent fever and neutropenia. National Institute of Allergy and Infectious Diseases Mycoses Study Group. N Engl J Med. 1999;340:764–71.
72. Ullmann AJ, Lipton JH, Vesole DH, et al. Posaconazole or fluconazole for prophylaxis in severe graft-versus-host disease. N Engl J Med. 2007;356:335–47.
73. Wingard JR, Carter SL, Walsh TJ, et al. Results of a randomized, double-blind trial of fluconazole (FLU) vs. voriconazole (VORI) for the prevention of invasive fungal infections (IFI) in 600 allogeneic blood and marrow transplant (BMT) patients. Am Soc Hematol Annu Meet Abstr. 2007;110:163.
74. Reboli AC, Rotstein C, Pappas PG, et al. Anidulafungin versus fluconazole for invasive candidiasis. N Engl J Med. 2007;356:2472–82.
75. Kuse ER, Chetchotisakd P, da Cunha CA, et al. Micafungin versus liposomal amphotericin B for candidemia and invasive candidiasis: a phase III randomised double-blind trial. Lancet 2007;369:1519–27.
76. Mora-Duarte J, Betts R, Rotstein C, et al. Comparison of caspofungin and amphotericin B for invasive candidiasis. N Engl J Med. 2002;347:2020–9.
77. Pappas PG, Rotstein CM, Betts RF, et al. Micafungin versus caspofungin for treatment of candidemia and other forms of invasive candidiasis. Clin Infect Dis. 2007;45:883–93.
78. Herbrecht R, Denning DW, Patterson TF, et al. Voriconazole versus amphotericin B for primary therapy of invasive aspergillosis. N Engl J Med. 2002;347:408–15.

79. Steinbach WJ, Addison RM, McLaughlin L, et al. Prospective *Aspergillus* galactomannan antigen testing in pediatric hematopoietic stem cell transplant recipients. Pediatr Infect Dis J. 2007;26:558–64.
80. Foy PC, van Burik JA, Weisdorf DJ. Galactomannan antigen enzyme-linked immunosorbent assay for diagnosis of invasive aspergillosis after hematopoietic stem cell transplantation. Biol Blood Marrow Transplant. 2007;13:440–3.
81. Wheat LJ. Rapid diagnosis of invasive aspergillosis by antigen detection. Transpl Infect Dis. 2003;5:158–66.
82. Petraitis V, Petraitiene R, Sarafandi AA, et al. Combination therapy in treatment of experimental pulmonary aspergillosis: synergistic interaction between an antifungal triazole and an echinocandin. J Infect Dis. 2003;187:1834–43.
83. Marr KA, Boeckh M, Carter RA, Kim HW, Corey L. Combination antifungal therapy for invasive aspergillosis. Clin Infect Dis. 2004;39:797–802. Epub 2004 Aug 27.
84. O'Shaughnessy EM, Meletiadis J, Stergiopoulou T, Demchok JP, Walsh TJ. Antifungal interactions within the triple combination of amphotericin B, caspofungin and voriconazole against *Aspergillus* species. J Antimicrob Chemother. 2006;58: 1168–76.
85. Smith J, Safdar N, Knasinski V, et al. Voriconazole therapeutic drug monitoring. Antimicrobial agents and chemotherapy 2006;50:1570–2.
86. Wald A, Leisenring W, van Burik JA, Bowden RA. Epidemiology of *Aspergillus* infections in a large cohort of patients undergoing bone marrow transplantation. J Infect Dis. 1997;175:1459–66.
87. Kotloff RM, Ahya VN, Crawford SW. Pulmonary complications of solid organ and hematopoietic stem cell transplantation. Am J Respir Crit Care Med. 2004;170:22–48.
88. Cornely OA, Maertens J, Bresnik M, et al. Liposomal amphotericin B as initial therapy for invasive mold infection: a randomized trial comparing a high-loading dose regimen with standard dosing (AmBiLoad trial). Clin Infect Dis. 2007;44:1289–97.
89. Marty FM, Lowry CM, Cutler CS, et al. Voriconazole and sirolimus coadministration after allogeneic hematopoietic stem cell transplantation. Biol Blood Marrow Transplant. 2006;12:552–9.
90. Redhead SA, Cushion MT, Frenkel JK, Stringer JR. Pneumocystis and *Trypanosoma cruzi*: nomenclature and typifications. J Eukaryot Microbiol. 2006;53:2–11.
91. Torres HA, Chemaly RF, Storey R, et al. Influence of type of cancer and hematopoietic stem cell transplantation on clinical presentation of *Pneumocystis jirovecii* pneumonia in cancer patients. Eur J Clin Microbiol Infect Dis. 2006.
92. De Castro N, Neuville S, Sarfati C, et al. Occurrence of *Pneumocystis jirovecii* pneumonia after allogeneic stem cell transplantation: a 6-year retrospective study. Bone Marrow Transplant. 2005;36:879–83.
93. Safrin S, Lee BL, Sande MA. Adjunctive folinic acid with trimethoprim-sulfamethoxazole for *Pneumocystis carinii* pneumonia in AIDS patients is associated with an increased risk of therapeutic failure and death. J Infect Dis. 1994;170:912–7.
94. Vasconcelles MJ, Bernardo MV, King C, Weller EA, Antin JH. Aerosolized pentamidine as pneumocystis prophylaxis after bone marrow transplantation is inferior to other regimens and is associated with decreased survival and an increased risk of other infections. Biol Blood Marrow Transplant. 2000;6:35–43.
95. Benson CA, Kaplan JE, Masur H, Pau A, Holmes KK. Treating opportunistic infections among HIV-infected adults and adolescents: recommendations from CDC, the National Institutes of Health, and the HIV Medicine Association/Infectious Diseases Society of America. MMWR Recomm Rep. 2004;53(RR-15):1–112.
96. Boeckh M, Erard V, Zerr D, Englund J. Emerging viral infections after hematopoietic cell transplantation. Pediatr Transplant. 2005;9 Suppl 7:48–54.
97. Ljungman P. Viral infections: current diagnosis and treatment. Hematol J. 2004;5 Suppl 3:S63–8.

98. Sandherr M, Einsele H, Hebart H, et al. Antiviral prophylaxis in patients with haematological malignancies and solid tumours: Guidelines of the Infectious Diseases Working Party (AGIHO) of the German Society for Hematology and Oncology (DGHO). Ann Oncol. 2006;17:1051–9.
99. Chakrabarti S, Pillay D, Ratcliffe D, Cane PA, Collingham KE, Milligan DW. Resistance to antiviral drugs in herpes simplex virus infections among allogeneic stem cell transplant recipients: risk factors and prognostic significance. J Infect Dis. 2000;181:2055–8.
100. Locksley RM, Flournoy N, Sullivan KM, Meyers JD. Infection with varicella-zoster virus after marrow transplantation. J Infect Dis. 1985;152:1172–81.
101. Weinstock DM, Boeckh M, Boulad F, et al. Postexposure prophylaxis against varicella-zoster virus infection among recipients of hematopoietic stem cell transplant: unresolved issues. Infect Control Hosp Epidemiol. 2004;25:603–8.
102. David DS, Tegtmeier BR, O'Donnell MR, Paz IB, McCarty TM. Visceral varicella-zoster after bone marrow transplantation: report of a case series and review of the literature. Am J Gastroenterol. 1998;93:810–3.
103. Rogers SY, Irving W, Harris A, Russell NH. Visceral varicella zoster infection after bone marrow transplantation without skin involvement and the use of PCR for diagnosis. Bone Marrow Transplant. 1995;15:805–7.
104. Boeckh M, Kim HW, Flowers ME, Meyers JD, Bowden RA. Long-term acyclovir for prevention of varicella zoster virus disease after allogeneic hematopoietic cell transplantation—a randomized double-blind placebo-controlled study. Blood 2006;107:1800–5.
105. Boeckh M, Nichols WG, Papanicolaou G, Rubin R, Wingard JR, Zaia J. Cytomegalovirus in hematopoietic stem cell transplant recipients: current status, known challenges, and future strategies. Biol Blood Marrow Transplant. 2003;9:543–58.
106. Hebart H, Einsele H. Clinical aspects of CMV infection after stem cell transplantation. Hum Immunol. 2004;65:432–6.
107. Boeckh M, Nichols WG. The impact of cytomegalovirus serostatus of donor and recipient before hematopoietic stem cell transplantation in the era of antiviral prophylaxis and preemptive therapy. Blood 2004;103:2003–8.
108. Junghanss C, Boeckh M, Carter RA, et al. Incidence and outcome of cytomegalovirus infections following nonmyeloablative compared with myeloablative allogeneic stem cell transplantation, a matched control study. Blood 2002;99:1978–85.
109. Holmberg LA, Boeckh M, Hooper H, et al. Increased incidence of cytomegalovirus disease after autologous CD34-selected peripheral blood stem cell transplantation. Blood 1999;94:4029–35.
110. Boeckh M, Gallez-Hawkins GM, Myerson D, Zaia JA, Bowden RA. Plasma polymerase chain reaction for cytomegalovirus DNA after allogeneic marrow transplantation: comparison with polymerase chain reaction using peripheral blood leukocytes, pp65 antigenemia, and viral culture. Transplantation 1997;64:108–13.
111. Ljungman P, Reusser P, de la Camara R, et al. Management of CMV infections: recommendations from the infectious diseases working party of the EBMT. Bone Marrow Transplant. 2004;33:1075–81.
112. Ljungman P, Deliliers GL, Platzbecker U, et al. Cidofovir for cytomegalovirus infection and disease in allogeneic stem cell transplant recipients. The Infectious Diseases Working Party of the European Group for Blood and Marrow Transplantation. Blood 2001;97:388–92.
113. Boeckh M, Leisenring W, Riddell SR, et al. Late cytomegalovirus disease and mortality in recipients of allogeneic hematopoietic stem cell transplants: importance of viral load and T-cell immunity. Blood 2003;101:407–14.
114. Hakki M, Riddell SR, Storek J, et al. Immune reconstitution to cytomegalovirus after allogeneic hematopoietic stem cell transplantation: impact of host factors, drug therapy, and subclinical reactivation. Blood 2003;102:3060–7.

115. van der Heiden PL, Kalpoe JS, Barge RM, Willemze R, Kroes AC, Schippers EF. Oral valganciclovir as pre-emptive therapy has similar efficacy on cytomegalovirus DNA load reduction as intravenous ganciclovir in allogeneic stem cell transplantation recipients. Bone Marrow Transplant. 2006;37:693–8.
116. Einsele H, Reusser P, Bornhauser M, et al. Oral valganciclovir leads to higher exposure to ganciclovir than intravenous ganciclovir in patients following allogeneic stem cell transplantation. Blood 2006;107:3002–8.
117. Wiltshire H, Paya CV, Pescovitz MD, et al. Pharmacodynamics of oral ganciclovir and valganciclovir in solid organ transplant recipients. Transplantation 2005;79:1477–83.
118. Goodrich JM, Bowden RA, Fisher L, Keller C, Schoch G, Meyers JD. Ganciclovir prophylaxis to prevent cytomegalovirus disease after allogeneic marrow transplant. Ann Intern Med. 1993;118:173–8.
119. Boeckh M, Gooley TA, Myerson D, Cunningham T, Schoch G, Bowden RA. Cytomegalovirus pp65 antigenemia-guided early treatment with ganciclovir versus ganciclovir at engraftment after allogeneic marrow transplantation: a randomized double-blind study. Blood 1996;88:4063–71.
120. Drew WL, Miner RC, Marousek GI, Chou S. Maribavir sensitivity of cytomegalovirus isolates resistant to ganciclovir, cidofovir or foscarnet. J Clin Virol. 2006;37:124–7.
121. Winston D, van Burik JA, Pullarkat V, et al. Prophylaxis against cytomegalovirus infections with oral maribavir in allogeneic stem cell transplant recipients: results of a randomized, double-blind, placebo-controlled trial. Blood 2006;108:179A-A.
122. Zerr DM, Corey L, Kim HW, Huang ML, Nguy L, Boeckh M. Clinical outcomes of human herpesvirus 6 reactivation after hematopoietic stem cell transplantation. Clin Infect Dis. 2005;40:932–40.
123. Seeley WW, Marty FM, Holmes TM, et al. Post-transplant acute limbic encephalitis: clinical features and relationship to HHV6. Neurology 2007;69:156–65.
124. Cone RW, Huang ML, Corey L, Zeh J, Ashley R, Bowden R. Human herpesvirus 6 infections after bone marrow transplantation: clinical and virologic manifestations. J Infect Dis. 1999;179:311–8.
125. Kojaoghlanian T, Flomenberg P, Horwitz MS. The impact of adenovirus infection on the immunocompromised host. Rev Med Virol. 2003;13:155–71.
126. Bruno B, Gooley T, Hackman RC, Davis C, Corey L, Boeckh M. Adenovirus infection in hematopoietic stem cell transplantation: effect of ganciclovir and impact on survival. Biol Blood Marrow Transplant. 2003;9:341–52.
127. Runde V, Ross S, Trenschel R, et al. Adenoviral infection after allogeneic stem cell transplantation (SCT): report on 130 patients from a single SCT unit involved in a prospective multi center surveillance study. Bone Marrow Transplant. 2001;28:51–7.
128. Lion T, Baumgartinger R, Watzinger F, et al. Molecular monitoring of adenovirus in peripheral blood after allogeneic bone marrow transplantation permits early diagnosis of disseminated disease. Blood 2003;102:1114–20.
129. Ljungman P, Ribaud P, Eyrich M, et al. Cidofovir for adenovirus infections after allogeneic hematopoietic stem cell transplantation: a survey by the Infectious Diseases Working Party of the European Group for Blood and Marrow Transplantation. Bone Marrow Transplant. 2003;31:481–6.
130. Erard V, Huang ML, Ferrenberg J, et al. Quantitative real-time polymerase chain reaction for detection of adenovirus after T cell-replete hematopoietic cell transplantation: viral load as a marker for invasive disease. Clin Infect Dis. 2007; 45:958–65.
131. Randhawa PS, Demetris AJ. Nephropathy due to polyomavirus type BK. N Engl J Med. 2000;342:1361–3.
132. Erard V, Storer B, Corey L, et al. BK virus infection in hematopoietic stem cell transplant recipients: frequency, risk factors, and association with postengraftment hemorrhagic cystitis. Clin Infect Dis. 2004;39:1861–5.

133. Erard V, Kim HW, Corey L, et al. BK DNA viral load in plasma: evidence for an association with hemorrhagic cystitis in allogeneic hematopoietic cell transplant recipients. Blood 2005;106:1130–2.
134. Bruno B, Zager RA, Boeckh MJ, et al. Adenovirus nephritis in hematopoietic stem-cell transplantation. Transplantation 2004;77:1049–57.
135. Williams JW, Javaid B, Kadambi PV, et al. Leflunomide for polyomavirus type BK nephropathy. N Engl J Med. 2005;352:1157–8.
136. Englund JA. Diagnosis and epidemiology of community-acquired respiratory virus infections in the immunocompromised host. Biol Blood Marrow Transplant. 2001;7 Suppl:2S–4S.
137. Nichols WG, Gooley T, Boeckh M. Community-acquired respiratory syncytial virus and parainfluenza virus infections after hematopoietic stem cell transplantation: the Fred Hutchinson Cancer Research Center experience. Biol Blood Marrow Transplant. 2001;7 Suppl:11S–5S.
138. Peck AJ, Corey L, Boeckh M. Pretransplantation respiratory syncytial virus infection: impact of a strategy to delay transplantation. Clin Infect Dis. 2004;39:673–80.
139. Boeckh M, Englund J, Li Y, et al. Randomized controlled multicenter trial of aerosolized ribavirin for respiratory syncytial virus upper respiratory tract infection in hematopoietic cell transplant recipients. Clin Infect Dis. 2007;44:245–9.
140. Williams JV, Harris PA, Tollefson SJ, et al. Human metapneumovirus and lower respiratory tract disease in otherwise healthy infants and children. N Engl J Med. 2004;350:443–50.
141. Englund JA, Boeckh M, Kuypers J, et al. Brief communication: fatal human metapneumovirus infection in stem-cell transplant recipients. Ann Intern Med. 2006;144:344–9.

Index

K

Printed in the United States of America